Chin Na In Ground Fighting

Chin Na In
Ground Fighting

Principles, Theory, and Submission
Holds for All Marital Styles

Al Arsenault & Joe Faulise

YMAA Publication Center
Wolfeboro, NH USA

YMAA Publication Center
PO Box 480
Wolfeboro, New Hampshire 03894
1-800-669-8892 • info@ymaa.com • www.ymaa.com

ISBN: 9781886969663 (print) • ISBN: 9781594391835 (ebook)

20250424

Copyright ©2003 by Alan D. Arsenault and Joseph Faulise
All rights reserved including the right of
reproduction in whole or in part in any form.
Illustrations coordinated by Ocean Silver/OSD tekographix
Edited by Susan Bullowa
Cover design by Tony Chee

Publisher's Cataloging in Publication
(Prepared by Quality Books Inc.)

Arsenault, Al.
    Chin na in ground fighting : principles, theory, and submission holds for all martial styles / Al Arsenault & Joe Faulise.— 1st ed.
    p. cm.
    Includes bibliographical references and index.
    LCCN: 2003103094
    ISBN: 1-886969-66-3

    1. Hand-to-hand fighting, Oriental. I. Faulise, Joe. II. Title.

GV1112.A77 2003   796.81
                          QBI03-200242

Anatomy drawings copyright ©1994 by TechPool Studios Corp. USA, 1463 Warrensville Center Road, Cleveland, OH 44121

Disclaimer: The author and publisher of this material are NOT RESPONSIBLE in any manner whatsoever for any injury which may occur through reading or following the instructions in this manual.

The activities, physical or otherwise, described in this material may be too strenuous or dangerous for some people, and the reader(s) should consult a physician before engaging in them.

Printed in USA.

Dedications

To Dr. Wong, Yuwa, my teacher, mentor and friend for life, for all that you have shared with me within the realm of the martial arts and even life itself. Your modesty, knowledge and skill constantly humbles me and gives me hope and strength as I scratch my way along the path.

—Al Arsenault

I dedicate this book to those martial artists who learn and train in the classical styles of martial arts. I urge you to develop an understanding of how to apply your knowledge in a practical way. Many martial artists today do not analyze or question the applicability or effectiveness of their own techniques. They simply have blind faith in the system in which they train.

There is no one supreme system or style of martial arts. There is however, a very small group of martial artists who constantly search for a better way to train themselves, borrowing from all styles of martial arts, in order to suit their own body types and complement their natural abilities.

I believe this is why my co-author Al and I get along so well. When we met in Vancouver through Liang Shou-Yu's Sanshou Dao program, we helped strengthen each other by sharing knowledge, techniques, and by questioning and researching many aspects of the martial arts, not just ground fighting. It has been said, "Let one technique become ten thousand." I think this sums up nicely what a true understanding of the principles behind martial art techniques can bring.

—Joseph Faulise

Table of Contents

Foreword by Dr. Yang, Jwing-Ming ix
Foreword by Master Liang, Shou-Yu xi
Preface by Alan D. Arsenault xiii
Preface by Joseph Faulise xvii
Romanization of Chinese Words and Terms xix
Acknowledgments xxi

Part One—General Concepts
Chapter 1. General History and Principles
    1-1. Introduction 3
    1-2. Comparative Histories of Qin Na and Ground Fighting 7
    1-3. General Principles of Qin Na 22
    1-4. General Principles of Ground Fighting 32
    1-5. Principles Common to Both Qin Na and Ground Fighting 46
    1-6. Physical Training Principles 51
    1-7. Training Considerations 54

Chapter 2. The Science of Technique
    2-1. Introduction 57
    2-2. Basic Principles of Physics 57
    2-3. Variations of the Straight Arm Bar 74
    2-4. Body Positions 85

Chapter 3. Pressure Points of the Fourteen Meridians
    3-1. Introduction 97
    3-2. Meridian Theory 103
    3-3. Pressure Points 105

Chapter 4. Body Tools and Vulnerable Points
    4-1. Introduction 143
    4-2. Body Tools 144
    4-3. Other Vulnerable Areas and Miscellaneous Tools 179

Part Two—Joint Locks
Chapter 5. Controlling the Arm
    5-1. Introduction 193
    5-2. Straight Arm Bars 195
    5-3. Bent Arm Locks 209

Chapter 6. Controlling the Leg
    6-1. Introduction 217
    6-2. Ankle Locks 218
    6.3. Knee Locks 228
    6.4. Knee Blocks 233
    6.5. Combining Ankle and Knee Locks 238

Chapter 7. Controlling the Head/Neck and Body
    7-1. Introduction 241
    7.2. Neck Locks 248
    7.3. Sealing the Vein 253
    7.4. Sealing the Breath 264
    7-5. Controlling the Body 271

Chapter 8. Fighting Sequences
    8-1. Introduction 273
    8-2. Fighting Sequences 274

Epilogue 303
Appendix A. Glossary of Martial Arts Terms 305
Appendix B. Glossary of Medical Terms 331
Bibliography 345
About the Author, Alan D. Arsenault, B.Sc., B.Ed. 349
About the Author, Joseph Faulise 351
Index 353

Foreword by Dr. Yang, Jwing Ming

All Chinese martial styles include four fighting categories: kicking (Ti, 踢), striking (Da, 踢), wrestling (Shuai 摔), and Na (Chin Na, 擒拿) Among them, wrestling is designed to oppose kicking and striking, Chin Na (Qin Na) is to counter wrestling, and kicking and striking are used against Chin Na. Therefore, these four categories are mutually supporting and conquer each other, thus completing a perfect martial style.

The main purpose of wrestling is to take the opponent down so killing techniques can be executed effectively. The reason for this is because almost all ancient soldiers wore armor and helmets in battle. As a result, when a soldier was standing, the vital areas of his entire body were usually well protected. In order to expose these vital areas so the killing techniques can be carried out, the first step was to take him down. With the heavy weight of the armor and helmet, it would take some time and effort for the soldier to stand again. And, when the soldier was on the ground, the vital areas would be exposed to attack.

Conversely, when it is necessary to take one's opponent alive after having taken him down, Chin Na techniques must be immediately applied to lock him in place. Except for Mongolian wrestling, most Chinese wrestling styles do not emphasize Chin Na control when the opponent is on the ground, for it was rare in ancient times that taking one's opponent alive was necessary. Most of the time, killing immediately followed wrestling. However, the situation in today's society is very different. First, we seldom use sharpened weapons such as knives in battle as in ancient times. Second, killing a person in a fight is to be avoided at all costs. For these reasons, there is a great demand for revealing existing ancient techniques and for further research into their applications.

Ground control techniques have become more effective and useful to the modern martial arts practitioner. Al Arsenault and Joe Faulise both have many years of experience in wrestling and Chin Na. They have revealed all of what they have learned and practiced. I believe that this book will be the beginning of a wider and deeper study of this field in all of martial arts society. I sincerely hope those who are interested in wrestling and Chin Na can benefit from this book and use these arts more effectively. I also hope that this book will stimulate further study and publications on this subject.

Dr. Yang, Jwing-Ming
President, YMAA International
April, 2003

Foreword by Master Liang, Shou-Yu

Fifteen years ago, the International Wushu Sanshou Dao Association (a.k.a. IWSD and Sanshou Dao) was established with the goal of integrating the essence of major martial arts systems and fostering well-rounded martial artists. The training contents of Sanshou Dao are very extensive, requiring all its members to be well-versed in various disciplines. These disciplines include barehanded and weapon routines, both from the Internal Styles and External Styles of martial arts. Members are required to consistently improve in their free-fighting, takedowns, Shuaijiao, Qinna, Dianxue, ground control and push hands skills, as well as, to improve their physical tolerance to attacks, attain greater physical and internal strength, train in many hard and soft Qiqong, and practice meditation.

Sanshou Dao members are expected to learn and understand a well-rounded theory and philosophy of the martial arts in addition to the technical abilities. The expectation and requirements are high for Sanshou Dao members. Having a black belt in another style of martial art is a prerequisite for Sanshou Dao.

There have been over twenty IWSD affiliate schools established around the world during the past fifteen years, yet the numbers of people who have been able to achieve black belt levels are less than one hundred. These black belts are experts in their respective martial art systems with the focus of their training being on the essence of the martial arts. It is the quality not the quantity of their attainment that is valued. Their tests are conducted with the utmost integrity. Ranks can't be awarded without true attainment. No amount of money or emotional debt can substitute for real ability. It is a pure integrated martial arts system.

Al Arsenault is the current and Founding President of IWSD. He has over 30 years of experience in many martial arts disciplines, including Karate, Judo, Jujitsu, Shuaijiao, Qinna (Chin Na, T'ai Chi Chuan and Qiqong). His training has given him a well-rounded ability and understanding of the martial arts. He is especially well-versed in police arrest and control tactics and Qinna.

Al has continuously enhanced his abilities by going to various places to learn new techniques and approaches. His travels have taken him to the United States, China, Japan, Australia, India and Thailand to research, train and teach martial arts.

Likewise, in 1992 Joe traveled here to Canada from Tok, Alaska, for nine months just to train in Sanshou Dao. He has trained extensively in Judo, Ju Jitsu, Aikido, Wrestling, Karate, Bagua, T'ai Chi (Taiji). Joe is the pioneer of Sanshou Dao in Alaska, having set up his own Sanshou Dao school there in 1993. His students have been regular tournament winners in all classes of competition throughout Alaska.

Al was the fighting coach for and a participant of the May '1994 North American Martial Arts Demonstration Tour' of China, a team that also included Joe. While on this tour, both Al and Joe were awarded gold medals at the Shanghai International Wushu Competition for their outstanding performances (our combined U.S./Canada team won 75% of the gold 56 medals so the 'Oberon Cup' was awarded to us for the best results from a field of 23 competing countries).

Al and I have been friends for over twenty years, and Joe as nearly as long as that. Both are strong, charismatic, sociable and friendly people. Al is an outstanding police officer in Vancouver, British Columbia, while Joe has done surveying and fire-jumping around the continent. In his twenty-three year career as a police officer, Al has been recognized many times for his valuable contributions and services for the people and city of Vancouver. One time in 1989, he even recovered a stolen Vancouver police radio near Beijing while returning from a Sanshou Dao mission in Harbin, but that is another story. His anti-drug work with the Odd Squad is renowned worldwide.

Ask Joe to tell you about the time he escaped the frozen jaws of death by digging himself out an avalanche (this took more than a day to do so), and also saving his work mate in the process. As with life, Joe has shown incredible determination and perseverance in his training. His ground fighting skills are exceptional and his technical contributions to this book shine through.

I rejoice about Al Arsenault's and Joe Faulise's book *Chin Na in Ground Fighting*. I believe this book will be a valuable learning reference for all martial artists.

Liang, Shou-Yu
Vancouver, B.C.
Canada
August, 2002

Preface by Alan D. Arsenault

At an early age I viewed myself as a diamond in the rough; I was a hard case, with a lot of potential. So I took to the martial arts, unwittingly as it turned out, to polish myself up. I am still at it today as I pass the half-century mark of my life.

This book has come about through my relationship with my teacher Liang, Shou-Yu, his martial arts brother Dr. Yang, Jwing-Ming, and Joseph Faulise, my martial arts brother. My martial arts background since the early 70's had been primarily in the striking arts of Goju Ryu and Okinawan Karate. Even as a novice, I was well aware of the shortcomings of karate as a complete fighting system (recently this has become painfully illustrated in the Ultimate Fight Championships). I dabbled in judo and eventually studied Qin Na (Chin Na) and Shuai Jiao with Master Liang. So strongly did I feel about being personally unable to address the missing portions of the fighting spectrum, I felt incumbent to bring judoka into the various karate dojo in which I trained. I did this in order to broaden the minds of fellow students and instructors who were open-minded and secure enough in their own art forms to allow such a different kind of training to take place. Over the last 24 years as a street policeman in the mean streets of Vancouver, I have come to realize the acute deficiencies of karate as a defensive art, or more practically as a controlling art, as my chosen vocation demands. For myself, Qin Na was like a 'Snap-On' tool: it allowed me to adapt my martial arts ability to suit the highly balanced needs of personal self-protection with controlling those I was empowered to arrest. I was entrusted to use only as much force as necessary, as prescribed by law. And so, I have mentally wrestled with the solutions to resolving problems that I encountered, or reasonably expected to encounter, on the street. I had to select and apply force options from the entire use of force spectrum: from mere presence, appearance and reputation, to dialogue, empty hand control, impact weapons and even deadly force.

My karate instructor Wong, Yuwa met Master Liang, Shou-Yu through his colleague Michael Levenston. Michael is Yuwa's longest-term student still in training. He always had a penchant for the Chinese internal martial arts. Yuwa encouraged his studies outside the dojo. It was in this garden of openness and enlightenment that our cross training began with Master Liang in the late 1980's: the seed of Sanshou Dao was planted. We all realized that each of our respective art forms failed individually to cover the entire fighting spectrum and that together we might synthesize a new, exciting and more complete martial arts system.

I first met co-author Joe Faulise when he came from Alaska to train in Wushu and ultimately in Sanshou Dao in 1992. I was immediately impressed with Joe's gentle nature, powerful throwing and ground fighting techniques, his insatiable thirst for martial arts knowledge and his indomitable will to survive (later put to the ultimate test after being entombed by an avalanche, several years ago). I realized that we complimented each other's knowledge and skills. Together as training partners and teachers, we were helping each other grow as well as lead our students in the

Sanshou garden so expertly tended, primarily by master Liang, Shou-Yu, with the help of masters Wong, Yuwa and Yang, Jwing-Ming. After training together here in Vancouver and Alaska, demonstrating together throughout the heart of China in 1994 (and even imbibing a few rounds together), I came to have a deep respect and caring for Joe, his family, friends and students in Tok, Alaska. A few years ago, Master Liang asked me to contribute a chapter on ground fighting in his book *San Shou Kuai Jiao* (1997) and I reluctantly complied. Master Liang and Dr. Yang then asked me to write an entire book on this topic. I agreed only if I could enlist the assistance of Joe Faulise, who has had considerably more experience rolling around on the mat than I. I was content knowing that painting this particular fence would be a lot easier when a more experienced painter was helping me to do a good job.

When struggling with this book's basic concept, I began to look at the relationship between Qin Na and ground fighting in the Police Judo classes that I continue to train in. From an intellectual stand point I used this knowledge of the biomechanical principles of Qin Na in order to understand the techniques that were being shown to me. But from the standpoint of survival on the mat, I was forced to fight back with Qin Na in order to strengthen whatever hold I could muster or to weaken my opponent's resolve with what feels and looks like just plain old 'dirty fighting'. I came to realize that I couldn't use too many Qin Na techniques, because attacking joints like those of the fingers and wrists, for example, are illegal in judo, with overt cranial and cervical pressure point attacks being forbidden as well. Many of these potentially harmful techniques, including leg locks, were taken out of the sporting forum so that healthy and safe competitions could take place. I did examine judo techniques through the filter of Qin Na and realized that I could hold some of the principles of judo within the conceptual framework of Qin Na. I also realized that the reverse should be true because we are dealing with only a limited number of biomechanical principles relating to the bending and twisting of the various body parts, mainly those of the extremities. It really does not matter if you are working the finger, arm, leg or even the entire body as a jointed and segmented unit; bend and/or twist the segment in an unnatural or extreme way and you can defeat your opponent. The resultant pain you create will give you the ability to control your opponent to some degree and if necessary break down his fighting machine. Certainly it takes a lot more strength to manipulate the torso than the pinkie finger, nor will bending this same little finger guarantee that your opponent submit, but both these kinds of techniques have their place in your ground fighting arsenal. Rather than just putting out yet another collection of interesting holds, we felt that we could make this book more useful and original by concentrating on the following three martial aspects:

1. the selection and preference of holding techniques which are capable of immobilizing or incapacitating an opponent with a limited danger to counterattack (that is to say you are not confined by, nor protected by, the rules of sport),
2. the relationship of these holds to the biomechanical principals used in Qin Na and the augmentation of these holds using Qin Na techniques,
3. the identification and use of pressure points for offensive and defensive purposes.

In Sanshou Dao there are no rules other than not to injure one's training partner. We are not bound by the limitations of sport rules, boundaries of an art form, or by organizational parameters that keep styles 'pure'. No style is really pure anyway. If you can trace martial roots back far enough, these 'pure' styles are usually a combination of several styles or are merely relatively minor variations of a given style. No style is 'better' than another. If you look at the differences long and hard enough, you will see common similarities that exist within each type of martial art. After all, there are only a limited number of biomechanical principles that are used in the martial arts, which have been creatively dressed up with a fancy or foreign name or with slight variations in form and function, to make up the myriad of martial art styles we see today. We have all borrowed from a wide variety of martial arts disciplines such as wrestling, judo, jiu jitsu, Qin Na, karate, aikido, etc.

We present a host of techniques to you in order to stir your creative juices. In no way however, are we attempting to offer an all-inclusive text on the grappling arts. Firstly we do not know all that there is to know. Our life-long study continues in earnest. Nor are we guaranteeing a lack of omissions of any major techniques within these styles. To do so would fill volumes. The techniques shown merely reflect our own personal interests and knowledge base. It is up to you, the reader, to take what suits you and your needs and toss the rest aside. We are offering a wide range of techniques, basic and advanced, simple and complicated, restraining and crippling.

The ease of application, reliability, and street effectiveness without the reliance of clothing were important considerations in the selection criteria for the techniques presented in this book, but these are loose guidelines. After all, what good is your headlock if the opponent can easily access your eyes and groin? Even the rough and tumble U.F.C. matches would change in strategy and technique deployment, if it were truly a 'no-holds barred' event, akin to a nasty street fight. We did not deal with throws, entrances, counters or striking finishes as these too are beyond the scope of this book. We did include a few fight sequences to show how take downs, positional changes and strikes can be interwoven from the body of static techniques outlined in this book. One can individually sense the relative combat viability and versatility of the techniques, so pick and choose those requiring further study and make them your own.

It is my hope that the Qin Na specialist can look at ground fighting with a familiarity that would invite him to expand his skills on the ground. Conversely, the ground fighter can gain an appreciation of the principles of Qin Na that would enhance his technique, be it for sport (if allowable or able to be done covertly) or street purposes (hopefully within the confines of the law).

One such improvement in the former scenario is exemplified by the tweaking up of *ude garumi* (see Chapter One). By grabbing the forearm to be controlled just above the wrist and twisting it inward to take out the slack in the forearm muscles and place extra pressure on the elbow joint prior to actually applying torque to the arm itself, the effectiveness of this technique was legally enhanced. (Figures 1-100 to 1-102) This has a similar effect on the elbow joint as grabbing the hand and doing an outside wrist lock, which is illegal in sport judo, during the application of *ude garumi*. Similarly, the Qin Na practitioner can readily make the transition of a figure-four arm lock to a figure-four leg lock or even a figure-four leg lock using the legs (or a figure-four arm lock using the legs for that matter). Take a principle and let your creativity make many techniques from it.

When I visited Australia in 1986, a martial arts instructor proudly expounded, "There are ten thousand techniques in my style". Rather than learn or teach ten thousand techniques, it is much easier to learn and teach the underlying principles common to all of those techniques. And so I advise the reader to peruse the material in this book with a view to understanding the underlying concepts. Keep an open mind and seek to improve your technique. You will polish yourself in the process and shine brilliantly on the mat and in life itself.

Finally: I would like to receive any comment that you may have regarding this book. Please send them to arsenault@telus.net. Do you have a rare or unusual martial arts book that needs a good home in my extensive martial arts library? Let's talk!

Preface by Joseph Faulise

There are many different styles of martial arts from many different countries. Some of them date back thousands of years. Regardless of where they came from or how long they have been in existence they have all gone through a process of evolution or change. Some, such as Tae Kwon Do, have specialized in kicking; some have specialized in throwing, such as Judo. Other martial arts moved in the opposite direction and expanded their theories to include other facets of fighting. One example of this would be Bruce Lee's conception of Jeet Kune Do.

It is my opinion that, in the last ten or so years, one of the most important innovations in the martial arts is the no-holds barred type of fighting. Matches such as the Ultimate Fight Championship, the Tude Vale or the Shoot Fighting matches in Japan have been well received by the public. These different events helped to break down the wall that kept many martial artists apart, due to stylistic differences. Now it is not uncommon to find people who study a grappling martial art, cross training with a person who studies a striking martial art and vice versa.

When Al asked me to help him with this book on ground fighting, it was our cross training together that helped us come up with how to approach the subject of ground fighting. For many months we debated what angle to approach this subject from. Should we look at it from a grappler's point of view? Or perhaps a person can look to fortify what ever striking art they currently study. The one thing Al and I had in common was our Qin Na (Chin Na) background. It was Al who came up with the idea that many of the people who study striking arts do, to some extent, have some sort of knowledge of locking techniques. They just don't do them on the ground. If we could relate the similarities between the locks used in stand up fighting to the locks used by ground fighters we could find a common ground to help bring the two groups together. As we went on to examine the relationship between locks executed in the standing position and locks used on the ground, not only did we cross-reference the position of the limb being attacked, but also the tools being used (pelvis, hand, shoulder etc.) to execute the lock, along with different principles involved.

When Master Liang, Shou-Yu and Dr. Yang, Jwing-Ming and Master Wong, Yuwa started Sanshou Dao, I believe they wanted the student to go through this type of cross-referencing of principles and techniques in the martial arts. In this way the student would learn to see the similarities between the different style of the martial arts, helping the student to keep an open mind to new ideas.

By writing this book, I feel that Al and myself have taken a true Sanshou Dao journey. We have taken techniques from many different styles and have tried to show the practical similarities, while not giving credit to any one art or style (although judo is highly favored).

I feel that Al and myself would like to give credit to the men of the no-holds barred fighting. It was, after all, these events that rekindled interest in this wonderful facet of the jewel that we call the martial arts. We both hope that maybe this book would inspire others to share their knowledge with other martial artists and to write books of their own.

Romanization of Chinese Words and Terms

This book uses the Pinyin romanization system of Chinese to English. There are two other systems currently in use. These are the Wade-Giles and the Yale systems. The cover of this book presents the Wade-Giles romanization without apostrophes in order to simplify cataloging

Some common conversions:

Pinyin	Also Spelled As	Pronunciation
Qi	Chi	chē
Qigong	Chi Kung	chē kŭng
Qin Na	Chin Na	chĭn nă
Jin	Jing	jĭn
Gongfu	Kung Fu	gōng foo
Taijiquan	Tai Chi Chuan	tī jē chüén

For more information, please refer to *The People's Republic of China: Administrative Atlas, The Reform of the Chinese Written Language,* or a contemporary manual of style.

The spelling of Chin Na is used in the title. In the book, The term Qin Na is frequently accompanied by Chin Na within parenthesis, i.e., Qin Na (Chin Na).

Comparison of Terminology for Acupuncture Points Used by Three Authors

The nomenclature of the points in this book is that of the standard numbering system used in China. The translations of the acupuncture point names follow the interpretations by Dr. Li Ding whose book, *Acupuncture, Meridian Theory, and Acupuncture Points*, is highly recommended to those seeking to know more about acupuncture points.

Li Ding (1992)	**Yang (1992)**	**Tedeschi (2002)**
DU 1 Changqiang	Gv-1 Changqiang	GV-1 Chang Qiang
REN 6 Qihai	Co-6 Qihai	CO-6 Qi Hai
Lung Meridian	Lung Channel of the Hand – Greater Yin	LU Lung Meridian
Lu. 2 Yunmen	L-2 Yunmen	LU-2 Yun Men
Heart Meridian	Heart Channel of the Hand – Greater Yin	HT Heart Meridian
H. 3 Shaohai	H-3 Shaohai	HT-3 Shao Hai
Pericardium Meridian	Pericardium Channel of the Hand – Lesser Yin	PC Pericardium Meridian
P. 6 Neiguan	P-6 Neiguan	PC-6 Nei Guan
L.I. 4 Hegu	LI-4 Hegu	LI-4 He Gu
S.I. 16 Tianchuang	ST-16 Tianchuang	SI-16 Tian Chuang
S.J. 3 Hand-Zhongzu	TB-3 Hand-Zhong hu	TW-3 Zhong Zhu
Stomach Meridian	Stomach Channel of the Foot – Yang Brightness	ST Stomach Meridian
St. 1 Chengqi	S-1 Chengqi	ST-1 Cheng Qi
Urinary Bladder Meridian	Urinary Bladder Channel of the Foot – Greater Yang	BL Bladder Meridian
U.B. 40 Weizhong		BL 56 Wei Zhong
U.B. 56 Chengjin	B-56 Chengjin	BL-56 Cheng Jin
Gall Bladder Meridian	Gall Bladder Channel of the Foot – Lesser Yang	GB Gall Bladder Meridian
G.B. 6 Xuanli	GB-6 Xuanli	GB-6 Xuan Li
Spleen Meridian	Spleen Channel of the Foot	SP Spleen Meridian
Sp. 11 Jimen	Sp-11 Jimen	SP-11 Ji Men
Kidney Meridian	Kidney Channel of the Foot – Lesser Yin	KI Kidney Meridian
K. 3 Taixi	K-13 Taixi	KI-3 Tai Xi
Liver Meridian	Liver Channel of the Foot – Absolute Yin	LV Liver Meridian
Liv. 13 Zhangmen	L-13 Zhangmen	LV-13 Zhang Men
EX-HN 2 Yingtan	-	M-HN-3 Yin Tang

Acknowledgments

I would like to thank Master Shou-Yu Liang for giving me the opportunity write an introductory chapter in his book *Chinese Fast Wrestling for Fighting* (my brother Gordon Arsenault and fellow Sanshou Dao student Craig Osmachenko deserve credit for serving as stand-ins during the preliminary photographic sessions needed to complete this initial work). It was the popularity of this sub-topic that lead to the writing of *Chin Na in Ground Fighting* at the insistence and support of both Master Liang and Dr. Yang Jwing-Ming.

I appreciated the initial editing assistance from Michael Holmes, who has been one of the most diligent and dedicated students that I have had the pleasure to teach. I extend my thanks to Sabra Sheldon for her work on the medical glossary.

I gratefully indebted to both my police/ judo partner Toby Hinton and our judo instructor Brian Shipper for their assistance in posing for some of the photos and for their solid judo training, instruction and friendship at the Vancouver Police Judo/ Jiujitsu Club. Marg Hewitt-Zaitlin truly has a wonderful instructional program in her 'Canadian Fitness Education Services Fitness Knowledge Course'. I enjoyed extensive use of her very informative manual (see www.canadianfitness.net). Susan Bullowa did a good job of cracking the whip on me, driving me to complete this book, and her fine editing skills were greatly appreciated. I appreciate the photographic expertise of Martin Hatfield of 'Photo Arcane' (horn@direct.ca) who shot the cover photo of myself and Toby Hinton.

Most importantly, I owe a huge debt gratitude to my special friend April Miller, who encouraged me to complete this book during a very hard time in my life. She is a master organizer who readily transforms frenetic chaos into simplicity and tranquility. And so it was, that from the ashes of personal hardship, the phoenix struggled and rose with this book on its back.

—Al Arsenault

Part One
General Concepts

CHAPTER 1

General History and Principles

1-1. INTRODUCTION

Definitions of Qin Na and Ground Fighting

Before we delve into the relationship between Qin Na (Chin Na) and ground fighting, let us define each of these aspects of fighting. *Qin (Chin)* means 'to seize or catch' and *Na* means 'to control or hold'. By law, a police officer that arrests a person must technically touch him/her and state the reason for his/her detention. For the combative criminal, a judicious application of force comparable with the amount of resistance offered by the arrested party is legally acceptable, hence Qin Na can be thought of in the way that a police officer 'seizes and controls' his suspect (Figure 1-1

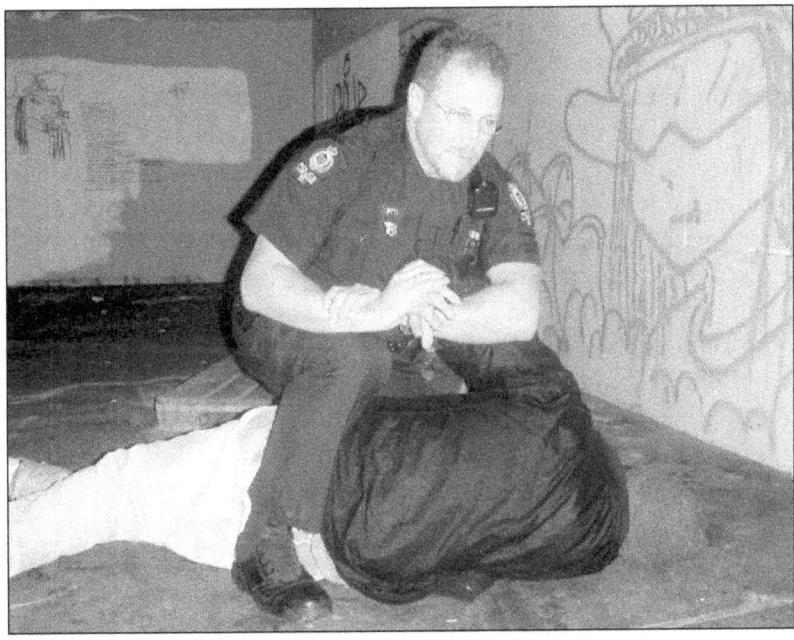

The Street Application of the Shoulder Crank
Figure 1-1 The author making an on-duty arrest on an assault suspect in the skids. The shoulder crank is a very effective hold down technique.

that shows the author making an on-duty arrest on an assault suspect. The shoulder crank is an effective hold down technique.). Although many martial arts claim to have a component of Qin Na in their style of fighting (often hidden within the kata), it is most highly refined in the Chinese martial arts where it is considered as one of four essential martial components. The components are: *Ti, da, shuai,* and *na. Ti* refers to kicking techniques; *da* refers to striking and punching moves; *shuai* refers to wrestling (stand-up grappling more closely associated to tripping and throwing); and *na* as just explained, refers to 'seizing' and 'controlling' a person's joints, muscles and/or tendons and includes pressure point attacks on body cavities.

We refer to ground fighting as an eclectic grouping of any wrestling and grappling techniques done on the ground. The focus of this book has been shifted away from counterattacking moves as well as kicking and striking techniques done from the ground against a standing opponent. We will look at the overlap or similarities between Qin Na and ground fighting.

Value of This Study

What value is there in studying the relationship between Qin Na and ground fighting? Succinctly, both fighting arts mutually augment each other. The Qin Na specialist can obviously benefit from cross training in ground fighting because he traditionally stays on his feet while applying his skills. For him, the ground is a foreign place from which to fight. Some of his arsenal cannot be applied due to lack of mobility. Some techniques can be done standing up or lying down. Apart from these obvious similarities, ground fighting techniques have the same principles behind them as used in Qin Na. If the Qin Na specialist were left to his own devices, he could discover parallel applications of his art to those needed to effect ground fighting submission holds because of his understanding of the biomechanical principles involved. The method of applying these techniques could be radically different, but it is not entirely a whole new endeavor. The ground fighter would be further ahead in the fighting game than the Qin Na specialist in this arena because of his familiarity in general with fighting on the ground, the kinds of submission holds used, and the type of conditioning required to win on the ground. What he could learn from cross training with the Qin Na specialist is the augmentation of his own technique outside the rules of sport. The judo practitioner can benefit from the knowledge of 'dirty fighting' techniques obtained from Qin Na. Dirty fighting techniques are nothing more than fighting outside the realm of sport rules. The only rule in street fighting is that there are no rules (other than rules of morality, which tempers those with a conscience not to indulge in the excessive application of force). Indeed street fighting is a matter of survival, not rules.

Book Outline

This book is divided into two parts: General Concepts (theory) and Joint Locks (application). The initial chapter deals with general introductory remarks about Qin Na and ground fighting styles, including their respective histories and common biomechanical principles underlying the techniques. Due to limitations in time and space, we will look briefly at the development of wrestling and Jujutsu (judo) as a part of the history of ground fighting, although there are other martial arts that incorporate ground fighting into their styles. Chapter Two deals with the principles and rules of physics that we are biomechanically bound by, with variations of the arm bar examined in this light. Understanding *why* techniques work will improve your technique and improvisational abilities. The types of relative body positions encountered on the ground and how some positional changes can be made are outlined. Chapter Three is an introduction into meridian theory and is included for those seeking information about the application of Traditional Chinese Medicine's acupuncture points as they relate to target selection and acquisition. Some of the more common pressure points (with details of the local anatomy) are outlined in relation to the fourteen meridians. These points are spread out all over the body and some are always be accessible to you during ground fighting. Chapter Four reviews the body tools that we can use in combative situations as well as relate how we can use these weapons effectively against these pressure points (and other miscellaneous vulnerable areas).

Part Two of the book takes you through a systematic analysis of joint locks, beginning with the arm (Chapter Five) and progressing to the legs (Chapter Six), and finally the neck/head and body. The final chapter shows a few fighting sequences to start the creative juices flowing as to how to apply the statically introduced techniques in the dynamic, three dimensional sense of fighting. It is left up to the individual to apply the techniques in the best way that they can. This book cannot take the place of a qualified and knowledgeable instructor who can provide you with good training partners in a safe learning environment.

SOME OF THE PRESSURE POINTS AND TECHNIQUES CONTAINED WITHIN THIS BOOK ARE DANGEROUS AND CONSIDERABLE RESTRAINT MUST BE EXERCISED WHEN PRACTICING WITH YOUR TRAINING PARTNER.

This text is fully indexed with almost encyclopedic and fully cross-referenced Martial Arts and Medical Glossaries to assist you in your study and reading enjoyment.

The Fighting Spectrum

It is important to remember that this book covers only a portion of what is known about ground fighting and that ground fighting (and Qin Na for that matter) only addresses but a portion of the fighting spectrum (Figure 1-2 which shows the range of attacking techniques that vary with the distance separating the opponents.). These aspects of fighting are not to be held in isolation. They overlap and complement other methods of fighting that move laterally along the fighting spectrum.

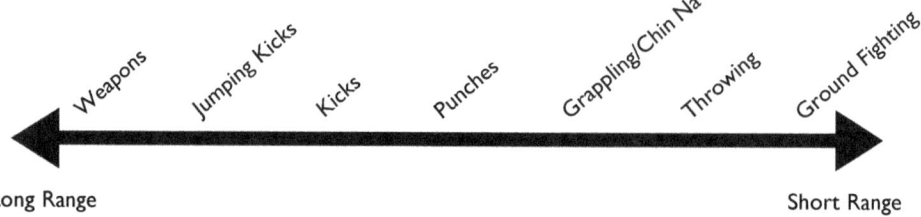

The Fighting Spectrum
Figure 1-2 The kinds of attacking techniques employed vary with the distance separating the opponents.

As the range between two combatants close, so do the kinds of techniques that can be applied change. Some styles have evolved techniques that lie only in a certain portion of the fighting spectrum with minor offerings to the rest. Judo for example, is a close-range sport that utilizes grappling (from both the standing and ground positions) and throwing techniques. It also has *atemi waza* (striking techniques) that are now very rudimentary and unsophisticated. Judo clearly places an emphasis on throwing and ground fighting techniques. Tae Kwon Do on the other hand (foot) specializes in kicking techniques: jumping kicks, turning kicks; kicks of every type and description. The kicks are so highly refined that some clubs have done little to work on their hand techniques and ground fighting is never attempted (or it entails just kicking from the ground). The limitations of these styles are entrenched in the rules that govern their individual sport, so there is little need to venture out into other areas of the fighting spectrum except to address self-defense concerns raised by the students.

Value of Cross Training in Martial Arts

Martial artists in some schools claim to teach 'self-defense', but often neglect realistic training geared for the streets, preferring to train their students to be highly proficient and competitive in their chosen form of sport. No clearer has it been shown what bitter defeat and a lack of well-rounded training can bring, than in the venues such as the Ultimate Fight Championship (UFC) and Extreme Fight Matches. Challengers, expecting to stay on their feet using a few well-placed punches and kicks, were taken to the ground and mercilessly choked out by experienced and well-conditioned ground fighters. It has been said that most fights end up on the ground (at least for one combatant). The best way to neutralize the ability of a puncher or kicker to do you harm is to smother his weapons by getting in close to him. Even overtired or injured boxers hug each other in the ring to keep from being hit. We saw that the ground fighters often triumphed in the UFC fights given the rules that were in effect. It is interesting to note that an evolution within the return combatants and first time fighters took place within a short period of time. By cross training, they managed to obscure the boundaries between pure styles for the sake of survival in the octagon.

Chapter 1: General History and Principles

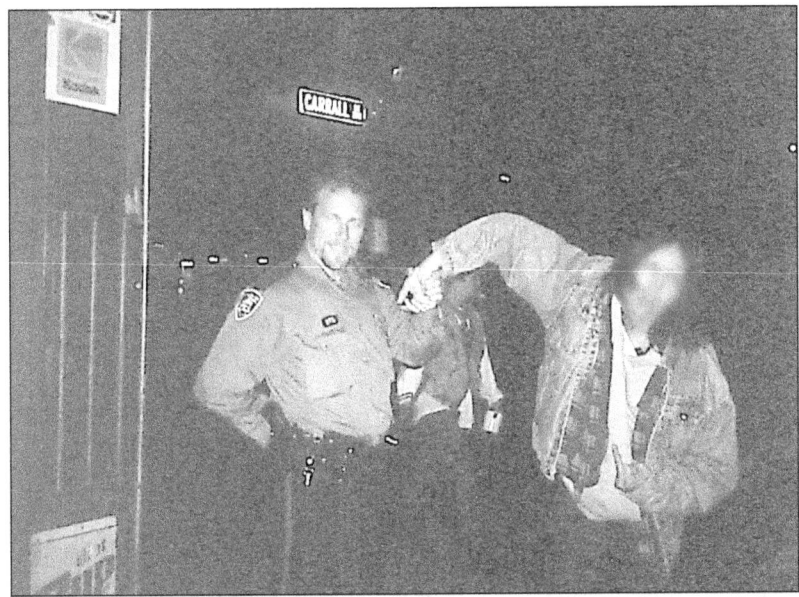

The Street Application of the Wrist Lock
Figure 1-3 The twisting wrist lock is an effective way to control a person's ability to move (the suspect rates the author's technique as '#1').

The winners were often ground fighters who learned to cross train in the striking arts. Losers went back to learn some ground fighting. So, is ground fighting the ultimate fighting form? Not so, if you change the rules to two or three opponents on one, for example. How would a person who knew only about ground fighting do in a swarming? In this domain, the strikers would do better than the grappler. A police officer is better off using Qin Na to seize and control his opponent in a hostile environment (potential for other assailants) as opposed to going to the ground to gain control (Figure 1-3 which shows the twisting wrist lock that is an effective way to control a person's ability to move.). Besides that, his uniform will stay clean and remain untorn if he does so! When confronted with multiple assailants, he is taught to use weapons, punch, kick, call for 'backup' or what ever it takes to overcome the odds and convert it into a winning battle. The kind of fighting that is done changes in accordance to the type of resistance (real or perceived) that is encountered.

1-2. COMPARATIVE HISTORIES OF QIN NA AND GROUND FIGHTING

Early History

Men have probably always engaged in fighting. Some say it is in our nature or even in our genes to fight and to engage in warfare. Whether we do so to acquire more resources to allow our race to thrive and perhaps to maintain genetic purity or whether we fight out of pugilistic pride is moot. Prehistoric man probably grappled with each other and wild beasts, the activity of which would have abated somewhat, when primitive weapons were invented. With each new class of hoplological advanc-

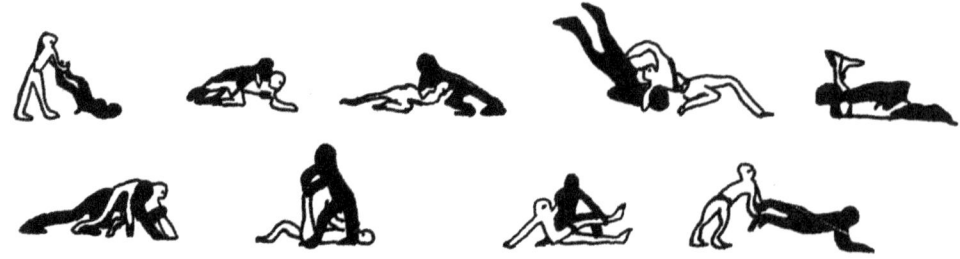

Drawings of Early Egyptian Wrestling Techniques

Figure 1-4 Modern free-style wrestling techniques are reflected in these ancient drawings from the Beni-Hasan wall paintings of early Egyptian bouts (circa 2000 B.C.).

es, so did the relative importance of hand-to-hand combat also diminish. Clearly, the advent of gunpowder changed the regimen of military training away from the emphasis of unarmed combat. From survival to sport, wrestling has remained a popular activity throughout the ages. Men have used wrestling to test their strength and skill against each other and even settle disputes, just as they do today. Virtually every country has some indigenous form of pugilism, often in the form of wrestling. Even in present day Nubia (lower Sudan), wrestling is the most important social focus for society. The beauty of it, is that no equipment or training hall is really required to partake in this sport, as most kids play-fighting in the school yard can attest.

Undoubtedly wrestling pre-dates the written language. The earliest recorded evidence of pugilism comes from the wall painting of wrestling groups from Beni Hasan in Egypt, where a series of wrestling holds had been drawn some 4000 years ago (Figure 1-4). It should not be surprising that these pictures look remarkably similar to wrestling of today, given that body mechanics have not changed throughout the millennia. Sometimes these scenes were painted together with military activities, suggesting that wrestling was a part of the military training at this early time. There has been much warfare throughout the ages. In fact, there has been 268 years of recorded global peace in the past 3,400 years. The three civilized empires based in Mesopotamia, Asia Minor and Egypt engaged in almost constant warfare for supremacy from the period of 2000–1000 B.C There have almost been about 14,500 wars fought since 3,600 B.C (2.6 wars per year). (*Genetic Seeds of Warfare*, Shaw and Wong. P. 3.)

The relationship between the pugilistic sports and military training was not always a positive one. Some detractors such as Plato (400 B.C) recommended these sports for youth, but not for military training. He felt that warfare was better served through team participation resembling battlefield situations. Even the gifted wrestler of this same era, General Philopoimen, learned that wrestlers did not make effective soldiers, hence he banned the troops from engaging in sport and he stopped engaging in it himself.

Chapter 1: General History and Principles

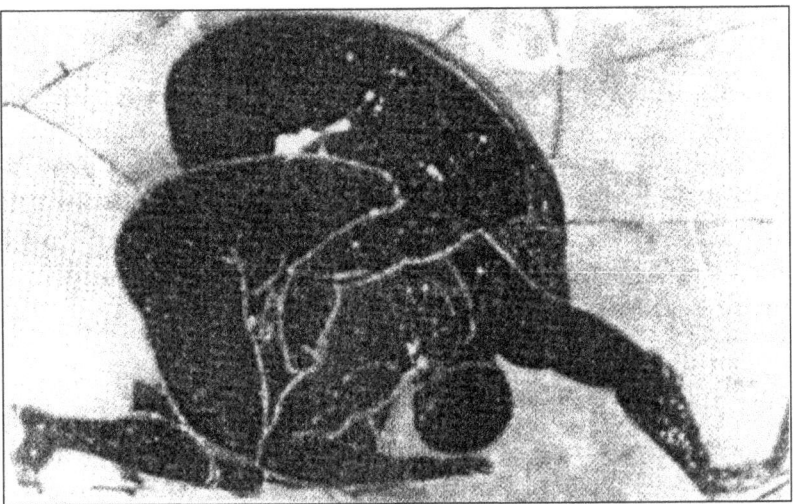

Greek Vase Painting of Wrestlers
Figure 1-5 This drawing was made from a photo of an ancient Greek vase (circa 360 B.C.). One wrestler is using his head to put pressure on his opponent's triceps.

Early Greek History

About 3000 B.C writing was invented in Sumer, so much of early history in general has had to be gleaned from hieroglyphics in tombs and on cultural artifacts such as pottery. Accounts of wrestling matches in Babylonia and Assyria date back to 2000 B.C After 1000 B.C., longer lasting forms for recording events were invented and used. Indeed the writings of the Homeric Era (700 B.C.) contained many important and honorable mentions of Greek wrestling heroes. The excavations at Eretria, on the Greek island of Euboea have yielded vases showing well-drawn scenes of wrestling and *pankration*, as well as some rare examples of ground fighting from 400 B.C. Figure 1-5 is a drawing that was made from a photo of an ancient Greek vase circa 360 B.C. One wrestler is using his head to put pressure on his opponent's triceps. In (Greek) Hellenic society, the educated and accomplished male adults practiced wrestling. Early Mesopotamian prose and poetry already refer to wrestling and sport as being entrenched in society by this time.

Wrestling was practiced in Rome as early as the 5th century B.C. having been influenced by Greek wrestling (the latter having been practiced at the 18th Olympiad for the first time in 708 B.C.). The Roman Empire expanded immensely, collapsing the Greek Empire during the Punic Wars (264-146 B.C.). In 186 B.C., a special contingent of athletes, including wrestlers and *pankrationists* from Greece, were brought to Rome for entertainment purposes. Gladiatorial fight to the death matches, complete with lions and panthers imported from Africa, were regularly held at this time. The non-athletic crowds of Rome were unimpressed by Greek wrestling (although of all Greek sports, their new found patriotism only allowed them to favor boxing, wrestling and *pankration*), so they combined elements of this wrestling with their Etruscan-based wrestling (that featured ground fighting) to form Graeco-Roman wrestling. Gone was the Greek upright style, tripping was forbidden, and more emphasis was placed on strength over agility. The Romans encouraged the Olympic Games, sans the sadistic Roman gladiatorial-style displays, to continue. The Romans even became more heavily involved in athleticism under the reign of Emperor Hadrian (A.D. 117), although this was now a time of professional tournament fighters. These fighters were bound together in powerful synods or trade unions that set up the tournaments and *gymnasia* to appease the huge interest in combative sports in Greece, the Roman world and in the east. The evils of professionalism, as today, brought in corruption such as fight fixing, which the public despised. Wrestling was no longer an honest sport. The Greeks claimed that the use of professional athletes was tarnishing the Olympic Games. The Romans denied the charges but the whole situation came to a head in 392 A.D. when a huge battle broke out between the Roman and Greek athletes at Olympia, which saw an almost total destruction of the stadium. The reigning emperor Theodosius abolished the Games (they were not re-opened until 1896) after the ruins at Olympia were re-discovered. Wrestling proved to be too entrenched to die with the Games, even with the defeat of the Roman Empire by the Barbarians in 476 A.D. Indeed, the Graeco-Roman style is still practiced today in a modified form at the Olympics.

No real clear distinction between Qin Na (Chin Na) and ground fighting has been made until recent history. Distinctions were made in the ancient Olympic games between striking and grappling arts, however *pankration* combined both martial arts of boxing and wrestling (the grappling sports had rudimentary elements of Qin Na that can be seen in the act of finger grabbing).

Pankrationis, a Greek word for 'complete strength' or 'total victory', referring to a victory being won by a brutal mix of wrestling, boxing, kicking, strangleholds and pressure locks. This must have been as close to an all out fight as could be imagined. It was almost the last event to appear in the ancient (33rd) Olympics in 648 B.C. and the first to be dominated by professionals (end of the 4th century B.C.) because of its crowd-pleasing spectacle.

> *Pankrationists must employ backward falls which are not safe for a wrestler. They must have skill in various methods of strangling; they also wrestle with an opponent's ankle and twist his arm, besides hitting and jumping on him, for all these practices belong to the pankration, only biting and gouging being excepted.*
>
> *Philostatos, 2nd century A.D.*
>
> *(from Judith Swaddling,* The Ancient Olympic Games, *1980, p. 60.)*

Pankration was filling a growing lust for blood sports that society wanted at that time. Only biting and gouging were disallowed (except by the Spartans). *Pankration* saw lots of ground wrestling because that is where the fight often ended up. Submissions could be more readily obtained from this position.

In ancient Greece, wrestling, *pankration,* and boxing were the heavy sporting events that saw no weight classes (although some had two to five age groups) and plenty of blood and death, particularly in the latter two sports. Wrestling greatly appealed to the ancients because of the role of skill and science used in this sport. Three falls were needed to win a match against one competitor, so a maximum of five rounds was needed to determine a winner. This demanded that the opponent be able to continue fighting the rounds, but the rules were remarkably tolerant to rough tactics nonetheless.

One pankrationist, Sostratos from Sikyon, was called 'Mr. Finger Tips' because of his skill in breaking his opponent's fingers in order to gain an early and quick submission. This technique was known as *ackrocheirismos*. Another Sicilian Greek fighter named Leontiskos, although a poor thrower, won at Olympia in the in the mid-fifth century B.C. by breaking his opponent's fingers. It was said that only contestants who were unable to throw down their opponent used this technique. This tactic was later banned lest the judges physically beat the offender, as prescribed by law.

Throwing or even touching a man's back and shoulders to the ground constituted a fall. Pinning, as the modern term of holding both shoulders to the mat for a period of time indicates, did not take place in ancient times. Completely proning the opponent out or tying him up as to control him from escaping were also winning techniques. It is interesting to note that the ancient Greeks used chokeholds to effect submission (as did *pankrationists*).

Wrestling was often referred to as a 'sport of craft' because of the large number of moves and holds that went with it. Most of us are happy today that, unlike early Greek wrestling practices, competitions were held at a *palaestra* (from the Greek verb *palaio* meaning to wrestle) in the nude. The use of olive oil was the norm (with a dusting of powder to allow for gripping). Upright wrestling took place in a leveled section of sand called the *skamma,* whereas ground-wrestling was staged in a specially prepared area called the *keroma* that had a muddy, sticky, 'beeswax' type of surface. The ancient Greek and Roman wrestlers wore their hair short, whereas Mesopotamian and Egyptian art depicts wrestlers with long hair, presumably because of contest rules. We all can appreciate the liability that long hair brings into a street fight because of its blinding effects and availability for use as a handle by an opponent.

Far East

Wrestling has flourished elsewhere in the Middle and Far East for at least three thousand years. In Mongolia and China, wrestling was practiced at religious festivals (not unlike the Greeks dedicating the Olympic Games to Zeus). Accounts of Japanese, Indian and Turkish wrestling matches predate the birth of Christ. The latter country is famous for its rich and successful wrestling heritage. Unlike the Ancient Greeks though, these wrestling styles generally were variations of the age old catch-as-catch-can, with a person losing if any part of his body touched the ground (some styles did require the pinning of a shoulder to win). The first recorded wrestling match took place in Japan, 23 B.C. A man named Sukune won the match by killing his opponent (with kicks). He became a national hero and is now the patron saint of all Japanese wrestlers. This contest was purportedly an early Sumo bout, but the kicking suggested a more ju jutsu type of fighting. The ninth century emperor Ninmyo highly supported wrestling festivals because of the benefit to military strength and the amusement of the people. Ground fighting evolved into some of these sports with time (Sumo stayed purely a throwing and pushing-out of the ring type of combat). For example, some historians believe that jiu jutsu originated in China. Imported in the 1600s by Chin Gen-Pin, it was then tempered and fused with indigenous Japanese martial arts and utilized by the samurai until their disbanding in 1867.*

Others believe that imported Chinese Kempo merely augmented the indigenous Japanese fighting skills, honed from centuries of feudal combat. In any case, there were approximately fifty different variations of ju jutsu from the Tokugawa period (1615-1867), such as Yawara, Kempo, Kugusuku, Taijutsu, Torite, Kumiuchi, Hakudo, Shubaku, etc. (all minor variants of the same principles) practiced in Tokyo alone in the late 1800s. These systems of fighting included throwing, striking, choking, joint manipulations and ground fighting techniques that were capable of rendering an opponent in painfully compliant holds, with broken bones, in an unconscious state or even dead. These ju jutsu styles, were pared down and made a hybrid by Jigoro Kano in 1882 to become the sport of judo, complete with a wide array of submission holds on the ground (he also established the judo headquarters, the Kodokan, in Tokyo). The nasty bone-breaking techniques and *atemi waza* (striking techniques), once required by the samurai for survival in combat, were removed for the safety of judo's participants. Like karate, judo was imported to the U.S. by G.I.'s returning from the Second World War. Japanese sole dominance in judo was broken in 1961 at the World Judo Championship at Paris and 1964 at the Tokyo Olympiad. A non-Japanese judoka (Anton Geesink of Holland) became the first foreigner to win gold medals in judo (ironically, this was the first time judo was included as an Olympic sport). Today judo is practiced around the world.

Wrestling

*The terms ju jutsu, ju jitsu, jiu jutsu, jiudo are partially derived from the words ju or jiu meaning gentle, soft, yielding or harmonizing; jutsu meaning methods or techniques, and jitsu meaning science or art. Do means path or way, indicating moral or spiritual connotations associated with a way of life and training. Thus, ju jutsu translates roughly to be 'gentle art' whereas judo means 'gentle way'. Ju jutsu and ju jitsu have often been used interchangeably and also with judo, it being the most modern form of these arts and ju jutsu being the older art.

Chapter 1: General History and Principles

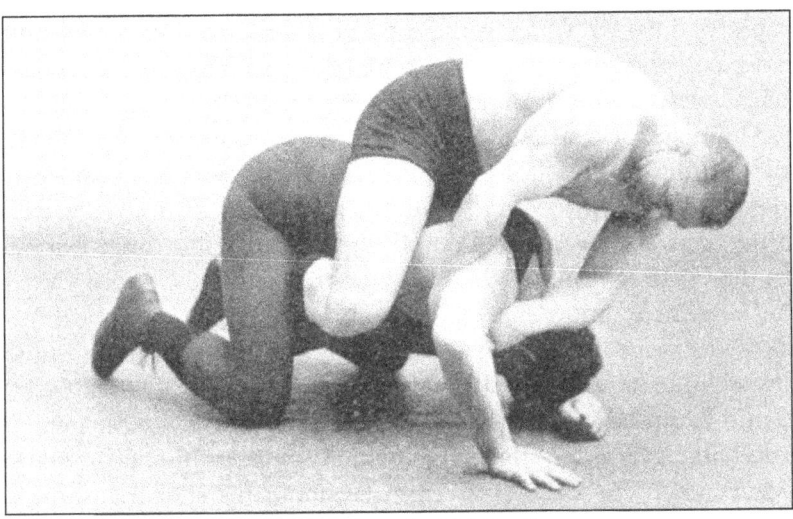

George Hackenschmidt Wrestling
Figure 1-6 This photo shows George Hackenschmidt trying to turn over his opponent with a bar-Nelson while applying the leg scissors to his torso.

Wrestling was thought to have been practiced in Europe even before the importation of the Graeco-Roman style by Roman soldiers. It was a popular sport in Europe, being the feature of many holiday events. During the Middle Ages, international wrestling matches were held frequently with traveling shows touring Europe until the 1900s. In America, wrestling had been popular with the Indians and the pioneers alike, the latter group bringing English wrestling like that of Cornish and Westmoreland styles with them from their motherlands. Abraham Lincoln was in fact the young wrestling champion of Sangamon County, Illinois. Wrestling was seen as a health and character building activity. Benjamin Franklin published a work in 1749 titled "Proposals Relating to the Education of the Youth of Pennsylvania" in which he advocated the establishment of a youth academy that promoted sports (including wrestling). But it was George Hackenschmidt, the 'Russian Lion', who indirectly stimulated international wrestling in America. Figure 1-6 shows Hackenschmidt scissoring and placing a Nelson bar on an opponent in preparation for turning him over. He turned professional in 1900 and toured Europe, thus bringing on the golden age of wrestling (until 1914). It was during these years that wrestling had the largest draw of any sport in the English-speaking world. An American, Frank Gotch defeated Hackenschmidt, in 1908. This win sparked much interest in wrestling. The first organized intercollegiate wrestling contest was held between the University of Pennsylvania and Yale in 1900 and wrestling has always had a place on the campuses since.

History repeated itself with claims of professional fight fixing (but not as much as with boxing). Gotch ruled supreme until he ran out of opponents. He was forced to retire at the onset of the First World War. Bizarre showmanship subsequently took over professional wrestling in the early post-war years. Vaudeville antics paled in comparison to the soap opera theatre-on-the-mat witnessed in today's professional arenas. Every country claimed their best wrestler to be the world champion, mostly due to a lack of centralized administration and organization that existed in the wrestling world. In 1940 for example, over twenty wrestlers claimed the heavyweight championship of the world.* Gimmicks abounded: masked men, wrestling bears, evil midgets and even female mud wrestlers all took turns entertaining the crowds. In the 1940s, wrestling was one of the first sports to receive TV coverage in California. 'Cavemen', 'murderers' and 'executioners' began to appear in tag team, ice and snow, and cage matches, as the spectacle continued to unfold in the 1950s. In 1961, wrestling reached its peak in popularity in the U.S. when 34,000 people crammed into Comiskey Park in Chicago to witness a wrestling match. Today the TV audiences are huge, as wrestling choreography, with its high degree of sophistication and excitement, approaches its zenith. Without the showmanship, few would care to watch these matches. This pugilistic ballet is a reflection of our society in some ways and delivers the need for pseudo-ultra-violence as good triumphs over evil, pretty boys over villains (or vice versa!). Today, serious wrestling matches take place in high schools, universities, and private clubs all across North America. The advent of the 'extreme fighting' matches have recaptured the need to see realistic fighting matches with relatively few rules. These fights often go to the ground for an eventual submission.

Ju Jitsu

Police and other law enforcement agencies have long used martial arts in their training. All Japanese police departments have a dojo in which to train as all recruits must have a black belt in judo. It is interesting to note that ju jitsu was replaced by judo in Japan after a contest was held on June 10, 1886 at the Tokyo police headquarters dojo between the head police ju jitsu instructor and one of Kano's judo students (who was also an aiki jutsu master). It was reported that the police ju jitsu master died from his beating and ju jitsu instantly lost credibility in Japanese law enforcement circles and it was echoed by the progression of Japan from a feudal era to modern times. This did not mean that ju jitsu became totally obscure, rather, the modernization of the peaceful society demanded modifications that was best presented in judo. Certainly, no holds barred jujitsu tournaments became less popular with students not willing to sacrifice life and limb, merely for sport. Judo eliminated almost all of the *atemi waza* (striking techniques) except for what was found in *kata* and other war-like, bone-breaking, joint-locking techniques basic to ju jitsu. The Japanese police and national defense forces retained some of these elements in the form of taiho jitsu, as they best filled their requirement for restraint and control techniques for use in arrest situations. The Chinese police similarly are well adept at Qin Na techniques, used to seize and capture criminals in order to control them

---

*A Pictorial History of Wrestling by Graeme Kent, 1968, p. 173.

without having to resort to the use of lethal force. These techniques are also popular with law enforcement agencies in North America. The amount of training dedicated to these pursuits by most officers is minimal, although they have never been more accountable for their use of force as they are today. What force they do use must be, therefore justifiable and reasonable to the courts and the public they serve.

Qin Na

Just as wrestling began in the dawn of mankind, so too did the seizing and grappling arts emerge. Qin Na (Chin Na) is a wonderful adjunct to any martial art. Recorded history indicates that, after 525 A.D., the Shaolin priests practiced the martial arts to fend off robbers through weapons disarming and controlling techniques, following the arrival of Bodhidharma from India. This Buddhist priest founded the Ch'an Buddhism in China (known as Zen Buddhism in Japan). It is believed that he taught the monks ways to strengthen the body to deal with bodily demands placed on them by the rigors of extended meditation training and possibly to deal with marauding bandits. This led to the development of martial arts techniques.* The Shaolin system came to be the premier martial arts organization in China. Qin Na became a well-developed component of their fighting arsenal. Almost every form of martial art has some form of Qin Na blended into the system, but no system is devoted solely to Qin Na. Knowledge relating to Qin Na, once secret, became available to the public by the end of the Ching Dynasty (late 1900s). These techniques became incorporated into the many fighting styles indigenous to China. The southern styles of Chinese martial arts generally have more highly refined and utilized hand skills for close combat than do the northern styles. Historical records reveal an influx into Japan of martial art skills and a consequent influence on indigenous Japanese martial arts, hence it is reasonable to assume that ju jitsu and aikido techniques were enhanced by Qin Na techniques. Books on the jujitsu or its predecessor ju jutsu, referred to the techniques as 'tricks', the trick being that a small man could catch an unwitting larger man's fingers, for example, and bring him to his knees grimacing in pain. The misinterpretation of the Japanese term *waza*, meaning technique, may have come about for several reasons. It may have occurred as the result of racial prejudices (inferred by the connotation that some form of 'trickery' was being employed) and/or misunderstandings of the Japanese martial arts and their underlying philosophies (putting a mystic view on that which was not readily understandable by Westerners).

Ju jutsu (and later judo) removed many of the Qin Na types of attacks from the art. Some practitioners, like S.K. Uyenishi, battled against misconceptions being propagated at the turn of the nineteenth century:

---

*Bodhidharma lived circa 448-527 A.D. and was an obscure figure in Indian and Chinese literature relating to the martial arts and Buddhism. He was also known as Bodai Daruma Daishi in the Japanese literature and Damo in Chinese literature. *Spiritual Dimensions of the Martial Arts* by Michael Maliszewski, 1996, p. 43.

> *Before preceding to tell you what ju-jutsu really is, I must mention a few of the things which it is not. And these, I regret to have to say, include the majority of those marvellous (sic) powers, etc., which are and have been so mysteriously referred to in most recent publications in ju-jitsu. The 'pinches' to which reference is so often made, are not only no longer used, but are not even permitted in any ju-jutsu contests at any of the important meetings held in Japan. I am afraid that any man who depended on one of these 'pinches' in order to secure a victory in a serious contest would find himself sadly disappointed. These 'pinches' are absolutely barred, together with hitting, finger gripping, and twisting or using the hand on an opponent's face, or similar movements whereby damage might be caused before the signal of defeat could be given (tapping out).*
>
> The Text Book of Ju-jutsu as Practised in Japan
> *by S.K. Uyenishi, circa 1918, pp. 18-19.*

Oriental Mysticism

Certainly the west was greatly mystified by accounts of almost superhuman pugilistic prowess possessed by the Japanese, who purposely kept their techniques guarded during the feudal era that just ended. Even their own commoners were not privy to these techniques as they were reserved for the nobility, samurai class bodyguards and later the police. Ju jutsu's beginnings were traced back to the period of the first half-century of the Tokugawa (Edo) period (1600-1867). The 'Golden Age' of ju jutsu was seen in the late seventeenth to mid-nineteenth centuries when there when hundreds of schools teaching variations of this fighting system, although it is believed that the first true ju jutsu style (Takenouchi Ryu) was started by Toichiro Takenouchi in 1532. As early as 1892, Rudyard Kipling wrote in the *London Times* about the superiority of the Japanese art of yielding over the British use of brute force (in reference to the punch-ups between the Japanese police and the visiting British sailors):

> *He has a grievance against the Japanese policeman (all Japanese policemen are required to have a workable knowledge of judo) who is paid a dollar for every strayed seaman he brings up before the Consular Courts for overstaying his leave and so forth. Jack says that the little fellows deliberately hinder him from getting back on his ship, and then with devilish art and craft of wrestling tricks- 'there are about a hundred of 'em and they can throw you with every qualified one'- carry him to justice.*
>
> Championship Judo *by Tamio Kurihara and Howard Wilson, circa 1965, pp. 16-17.*

Ju jutsu was on a road of continuing misunderstanding that was not always kept in check by the experts. On one hand, superhuman feats of pugilism helped create interest in the arts. But the common ignorance about sealing the vein (neck restraint) and the subsequent revival techniques (*katsu*) created a "death touch' and 'bringing back from the dead' nonsensical, occult-like following with a public hungry for such sensationalism.*

A degree of ethnophobic distrust brought on historically by isolationist and feudal attitudes, and later racial skepticism, fueled by mystic and spectacular claims were not uncommon at this time. This attitude is best described and put into a balanced perspective by E.J Harrison, a journalist who spent twenty years in Japan (and practiced judo in police dojo) around the turn of the century. His accounts, unfortunately, were not published until just prior to the second World War, when anti-Japanese sentiment was at its highest:

> *It must frequently have puzzled and bewildered a big and brawny bluejacket (sailor) to find himself easily mastered by a little Japanese policeman half his size. Let me hasten to add that it is not every Japanese policeman who is skilled in judo, though at home the conviction has apparently gained a firm foothold that the most anaemic (sic) and attenuated native of Dai Nippon has but to touch the most herculean (sic) Westerner with his index finger in order to bring his victim to the ground a shuddering piece of helpless, shattered humanity. On the contrary, the average efficiency of the Japanese police in this regard is not very great, and as a general rule, man for man, the Japanese policeman had in my day fared but second best at the hands of American and British Jack Tars (sailors) in those not infrequent 'scraps' between 'liberty men' (sailors on shore leave) and the junsa (Japanese policeman) of Yokohama Nagasaki and Kobe. Elsewhere in these pages I shall have occasion to describe a class of Japanese judoka (exponent of judo) whose skill and strength combined, I make bold to say, could not be equalled (sic), much less excelled, in any part of the world.*
>
> The Fighting Spirit of Japan, *by E.J. Harrison, 1955, pp.32-33.*

East Meets West

This air of secrecy and sinister mysticism should have lasted only until the turn of the century when Japan eagerly embraced the ways of Western modernization during the Meiji Restoration (1868–1912). The Japanese were very keen on intercultural exchanges as social changes swept the country. In the dojo, martial practices changed from that of *bugei* (military oriented training arts) to that of *budo* (way of martial arts). Just as the military leadership of the Tokugawa shogunate ended, marking a period of peace, personal freedom and enlightenment, so too did the bugei give way to budo.

---

*Hiagashi and Hancock did put these techniques into proper perspective in their book, however, the author's 1961 "unabridged and unaltered replication of the first (1905) edition" has 26 pages dealing with "serious and fatal blows and kuatsu (sic), dealing with the restoration of life "omitted. This was "because their value to the public is questionable and they do not contribute to the over-all value of the book".

Japanese ju jitsu masters/emissaries of the martial arts, like Professor Yukio Tani and Sadukazu K. Uyenishi came to England. People such as William Barton-Wright (1860–1951) beckoned such masters (and managed them) to teach their martial arts and to write on the subjects. Barton-Wright wrote a series of articles in 1899–1901 in Pearson's Magazine, expounding the virtues of self-defense, making him the first pioneer of ju jutsu in England as well as a pioneer of cross-training for complete (eclectic) self-defense training. As such, he founded his own style Bartitsu.*

Uyenishi expounded:

> *If it in any way helps to bring Ju-Jutsu into a more prominent position among English Athletic Sports (and this I may say appears to me to be a matter of supreme and even of National Importance) I shall then be able to feel that my labours have not been altogether in vain.*
>
> *The Army authorities have included the science in the curriculum of their Gymnasia. The Police have adopted many tricks, locks, holds, and throws from Ju-jutsu and have included these in their system of training.*
>
> The Textbook of Ju-jutsu as Practised in Japan
> by S.K. Uyenishi, circa 1918, p. 11.†

A number of books were published at this time with the assistance of other British martial art pioneers such as E.J. Harrison and Percy Longhurst. Indeed, ju jutsu was being introduced to westerners just as catch-as-catch-can wrestling was approaching its zenith, and well on its way to being accepted as collegiate and Olympic sports and forming the basis of the ring ballets seen later in professional wrestling. In 1918, Gunji Koizumi founded the Budokan in London under the watchful eye of E.J. Harrison. This judo headquarters, to which the European clubs reported, was directly affiliated to the parent headquarters, the Kodokan in Tokyo.

Similarly, B.H. Kuwashima and Katsukuma Higashi came to America to teach and co-author Jiu-jitsu (sic) books with Capt. Harry H. Skinner (1904) and H. Irving Hancock (1905) respectively. The latter ju jutsu practitioner Higashi, was only twenty-three years old when he arrived in America to successfully demonstrate the practicalities of his art to the New York City Police Department's finest. He performed his 'tricks' on a sizeable and unsuspecting cop.‡ But the mystique of Japanese martial arts was not to die an easy death.

President Theodore Roosevelt, a sports and pugilism buff, was responsible in some ways for both the interest and decline of ju jutsu in the U.S. In 1904, he

---

*An Introduction to W. Barton-Wright and the Eclectic Art of Bartitsu, by Graham Noble, Journal of Asian Martial Arts, Vol. 8, No. 2, 1999, pp.51-61.

†Early British publishers had a common practice not to date their books for some unknown reason. Sometimes writing styles or references to dates or events could help fix approximate dates.

‡"Jujutsu: The Gentle Art and the Strenuous Life" by Joe Long in the *Journal of Asian Martial Arts*, Vol. 6, No. 4, p. 72.

brought Yoshiaka Yamashita to the White House (and other high-ranking judoka into the U.S.) to augment the instruction given to him by James J. O' Brian, a police officer who may well have been the first ju jutsu pioneer in America.* Roosevelt could have been as outspoken for ju jutsu as he was for Western wrestling and in particular, amateur boxing, yet he was not, possibly because of its political ramifications (for example, the Russians and Japanese fought the Russo-Japanese War in 1904-5). This was in spite of the fact that he used Yamashita to develop a judo program (ten years before the collegiate wrestling program was established) for the U.S. Naval Academy in Annapolis in 1905, whose resulting judo club is still in existence today.

As for Higashi, his fame was to be short-lived, ironically by his own doing along with the unforeseeable assistance from judo. Although Higashi was mainly a jiu jitsu practitioner, he was heavily influenced by Kano's adoption of judo (1882) whose modification was in turn influenced by Western style of physical education.† Safe physical education for schools to keep America's youth healthy and fit became a goal. Kano not only had taken out the more dangerous techniques for the betterment of its practitioners, but he also made rules for the sport so that the techniques could be practiced with speed and power again at minimal risk to the competitors. These new rules no doubt led Higashi, first to compete in this match, and second, to lose as a result of the hindrances that the rules imposed on his style of fighting (as well as how the match was scored). This is what happened in this match. In 1905, the year his book *The Complete Kano Jiu-Jitsu (Judo)* was published, the 110-pound Higashi set up a contest at the Grand Palace in New York City with the United States lightweight wrestling champion of the time, George Bothner. There was no clear winner due to contention in the contest rules (pins versus throws for points); however, the media extolled the virtues of All-American Wrestling over Oriental trickery. Bothner was touted as the winner leaving ju jutsu to a destiny of floundering and continued misunderstanding that grew until after the Second World War was over.

Post-War Years

Certainly the Second World War dealt almost a deathblow to the Japanese martial arts, as suspicion and disrepute for such martial heritage dominated contemporary thought. Indeed, 72,000 people of Japanese ancestry had been rounded up and placed into relocation centers. Judo was officially banned (along with Kendo) at least temporarily (later practice was allowed on a limited basis). In Japan, judo instructors were ordered to teach *atemi waza* (striking techniques) and other harmful techniques previously removed from ju jutsu. This compromised the moral fiber of judo as laid out by Kano, in preference to the needs of the Japanese war machine. Forget the sport; this was war.

Post World War II publications, while denouncing the Japanese for not adhering to the Bushido code during the war, upheld the value of judo. A pocket book

---

*Long; Kurihara and Wilson (ca. 1965) cite 1902 as Yamashita's arrival date.

†Clark, 1992:138 in "Jujutsu: The Gentle Art and The Strenuous Life", by Joe Long in *The Journal of Asian Martial Arts*, Vol. 6, No. 4, 1997, p. 65.

(propaganda) author on judo during the latter part of the Second World War, referred to the Japanese as "little, evil brown men", yet he held this science of judo in high regard:

> *Foolish would it be indeed, for us, to sneer at everything the enemy possesses. Criminal, if we cannot learn from a foe how to 'blast' him with his own weapon. If judo is good for the Japanese then it is doubly good for Americans to use against the Nipponese. It is sort of retributive justice for us to learn what they know and confound them with that knowledge.*
>
> American Judo *by Arthur Hobart Farrar, 1943, p. 6.*
>
> E.J. Harrison's post-war postscript to his book stated:

> *The dismal failure of the Japanese to live up to the lofty claims of their vaunted bushido (warrior code), or 'Way of the Warrior', and to the alleged moral precepts underlying bujutsu, or martial arts. 'O! what a fall was there, my countrymen!' Rarely has practice lagged so far behind in theory as in the record of Japanese militarism during the last war. Unhappily for too many victims, the Japanese warrior's 'Way' was all too often anything but a great exemplar of chivalry.*
>
> The Fighting Spirit of Japan, *by E.J. Harrison, 1955, p. 248.*

Certainly, the post-World War II era was the real beginning of significant influx of martial arts into North America by trained American soldiers who had been stationed in the Far East. Although the ban on judo and other martial activities in Japanese schools was not lifted by the occupying forces until 1951, it was taught privately, in police schools and to the occupying G.I.'s. The anti-Japanese sentiment and prejudice was short-lived in the U.S. Judo circles. This was evidenced by the number of judoka competing (and advisory judo club members) of Japanese ancestry who competed harmoniously against the many American military judoka. These groups dominated the competitions by virtue of their cultural and professional interests in judo, although Harrison decried the qualifications of the G.I. 'experts' returning from service:

> *Thus it is difficult to resist the impression that since the war the grading panels of the Kodokan have been consistently more lavish in their bestowal of Dan grades to foreign pupils drawn more particularly from the ranks of the forces of occupation than were the grading panels of the Meiji era (1868-1912) during which I practised at the Kodokan. Doubtless the tendency to curry favour with representatives of the victorious allies is a natural weakness, but it must not be allowed, for that reason, to cloud our objective judgment of the facts. In light of this evidence all a priori assumptions that modern judo is impeccable in all its manifestations are untenable*

and must be abandoned and in their stead substituted a wholesome respect for eternal verities. "Tell the truth and shame the devil."

The Fighting Spirit of Japan, *by E.J. Harrison, 1955, p. 249, (Postscript).*

Judo was particularly popular in the 1950s and 1960s as evidenced by the number of judo articles appearing in the early Black Belt magazines. Its first volume, for example, was a special "Judo issue" reporting on the 9th National Amateur Athletic Union (A.A.U.)* Finals:

Growing American interest in judo was dramatically demonstrated at the national A.A.U. championships in Fresno, California, April 14-15 (1961), where an enthusiastic crowd of 8,000 packed the San Jose Sate College Auditorium to witness the event.

Team winner was the United Sates Air Force, which exercised its chosen role of deterrence through strength by triumphing over top representatives of judo clubs from across the nation. Over 150 skilled contestants took part in this two-day exhibition of this growing sport.

(Black Belt Magazine, *Volume 1, Number 1, 1961, p. 28*)

This same magazine, though dedicated to all of the martial arts, had five of the nine articles dealing with judo and half of the six magazine consultants were judoka. Over time, the promises of quick fixes to combat crime and evil disappeared (albeit, memberships and the numbers of pistol-shooting clubs no doubt have risen accordingly).

Recent History

The cloud of mysticism surrounding judo evaporated and flashier new forms of self-defense came into vogue, once again putting judo in the shadows. Judo appeared to decline, or rather, the popularity of karate and Kung Fu (Gong fu) exploded with the phenomenon of the Bruce Lee craze of the early 1970s. For decades, hardly a cover of Black Belt appeared without some reference to Bruce Lee on it (despite his untimely demise in 1973). The proportion of judo articles is accordingly small in comparison with the plethora of striking arts that are now in print. Judo just did not, and still does not have the flash that the striking arts have. Judo and grappling styles have recently enjoyed a resurgence in popularity (at least from the spectator's perspective), as a result of the airing of the 'extreme fighting' types of contests that pits all styles against each other in forums like the Ultimate Fight Championship's 'octagon'. What transpired was a rash of impressive ground fighting wins over all

---

*The A.A.U. appointed a committee on judo in 1955 and in this same year, the Amateur Judo Association of America was formed. Strategic Air Command's General Curtis Lemay adopted judo into their program of physical fitness around this time "to relieve tension and pressure of the men". Some 350 judo dojos were in existence with San Jose State College being one of the more active centers of judo in the U.S. *Championship Judo* by Tamio Kurihara and Howard Wilson, pp. 18-19, circa 1965

styles by the Gracie ju jitsu clan. Mitsuyo Maedakama taught judo to senior Carlos Gracie, who mixed it with other forms of pugilism. He then taught his Brazilian Jiu Jitsu to his younger brother Helio, who in turn passed it onto his sons Rorion, Royce and Rickson. In any case, the undervalued appreciation of the importance of having ground fighting skills quickly became very clear when the Gracies took most of the fights to the ground to effect submissions. Urgent cross training was undertaken by repeat contestants (even those initially victorious) in efforts to make them more competitive on the ground. Between these matches and the dramatically exaggerated spectacles put on by organizations like the World Wrestling Federation, wrestling is certainly seeing a lot of television airtime. Wrestling still remains popular at the Olympic Games and at some collegiate venues across North America. It appears, however, that society has once again indicated a preference or blood thirst for pugilism, real or choreographed. The stark cinema of violence has been in full swing for decades and it shows no sings of abatement.

1-3. General Principles of Qin Na

Components of Force in Qin Na

When applying any Qin Na (Chin Na) technique, there are several considerations about force that should be evaluated:

1. The amount of force to be used.
2. The direction of the applied force.
3. The type of force, applied to best suit the situation.

The first consideration will depend on variables such as the level of the perceived threat (for example, weapons, deadly force situation), the relative size, strength and skill of the assailant as well as situational factors (for example, multiple assailants, hostile crowd). The direction of the force used will depend on the type of technique chosen and allow the user to reposition the assailant anywhere he chooses (for example, to an inferior position, out of a room, and so on). The type of force applied will depend on the degree of control and damage the user wishes to inflict upon his opponent. These force considerations are interrelated (not mutually exclusive), but it is the type of application that may be the most critical and difficult determination to make in combat.

Types of Qin Na Applications

Qin Na can be used to distract, control, injure, immobilize or even kill your opponent using several different kinds of force applications.

1. Grabbing techniques that include joint lock maneuvers and muscle/tendon stretching. Figure 1-7 shows Grey applying a painful wristlock to White's right arm in preparation for applying clockwise torque to effect a shoulderlock. Both tech-

Chapter 1: General History and Principles

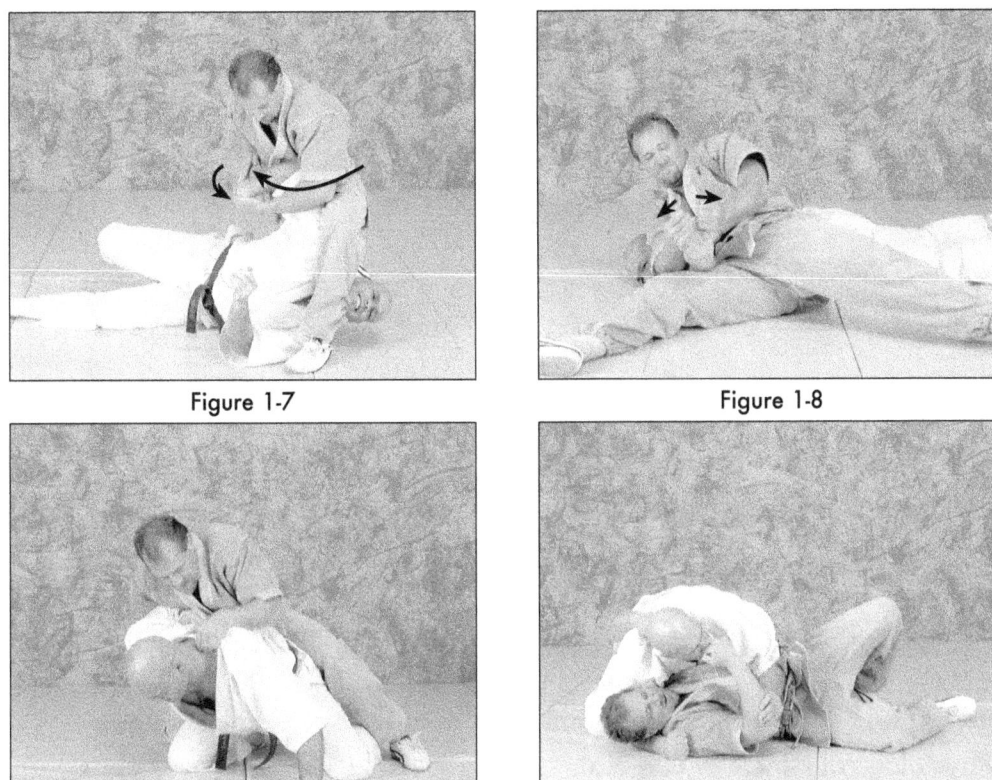

Figure 1-7

Figure 1-8

Figure 1-9

Figure 1-10

niques are examples of joint lock maneuvers. In Figure 1-8, Grey is using a muscle/tendon splitting technique by splitting the fingers of White's left hand in order to better control White on the ground. Grey already has White's left arm in an arm bar and wristlock (refer to Part Two of this book dealing with 'Joint Locks').

2. Pressing techniques that include pressure point attacks on Chi cavities and nerves. Figure 1-9 shows Grey attacking White's brachial plexus in the clavicle notch (St 12 Quepan). By gouging deeply into this point, in the hollow, well-like formation behind the midpoint of the clavicle, paralysis of the arm, mental stunning, and possibly unconsciousness could result. This should keep White from scooting forward to escape the hammerlock Grey has on his right arm. Figure 1-10 shows Grey using his fore knuckles to grind the soft spot under White's nose, in the nasalabial groove (DU 26 Renzhong). The loose protective skin of the philtrum can be stretched downward by using a pressing and rolling action with the knuckles to reduce the thickness of this upper lip area, and thereby allow optimal pressure penetration on the infraorbital nerves. This pressure point is quite painful, causing watering of the eyes, mucous discharge from the nose, and low level stunning. It is a good place to apply pressure as a means of creating distance or as a tool of distraction (see Chapter Four for more on pressing techniques).

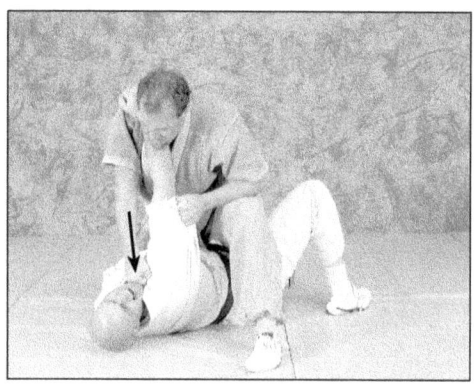
Figure 1-11

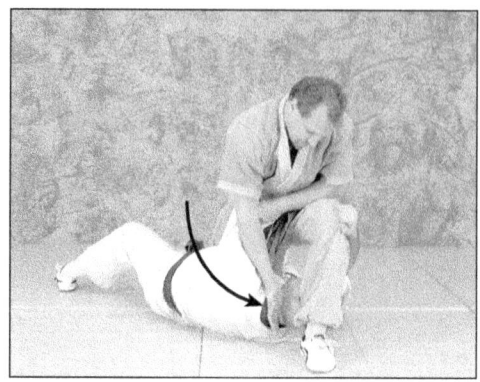
Figure 1-12

3. Striking techniques that include blows to vital points. Figure 1-11 shows Grey kneeling over White and punching the point of his jaw because he failed to tie up Grey's right arm. A heavy punch like this, with the head fixed against the floor, could break White's jaw and knock him unconscious. In Figure 1-12 Grey attacks a pressure point-rich target (side of White's neck) with a knife-hand strike. Such a blow can be devastating (see Chapter Four for more on striking techniques).

These kinds of techniques all serve to neutralize your opponent's ability to fight and to resist your attempts to control him via the use of pain compliance, structural breakdown of the body, unconsciousness, or in extreme cases, even death.

Physiological Effects of Qin Na

Qin Na techniques can be categorized more specifically by the physiological effect the applications of force have upon the body:

1. *Fen Jin* refers to the splitting or dividing of the muscles or tendons (muscle/tendon tearing). Figure 1-13 shows Grey bending White's baby finger backward in order to gain an extra measure of control over this arm (refer to Part Two of this book dealing with 'Joint Locks').

2. *Cuo Gu* refers to the misplacing of the bone(joint dislocation). Figure 1-14 shows Grey cranking White's left bent arm upward, applying extreme pressure on the shoulder joint. Grey's prying arms can easily break this joint (refer to Part Two of this book dealing with 'Joint Locks').

3. *Bi Qi* refers to the sealing of the breath (choking to unconsciousness by restricting airflow to the lungs or otherwise impair respiration). Figure 1-15 shows Grey choking White, having placed the *radial* edge of his right wrist across White's throat. White will fight back as long as the air lasts in his lungs, providing the windpipe is completely sealed. He will then fall unconscious (see the section "Sealing the Breath" in Chapter Seven for the physiological reasons for this response).

4. *Dian Mai* refers to the pressing of an artery (vascular neck restraint restricting blood flow to the brain). Figure 1-16 shows White applying pressure to both sides of Grey's neck on the posterior side of the carotid artery (where it splits into the internal and external carotid arteries) in front of the sternocleidomastoid muscle

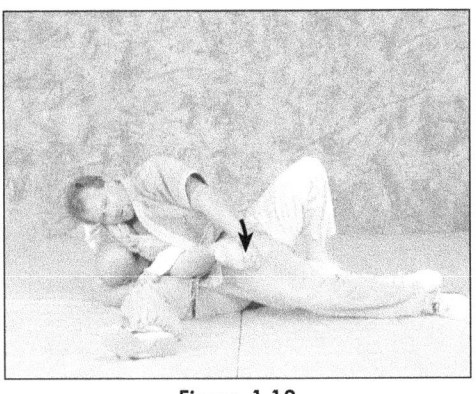

Figure 1-13

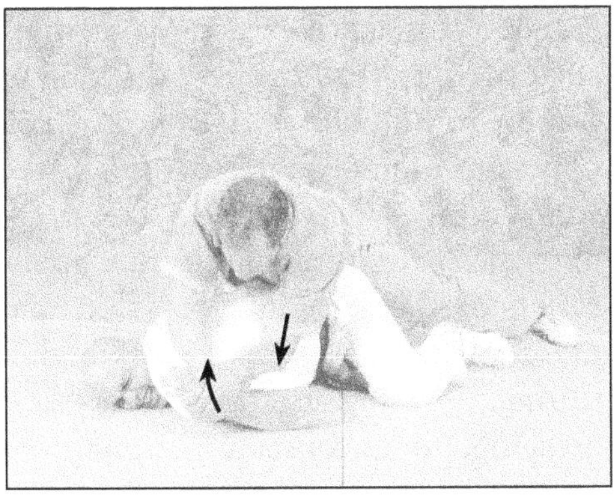

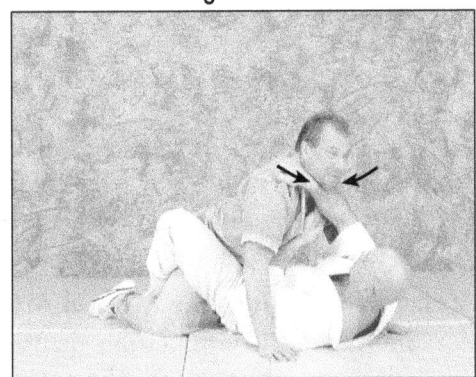

Figure 1-14

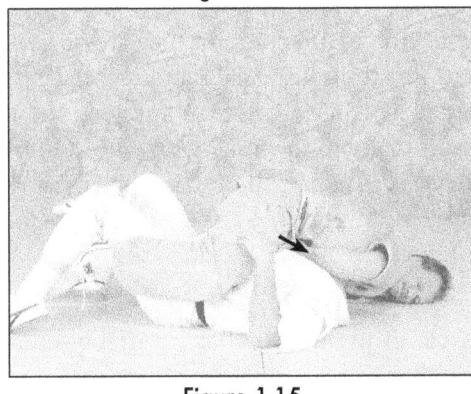

Figure 1-15

Figure 1-16

(St. 9 Renying). White has anchored his right hand on Grey's right shoulder and he pries his ulnar edge of his forearm into the front side of Grey's neck. White has also grasped Grey's left lapel so that he can lever this side of Grey's neck into it with his right arm. This in effect scissors Grey's neck from both sides to seal both of his jugular veins and underlying carotid arteries. The cessation of blood flow to the brain will render him unconscious within seconds as the brain is quickly starved of oxygen. A punch, slap or pressure point attack here can also cause unconsciousness (see section 'Sealing the Vein' in Chapter Seven for the physiological reasons for this response).

5. *Dian Xue* refers to the pressing of a Chi cavity (pressure point attacks of acupuncture points on the Chi meridians corresponding to organs of the body). Figure 1-17 shows Grey fighting back from an inferior position by attacking White's jugular notch (Ren 22 Tiantu). Grey has inserted his first two fingers into the depression at the upper border of the sternum in order to affect the supraclavicular nerve. Even light finger pressure will cause discomfort and coughing because of the presence of the underlying trachea (windpipe), making it a favorite pressure point attack to push someone back away from you. Pushing straight inwards or upwards interferes with the trachea that could cause swelling and subsequent suffocation.

The first three categories are relatively easy to understand and master. All that is required is practice exerting your muscular strength (*Jin*) to effect the kind of control or amount of damage to your opponent. This could range from the stimulation of nerve endings resulting in acute pain throughout the application of the technique, to skin and muscle bruising, muscle and tendon tearing, joint dislocations and bone breaking, to unconsciousness or even death. The latter two categories require a more sophisticated knowledge about

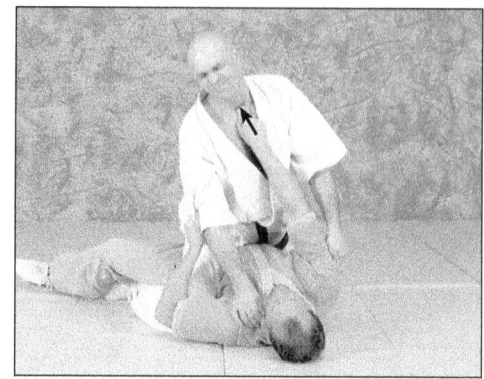

Figure 1-17

the exact location of the target areas (and even timing of attacks as in the case of *Dim Mak* theory) and feeling (sensitivity of application through special hand techniques) which is best taught through a qualified master. The consequences of applying these techniques can be fatal so they are not passed on freely to those persons who do not hold themselves accountable for the force they use. Indeed there have been many accidental deaths associated with the improper or unintended use of these techniques (as well as non-existent or inadequate revival treatment).*

Value of Qin Na in the Martial Arts

Any physical confrontation that leads to close quarter combat invariably ends up with the combatants grappling each other either to set up a throw or resist being thrown; to deliver strikes or prevent strikes from being executed; or to apply some kind of controlling move such as a joint lock and avoidance of the same. Those who know not about the ways of pugilism, effect a hold that may not protect themselves or further their own ability to attack his opponent (Figure 1-18). Those knowledgeable in the grappling arts are able to tie up their assailant, often by controlling a limb, and force them to submit through the principles of pain compliance (Figure 1-19). The extremities of their body may be broken down if they do not comply. So valuable a skill is that most Chinese martial arts styles have Qin Na fused into the system. Many oriental martial arts forms have at least a rudimentary treatment of Qin Na in their systems as well, particularly in countries such as Japan and Korea that have been influenced by the Chinese.

Qin Na is an excellent tool for modern police as it offers a non-violent looking way to use minimum force while offering maximum pain to gain control over resistive perpetrators. All police departments teach some form of 'restraint and control' techniques as an adjunct to the process of handcuffing. Police trainers have a saying that "you can't handcuff someone who doesn't want to be handcuffed unless you **own** them". Many suspects have run amok because a poorly trained officer tried to handcuff someone without the prerequisite limb control (and concomitant body

---

*For an excellent look into the art of refer to *Comprehensive Applications of Shaolin Chin Na* by Dr. Yang Jwing-Ming.

Chapter 1: General History and Principles

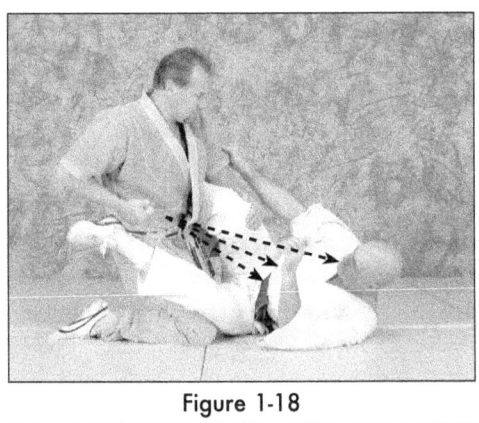

Figure 1-18

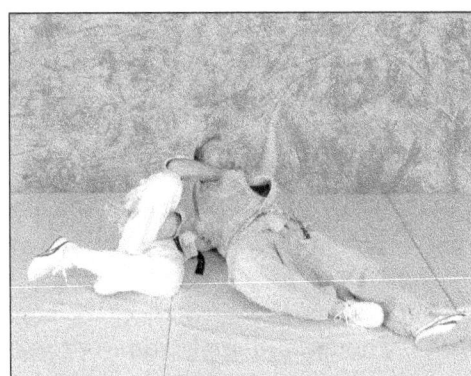

Figure 1-19

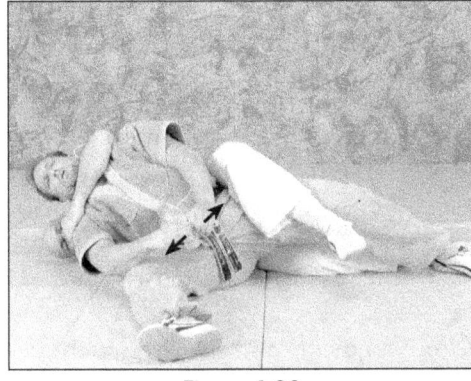

Figure 1-20

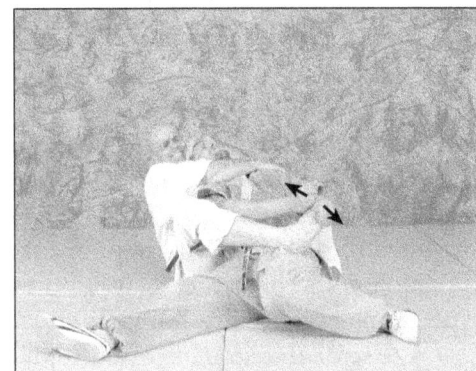

Figure 1-21

control) prior to the attempt.

Qin Na is also an excellent means by which you can disengage yourself from a ground fighting situation in which you are in control without having to trust your opponent's assertions that the fight is actually over. Otherwise, you would have to break a part of your opponent's body or take your chances on a truly peaceful disengagement while getting up off the ground (see Figures 1-27 through 1-31).

Important Points

When applying Qin Na it is important to remember several key points:

1. Go for abnormal movement: Bend and/or twist a joint in a direction opposite to its normal function or to such a degree that the joint is structurally compromised. Any joint bent beyond its natural range of motion will result in ligament and joint capsule damage. Splitting the fingers is a common Qin Na technique (Figure 1-20); slitting the toes (Figure 1-21) and even the legs (Figure 1-22) are not. These latter applications may be uncommon; the principle of the technique is not.

2. Apply pressure/counterpressure: When applying pressure to a joint through an attached appendage, be it a finger, hand or arm, be aware of the source of the counterpressure needed to trap the opponent to prevent him from moving away from your controlling force and thereby escaping. This counterpressure may be from the person's own body weight after he is up on his 'tippy toes' (in the stand up situation). Or it could be obtained from a solid object such as a wall or floor, or simply the counterpressure exerted by your own body (opposing hand, armpit, etc.) as shown in Figure 1-23.

3. **Use your whole body:** It is best to use your entire body to apply Qin Na, right from your rooted stance and body movements integrated into your Qin Na technique. In the standing situation, this may be accomplished in any of these ways:

a) Lowering your stance, thereby dropping your center of gravity to enhance a downward application of force.
b) Side stepping to improve your angle of attack simultaneously minimizing his ability to counterattack.
c) Or more simply and directly, by using your hands in combination with your hips.

On the ground, these principles are more difficult to apply, but total body control is imperative. Going to the ground does make it possible to use your legs and involve your whole body to apply your technique since your legs may not be required for balance purposes. For example, you may use your leg and back in conjunction with your arms to peel off a defensive arm that would otherwise prevent you from applying a reclining arm bar (Figure 1-24).

4. **Use distraction/surprise:** Apply your Qin Na quickly and accurately, 'softening up' your opponent with distracting blows and pressure point attacks, to take him by surprise and weaken his resolve. By doing so, your opponent's attention and focus will shift away from the limb you wish to control or away from the limb of yours he is controlling. In the latter case, you must move decisively or your opponent will force you to cease resistance by increasing the pressure of his hold. In Figure 1-25 White is attacking the mandibular angle (S.J. 17 Yifeng), the point in the depression under the ear lobe between the mandible and the mastoid process. Pressure attacks directed inward and forward towards the nose will cause low level stunning and extreme pain.

5. **Speed and strength of application:** Do not apply your Qin Na technique in increments to the point of being effective because it will allow your opponent to sense your intention and allow him to take evasive action or counterattack you. Decide whether you need to merely control your opponent's movements (as with an ineffective assaultive drunk) or in the case of a more serious encounter (such as with a knife attack), to break the knife-wielding arm. Apply a judicious amount of force needed to get the job done.

6. **Be aware:** Look at the big picture. Be aware of your surroundings and other possible assailants should you need to break off and disengage from your assailant and engage others with striking techniques (or RUN if tactically sound to do so). If you go

Chapter 1: General History and Principles

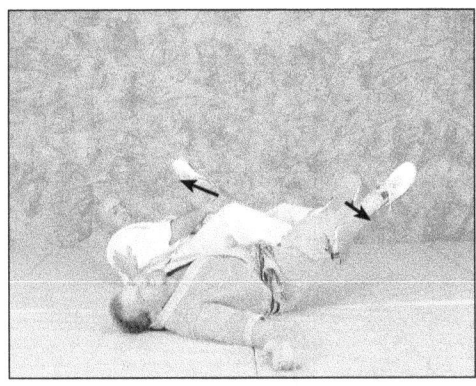

Figure 1-22

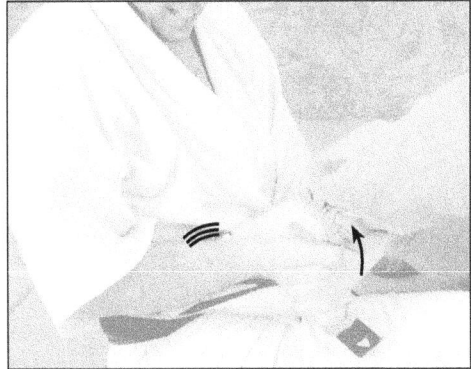

Figure 1-23

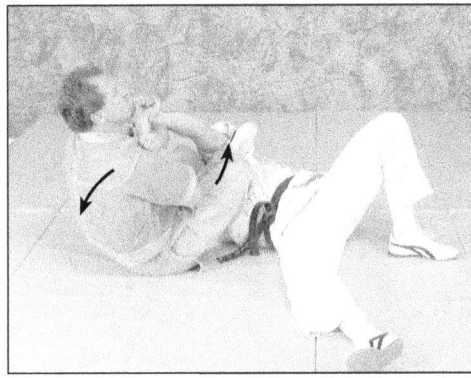

Figure 1-24

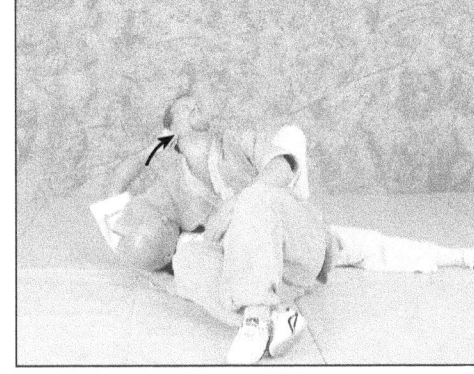

Figure 1-25

to the ground, then look around (Figure 1-26) as your biggest threat may be looming near you. Choose a hold-down technique that can offer you the safest position that you can adopt, depending upon the circumstances in which you find yourself.

7. **Move to superiority:** Use the direction of Qin Na techniques and your ability to flow from one technique to another in order to place your opponent in an increasingly inferior position, preferably in the prone position where his ability to counterattack is severely limited. You may want to stand up because of some other threat in your vicinity (other attackers) or because your opponent has given up. But why trust him? Instead, maintain control over him as you get up, and then decide if you should relinquish control. For example, Grey has White in a hammerlock and White gives up fighting, wishing to call the fight off

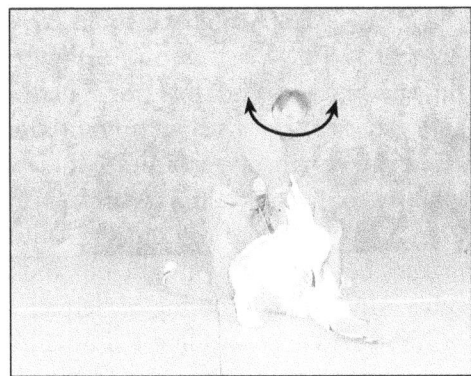

Figure 1-26

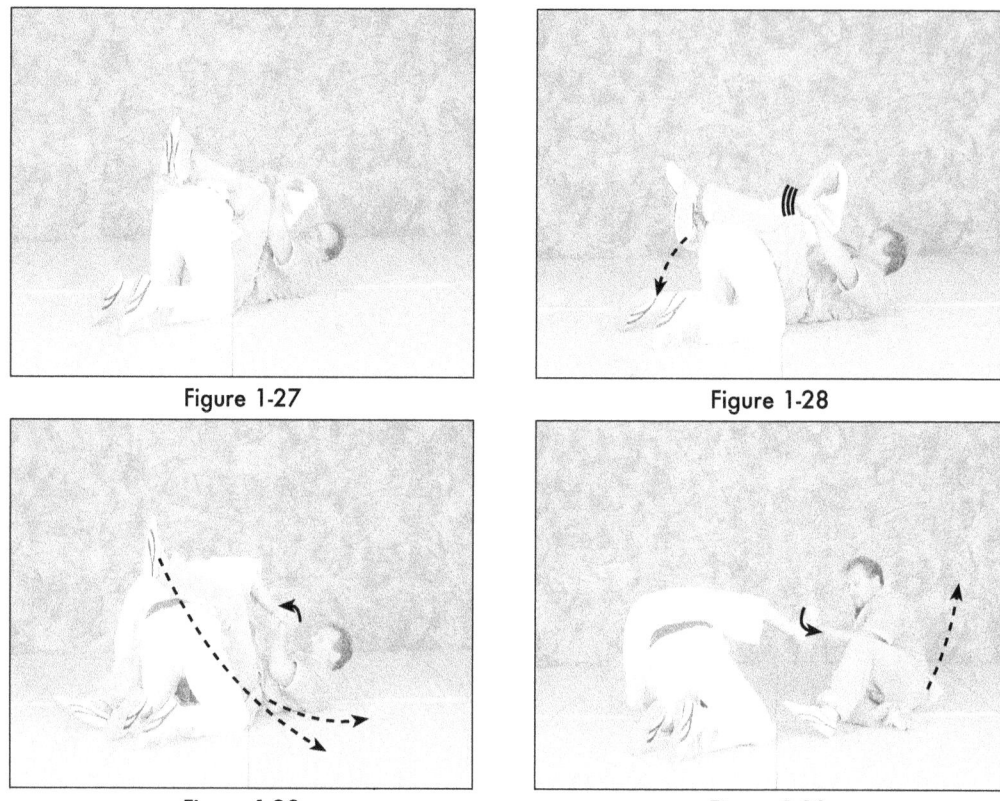

Figure 1-27

Figure 1-28

Figure 1-29

Figure 1-30

(Figure 1-27). It would be foolhardy to just let him go unless perhaps you broke his arm and he has passed out. Figures 1-28 and 1-29 shows Grey grabbing a few fingers. The pain and directional nature of the chosen finger lock keeps White down and under control without any interference from White (Figures 1-30 and 1-31).

8. Leave no opportunities for escape: Just holding onto someone is not the same as controlling him. Figure 1-32 shows that White has ineffectually controlled Grey so he is able to roll out of White's grip to quickly do a reversal on him. Grey reaches behind his own right hip and inserts his arm under White's right leg as he spins into him by shooting his left leg underneath himself. Grey, knowing the value of immediately controlling a limb, also grabs White's right hand with his left hand as he completes his reversal (Figure 1-33). Grey levers down on White's arm and drops his weight on White's shoulder and upper arm to force him to the mat. Grey improves his control over White's arm with a bent wristlock (Figure 1-34).

Once you gain the upper hand with a Qin Na technique, keep the pressure on the joint/pressure point fixed as to not allow an opportunity for escape. You must give his brain an opportunity for minimizing pain: it should be presented as an option that it cannot pass up. The more a person resists, the more pressure is applied. If a person complies with your commands, take some of the slack out of

Chapter 1: General History and Principles

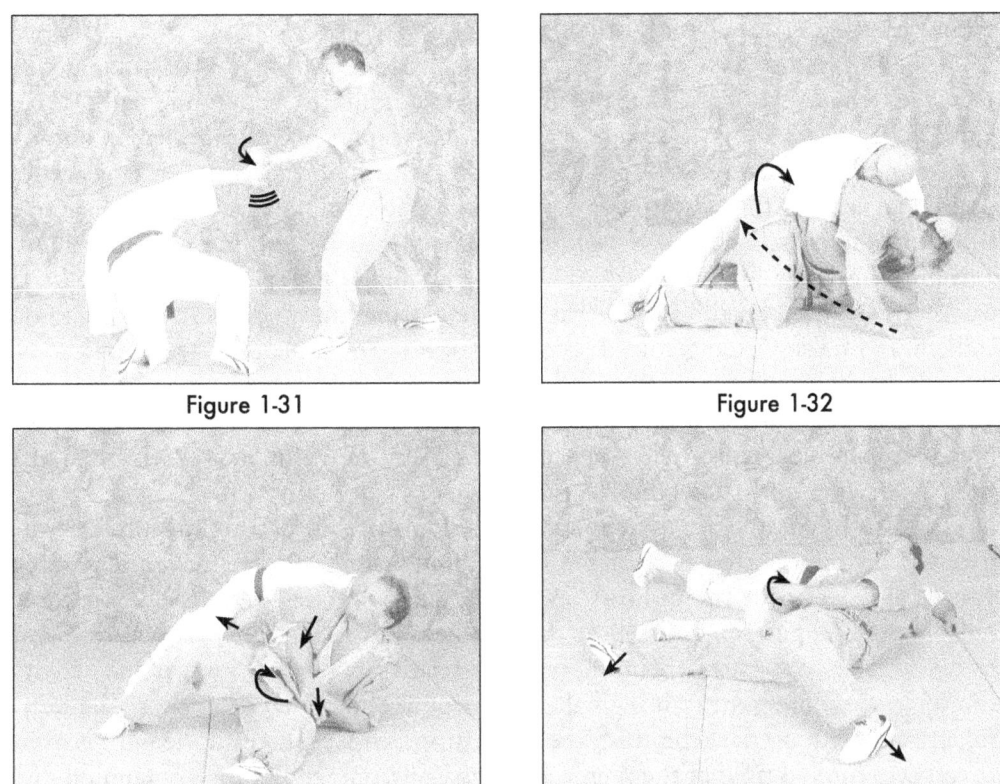

Figure 1-31

Figure 1-32

Figure 1-33

Figure 1-34

the technique, but do not relinquish your control over him ('tapping out' should not mean letting go of your opponent entirely). It's a pain/reward system. Use the directionality of the technique itself to move the person in the direction you wish to take him. If you cannot accomplish this with the hold that you have on him, use transitional moves to get the required hold on him. Be sure never to lose control over your opponent as you do so because he will sense this lapse of control and escape.

9. Let him help you: If at any point during your control over him, he begins to resist, tries to counterattack, or escape your grasp, try cranking the pressure back up to effect the desired level of compliance. Get him to assist you in your endeavors to move him from one position to another by using the subtle art and craft of applying pain.

10. Tell him what you want: Be firmly vocal in your treatment of your opponent so that he knows exactly what it is that you want him to do. Loud, repetitive verbal commands can cut through the anger, confusion, panic and pain that your opponent may be experiencing. Keep your commands simple, direct and assertive to show him and others, who may be listening, that your intention is simply to control his resistive or assaultive behavior, not to punish him. You must control the fight scene by not appearing to be heavy-handed once he is under control. Otherwise, others may jump to his aid or you risk the possibility of providing your opponent with witnesses regarding your 'brutality'.

11. Do not use excessive force: Apart from legal problems that you may be incurring, there is a real danger of bystanders coming to your opponent's aid if you 'beat the person up'. Or your opponent may experience an 'adrenaline dump'. This latter phenomenon is the result of the 'fight or flight' response in which your opponent, sensing that his arm, for example, is about to break, will muster almost superhuman strength supplied by the introduction of adrenaline into his bloodstream from the endocrine glands. This is a physiological response to stress (in this case, the threat of bone breakage) that you are placing him under. He may try to do something foolish or dangerous in order to escape. Some people have been known to fight through severe injuries in order to survive a critical incident.

12. Tapping out: When training with a partner, you may incrementally apply pressure when you sense that you are near his full range of motion or otherwise near his personal pain tolerance level. He can let you know when your technique has come to its completion by tapping out to submit. Your partner must **release the pressure on the affected part of the body immediately, but we recommend that you do not let go of the hold.** A few quick taps on your partner's body is more reliable than tapping on yourself or the mat because your partner may not be able to see or hear your taps depending on your relative body positions or the activity (noise) level within your training hall. It is recommended that you release the hurting pressure, but do not relinquish the hold, for practice sake, until the fight is over. If you ever find yourself at the mercy of a classically trained fighter, try tapping out! Remember that under stress, people will most likely react the way they were trained.

1-4. GENERAL PRINCIPLES OF GROUND FIGHTING

Going to the Ground

Some martial artists train solely for stand up fighting situations because they feel that if they train properly, then they will never end up on the ground. They feel that they are wasting their time studying a skill that they would never use. Realistically, there is a probability that if you engage in a physical altercation with someone, you may end up on the ground. The fight there is radically different from the stand up fight. Many untrained fighters enter the grappling stage very quickly as a matter of self-preservation, as opponents try to smother each other's ability to attack or do so for a lack of a better fighting strategy. We have all seen it happen in real life. We believe that it is more important to be a well-rounded fighter with some highly honed and specialized skills than it is to be highly skilled in many techniques limited to only a small portion of the fighting spectrum. After all, the street offers a whole host of unpredictable variables like getting sucker-punched by another party, losing your balance on uneven or slippery surfaces or being taken down when your back is turned, to name a few situations that do not take place in the training hall. The

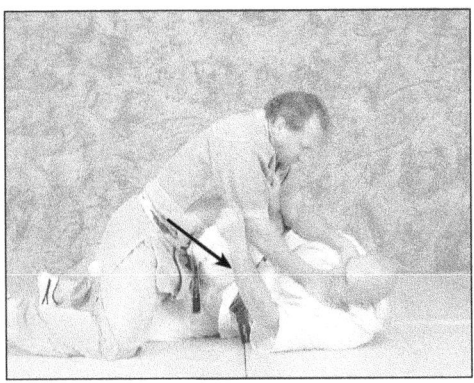
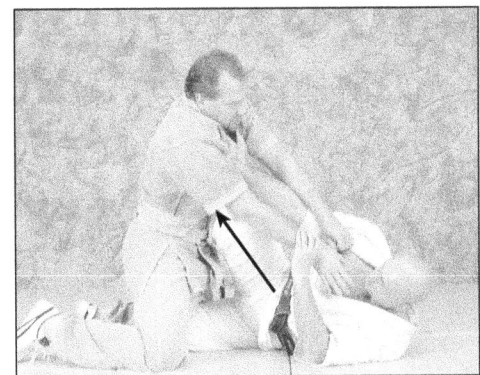

Figure 1-35   Figure 1-36

problem does not necessarily lie in getting into a bad situation, but awareness is the supreme key to avoidance; it lies in successfully knowing how to get out of it.

Fight Control Factors

In order to win on the ground, you must be able to control your opponent in several important ways. These are not the only variables or factors involved in a physical altercation. There are many others such as size disparities, differences in skill, stamina, strength, etc. but we will look at these six briefly:

1. Controlling the distance.
2. Controlling (protect/attack) the vitals.
3. Controlling the body positions.
4. Controlling the limbs.
5. Controlling the body weight.
6. Controlling the mind.

1. Controlling the Distance. Controlling the distance is one of the most important aspects of ground fighting. The distance determines the quality and types of attack (or defenses) and the kinds of positional changes that we can do. A stand up fighter relies on footwork to control the distance to his opponent, whereas the ground fighter can use his arms and legs, singly or in any combination of the four limbs to vary the distance from the opponent. When the people are ground fighting it is important to remember these general rules regarding the relative closeness of the hips:

a) Keep the hips in close when attacking. (Figure 1-35)
b) Keep the hips away when defending. (Figure 1-36)

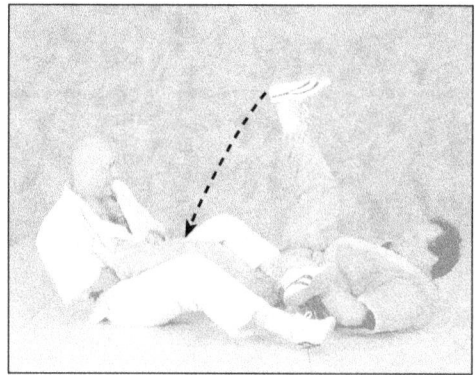

Figure 1-37

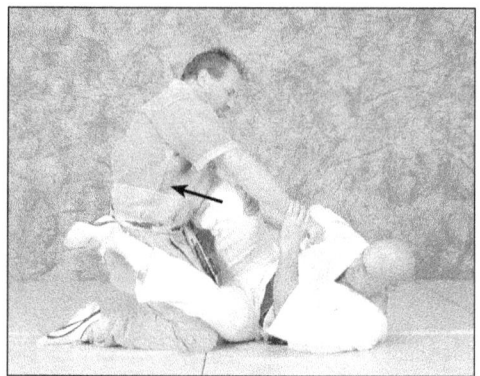

Figure 1-38

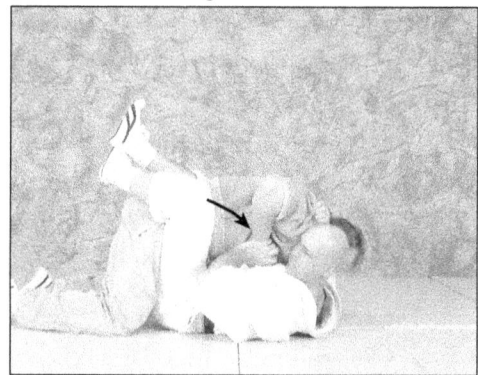

Figure 1-39

c) Don't give your opponent room or an opportunity to attack with his body tools. (Figure 1-37)

d) Keep your opponent close (like executing a throw) when changing positions, unless you need room to move into a different position.

If you can push your opponent's hips away from you using your feet while he tries to climb on top of you while in the guard or half-guard (assuming that he is not going for a leg lock), then his ability to attack you is greatly diminished (Figure 1-38). If you pull him into you with your legs or arms, then you can take the attack to him (Figure 1-39) or smother his attacks if he is on the offensive.

These general rules also apply to stand up fighting. The proximity of the hips for the boxer, who normally does not clinch, would be close (within jab reach) to attack and at least arm's length away to avoid being punched. Of course, a boxer's defense will continue within all striking ranges, but these are generalities.

2. Controlling the (Protect/Attack) the Vitals. As in a stand up fight, it is essential to protect your vital areas of your body and have the ability to attack your opponent's in order to neutralize him as quickly as possible. It is difficult to protect your vital areas using your arms alone, so you must rely on your body positioning, body movement, and positioning, using your other appendages to assist. Even being able and aware enough to keep your chin to your chest and to shrug your shoulders may mean the difference of fighting on or being choked out. If you sense that your opponent is setting up to strike a vital area, move to protect that spot, while looking to attack his vital areas. A few general rules are:

Chapter 1: General History and Principles

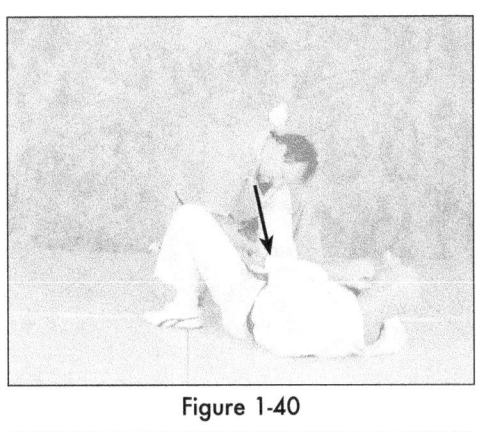

Figure 1-40

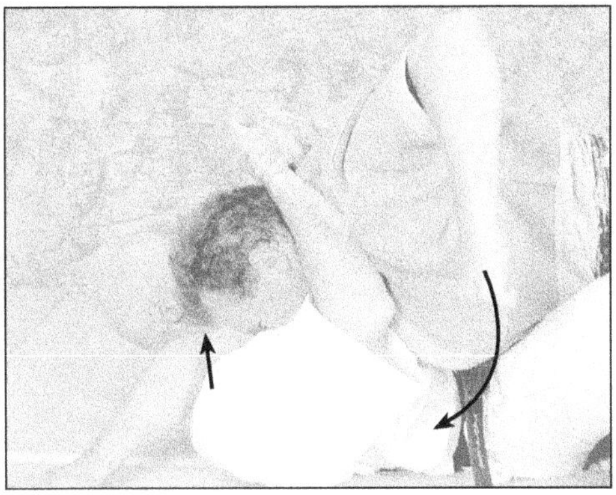

Figure 1-41

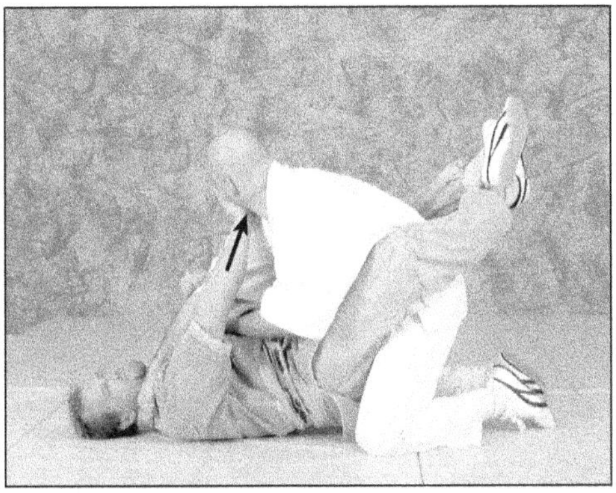

Figure 1-42

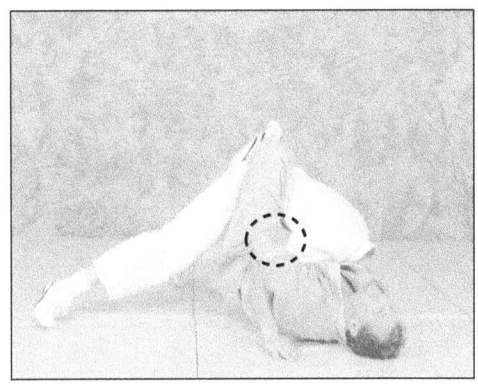

Figure 1-43

a) Do not expose your vitals to your opponent's uncontrolled body tools. (Figure 1-40)

b) Strike your opponent whenever and wherever possible using all of your body tools. (Figure 1-41) For example, Grey can use his left free arm to punch White's midsection as well as use his right elbow to gouge into the right side of White's neck.

Strike a balance between attack and defense. You must limit your opponent's ability to punch, lock or choke you while you look for a way to do the same to him. For example, if a person has you in the mounted position (straddling on top of you) and moves to choke you (attacking your vital carotid arteries), you can thwart him by palm-heel striking his chin (Figure 1-42) or by attacking his eyes with a finger jab. If you need to seal his breath from this same bottom position, you must include his free arm in your reclining guillotine to prevent him from gouging out your eyes (Figure 1-43).

3. Controlling the Position. Use positional changes to alter your ability to attack, defend or escape from your opponent. This is the real skill in ground fighting, having the ability to go from one position to a superior position smoothly and

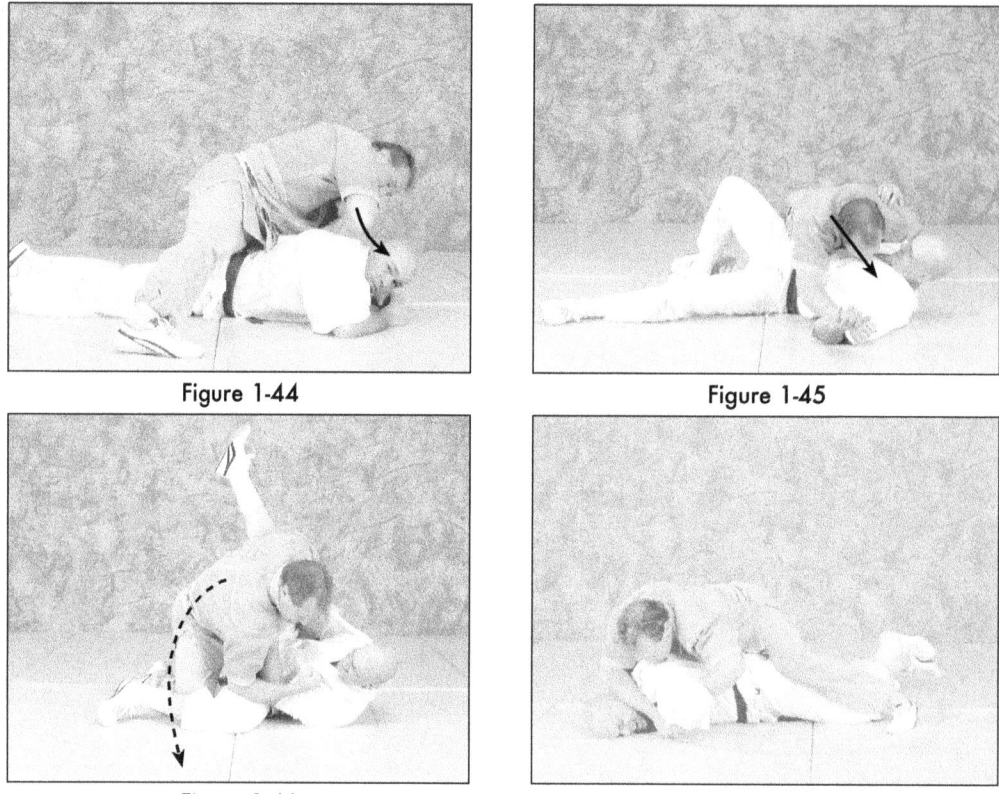

Figure 1-44

Figure 1-45

Figure 1-46

Figure 1-47

efficiently, without giving up anything to your opponent. Each position gives you different options of attack and defense. A few rules to remember are:

   a) Never expose your back to your opponent in any position (prone, on all fours or seated). White is almost defenseless against Grey's assaults when when in a prone position and he is also totally unable to attack Grey from this hugely inferior position (Figure 1-44).
   b) Keep your head near the center of his torso (his leg, arm and head tools are difficult to use against you when you are here). Grey is in a safer, more stable and therefore in a more dominating position in Figure 1-45 than in Figure 1-46.
   c) Maximize your ability to attack and minimize his ability to defend (e.g., when Grey puts him in the prone position, he does both in Figure 1-47).

During the transitional phase of a positional change, try to formulate your next move in advance of moving so that you can gain the advantage immediately. For example, Grey has mounted White who finds himself in an inferior position on the bottom (Figure 1-48). Grey tries to choke White who decides to make a positional change. White steps over Grey's right foot with his left leg and controls Grey's arms (especially his right arm) in order to keep Grey from using the appendages on his

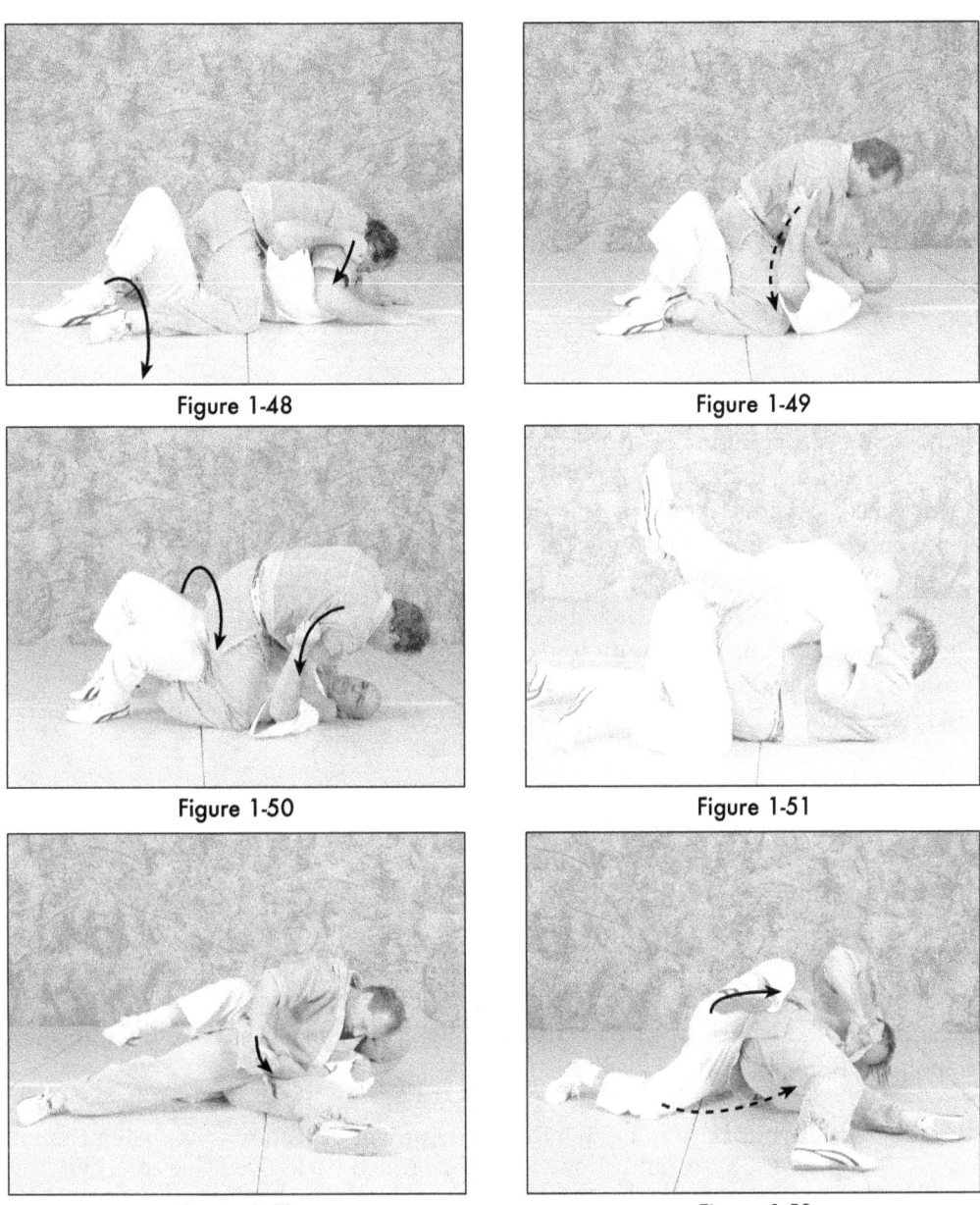

Figure 1-48

Figure 1-49

Figure 1-50

Figure 1-51

Figure 1-52

Figure 1-53

right side to thwart the rollover (Figure 1-49). White now bridges off his left shoulder while pulling Grey's right arm to the outside and downwards to effect the rollover (Figure 1-50). White uses the rolling momentum to bring him on top of Grey (Figure 1-51).

Another example of a positional change shows Grey holding down White in a scarf hold (inclined left headlock) while trying to effect a right arm bar using his left thigh as a fulcrum (Figure 1-52). White rolls into his opponent to free himself from the arm bar (Figure 1-53) and encircles White's torso with his arms in a bear

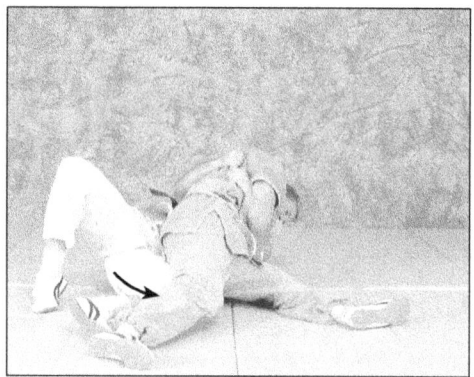

Figure 1-54

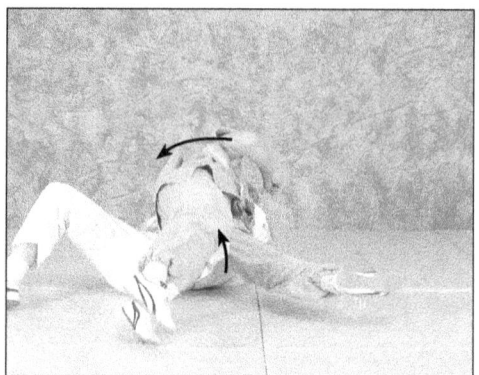

Figure 1-55

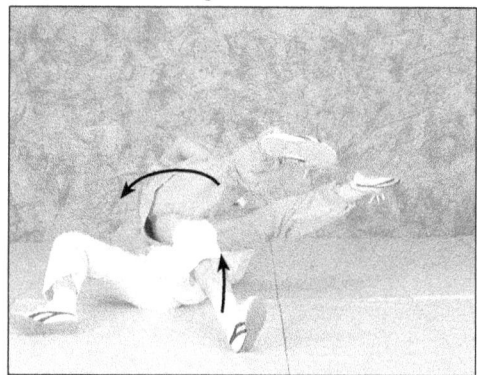

Figure 1-56

hug, taking care to slide his knee under White's right leg (Figure 1-54). White then quickly reverses direction (Figure 1-55) and pulls Grey over onto his back (Figure 1-56).

Or you may wish to switch from the guard position to the mounted position by scissoring him onto his back (see Figures 2-76 through 2-79). Or perhaps you want to prevent him from punching you in an arm-included headlock while in his guard by rolling onto your side that traps his free arm.

4. Controlling Your Body Weight. You want to use your body weight to maximum advantage in order to sap your opponent's strength, make it difficult for him to breathe, reduce his ability to move freely, create a sense of doubt, fear or panic in his mind while enduring crushing pain. While you control your center of gravity, it helps you to stabilize your own technique as you 'spike' your weight into your opponent. Remember this advice:

- a) Lower your center of gravity to maintain your position (e.g., being too high in the scarf hold allows you to be rolled backwards (Figure 1-55); being too high in the mount allows you to be bucked off) (Figure 1-69).
- b) Transfer maximum body weight onto your opponent (e.g., spike your weight through your chest onto his chest by keeping off your knees and butt) as in (Figure 1-58).
- c) Sense his center of gravity for your strategic advantage.

Chapter 1: General History and Principles

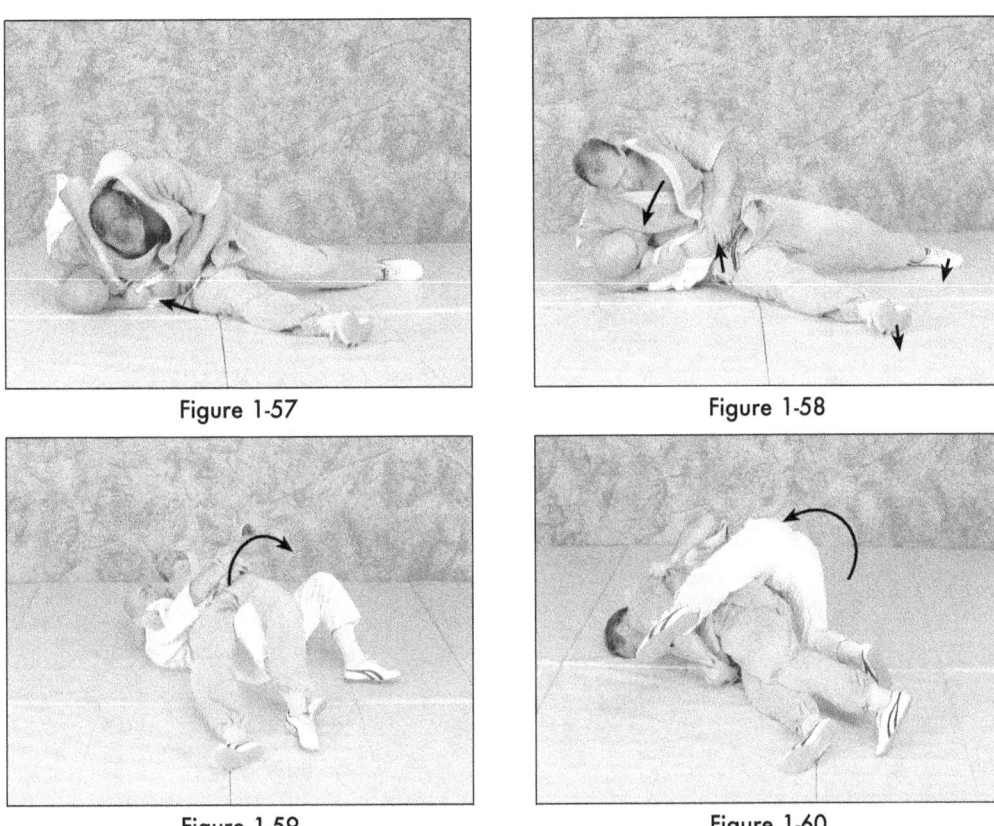

Figure 1-57

Figure 1-58

Figure 1-59

Figure 1-60

For example, if you sit on your buttocks while executing the scarf hold, you are going easy on your opponent for the reasons mentioned above (Figure 1-57). Make your opponent work for everything he does by rising your buttocks off the mat slightly thereby bridging from the edges of your feet to your ribs, anchoring your weight through his torso (Figure 1-58). It is not merely a matter of putting your weight on top of your opponent. For example, if you lean back a little too far, your opponent can easily tip you backwards (Figure 1-59). Lean too far forwards and your opponent may rise up and roll you over into the prone position (Figure 1-60). It is amazing what a trained ground fighter can do in these regards even though he may be significantly lighter than his opponent.

5. Controlling the Limbs. You must control your opponent's ability to attack you as well as to put yourself in a superior position in which to attack him. When two boxers get overly tired, they get into a clinch (controlling the distance), they tie up each others arms (controlling the limbs), and even drop and press their heads together to prevent (accidental) head butts (protecting the vitals). This can happen in the ground fighting situation to buy yourself some rest time (Figure 1-71). Here are some important tips to heed:

Chin Na In Ground Fighting

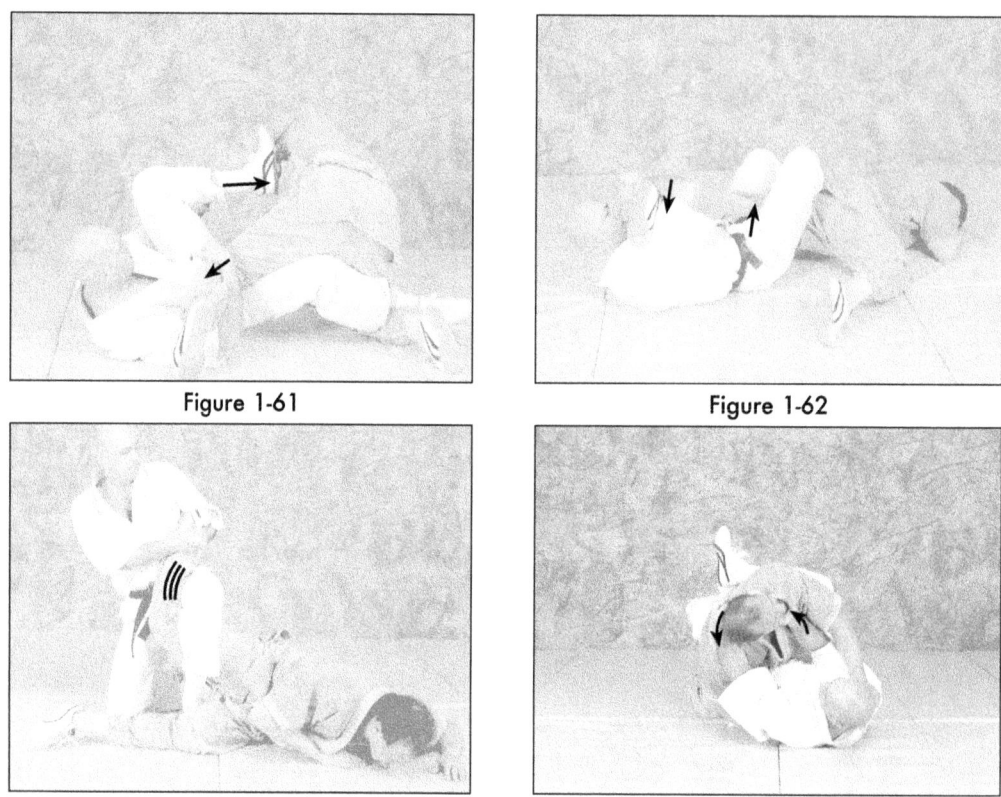

Figure 1-61

Figure 1-62

Figure 1-63

Figure 1-64

a) Take and use what your opponent gives you (e.g., White takes Grey's left leg in preparation for a leg lock as in Figure 1-61).
b) Limit his ability to fight back by taking a limb or two (White completes the leg lock as in Figure 1-62).
c) Control one of the five major body supports and you control your opponent (Figure 1-63).
d) Here we will consider the head/neck to be an appendage. Wherever the head goes the body will follow (Figure 1-64).
e) Sense your opponent's intent by his subtle body movements by relaxing and feeling loose.
f) Be aware of his attacking appendages and your own vulnerabilities.

By failing to control a key limb (you cannot always control all limbs simultaneously), you can put yourself at risk of being attacked (Figure 1-65). White can force Grey to stop punching by bucking him forward (Figure 1-66), thereby forcing Grey to use his attacking limbs for support (Figure 1-67). If you can control a limb or two, you will be in a very strong position for an attack, even if you are in

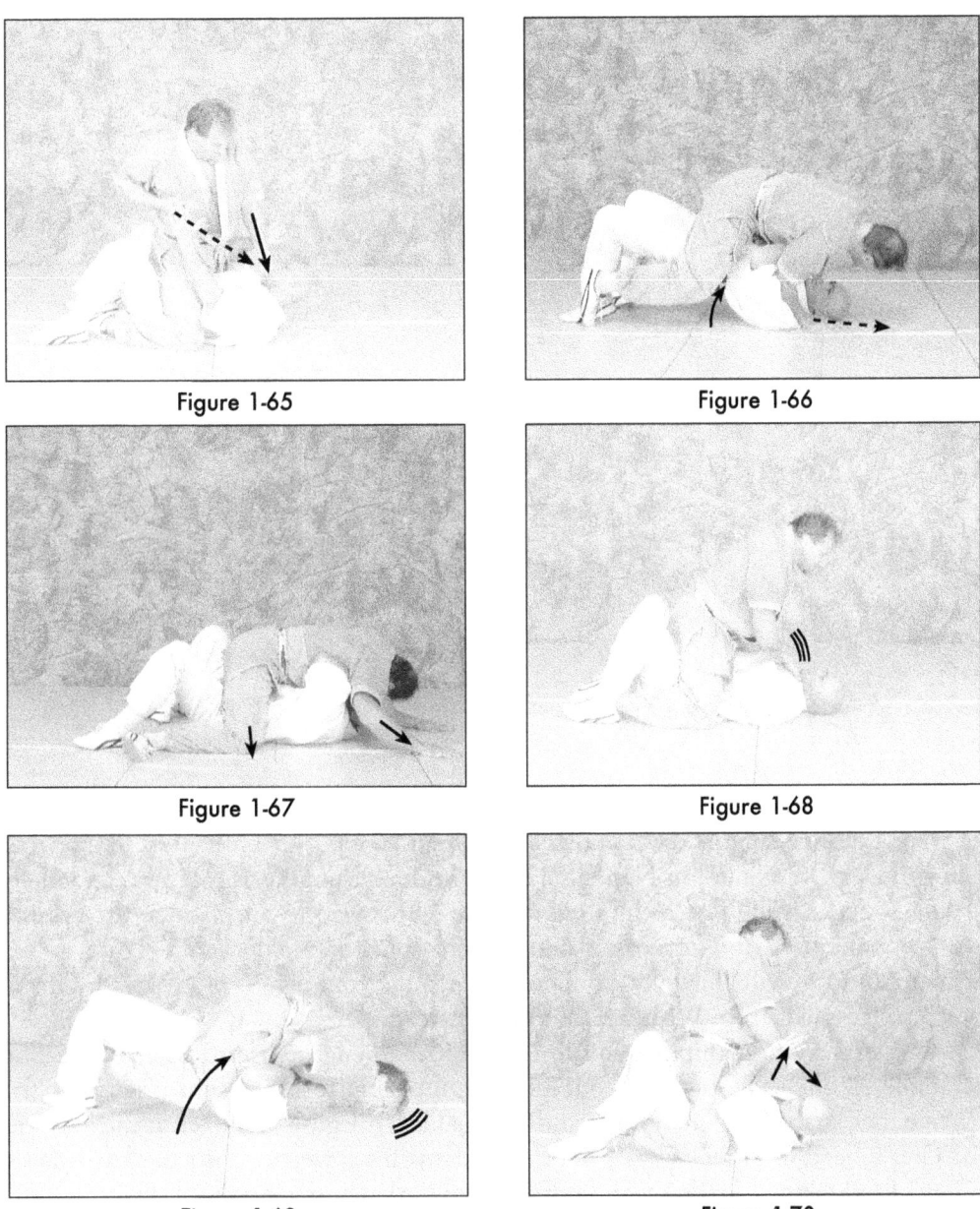

Figure 1-65

Figure 1-66

Figure 1-67

Figure 1-68

Figure 1-69

Figure 1-70

a disadvantageous position. White grabs both of Grey's wrists to prevent him from bracing against his bucking (Figure 1-68) which causes Grey's head to strike the mat (Figure 1-69)

If your opponent attacks you with a limb (Figure 1-70), try and seize it or minimize the distance between you as to smother his attack so that you do not have to repeatedly be struck (Figure 1-71). You may also neutralize an attack before it begins by doing something as simple as bridging the body (Figure 1-72).

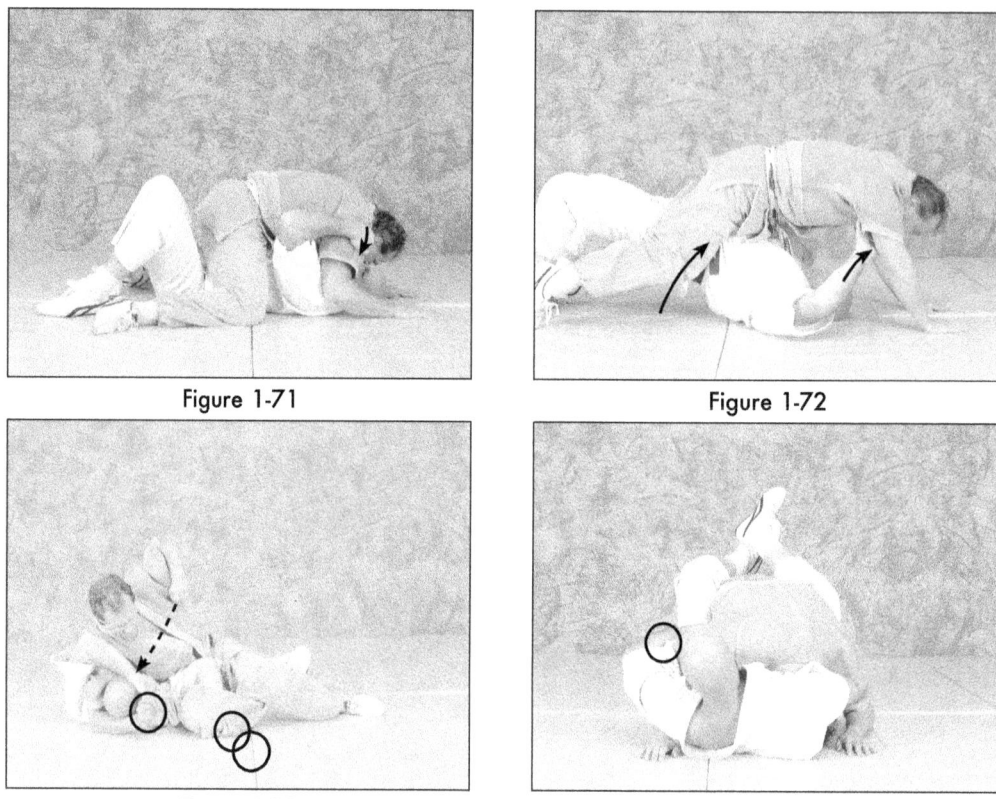

Figure 1-71

Figure 1-72

Figure 1-73

Figure 1-74

For example, Figure 1-73 shows that Grey has tied up both of White's arms using finger Qin Na (Chin Na) and a bent arm lock using his legs. Grey can punch White's face at will. The reclining guillotine works well if you include the arm of your opponent on the side of his body where your torso is located (Figure 1-74). Failure to do so will allow your opponent to gouge your eyes (Figure 1-75). Grey's left arm is too far from White's face to be a threat.

Use strategy to manipulate his limbs in order to engage it into a joint lock. For example, White lets Grey reach out and lean into him to choke him (Figure 1-76). White then grabs Grey's left wrist and swings his left leg up and over to the left side of Grey's head (Figure 1-77). White then slams his lower leg into the left side of Grey's head taking him down and putting him in the cross-mark hold (Figure 1-78). Conversely, you must not let your limbs get locked out while attacking your opponent. Figure 1-79 shows White lying in a supine position trying to pull Grey down by encircling his neck to effect a headlock. Grey seizes the opportunity to apply a kneeling arm bar to his outstretched right arm (Figure 1-80). Notice how Grey uses his right knee on White's neck to help keep him from moving around and escaping. Basically, you must simultaneously control the distance, body position, and body weight in order to effect a good joint lock and prevent attacks to your vital areas.

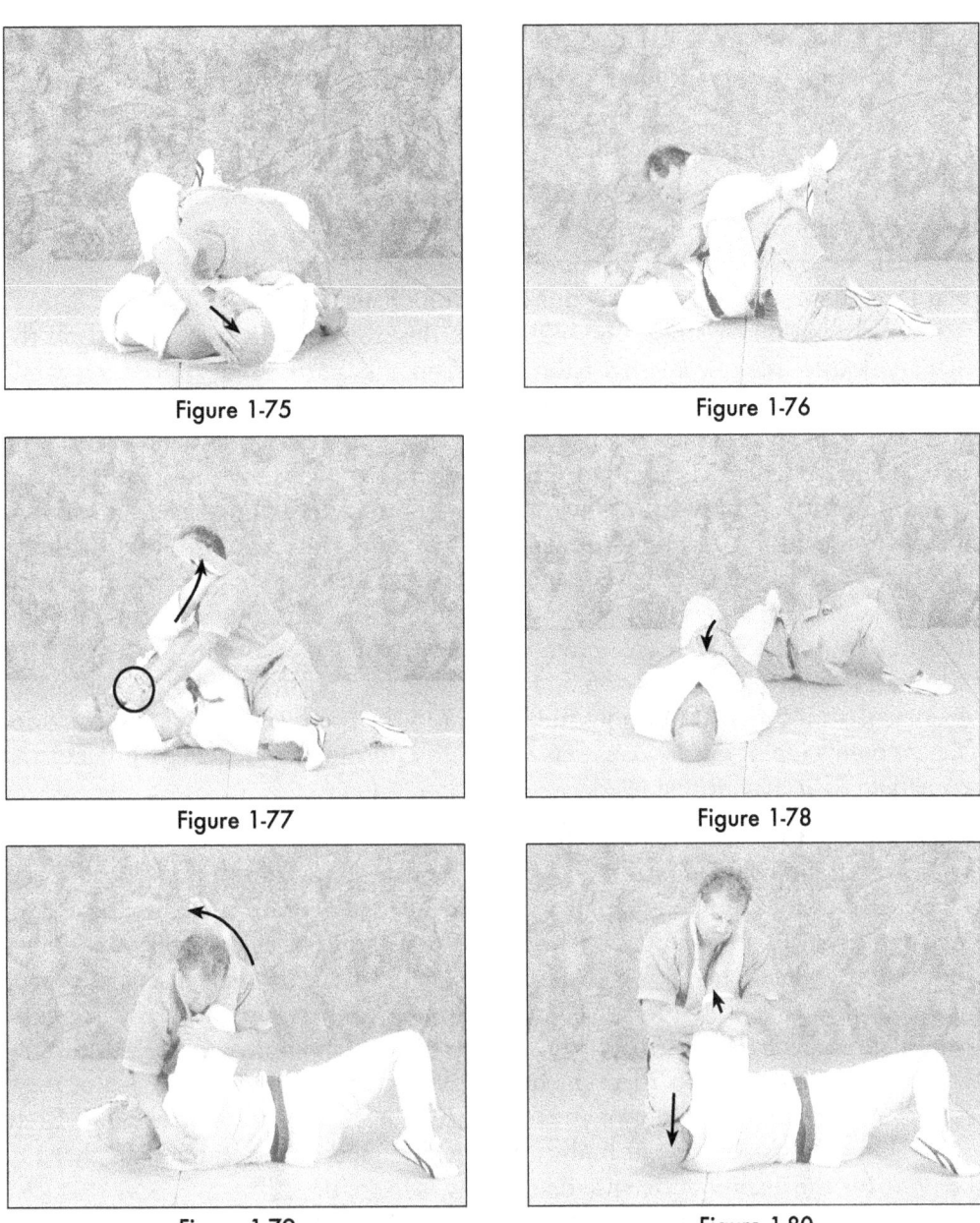

Figure 1-75

Figure 1-76

Figure 1-77

Figure 1-78

Figure 1-79

Figure 1-80

6. Controlling the Mind. Develop a winning mindset and you will have better odds at beating your opponent physically. Be confident that you can fight and win from the ground and even from the bottom (inferior) position. Conversely, try to infect his mind with doubt, fear, anger and/or loss in order to cloud his mind to your advantage. Some mental keys to winning are:

a) Have a winning mindset (will yourself to win at all costs).

b) Instill fear, panic, and doubt to cloud your opponent's mind.

c) Keep a calm, clear mind that is capable of strategically thinking ahead.

We will not begin to delve into this topic, because it is a book onto itself. Suffice to say that keeping a positive and winning training attitude will be more beneficial to you than a negative one. Know your limitations though and try to overcome them. Hard training toughens the body but it also toughens the mind.

Remember, under stress, you will do on the street as you were trained on the mat. A deadly example of this falling back onto basic training procedures while under high stress situations comes from shootouts. Police officers have been killed in gunfights while picking up spent shell casings. Why? Because this is how they were trained and under stress the mind shuts down and you go into auto pilot mode in order to survive. 'Empty your gun and pick up the spent casings before moving to the next stage of fire before reloading.' The range remains neat; but officers die in combat. These hard lessons have resulted in many changes to shooting training, such as never touching casings until the end of shooting and reloading anytime a shooter feels it is appropriate. Here is a minor example. If you get up off the mat using your hands for support, so too will you do so in a real fight, possibly with negative consequences if your opponent decides to kick you in the head while you are getting up. What about tapping out? We say to release the pressure immediately, but not the hold. The fight may not be over!

Relationship of Fight Control Factors

These fight control factors can be summed up as shown in Figure 1-81. Distance, position, and body weight are interdependently linked together. By changing your distance with your opponent relative to his/your body position, your ability to attack or defend changes (vulnerability). The relationship with distance to your opponent and your ability to apply your body weight onto him affects the degree of control you can have over his body movement (controllability). Vary the positioning with body weight and you affect the quality of movement (mobility). Each of these factors also affects the nature of your attack (or defense) that you can offer. Body positioning affects the type of limb (joint locking) and vital point attacks that can be done (or the quality of defense that can be delivered).

Similarly, distance influences the type of attack or defense that can be initiated. How you apply your body weight determines the efficiency (and possibly the effectiveness) of your technique. Whatever the relationship is, the same or the opposite relationship may hold true for your opponent. For example, if your hips are not close to your opponent's hips, you may be limited to striking techniques or leg locks. So too is it for your opponent. If you are maximizing your body weight onto your opponent, your opponent may not be able to use his at all because he is in an infe-

Chapter 1: General History and Principles

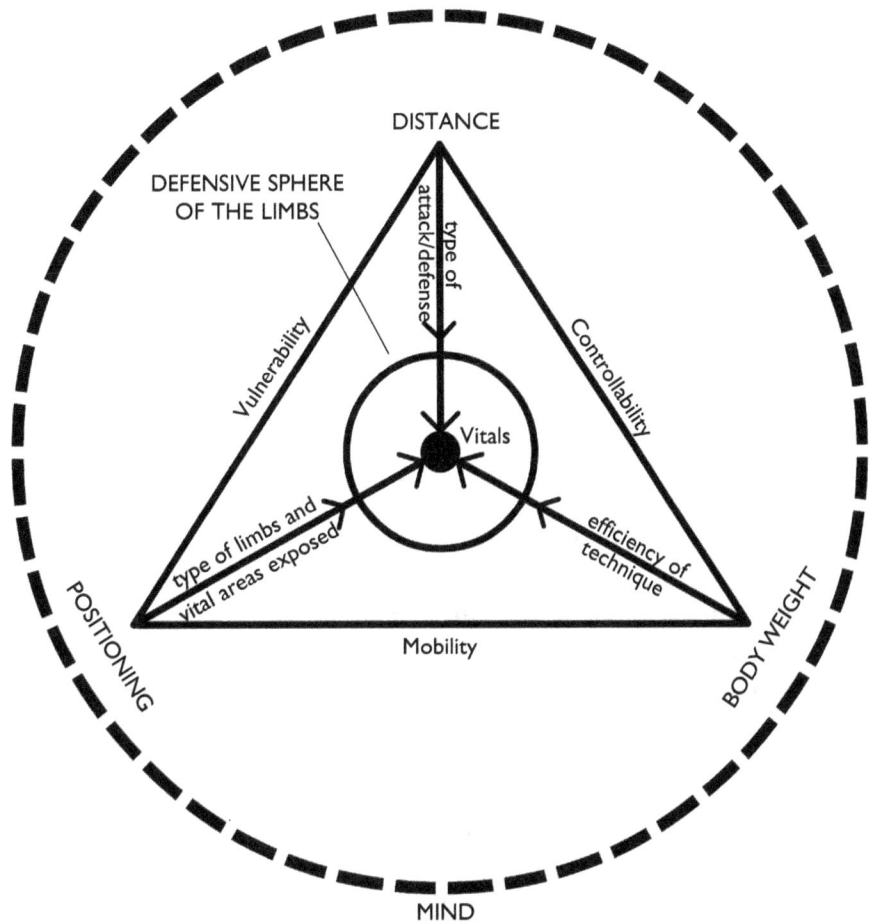

Fight Control Factors
Figure 1-81 The various interdependent fight control factors affects the nature of the attack or defense that can be offered

rior position to do so (underneath you), but your mobility may suffer. Being in an all fours position may give you mobility but less chance to apply your body weight onto him (making the same hold true for your opponent).

All of these variables (and others) are controlled by the mind. So the game of chess is in flux with every positional change, hold taken, weight shift and attack or defense made. Whether you are skillfully helping or unwittingly hurting your chances at beating your opponent with each move you make is clarified with practice. So too does your ability to read your opponent's attack and to capitalize on the opportunities he presents to you. And so the question remains, is the offering you see before you a trap? Will it be 'check mate' or victory?

1-5. Principles Common to Both Qin Na and Ground Fighting

Leverage

A lever is the simplest of machines, which utilizes a rigid bar to rotate around a fixed pivot point called a fulcrum in order to exert force on an object (load). If the resistance or load exceeds the strength of the bar, the bar will break. Biomechanically speaking, the arm is a bar, and when the fulcrum is at or above the joint, breakage can easily occur. There are 206 bones in the adult human body some of which, mostly those of the extremities (126 bones), are susceptible to the effects of external leverage for Qin Na (Chin Na) and ground fighting purposes. During the normal operational state of the body, the muscles provide the force that makes the levers operate to produce motion (movement chains) within the functional range of the joint.* In the context of applying joint locks, we use the principle of leverage to effect control over our opponent. Qin Na techniques tend to use leverage often as a means of pain compliance. This may mean bending a finger or two to such a degree as to give the pain-receiving brain an offer it cannot logically refuse. It is important to remember that joints can be more readily damaged through torsion than hyperflexion (or hypercontraction). Combining the two stressors is best particularly if there is tension in the movement chain as well. The opponent must submit and comply with the person applying the painful technique or suffer continuing and even increasing pain and possibly even risk breakage of the seized appendage or related joint. Ground fighters also use the principle of pain compliance, adding the use of leverage as a means to restrict the ability of a person to move ('pinning' him), often using body weight as the driving force (Figures 1-82 and 1-83). Qin Na practitioners may use the ground as a place of positioning, but normally they themselves do not go to the ground ahead of their opponent. Rather, they are more reliant on applying the direction of a technique against such a fixed object (such as the ground) in order to create an overwhelming pressure to make the technique work and to restrict a person's mobility by pressing him into such a fixed object (Figures 1-84 and 85).

How do these principles of physics work for us in fighting situations? Firstly, we apply pressure on our opponent's finger, hand, arm, leg, and so on or whatever part of his body we can use as a bar. We use our own body to provide a fulcrum (pivot point) against the anatomically weak link between two bones, that being the joint (Figures 1-86 and 1-87). We use a load that either exceeds the strength of these bars causing the bone to break or, more commonly, produces painful stretching and tearing of the muscles, tendons and ligaments associated with that joint under pressure (Figures 1-88 through 1-90). The body has over 650 muscles, which are relatively elastic and are only capable of forcefully contracting (pulling), the coordinated result of which is movement of the body. A tendon attaches a muscle to a bone. Tendons are made up of strong somewhat elastic tissue. Over-stretching these results is a strain. A ligament attaches a bone to another bone. Ligaments are non-elastic and

---

*Zhao Da Yuan's *Practical Chin Na: A Detailed Analysis of the Art of Seizing and Locking* (1993) offers a wonderful account of body dynamics relating to Qin Na (Chin Na).

Chapter 1: General History and Principles

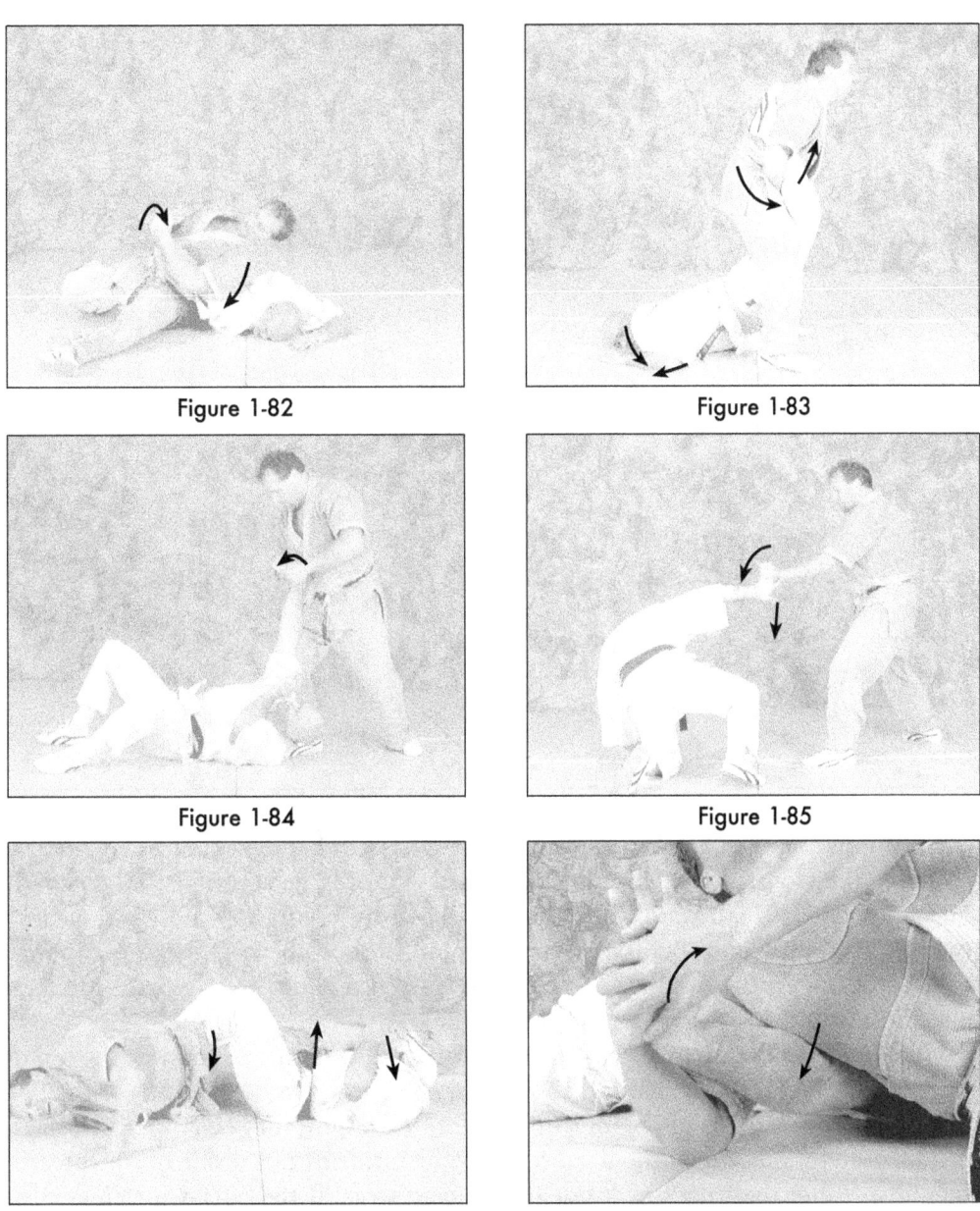

Figure 1-82

Figure 1-83

Figure 1-84

Figure 1-85

Figure 1-86

Figure 1-87

a sprain results when they are stretched. If the amount of attacking force generated causes the range of mobility of the joint capsule to be exceeded, the structural integrity of the joint is compromised. For example, in the case of applying *ude garumi*, Grey's right forearm is twisted inward to take the slack out of the joint prior to the actual application of the technique that assists in overloading the joint capsule (see Figures 1-100 through 1-102).

47

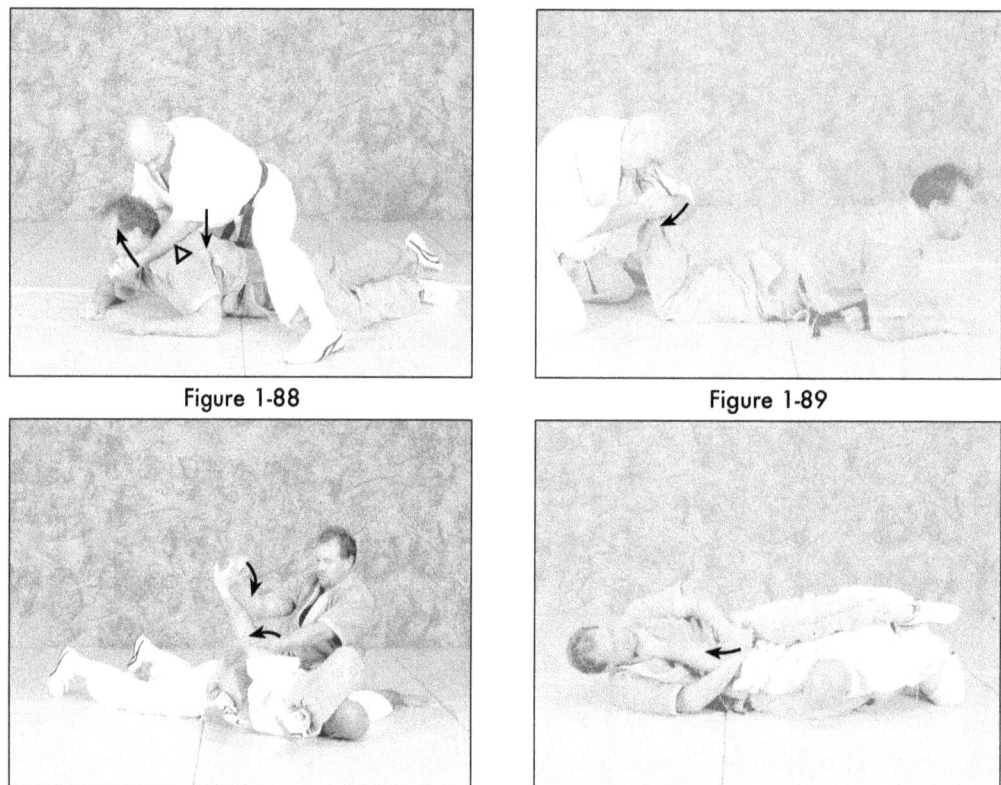

Figure 1-88

Figure 1-89

Figure 1-90

Figure 1-91

Secondly, we apply pressure to the body bar as to bend the appendage in the opposite direction(s) to which it is accustomed. This can be accomplished by bending an appendage 'backward' (extension, as shown in Figure 1-91), 'sideward' in a twisting fashion (Figure 1-92), or even 'forward' (flexion) beyond its' normal range of motion (Figure 1-93 shows White using Grey's shoulder as a fulcrum to crank his head forward).

The wrist for example can be bent backwards (back of fingers towards the top of the forearm, Figure 1-94). Also, the wrist can be bent forwards (bottoms of the fingers towards the bottom of the forearm, Figure 1-95). Or it may be twisted sideways, bending the thumb side of the hand towards the inside or radial side of the forearm (Figure 1-96) or the baby finger side of the hand towards the outside or ulnar edge of the forearm (Figure 1-97).

Later in this book (Chapter Two), we will look at the straight arm bar for example in detail to show how the same biomechanical principles can effect the same results by using different fulcrums and methods of applying force to the lever arm.

Sensitivity

Having an understanding of the anatomy of the human body is helpful when thinking of techniques needed to break it down. Indeed the study of biomechanics

Chapter 1: General History and Principles

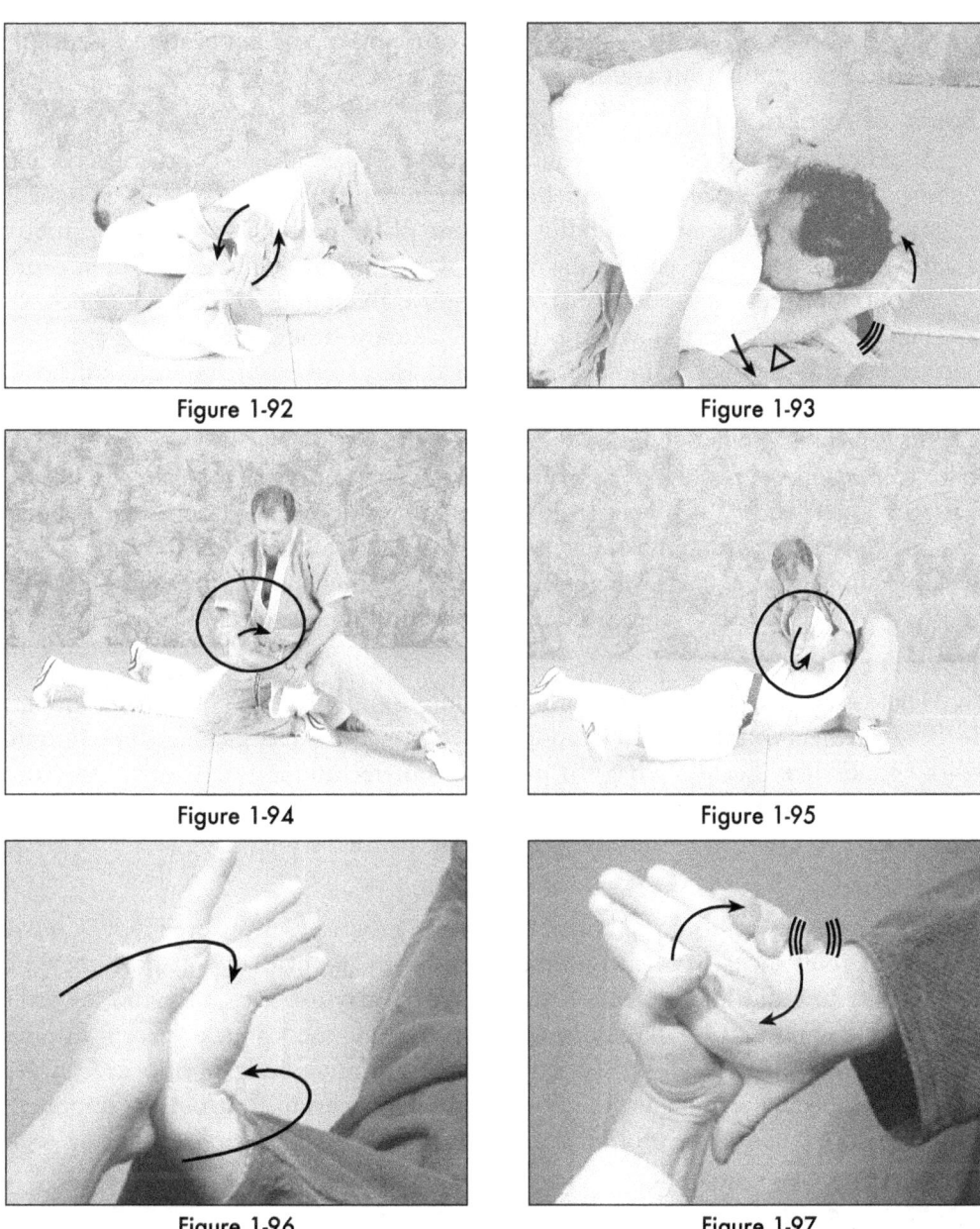

Figure 1-92

Figure 1-93

Figure 1-94

Figure 1-95

Figure 1-96

Figure 1-97

can lead to more smooth direct and transitional applications of techniques. Experts in both Qin Na and ground fighting can feel only a part of a person's body to know the structural orientation of that body. Blind judoka are the ultimate proof of this. The study of push hands offers excellent training for stand up grappling, throwing, and even ground fighting, though the traditional 'root' through the feet has been lost with the latter fighting style. Certainly sensitivity is gained naturally from seizing thousands of appendages and from countless hours grappling on the mat, but

Speed of Application

Speed of application is more a concern and a necessity in Qin Na than in ground fighting, although one can strive to seize opportunities to attack (or defend) as quickly as possible as they arise, being mindful of course of the possibilities of set ups (traps). To the Qin Na person, speed is of the essence when initially grabbing your opponent's appendages because your opponent is free to move about and is capable of punching, kicking, and throwing you down or otherwise taking you out with blinding speed. In encounters with such skillful fighters, attempts at using Qin Na are not recommended. Never underestimate your opponent. Apply your Qin Na with as much speed and conviction as possible. Follow-up techniques on the other hand, may be done in a slow and calculated manner if desired, once seizing contact has been made and pain compliance has been established. When you do ground fighting with a skilled opponent, you are generally locked up with him, and are fighting to establish a defensible position. It can be likened to a game of chess, where you may have to think a few moves ahead in order to get to where you want to be in order to effect your intended technique.

Need for a Partner

There is an absolute necessity for both Qin Na and ground fighting practitioners to have partners to train with because, unlike punching and kicking, there are no training aids like the heavy bag, to practice your technique on. Your partner can assist you with the refinement of your own technique if he provides meaningful feedback to you (hopefully not by screaming in pain).

Joint Attacks

The principles common to both Qin Na and ground fighting are many. Clearly the use of joint locks to effect submission in both are evident but how they are applied can be radically different. Ground fighters may use neck, arm and leg locks whereas the stand up Qin Na fighters do not generally use leg locks (except in cases where a kicking leg is grabbed) because of their relative body positions. Qin Na fighters prefer smaller appendages using mostly their arms to control their opponent (Figure 1-98), whereas the ground fighter is free to take on larger limbs, using their entire body weight, strength, and their legs to defeat their opponent (Figure 1-99).

Removing Slack

There are several ways in removing the slack from a joint. One way is to twist the bone leading to the joint (Figure 1-100) so that any rotational force applied to it will diminish the natural range of motion. Figure 1-101 shows White inserting his left arm under Grey's twisted right forearm. White pulls on Grey's wrist to apply further stress on his elbow joint (Figure 1-102). Pulling not only can remove slack from a joint, but this action can also be used to draw in your opponent tight to your body, so that you can apply your technique more effectively (Figure 1-103).

Chapter 1: General History and Principles

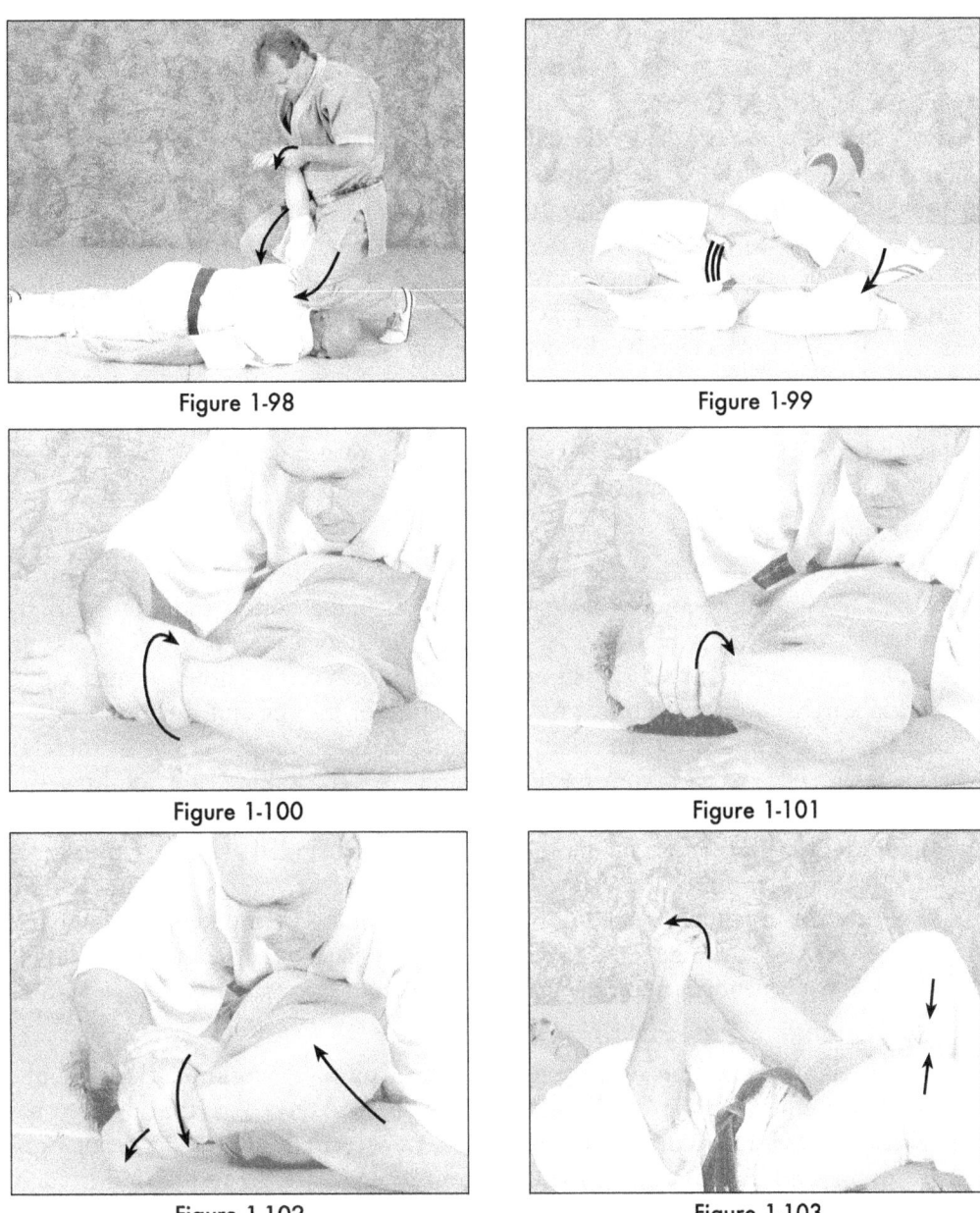

Figure 1-98

Figure 1-99

Figure 1-100

Figure 1-101

Figure 1-102

Figure 1-103

1-6. Physical Training Principles

Specificity of Training

Developing a strong and supple and physically enduring body is important to your development in the martial arts. There are a number of master training principles that you should make a note of when training.* The closer you follow them,

---

*The Canadian Fitness Educational Services, Fitness Knowledge Student Resource Manual (3rd edition) by Margaret Hewitt-Zaitlin, 1996, pp.3-4, 3-5

the larger the training benefit you will receive.

First, one should undertake a training program that mirrors closely the demands your martial art puts on you as possible. Of course, just as fighting with a training partner approximates the demands that may be placed upon you in a real fight, so too can training regimens prepare you physically for fight training sessions. Body conditioning is much more important for ground fighters than it is for Qin Na (Chin Na) practitioners, but that is not to say that aspects of strength, agility and flexibility are to be neglected by them. Adaptation of the various physiological systems to the stress that exercise places on them takes place during the resting intervals between training sessions. If one trains anaerobically over a period of time, the anaerobic system will become fitter. If the training is relevant to the type of martial art being practiced, then maximal gains may be seen from such specificity. One should take notice of the types and speeds of movements being done, ranges of motions, the energy systems utilized, and the neuromuscular pathways being trained.

Progressive Overload

In order to train the body to be superior to be what it is now, you have to incrementally challenge it to move more quickly, with more strength, stamina and suppleness. By progressively overloading the body, the necessary physiological adaptations will occur. We all have a genetically predisposed capacity to perform certain fitness-related activities. Flexibility is ultimately limited by the looseness or tightness of the joint capsule; speed may be controlled by the relative percentage of fast and slow twitch muscles, etc. Once you have reached your maximal training effect, nothing short of drugs will improve your performance (and this is not recommended). The further you are away from your peak performance, the more rapid will be your initial gain. Maximizing for physical potential may require much work. Once you are there, you do not have to train as often provided the intensity and duration of the training sessions are maintained. If you do not exercise at all, the training benefits that you have acquired will be lost in one or two months, depending upon the consistency of your past training regimen.

Recuperation

When the body has been subjected to a hard physical workout, the catabolic (break down) effect is observed. It takes time for the body to rest and heal. The anabolic (building) effect occurs in variable periods in accordance to the degree of stress placed upon the body. The harder the workout, the greater the rest period needed. The following guideline can be used to schedule your training sessions:

Component	Rest Needed
Cardiorespiratory Endurance	12-24 hours
Muscular Endurance	24-48 hours
Muscular Strength	48-72 hours
Flexibility	unknown

Threshold of Training

This refers to the minimum amount of physical training needed in order to have a positive training effect on the body. This requirement will vary from person to person and will be dependent upon the fitness level of the individual. If a person works out at an intensity level exceeding this threshold, then you have a progressive overload situation and the body will adapt to the change in work. Too much intensity in training and inadequate rest will be detrimental to the body.

Target Training Zones

If a person works out at the intensity of the threshold limit of training, no positive training effect will be experienced. This is a maintenance program and there is a corresponding heart rate associated with this training level intensity. This is about 60% of the theoretical maximum heart rate. If a person trains too hard and pushes the heart past 85% of the maximum heart rate, then a detrimental or negative training effect will be experienced. The training zone for the heart should be in this 60-85% of your maximum heart rate (220 – age = M.H.R).

Exercise Parameters

One should create a training program that will allow you to meet your training goals, bearing in mind the principle of specificity. Remember the acronym F.I.T.T. to stay fit:

>   Frequency: the number of workouts per week
>   Intensity: how difficult the workout is (heavier, faster, longer workouts)
>   Time: The length of the workout (total work out times or shorter interval times)
>   Type: the kind of workout being performed

Muscle Fiber Types

Muscles are composed of varying percentages of three fiber types: 1) slow twitch, 2) intermediate twitch, and 3) fast twitch. These percentages can be different within single muscle strands, between groups of muscles and between individuals. The slow twitch muscle fibers will be activated regardless what kind of activity you are doing, but these are well suited for performing slower, longer, less powerful aerobic activities like maintaining your stance and posture, and walking. Fast twitch fibers are larger in size and are reliant on anaerobic energy to generate speedy, explosive contractions that one uses in throwing, punching, kicking, etc. Intermediate twitch fibers have, as the name suggests, characteristics between these two fiber types. Although the percentage of fiber types does not change during training, the muscle's ability to use different energy systems can be enhanced. If you want to move about quickly and for an extended period of time, do aerobic training, whereas if you want to do well on the ground, train anaerobically.

1-7. Training Considerations

Instruction

There is simply no substitute for training under a qualified instructor, and with training partners you can trust when learning or developing any combative skills. This book can be used to give every martial artist ideas and techniques that will be useful in expanding his/her martial arts arsenal. For those who have limited access to a martial arts school, a heavier reliance on this book is necessary. These persons need only a partner, a place to train, and preferably a mat. The beauty of ground fighting techniques is that if they are not properly applied, you get the necessary feedback—your partner keeps fighting!

Safety

It is important not to over-apply the moves in training. An injured partner may not wish to train with you anymore or worse, he may sustain a permanent injury preventing him from continuing his training. A good martial artist is constantly striving to gain consummate control over his body from which his power will spring. Be sure to 'tap out' when the technique begins to cause some discomfort, but not before discomfort ensues because this will give your partner a false sense of the application being administered. Applying smooth and steady pressure incrementally is most wisely used in the training hall for obvious safety reasons.

Use of Force

Combative situations may require a more aggressive and dynamic use of force. The legalities about the decision to break a joint or to control a limb depend on many variables. Each situation will be judged on their own individual merits (number of assailants, size/skill disparities between combatants, threat level, etc.). If one chooses not to break a limb or joint, there is always the dilemma of release: Is the fight really over when your opponent insists that he has had enough? In policing, we must take control over a combative suspect (to 'own' him) prior to attempting to handcuff him. This control must exist throughout the handcuffing procedure or else the suspect may (re-)initiate the fight. This book will give you some ideas on how to maneuver a person around on the ground. Maintaining continuous control over him will allow you to move into superior positions, even to stand up while your opponent remains grounded.

Practice

As the old adage goes 'practice makes perfect', so practice the techniques often. The more they become second nature, the more available and effective they will be when you need them. You need to develop a feel for the techniques and understand the principles involved so that you can fight creatively. That is why having a number of different training partners is so beneficial. New situations and styles of fighting constantly challenge your ability to adapt.

Counters and Escapes

There are several important aspects of fighting that are not covered in this book, such as counterholds and escapes. Just as it is important to know how to heal in order to kill, it is even more important to know how to escape from a hold or thwart a technique in order to better successfully apply your own attack. Obviously, if you know how to escape from a hold, you can better prevent such a counter from happening to you and you would have a deeper understanding of the effectiveness and reliability of a given technique. All moves can be countered in their formative stages. Most of the techniques shown in this book, once applied, have a relatively low chance of being countered with any kind of striking techniques and are relatively effective in maintaining control over a person through joint breakage or the judicious application of pain.

CHAPTER 2

The Science of Technique

2-1. Introduction

Conceptualizing Techniques

The purpose of this chapter is to entice the reader to think of how the various joint locks used in ground fighting are applied in conceptual terms rather than as individual techniques. It is far easier to remember a few physical principles rather than to try and remember ten thousand techniques. In the situation of the arms or the legs, you may take control of these appendages as they are given to you in either the bent or straightened form. In the latter case, the physics of applying an arm or a leg lock to a straightened appendage is identical to the bent appendage techniques. What is different is *how* the techniques are applied. Through the proper understanding of the basic principles of biomechanics, one can use the least amount of force to affect the greatest results. In addition to the amount of force being applied, you must consider the direction of force and the point of application of this force in order to attain the desired results. These force components must be considered for the most effective and efficient results, whether it is applying a submission hold, attacking a pressure point, or even applying a punch or a kick for that matter. Invariably you are moving your opponent and/or applying pressure on joints and against his pressure points to cause pain and/or break structures of the body. In order to accomplish this, one further needs to understand the biomechanics of the body. Let's examine the basic physical principles relating to leverage, center of gravity and angles of force, and then apply them to the straight arm bar. Further, we will look at body positions and how they relate to your ability to fight on the ground.

2-2. Basic Principles of Physics

Levers

Central to joint lock manipulation is leverage. What is a lever? A lever is a rigid bar that is moved with force around a fixed point called a fulcrum (axis of rotation or motion). Levers allow us to greatly magnify the force we apply to our opponents,

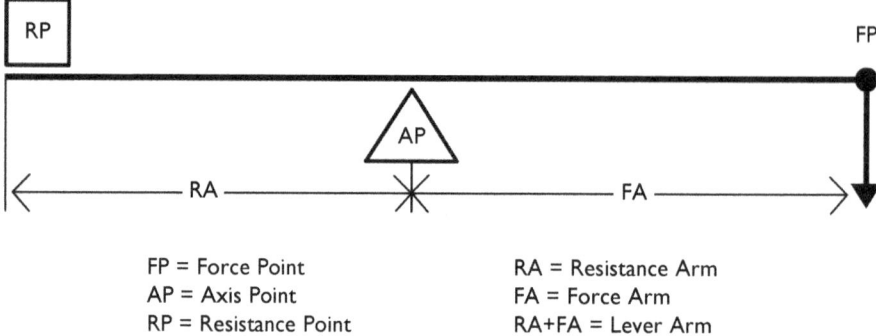

FP = Force Point
AP = Axis Point
RP = Resistance Point

RA = Resistance Arm
FA = Force Arm
RA+FA = Lever Arm

Force lever when FA > RA
Speed lever when FA < RA

Parts of a Lever
Figure 2-1 The relative positioning of the force point (FP), resistance point (RP), and axis point (AP) defines three classes of levers. The relative lengths of the arms determine what type of lever exists.

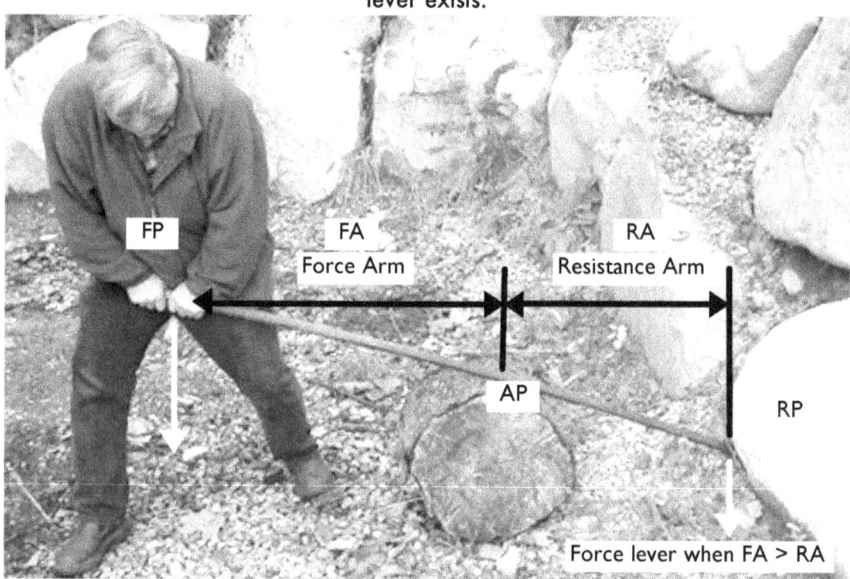

First-Class Lever—Pry Bar
Figure 2-2 A prybar is an example of a first-class lever. It is also a force lever because FP AP > RP AP.

thereby overcoming brute strength. The relative arrangement of the force point (FP) or point of force application, resistance point (RP) or load, and the axis (pivot) point (AP) or fulcrum, defines three classes of levers (Figure 2-1). The lever arm is that part of the lever between the resistance point (RP) and the force point (FP). Making up this lever arm is the force arm (FA) and the resistance arm (RA). The force arm is the length between the axis point (AP) and the force (application) point (FP). The resis-

Chapter 2: The Science of Technique

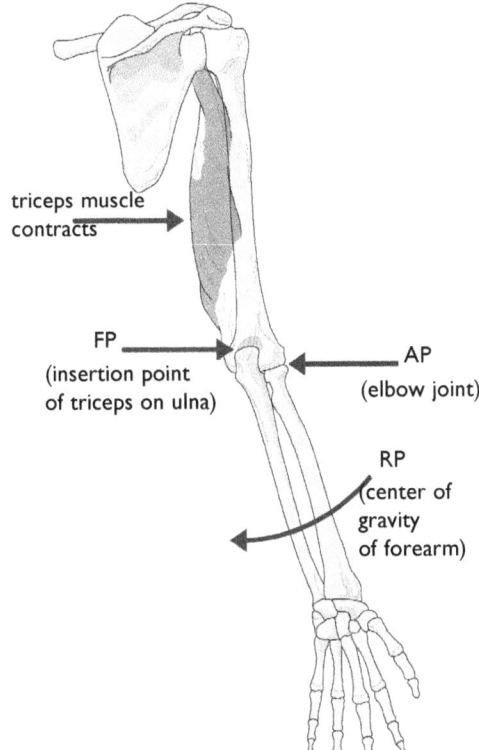

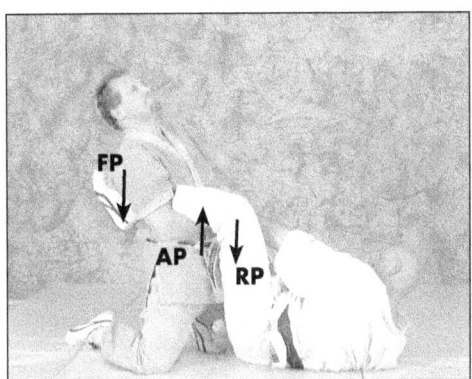

Anatomical First-Class Lever
Figure 2-3 (left) When the triceps tendon contracts to straighten the arm, it acts as a first class lever because the axis point (AP) is between the force point (FP) and the resistance point (RP).

Figure 2-4

tance arm (RA) is that part of the lever between the axis point (AP) and the resistance point (RP). For ground fighting purposes, the load is your opponent's body weight or the resistance offered by pressing his body against a fixed object. When the force used exceeds the load, your opponent must move away from the direction of the applied force or a result ranging between pain and breakage will occur.

The simplest lever is a first-class lever as exemplified by a pry bar (Figure 2-2) or a see saw. The greater the ratio between the force arm and the resistance arm is, the more effective this simple machine is. This is referred to as mechanical advantage. This type of lever is represented in the human body as the triceps muscle acting at the elbow joint (Figure 2-3). Figure 2-4 shows an example of a first-class lever in wrestling. Grey is using his armpit to press downward on White's lower leg while using his right forearm as an upward rising fulcrum. The load (White's body) is obviously too great for the lever to lift and this translates into pain at the axis point (fulcrum). If the force could be sufficiently great, the lever (lower leg bones) would break because of the excessive load. The same principles apply to an ankle lock where the fulcrum is placed at the ankle joint (Figure 2-5) or an armlock where the fulcrum is placed at or near the elbow joint (Figure 2-6).

A second-class lever is a force lever because the length of the force arm is greater

Chin Na In Ground Fighting

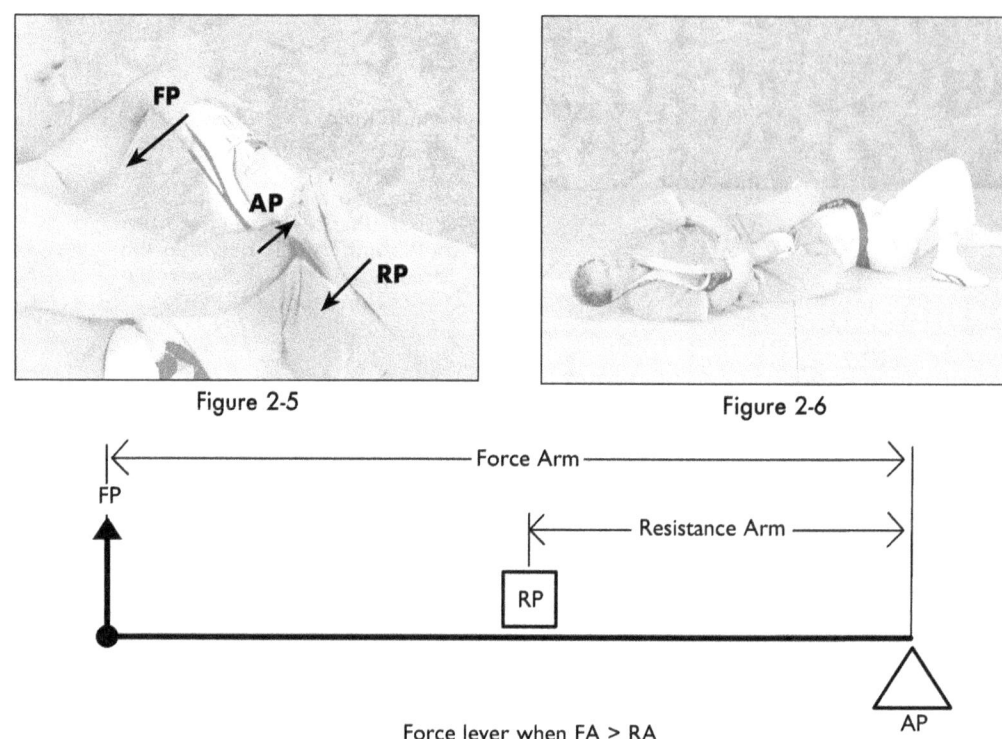

Figure 2-5

Figure 2-6

Force lever when FA > RA

Second-Class Levels

Figure 2-7 Second-class levers are force levers because the load or resistance point (RP) lies on the force arm (between FP and AP).

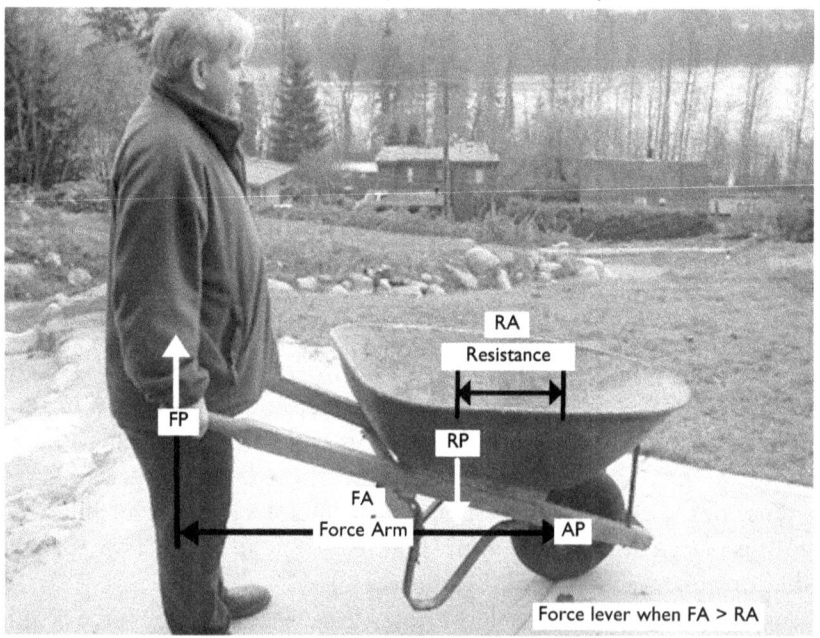

Second-Class Lever—Wheelbarrow

Figure 2-8 A wheelbarrow is a second-class lever, as is the bottle opener and nutcracker. The force arm (FA) is greater than the resistance arm.

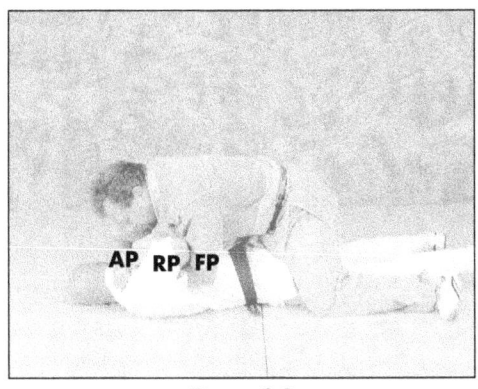 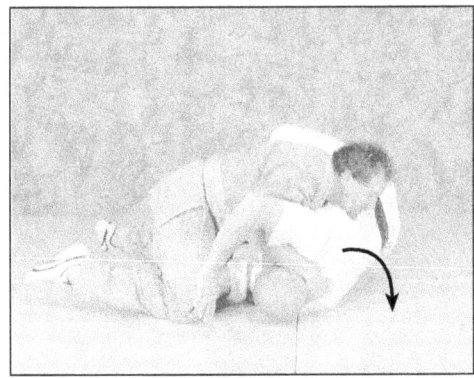

Figure 2-9 Figure 2-10

than that of the resistance arm. It has its resistance point between the force point and the axis point (Figure 2-7) such as in the case of the wheelbarrow (Figure 2-8), nutcracker or a bottle opener. It is not clear if this type of lever exists in the human body, but the principle underlying this type of leverage can be used in groundwork. For example, this type of lever is shown in Figure 2-9. Grey has pinned White prone to the ground from behind and has threaded White's left bent arm with his own left arm (hammerlock hold). Grey has established an axis point with his left hand (securing his own right pinning arm) and uses his left forearm as a second-class lever to work against White's upper forearm at the elbow. Grey can now use his whole body to lift upwards against White's bent arm to easily bend or break it. Another example is shown in Figure 2-10. This time Grey has grabbed White's neck (or collar) with his right hand to establish an axis point while kneeling beside White who is on all fours. Grey pushes sideways against White, lifting his right forearm upward thereby using this arm as a second-class lever against White's right armpit, causing him to roll over onto his back.

Third-class levers are also known as speed levers, as the length of the resistance arm is greater than that of the force arm (Figure 2-11). An anatomical example of this is an arm lifting a weight. The biceps and brachialis muscles act on the lower arm

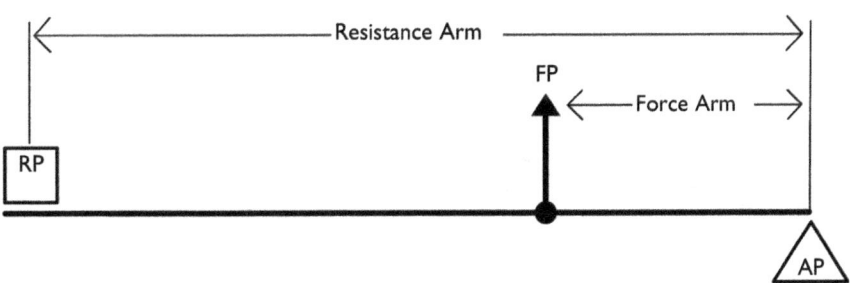

Speed lever when FA < RA

Third-Class Levers
Figure 2-11 A third-class lever has its force point (FP) between the resistance point (RP) and the axis point (AP). Speed levers are the most common type of lever in the body.

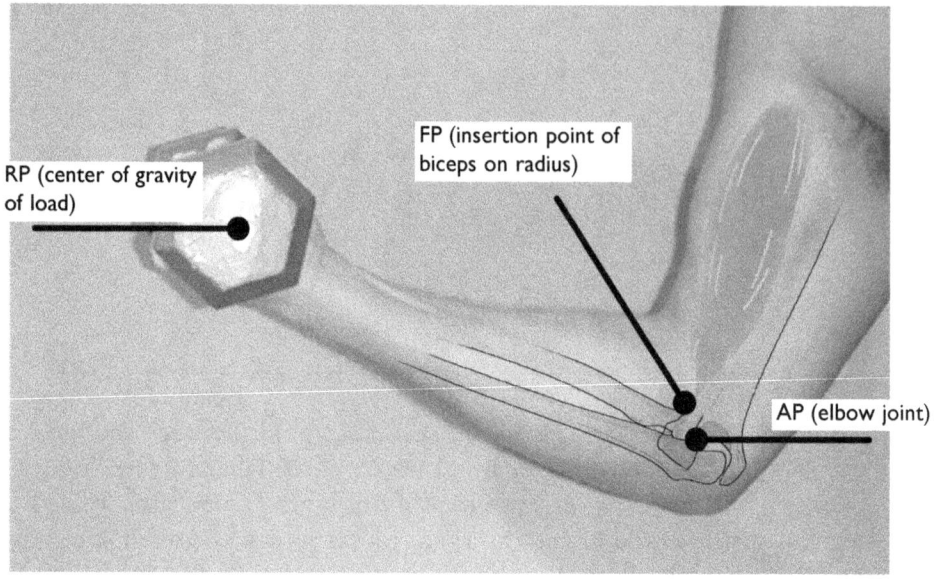

Anatomical Third-Class Lever—Arm Curl
Figure 2-12 The insertion of a muscle close to a joint ensures distance and speed of movement. The resultant speed levers sacrifice force of action.

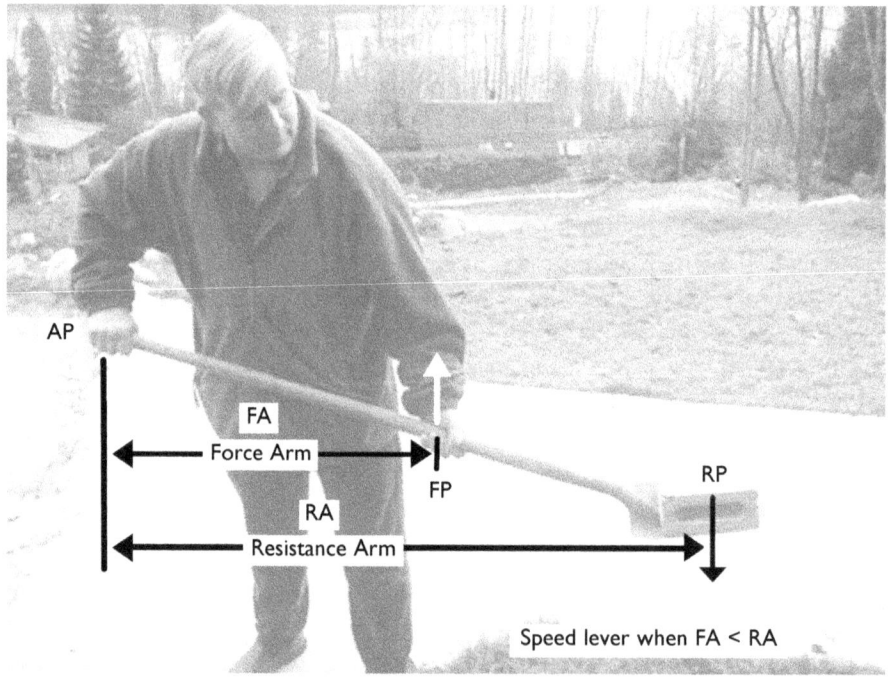

Third-Class Lever—Shovel
Figure 2-13 Third-class levers are always speed levers because the resistance arm (RA) is longer than the force arm (FA). Speed levers favor speed and range of motion over force.

(radius and ulna respectively) causing it to behave as a third-class lever (Figure 2-12). This is because the force point (point of insertion of the muscle to the bones of the forearm) is between the axis point (elbow joint) and the resistance point (load). An example of this is that of the shovel (Figure 2-13). Most of the levers in the human body are third-class levers, which allows for speed and range of movement at the expense of force of application. An example of a

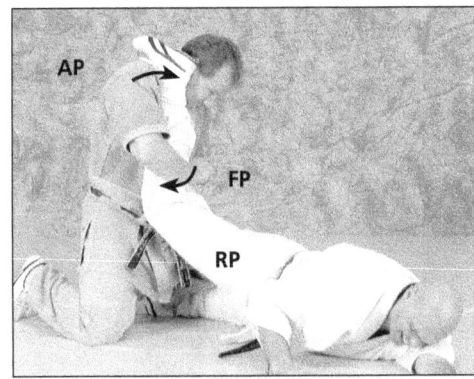

Figure 2-14

third-class lever in use in a ground fighting situation is shown in Figure 2-14. Grey has acquired a leg lock on White. By using his shoulder as the axis point and forcing the radial edge of his arm into White's calf muscle, Grey is using White's leg as a third-class lever to work against an unmovable load (White's body against the mat).

Mechanical Advantage

Mechanical advantage is the ratio between the lengths of the force arm over the resistance arm (MA = FA/RA). Mechanical advantage is enhanced when the force arm (FP–AP) is increased in length relative to that of the resistance arm (AP–RP). These levers can be classified as being either force levers or speed levers in accordance to the relative lengths of their force arms and resistance arms. A force lever exists when the force arm is longer than the resistance arm. Force is favored over speed (Figure 2-15). Conversely, when the force arm is not as long as the length of the resistance arm, a speed lever is created (Figure 2-16). This type of lever favors speed

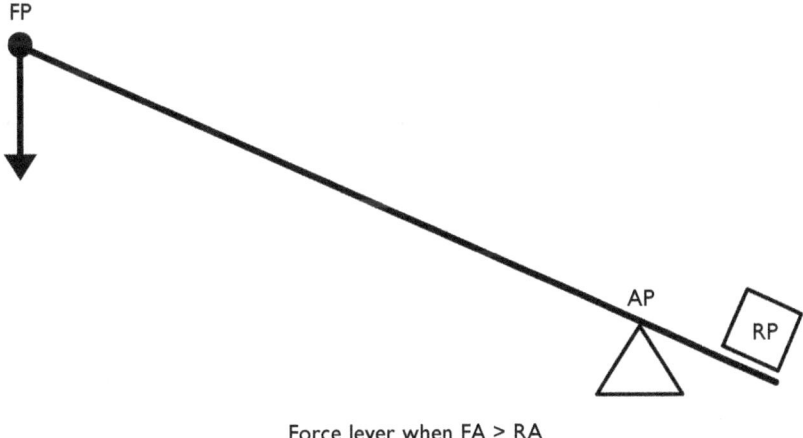

Force lever when FA > RA
(FP AP > AP RP)

Force Lever
Figure 2-15 When the force arm is longer than the resistance arm (RA), there is mechanical advantage that favors force over speed.

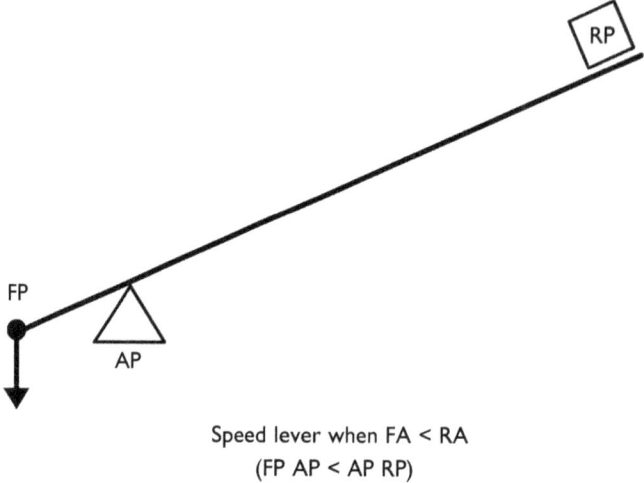

Speed lever when FA < RA
(FP AP < AP RP)

Speed Lever
Figure 2-16 When the force arm (FA) is shorter than the resistance arm (RA), speed and distance is favored over force.

and range of motion over force. Imagine a teeter-totter with a moveable fulcrum on which two people of equal mass are seated opposite from each other. Move the fulcrum closer to one party, and that party has a speed lever to work with. A minimum of movement on his part creates a faster and longer range of movement for his playmate, but more force is required to do this work because of the mechanical disadvantage involved. From the other's perspective, a force lever exists. Less force is needed to move his playmate but this movement is relatively slow because of the distance that he must cover to effect movement of his playmate.

First-class levers can be force levers or speed levers depending on the placement of the axis point relative to the force point and resistance point. For a pry bar to be very strong, the ratio between the lengths of the force arm and the resistance arm must be large. Clearly then if the force acting on the force arm of the lever is greater than that of the resistance arm (as offered by the load being pried), the lever will move making the attempt at prying successful.

Second-class levers always have a force arm greater than the resistance arm, making them functionally always force levers. Third-class levers have a force arm that is not as lengthy as the resistance arm, making them speed levers.

Center of Gravity

The term center of gravity refers to the approximation of mass (weight) to one point in a body. It is the central statistical center of the object's weight. The human body has a center of gravity that is close to that of the tanden in the lower torso. The X Y and Z axes (frontal, median, and transverse planes) are all balanced and intersect at this point (Figure 2-17), that is to say that if a person were skewered along these three axes individually, then the person would hang in balance. The

Chapter 2: The Science of Technique

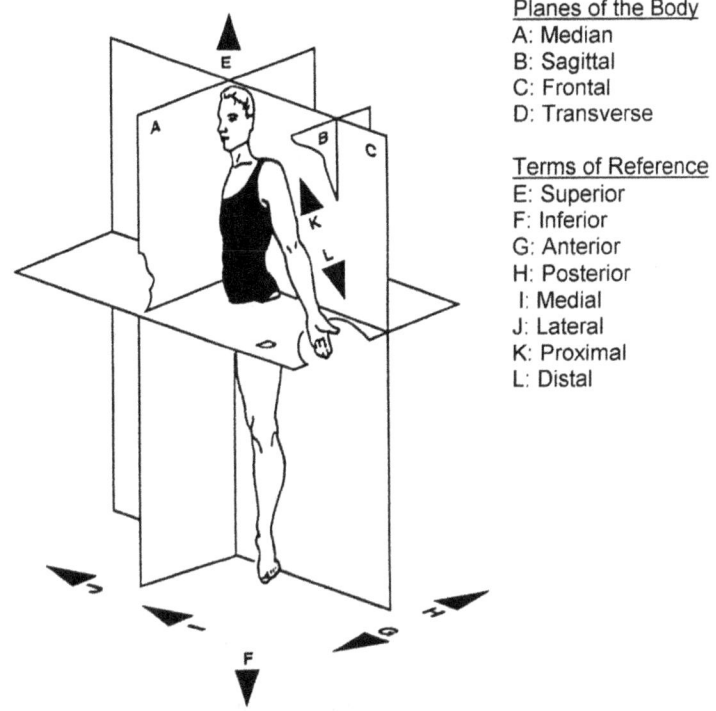

Anatomical Terminology
Figure 2-17 This is the universally recognized reference position when discussing body parts or planes of motion (see 'Medical Glossary' for definitions).

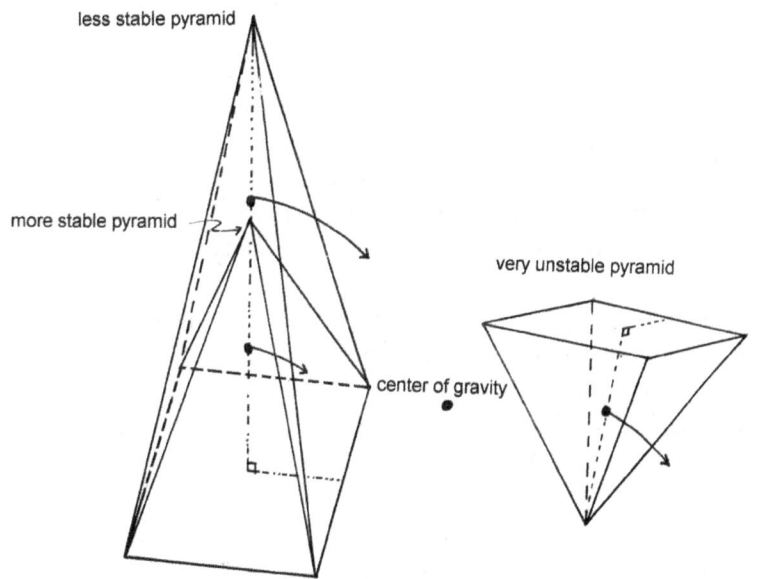

The Relative Stability of Objects
Figure 2-18 The greater the basal area and lower the center of gravity, the more stable an object will be. The inverted pyramid is the least stable object.

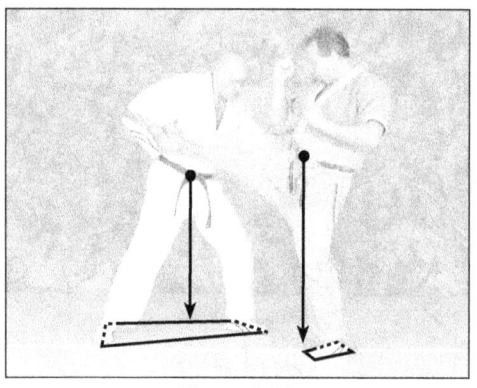
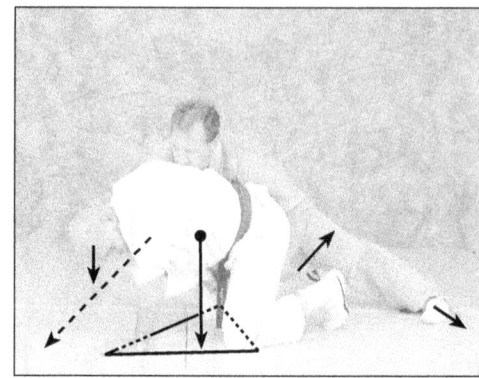

Figure 2-19   Figure 2-20

higher the center of gravity is from the base, the less stable it is. Consider the relative stability of three pyramids in Figure 2-18. The tall pyramid is less stable than the short pyramid with the same base and weight because the center of gravity is higher in the taller one. Both figures are relatively stable because the downward projection of the center of gravity lies in the middle of the base. An inverted pyramid is highly unstable because the base has been reduced to a single point over which the center of gravity must rest to remain in that position. Once the center of gravity moves beyond the base, it must topple from the lack of basal support. Your opponent will roll over once you move his center of gravity beyond his base.

As your base of support changes with your body postures, your center of gravity also undergoes change. Standing on two legs is more stable than standing on one leg with the other leg extended at waist level (Figure 2-19). You become unstable in the gravitational field and fall over when the downward vertical projection of your center of gravity lies outside your base of support. That is why you must transfer this projected gravity point (by changing your body posture) to within the base made by your supporting foot in order to keep from toppling. You can see White pulling on Grey's extended leg to further bring his center of gravity beyond his small base of support (the left sole of his foot) thereby unbalancing him. White's stance is stable (and his stance is strong) because his center of gravity is slightly lower and it lies within his greater base of support.

How does this knowledge translate to the mat? If your opponent is on all fours and you remove one arm, the center of gravity is brought closer to the truncated edge of the former rectangular base (now a triangular base). Therefore the person can be readily tipped in this direction (Figure 2-20). Grey uses White's right arm as a second-class lever by pulling up on this arm (like a wheelbarrow with his own body as the load).

The lower the posture and the larger the support base, the more stable you are. Being on all fours (Figure 2-21) is more stable than other stances, but it is less stable than lying prone (Figure 2-22), because of the very wide base of support and very low center of gravity that is central to this base. In the all fours situation, Grey again top-

Chapter 2: The Science of Technique

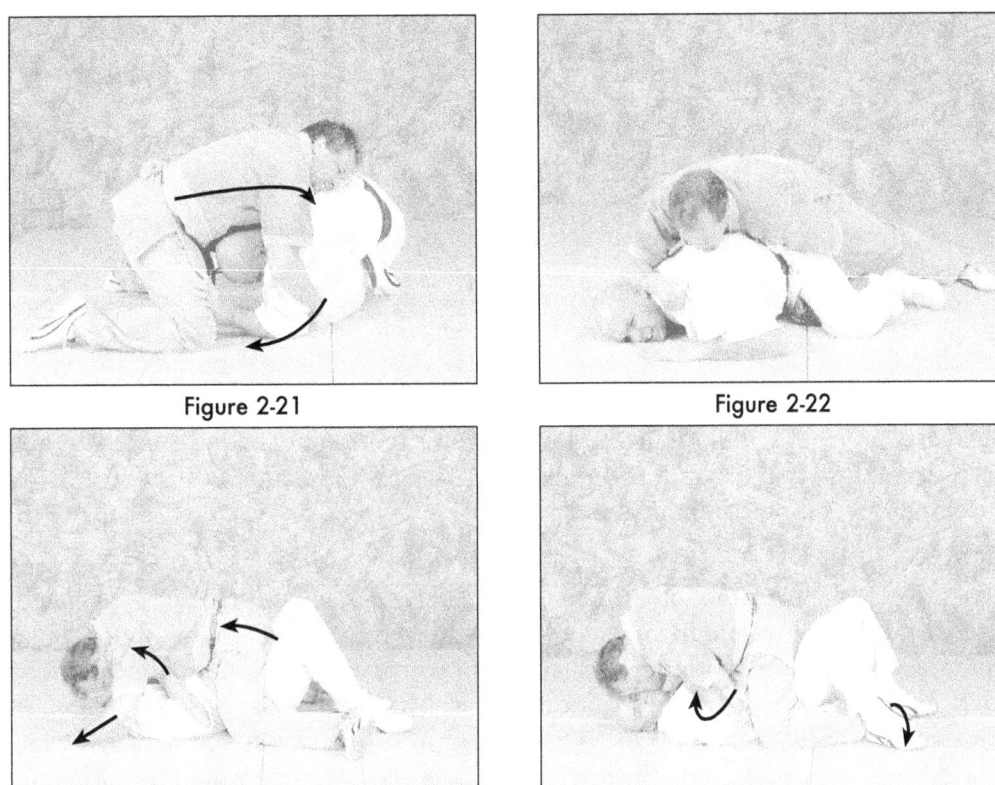

Figure 2-21

Figure 2-22

Figure 2-23

Figure 2-24

ples White by neutralizing White's ability to use his (left) arm as a stabilizer, allowing Grey to push him over in this direction. Lying flat out in a spread-eagled position is more stable (and more difficult to become mobile) than lying prone with your arms and legs by your sides because of the increased base of support that the spread-eagled position gives (centers of gravity are the same for both postures). The difference is like rolling a piece of plywood as opposed to a log weighing the same amount.*

Grey is mounted on top of White, who tries to tip Grey forward over his head (Figure 2-23). Grey shoots out his arms (outrigging appendages) to block his projected movement by increasing his base of support. His outstretched arms increase his base of support to include his center of gravity. White then changes his effort to free himself from the mount by trapping Grey's left leg with his right foot while scooping Grey's left arm with his right arm (Figure 2-24). White then bridges to his right, thereby toppling Grey who cannot use either appendage on his left side to prevent the turnover (Figure 2-25).

As in most acts in this balanced physical universe, when you change one physical parameter, you alter something else. For example, when you increase your base of

---

*The police use this prone spread-eagled position with the palms turned upward because it is very difficult for the suspect to become mobile (access weapons, fight, or flee) without making large, time-consuming movements with the arms and legs.

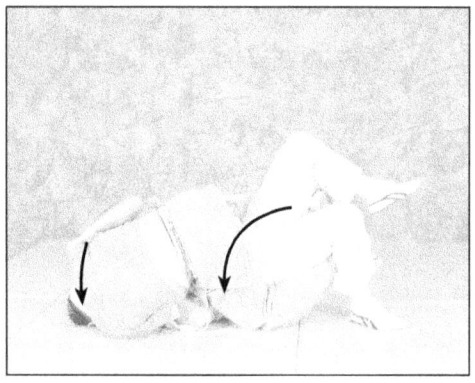
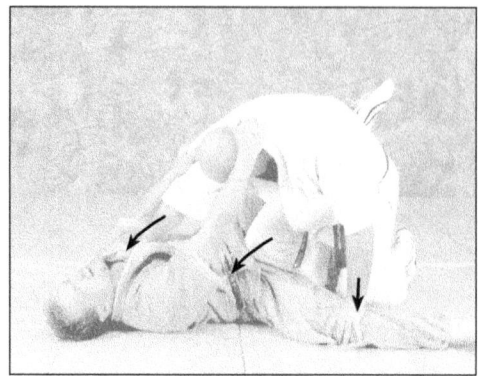

Figure 2-25   Figure 2-26

support, you gain stability but you lose mobility as a result (the difference between being on all fours and standing on both feet). Drop your center of gravity and you gain stability, but lose mobility, and so on.

Surface Contact

It is also important to understand that the larger surface area used in your base of support, the less pressure (penetration) you will have on the contacting (underlying) surface. Generate penetration by reducing your contact area on your opponent's body and you lose stability and control at that point. Just think of the pressure differences between identical pyramids. One is positioned to sit the way it was designed while the other is inverted. Clearly the inverted point of the latter one would have a greater penetrating ability (greater pressure per unit area). This is important to understand which of your body tools will give you the desired results when attacking pressure points of the body. It is also important to use this principle of applying force over a smaller surface area to maximize penetration when making body contact in ground fighting. Just reducing the contact surface area of your torso (spiking) can have debilitating effects on your opponent. In quicksand, you will have an easier time staying afloat if you lie down rather than try to stand up because you are spreading your body weight out over a larger surface area. When on the mat with your opponent, generally you want to maximize your stability and place your center of gravity over or as close to your opponent as possible while using his body as a base of one of your points of supports (making you lean on him). If you want to hurt him, transfer your weight onto your elbow so that your weight really penetrates your opponent.

An example of this is shown in Figure 2-26, which shows White kneeling on Grey's groin. He is further using his arms to pin Grey's right leg and chest to the mat while using little strength of his own (only body weight). If you need more control over his movement, widen your contact surface with him and broaden your base.

Torsional Movement

When dealing with rotational (torsional) movement, the axis of rotation and center of gravity may be considered as an equivalent point. The radius of a turn-

Chapter 2: The Science of Technique

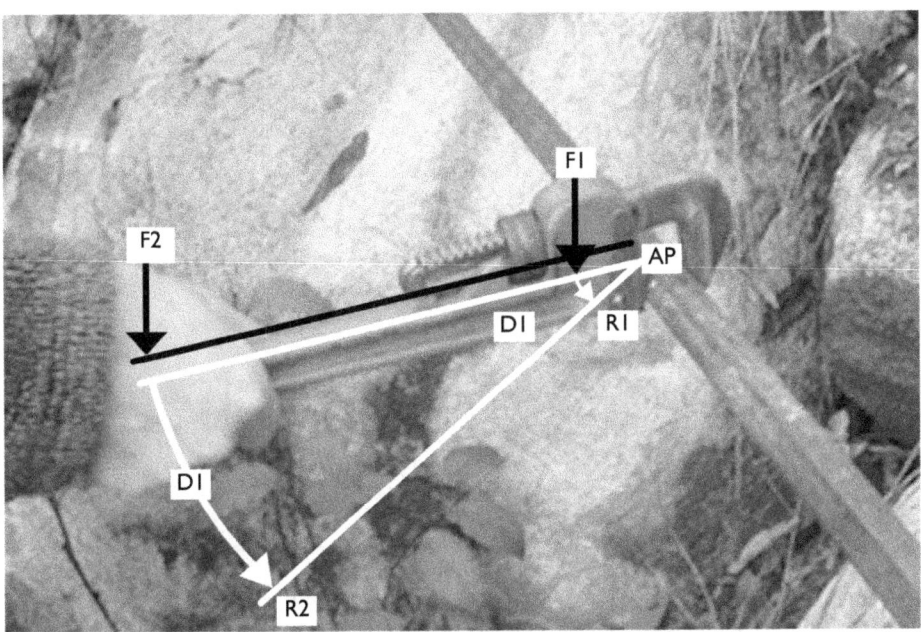

Mechanical Advantage of the Pipe Wrench
Figure 2-27 It takes far less force (F) to turn a pipe using a pipe wrench handle than at the head of the wrench (R2 > R1) because of mechanical advantage. This lesser force (F2) must be applied over a greater distance (D2 > D1).

ing cylinder (R) is the distance from the axis (turning) point (AP) and the point of application of force (F). This latter force is applied at a tangential direction, ninety degrees to the line of the radius line as in Figure 2-27. The turning of the finger, wrist, arm, leg, head or torso, follow certain laws of physics. Firstly, there is a greater mechanical advantage to applying torque pressure to a cylinder with a larger radius (R2) than a smaller radius (R1). There are greater counterrotation abilities associated with larger body parts though and smaller body parts can be grabbed more effectively. Nonetheless, it is mechanically more efficient to torque the arm at the forearm than the wrist or the finger (Figure 2-28), just as it is easier to turn a large steering wheel than a small one. Second, the larger the radius, the further/faster the points move at that given radius in a given interval of rotation (larger arcing distance: D2>D1). Finally, the greater the radius, the greater is the power. This means that a spinning back fist strike is easier to block at the shoulder where the strike is less powerful than at the wrist.

There are many Qin Na techniques that employ this type of movement as it tends to remove slack from joints allowing a more immediate manipulation. This type of movement also causes a significant augmentation of stress to the structure being attacked. A first-class lever may be used as a means of doing the shoulder crank for example. The force arm is the portion of the forearm selected to do the work (torque). The axis point is the center of rotation of the upper arm. The load is the resistance offered by the structure of the upper arm. The further up the forearm you place your

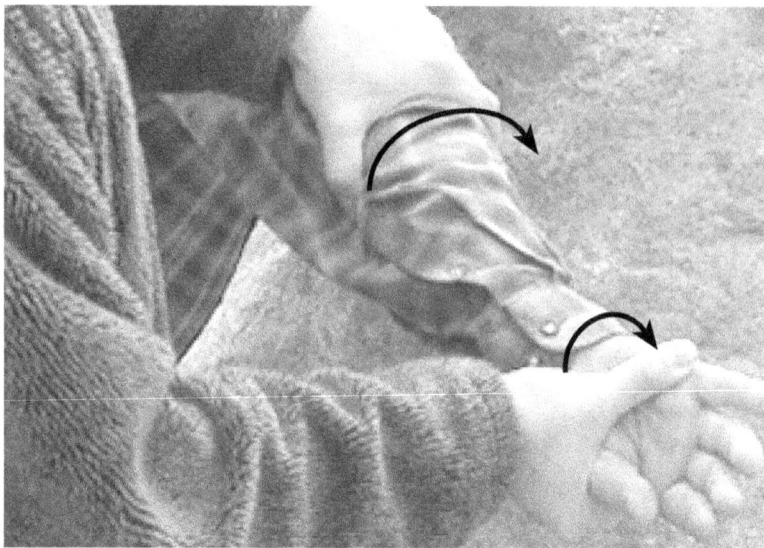

Preparing the Arm Bar
Figure 2-28 Torque on the arm can be generated at the elbow and/or the wrist. Although there is more mechanical advantage at the elbow, the wrist may be easier to grab, or the blade of the hand can be utilized to more readily affect torque.

force point, the greater the mechanical advantage (purchase) you have and the easier it is to perform the technique. The efficiency of Grey's ability to apply torque in Figure 2-29 is less than that of Figure 2-30 because of the maximum use of White's forearm as a lever to rotate (crank) the upper arm in the latter situation, thereby locking White's elbow and shoulder joints. Grey further locks White's wrist by applying pressure to the back of White's left wrist with his right hand while applying counterpressure with his left hand (Grey's left hand serves as the axis point for the shoulder crank as well).

Inertia and Momentum

Understanding the concepts of inertia and momentum are more important to stand up fighters because ground fighting is less dynamic in terms of large body movements and speeds of techniques. Whatever aspects do come into play must be capitalized on. Inertia is the physical tendency of a body to resist a change in motion, be it from a resting position to motion or from moving in one direction to changing its course. An external force must be applied to any body to overcome the effects of inertia; otherwise the body will remain stationary or on course (in a frictionless situation). Momentum is the quality of physical movement as determined by the product of its velocity (speed) and its mass (weight). The faster and heavier an object is, the greater the momentum it will have. The inertial force required to stop it will be greater once an object is moving than when it is moving slowly or at rest, as anyone who tries to stop a rolling car can attest. A faster thrown punch has more impetus, so that it will be harder to stop with a person's head, than with a slower moving punch,

Chapter 2: The Science of Technique

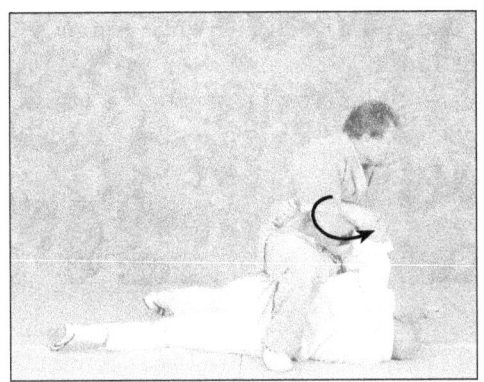

Figure 2-29

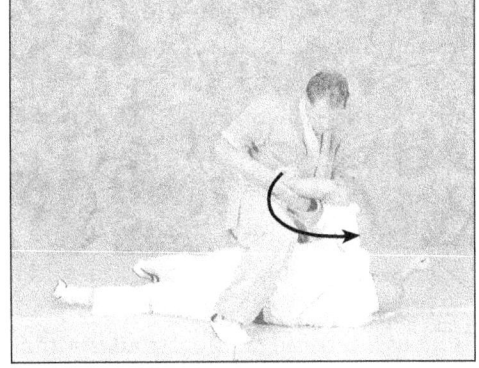

Figure 2-30

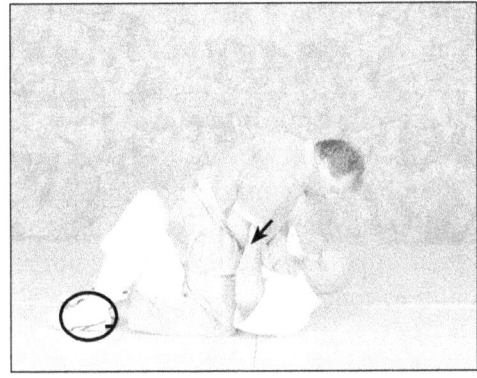

Figure 2-31

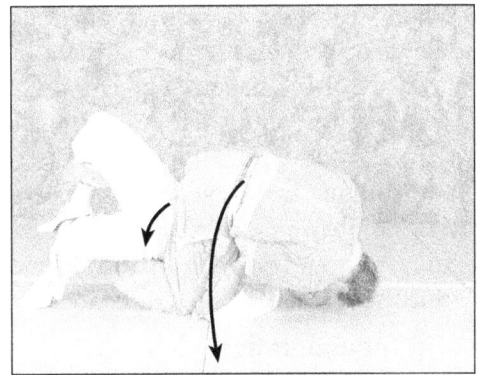

Figure 2-32

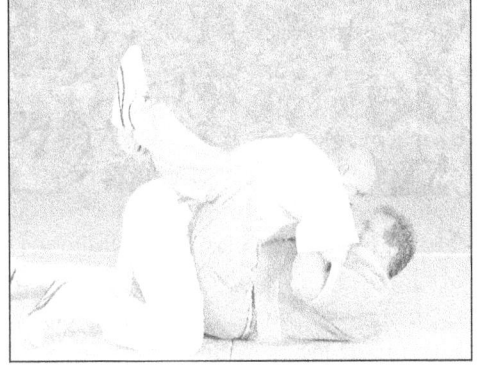

Figure 2-33

making it a 'harder' punch. We know that we can use the effects of gravity by bringing a person's center of gravity beyond his base of support, because he will fall over due to the instability that this position causes. Conversely, we can also make use of a person's momentum when we roll him over by riding him up (joining your body with his) so that his momentum carries you with him. For example, Figure 2-31 shows that Grey has mounted White who immediately controls Grey's arm, especially his right arm, while placing his left foot on the outside of Grey's right foot in order to trap it. White then bridges above his head and to his left, causing Grey to topple, having taken away his ability to extend a right-side appendage to prevent the rollover (Figure 2-32). By keeping his body close to White's, he couples with White's rolling momentum thereby riding up on top of Grey into his guard position (Figure 2-33). Once a person begins to move, it

71

is easier to keep him moving. Once you feel that you have broken your opponent's resting inertia, total effort should be brought into play to complete the move. Of course, applying force to your opponent should not be done incrementally. Rather, an explosive (plyometric) type of power should be used for best results; otherwise your opponent will move to block your attempts.

Dead Weight

It is important to develop sensitivity to your opponent's movements. Beginners in ground fighting often tense up and tire out quickly. A tense body is a more readily movable body. It's like trying to tip a rigid chair over as opposed to a beanbag chair. The use of 'dead weight' (making the body go limp as if dead) to thwart or hinder a parent from picking up their uncooperative child is an example of how softness of body can assist in making one seemingly immovable. A tense body can also be more predictable in terms of where the resistance is being offered by an opponent and when this resistance changes, it is easily recognized. A relaxed opponent offers as little telegraphing tension as possible until the move is made. Again, think of what it would be like to remove the two types of chairs off of your body. Clearly, the nebulous free flowing softness from the beanbag chair makes dealing with it more cumbersome than from the fixed rigidity of the regular chair. By relaxing, one can also better respond to the movements of your opponent because you are not all unnecessarily tensed up and fixated on maintaining your ground.

Grip Augmentation

Whenever you feel that your opponent is gaining advantage in acquiring a limb or is moving to defeat a hold you have on him, you should try to defeat his superior strength or mechanical advantage by doing any of the following: grab onto a body part; grasp clothing; or intertwine or trap your own arm/leg as to anchor the dominated limb. By doing any of these things, your opponent must use much more strength to overcome you. After all, it is far more energy consuming to hang a weight off of your wrist with the arm extended straight out than it is to hold it while grabbing onto a fixed object with the hand of the load-bearing wrist. Thus, the rule is to latch on whenever you can to anchor or fix your grip. The most obvious example of this is grasping your own two hands to effect a lock. Figure 2-34 shows Grey anchoring his right hand onto his left inside thigh by grabbing his *gi* pant leg as White has managed to slip out of Grey's initial around the waist hold. This will prevent White from attacking Grey's face with his left hand. An example of grip augmentation being used in a more active fashion can be seen in Figure 2-35. Here, White has managed to raise his right leg up while bringing his right arm under the crook of his own right knee. He then grabs Grey's collar and pulls downward against his own right arm, assisting with his leg, in order to try and unbalance White.

Chapter 2: The Science of Technique

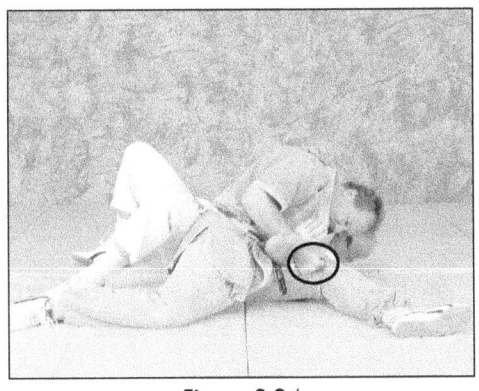

Figure 2-34

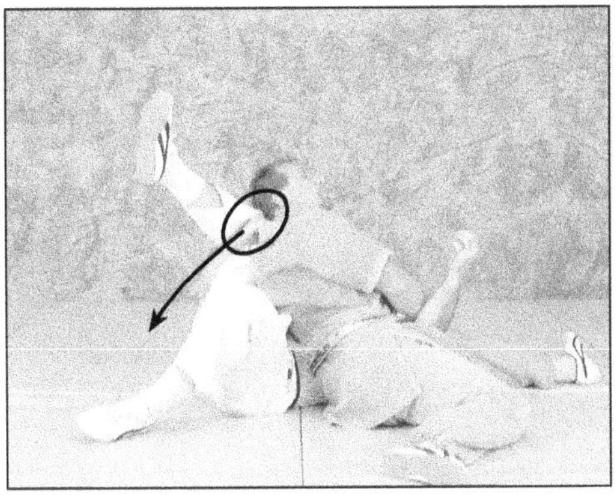

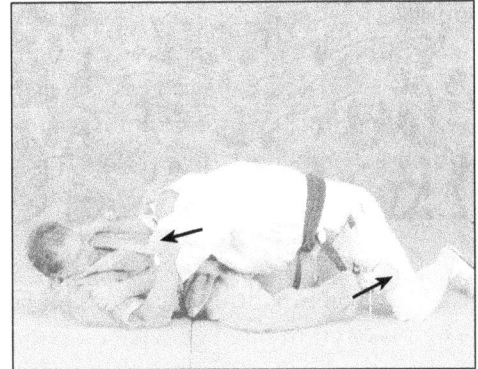

Figure 2-35

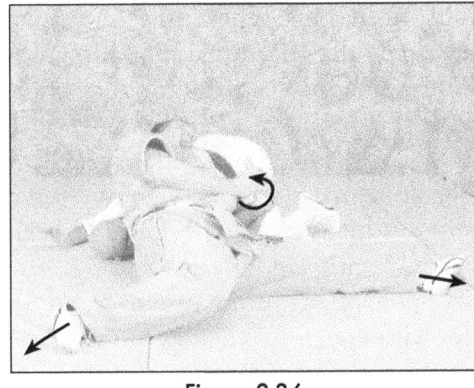

Figure 2-36

Figure 2-37

Using Your Whole Body

It is very important to have control over your whole body when ground fighting. Use as many muscles as possible when applying your technique. You need your arms to apply the actual hold, but you need to use your legs to provide stability. In Figure 2-36, Grey has White in an arm bar (reverse *waki gatame*). Grey has also applied a wristlock onto White's fully extended left arm. Notice how important it is for Grey to control his center of gravity and to maintain a wide base of support using his legs in order to drive backwards and onto White's upper body (using his legs and back muscles to arch backwards) in order to assist in immobilizing White. This pinning action keeps White where Grey wants him to be so that the arm bar can be best applied by Grey transferring his weight towards White's upper arm, placing an overbearing load on White's elbow and shoulder joints. White's arm then becomes effectively locked at his wrist, elbow and shoulder. Figure 2-37 shows Grey using his arms to control White's arms. Grey's left leg is used as a stabilizer as he uses his right leg to push against White's left leg in order to de-stabilize him. Grey is optimizing his leg push by pulling on White's arms in the opposite direction. Further to these actions, Grey can use his back muscles by arching backwards, adding significant force to his efforts. Another example of whole body action can

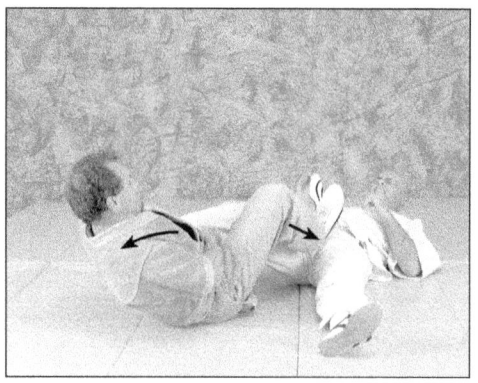 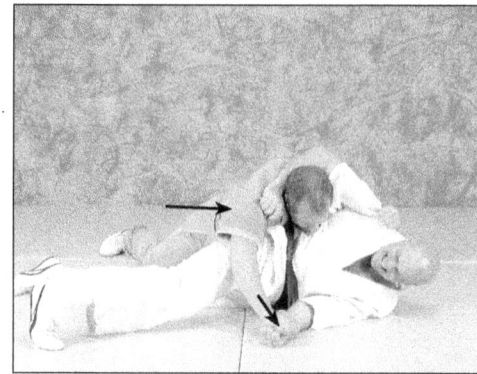

Figure 2-38   Figure 2-39

be seen in Figure 2-38. Grey has White's right leg in a heel hook using the radial edge of his left arm. Grey uses his right arm to secure the grip by clasping his hands together and he has placed his legs against White's right hip in order to create additional tension at White's Achilles tendon. This action produces a stronger base from which to apply his backward arching motion that is the key to the effectiveness of this technique. Just the lifting action of the arm alone may not be enough to effect a submission from White. Grey can also heel strike White's groin with his right heel.

Suffice to say that using the whole body is imperative in ground fighting, particularly when fighting a bigger and stronger opponent. As in the case of stand up Qin Na, an unwanted grab is best removed, not with one or two hands, but with the combined action of the hand(s) and body movement. The sum of the forces of all the muscles used to protect yourself will usually be greater than that of an attacking limb. The strategy of your opponent will be to maximize his power potential, as well as to neutralize your power base. For example, in Figure 2-39, White has Grey in a headlock with his right arm. Grey uses his own right arm to grab White's left wrist in order to keep him from securing his grip on his neck. At the same time, Grey is driving with his legs in order to roll White onto his stomach to further limit his abilities to attack him.

2-3. Variations of the Straight Arm Bar

Anatomy of the Elbow Joint

It is important to understand the anatomical structure of the arm, especially since over half of the Qin Na (Chin Na) techniques lock the elbow in some form.* Figure 2-40 shows the bones of the arm. The elbow is the joint between the upper and lower arms, skeletally comprised of the humerus and the paired bones of the radius and ulna respectively. The elbow joint is really three joint connections between these bones, all contained in a single joint capsule. The triceps tendons insert at the olecranon (top of the ulna) and run upward across the joint to the medial head of the triceps (Figure 2-41). Applying pressure with a bony part of your body on this tendon, several inches above the elbow, can cause considerable pain. This pressure

*Practical Chin Na by Zhao Da Yuan, (1993, p. 119).

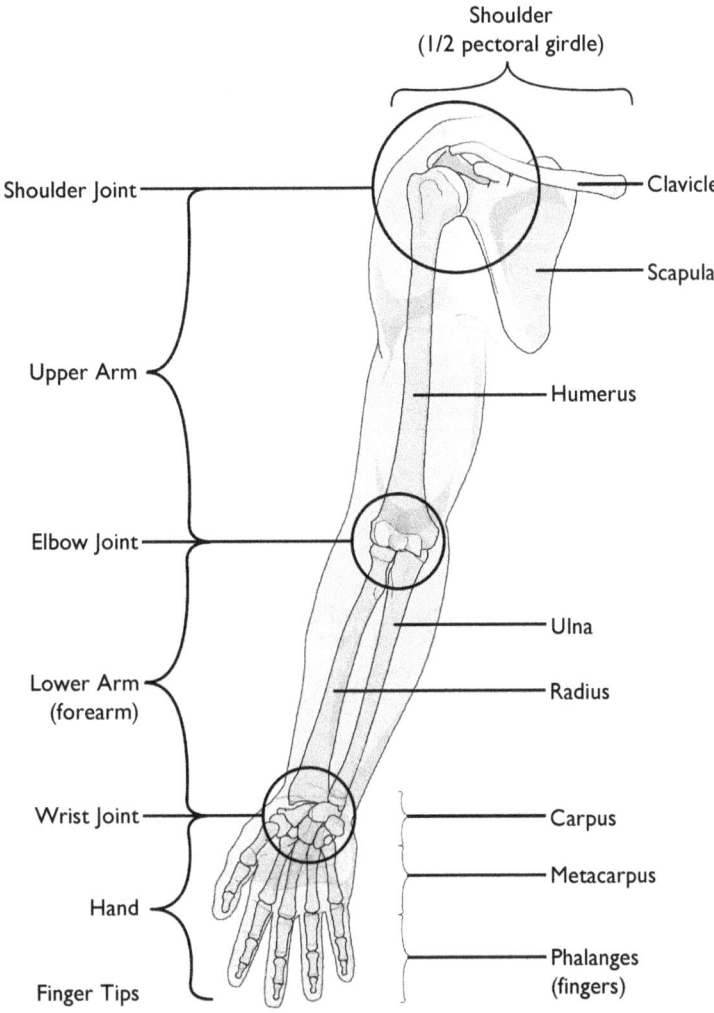

Segments and Bones of the Arm
Figure 2-40 Anterior view of the upper limb showing the anatomical segments and the bones contained within.

will make your opponent believe that you are applying considerably more force than you are and will assist you in keeping his arm straight or in distracting him. The radial nerve (Figure 2-42) innervates the triceps (lateral, long, and medial heads) and is the transmitter of this pain. The elbow allows 140-degree flexion and extension of the lower arm, mainly through the humerus-ulna joint and assisted by the humerus-radius joint. Because of the joint structure, extension of the arm backwards is not possible to a large degree, although women do have a slightly greater ability to do this than men. Strong pressure to the back of the elbow can move the humerus forward while the ulna moves backwards resulting in a rear dislocation of the elbow.

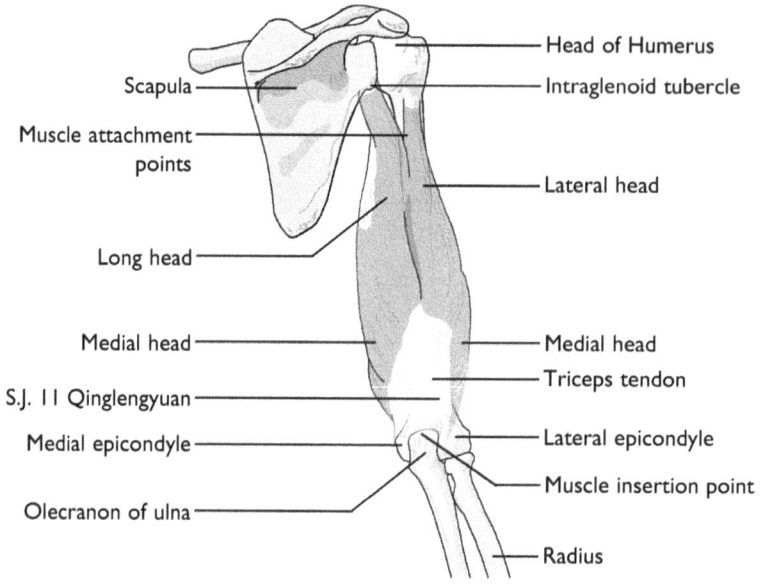

Muscles of the Posterior Arm
Figure 2-41 Note the positioning of the triceps muscle and the triceps tendon.

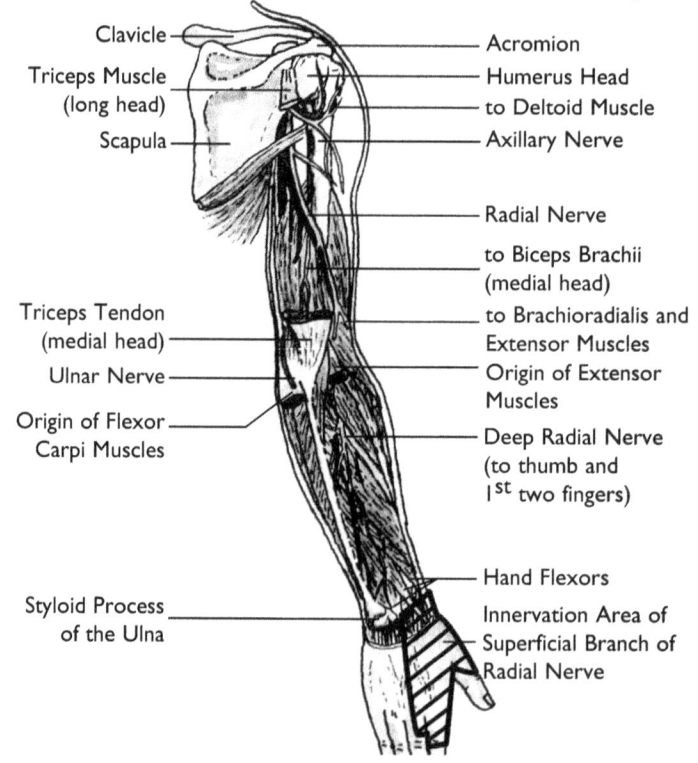

Nerves of the Posterior Arm
Figure 2-42 Note the innervation of the triceps muscle via a branch of the radial nerve. This nerve passes under the scapula and originates from the lower cervical vertebrae (C5, C6, C7).

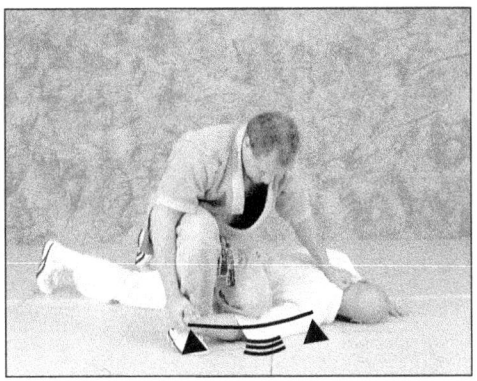 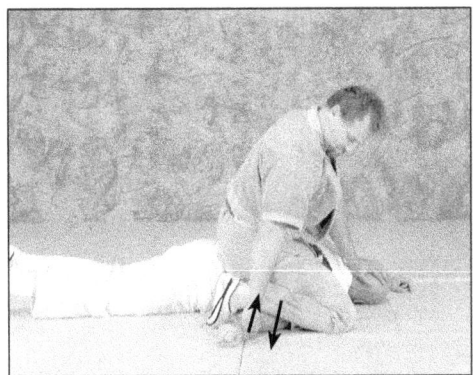

Figure 2-43   Figure 2-44

This hyperextension will damage the joint, ligaments and muscles with concomitant nerve damage. When the arm is placed under tension and the hand twisted to the outside, the smaller head of the radius can be more readily dislocated. Note also that the rotation of the arm is a function of the shoulder joint. The wrist locks the elbow, which in turn locks the shoulder joint. It is through this movement chain that the whole body can be physically controlled, like twisting links on a motorcycle chain.

Arm Bars in General

We will now examine how these physical principles and this knowledge of anatomy can be put into practice. Rather than memorizing each technique as a separate entity, we will look at the common biomechanical principle of overextending the arm and let you choose which body tool (see Chapter Four) to effect pressure on the elbow joint. Since the elbow only has movement around one axis, it can be stressed by twisting and/or hyper-extending/hyper-flexing it. We will look at the hyper-extension of the elbow. The premise is simple: find out which way the arm bends and bend it in this plane beyond its extension limit in order to inflict pain or break it.

In Figure 2-43 Grey demonstrates this principle of the arm bar. Grey places White's straight right arm so that the plane of flexion is directly downwards. He creates a bridge, from White's right shoulder that is tight against the mat to the top of his right foot. Grey merely has to kneel on the elbow joint to break it. Grey is controlling White's right wrist in a wristlock as he raises his wrist off the ground. The larger the wedge Grey inserts (his foot), the higher the bridged arm span will be and the greater the (hyper-) flexion will be experienced by White. It matters not how force is brought to bear against the elbow. Grey could put his shin across White's elbow and pull up on White's right wrist to create the same breakage, although the latter case involves physical strength as opposed to just using body weight (Figure 2-44).

If your opponent is very strong, you may decide to take his arm however he gives it to you: bent or straight. You may be able to straighten a bent arm if conditions are favorable to do so. We have already seen an example of this in Figures 1-32 through 1-34 that saw Grey using his whole body to straighten out White's hugging arm as he escaped his hold.

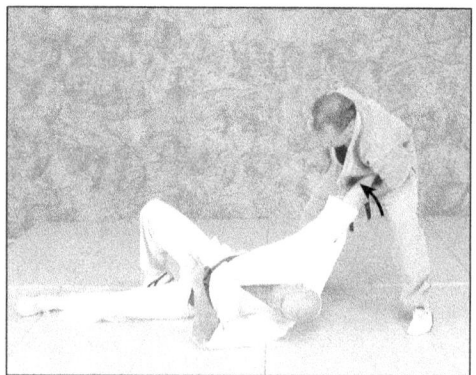

Figure 2-45

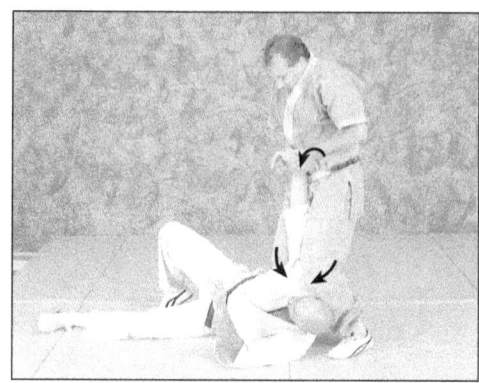

Figure 2-46

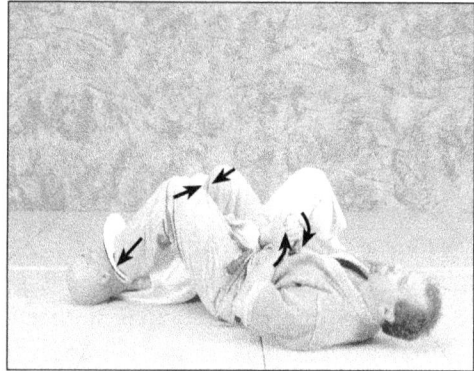

Figure 2-47

An arm bar can be applied in the stand up situation by using the arm as a first-class lever. Many Qin Na techniques can be applied on the ground. As well, (Figure 2-45) shows that Grey has taken hold of White's right arm as he slides his left forearm under White's elbow as a fulcrum. By lifting upward with his arms and back muscles, he can apply pressure on White's elbow. Grey uses this pain to roll White onto his left side where he transfers the pressure on the elbow from his arm to his knees or lower thighs (Figure 2-46). Grey now secures White's right wrist in a wristlock. Grey is also free to go to the ground and apply *juji gatame* (cross-mark hold) if he chooses, replacing his knees with his pelvis as the fulcrum (Figure 2-47). The technique is the arm bar; only the tools are different in order to create a fulcrum and/or apply pressure to the elbow. Let's look at a few ways to accomplish this task using different body parts. Keep an open mind about the *means* by which the hold can be applied and through your own creativity. Then you will be able to adapt the tools you have for the position you are in to effect the lock. Don't memorize the moves; learn the principles.

Hugging with the Forearms

One way to apply the arm bar is to hug the straight arm (*ude gatame*) as shown in Figure 2-48. Grey may trap White's right hand by shrugging his left shoulder and tilting his head in this direction. Notice how Grey kneels on White's head to further control him. Using his shoulder as a bridge, Grey can apply pressure on his upper arm and elbow with his augmented grip. Grey can selectively use the radial edge of his wrist to apply this pressure on the triceps tendon a few inches above the elbow. It matters not what position you are in to apply this technique. Figure 2-49 shows Grey applying it while reclining on his side.

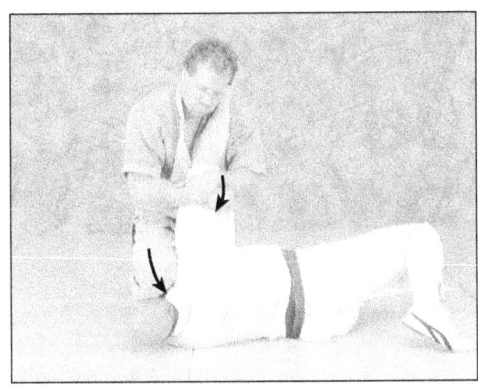

Figure 2-48

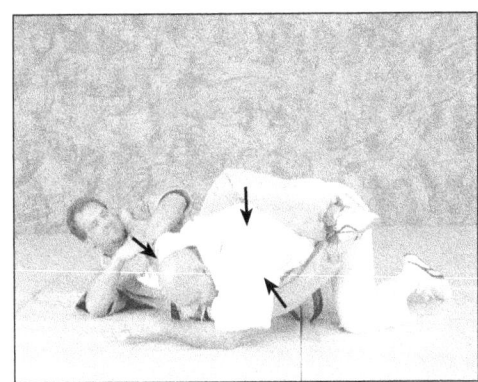

Figure 2-49

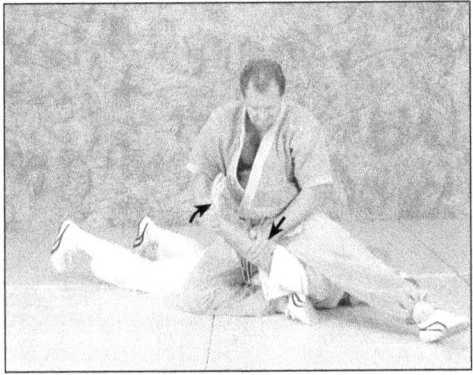

Figure 2-50

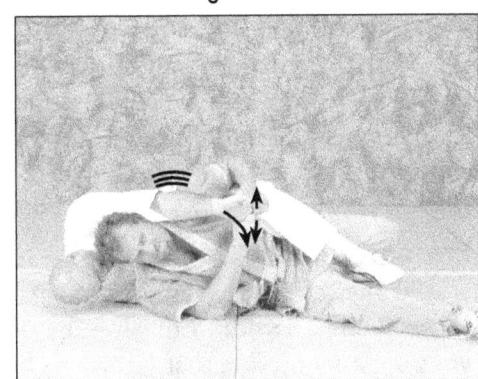

Figure 2-51

Pressing the Elbow

Figure 2-50 shows Grey pressing the back of White's right elbow while seated on him. Grey can further apply a wristlock to create the counterpressure needed to stress White's arm as well as to help subdue him. You may never end up in this position, but the point is that arm bars can be applied from a wide variety of relative body positions using many body tools.

Levering Over the Shoulder

In Figure 2-51, Grey has managed to grab White's left arm while seated in front of him. Grey rolled over to trap White's right arm under his body leaving him free to lever White's left arm over Grey's left shoulder, thereby putting him in an arm bar.

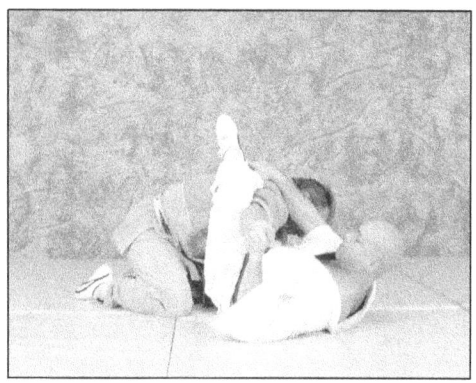
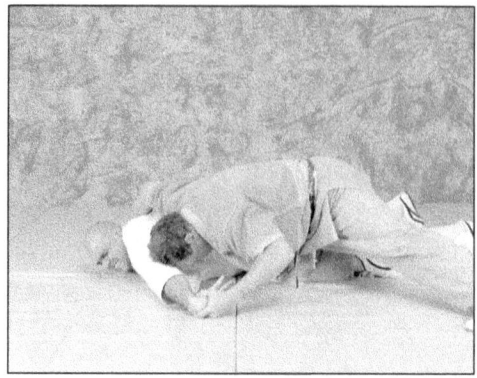

Figure 2-52   Figure 2-53

Levering Against the Lower Thigh

Another way of levering the arm is to use the leg (Figure 2-52). White is using his own left lower leg to act as a fulcrum on Grey's elbow. White grabs his own lower left pant leg with his right arm to stabilize this leg and hold Grey down while simultaneously applying countertorque to the right side of Grey's neck to keep him from advancing in a clockwise direction that would allow him to escape.

Pressing with the Head

Figure 2-53 shows Grey bulldogging White's left arm at the elbow with the top of his head. The head can often be used in novel ways to apply bony pressure to your opponent. Note that Grey also has applied a wristlock to White's left arm for an additional measure of control.

Figure Four

In Figure 2-54, Grey has White's right arm in a figure-four lock. The crook of Grey's right elbow is placed near White's right elbow. The radial edge of Grey's right arm can dig into White's upper arm. Notice that Grey is using his extended left arm to push against White's jaw downward as to create additional tension in White's trapped right arm.

Knuckle Digs

The fore knuckles can be driven into the triceps tendons of straightened arms (Figure 2-55). Here Grey grabs White's gi at the elbows and rolls his fists into White's tendons in order to break out of the choke hold White is applying. Grey can shrug his shoulders to help keep White's arms trapped if he chooses, but this is not a reliable trap for both hands.

Chapter 2: The Science of Technique

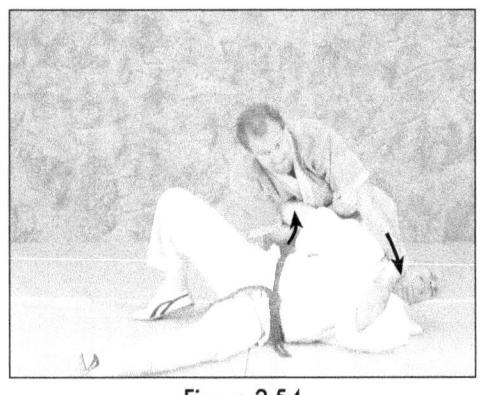

Figure 2-54

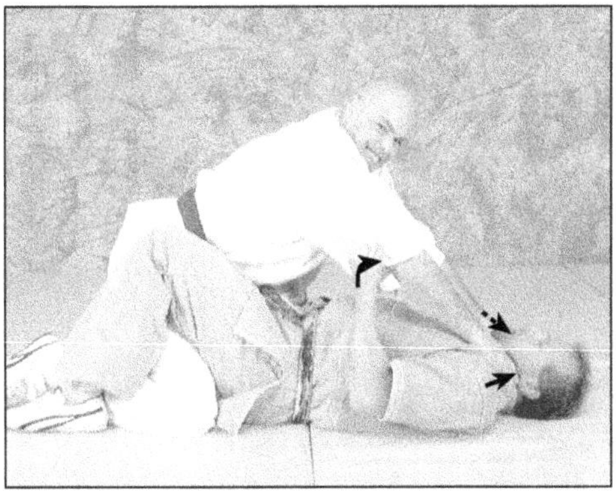

Figure 2-55

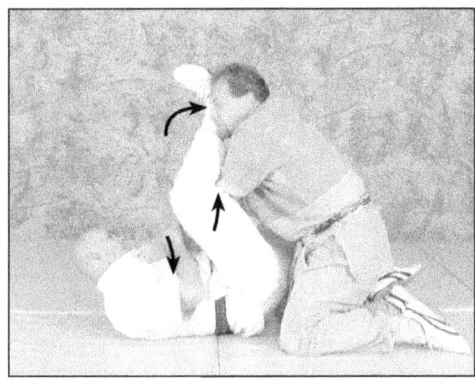

Figure 2-56

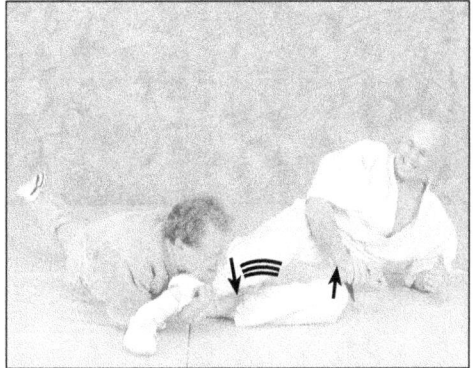

Figure 2-57

Scissoring the Arms

In Figure 2-56 Grey was in White's guard until Grey tried to choke him with both hands. White responded by grabbing both of Grey's wrists and swinging both of his legs up in front of Grey. By trapping Grey's hands onto his chest, palms facing each other, Grey can then scissor his legs against Grey's arms, effectively applying double arm bars on him. A single arm bar can be applied, again using the scissoring action of the legs (Figure 2-57). White is using his left inside thigh as a bridge between Grey's shoulder and he uses his right leg to apply pressure to Grey's extended left arm.

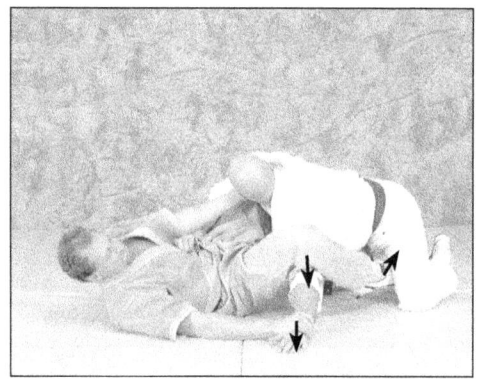

| Figure 2-58 | Figure 2-59 |

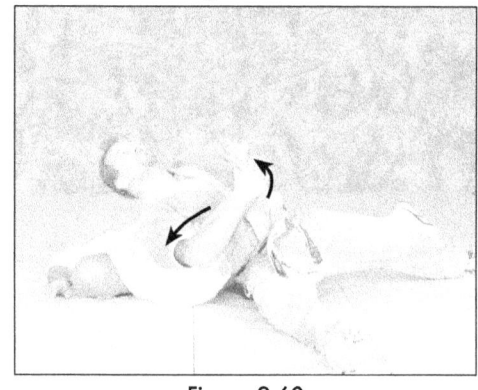

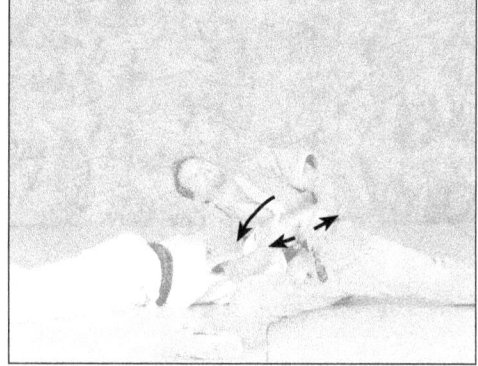

| Figure 2-60 | Figure 2-61 |

Pressing with the Back of the Knee

The reader should be getting the idea by now never to offer your opponent a straight arm. In Figure 2-58, Grey intercepts White's left arm as he tries to pass in under Grey's right leg. Grey traps White's arm and inserts his right foot into the left inside hip area of White's body. In order to strengthen the hold, Grey levers his leg downward by straightening it, using White's own body for counterpressure. Grey also elects to grab White's left wrist with both hands in order to lift up on this wrist to put White's elbow under even more stress (Figure 2-59).

Using the Armpit Hold

Figures 2-60 and 2-61 shows *waki gatame* being applied to White's arms, although the first hold is stronger because of the fact that Grey can better shift his center of gravity to hold White down. Grey applies wristlocks to the controlled arms in both cases. More pressure can be applied to White's elbow if Grey slides down onto White's arm somewhat, although this weakens his pinning pressure on him.

Chapter 2: The Science of Technique

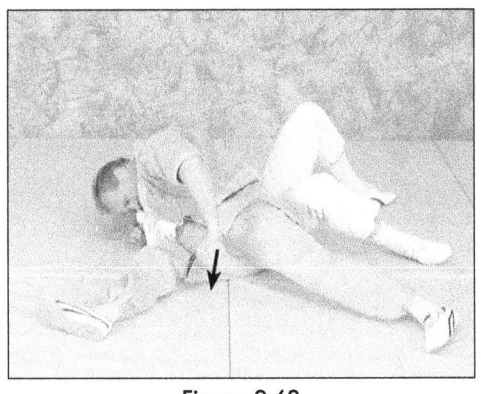

Figure 2-62

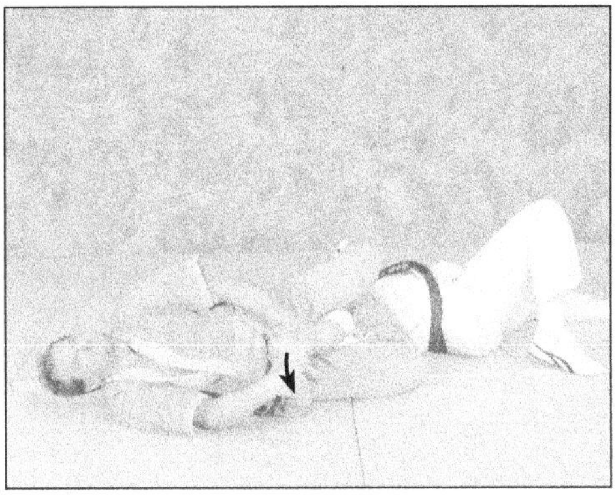

Figure 2-63

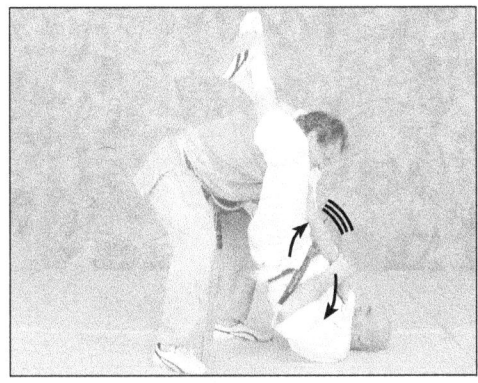

Figure 2-64

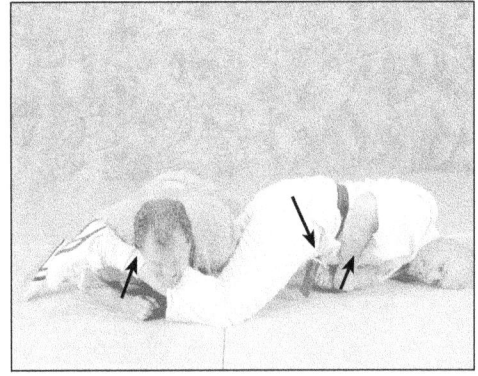

Figure 2-65

Using the Upper Thigh

Grey is seen applying *kesa gatame* (scarf hold) on White (Figure 2-62), but he elects to place White's right arm in an arm bar using his own right upper thigh as a fulcrum. Grey bears down on White's right wrist with his left arm in order to hyper-extend White's arm.

Levering with the Pelvis

There are numerous ways to apply *juji gatame* (cross-mark hold). In Figure 2-63, Grey scissors his legs as he applies pressure against White's right elbow using the upward action of his pelvis against the downward action of Grey's hands on White's wrist/hand. Note that Grey is augmenting his hold by bending a few fingers backward. This same technique can be done in a near vertical position (Figure 2-64 shows it is White who applies this hold possible as a result from his failed triangle choke) or from the prone position (Figure 2-65) shows White levering up against Grey's head and he presses his own pelvis downward to break Grey's arm).

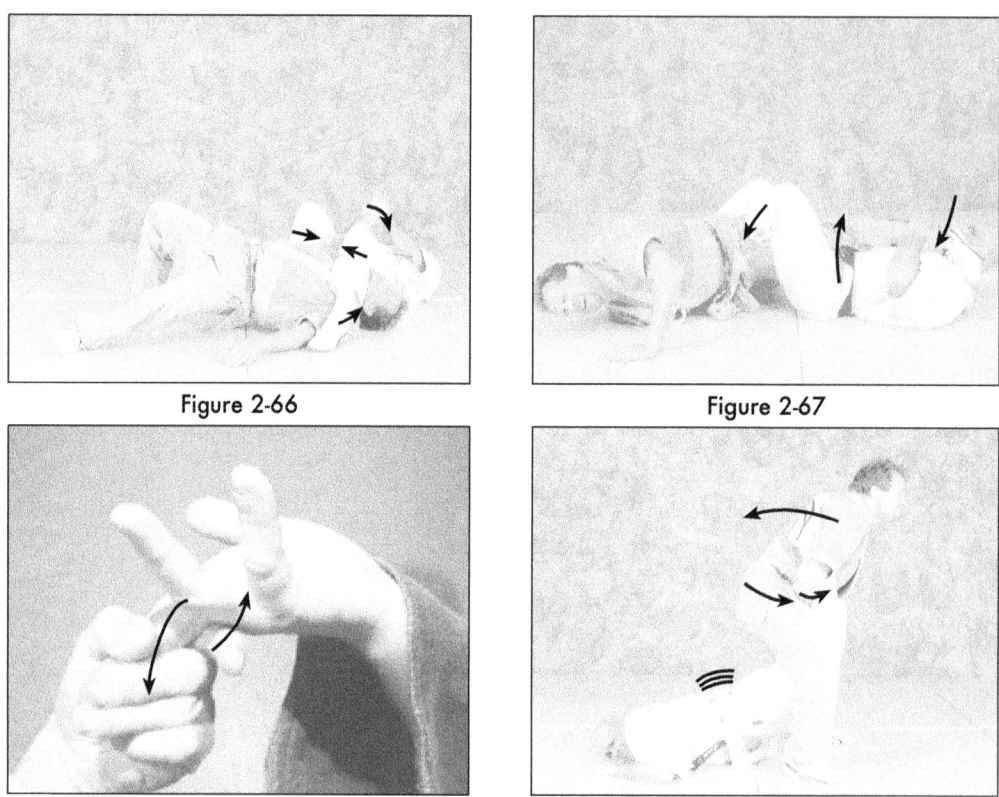

Figure 2-66

Figure 2-67

Figure 2-68

Figure 2-69

After looking at some of the many ways of putting on an arm bar, clearly it is easier to comprehend and apply the principles behind it rather than memorizing each technique. It does not matter whether we attack the arm position (Figure 2-66), leg position (Figure 2-67), finger position (Figure 2-68), or body position (Figure 2-69), other than the strength factor; the same principle applies to all. They are all segmented units, so bend them all up to or beyond their limits of flexibility.

Chapter 2: The Science of Technique

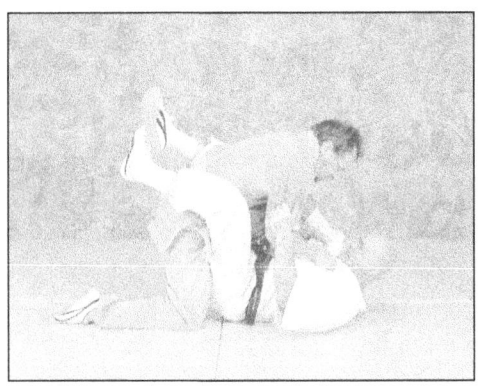

Figure 2-70

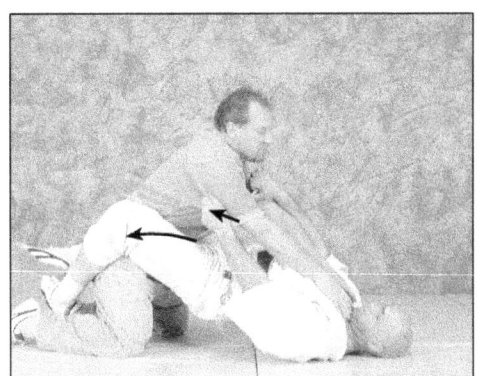

Figure 2-71

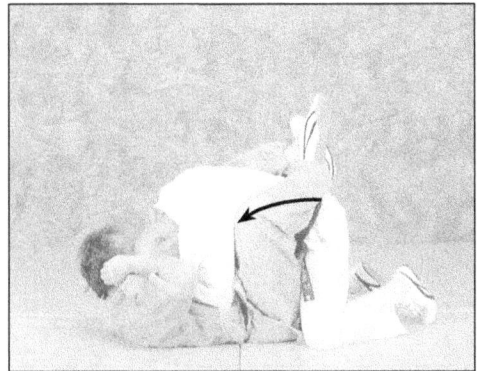

Figure 2-72

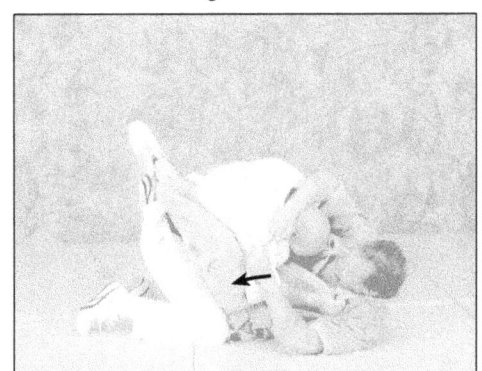

Figure 2-73

2-4. BODY POSITIONS*

The Guard

Figure 2-70 shows Grey in White's guard position. White may elect to lock his ankles to scissor Grey or use his legs for other purposes. It is of obvious importance to control Grey's arms and to defend against head butts. Using the guard, we have the ability to ward off striking attacks because we are facing our opponent and can see what's going on. By pushing him away (Figure 2-71) or pulling him in (Figure 2-72) with the legs, we can control the distance. We also have the ability to choke or lock our opponent, strike and even kick him. This is a good all around defensive position to be in on the ground because we can use all of our limbs for attack and defense.

Conversely, if we are in our opponent's guard, we can strike and block striking attacks, but locking our opponent's arms is more difficult from this position. Likewise, he may lock our arms or choke us if we are not careful. His legs are vulnerable to locks because they are relatively accessible. Figure 2-73 shows White beginning to break out

---

*When ground fighting it is essential to consider what limbs are available to you in each position. Each position has varying opportunities for attack, defense, and positional changes. We will not outline a detailed look at these basic positions nor offer strategies regarding them, as they are beyond the scope of this book.

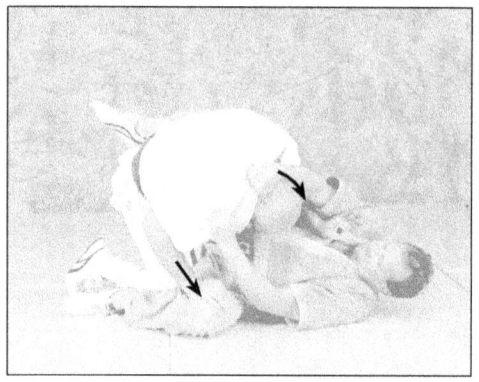

| Figure 2-74 | Figure 2-75 |

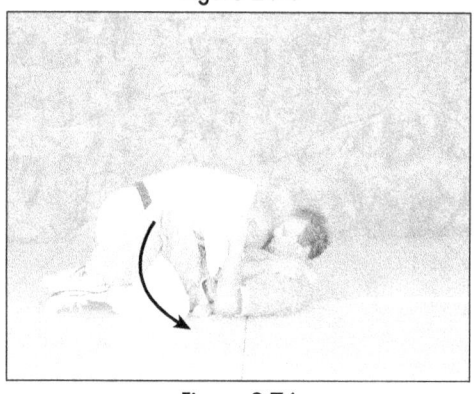
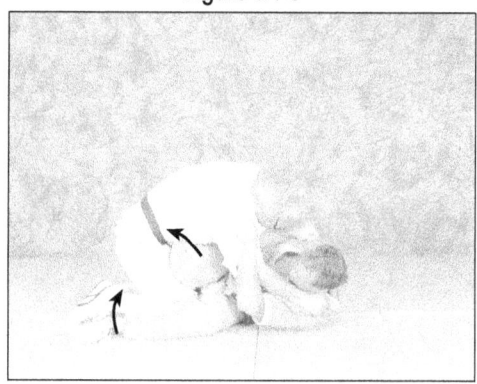

| Figure 2-76 | Figure 2-77 |

of Grey's guard by applying pressure to his thigh with his elbow. He eventually gets his elbow to bear down on Grey's inner thigh as to get him to release Grey's scissor lock on him. White then presses his hand onto Grey's left leg as he moves into a semi-kneeling position (Figure 2-74). White reacts by swinging his own left leg up and over Grey's right leg, placing it between his legs to effect a leg lock (Figure 2-75).

Although you can defend yourself and even attack the opponent in your guard, you may wish to take a more aggressive position with him. An example of a positional change from the guard position to that of the mounted position can be seen in Figures 2-76 through 2-79. Grey has White in his guard (Figure 2-76). Grey grabs White by the shoulders in preparation for applying torque to his upper body. Grey slides his hips out to his right and rolls over onto his left hip (Figure 2-77). He slides his right bent leg in between himself and White so that Grey's right shin lies across White's belt line, while his other leg drops to the mat. In an explosive burst, Grey scissors his legs while he twists White's upper body counterclockwise, causing White to topple (Figure 2-78). Grey pulls himself tightly into White's rolling body, coupling with his momentum in order to bring himself up on top of White's now supine body (Figure 2-79).

Chapter 2: The Science of Technique

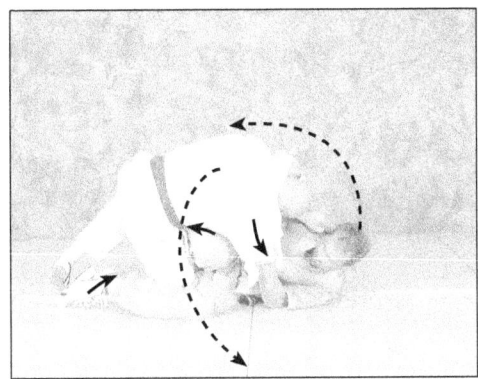

Figure 2-78

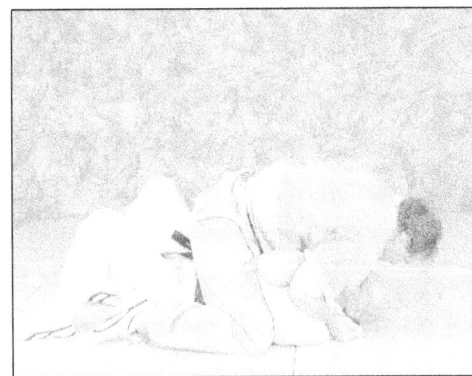

Figure 2-79

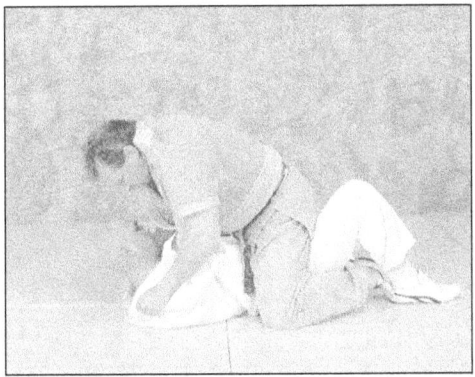

Figure 2-80

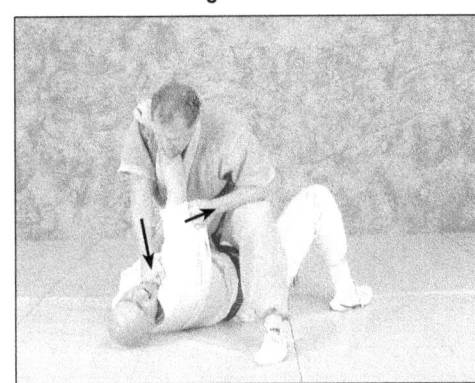

Figure 2-81

The Mount

Figure 2-80 shows Grey in the mounted position, straddling White's torso with his knees on either side of him. White can do relatively little offensively from this position, so it should be avoided. Figure 2-81 shows that he who has the upper hand has the strongest punch. White cannot put his body behind the punch nor can he draw his punching arm back very far because of the contact his elbow makes

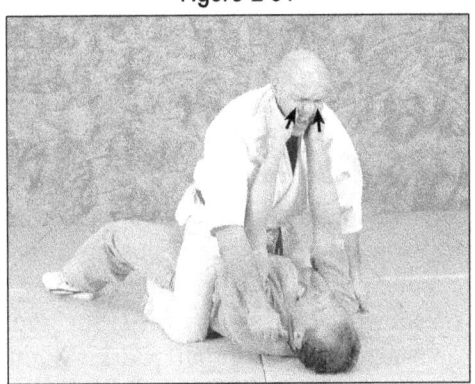

Figure 2-82

with the mat. This does not mean that the bottom man is defenseless. Figure 2-82 shows Grey attacking cranial pressure points (S.I. 18 Quanliao-zygomatic crevice) from the bottom position. It is better to make a positional change. Not only is there the threat of a barrage of strikes to defend from but also our opponent may choke or lock our arms from this position with little threat of being strongly countered if you are mounted. The easiest way to do this is to simply raise your hips quickly off of

Chin Na In Ground Fighting

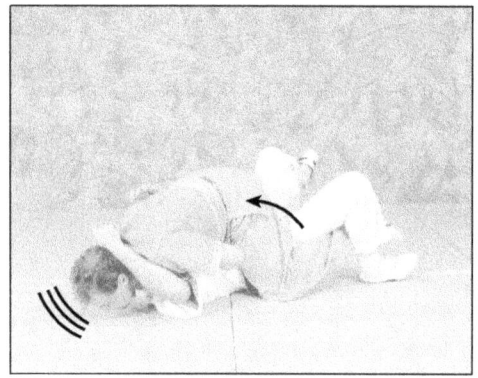

Figure 2-83

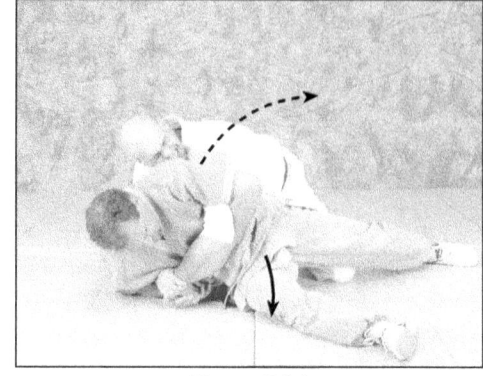

Figure 2-84

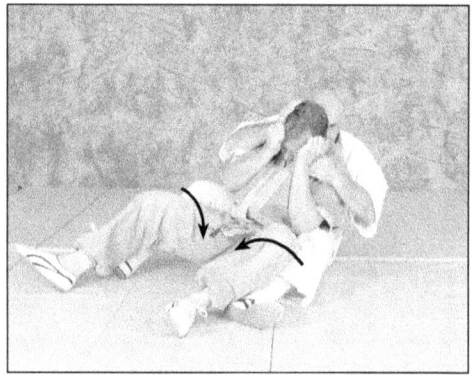

Figure 2-85

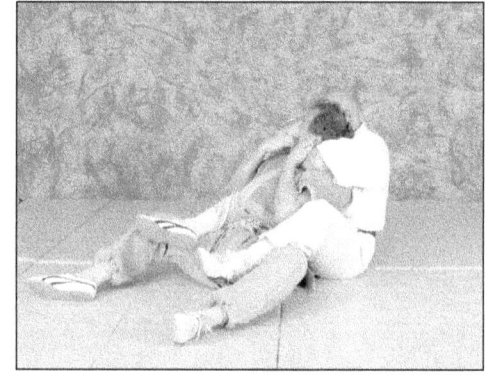

Figure 2-86

the mat to buck him off you as White has done to Grey (Figure 2-83). If his arms are controlled or trapped, he can be launched face-first.

The Rear Guard

Although not a common position to be in, the rear guard position does occur in ground fighting, be it from a takedown or a breakdown from your opponent being on all fours. White has bear-hugged Grey on all fours, but Grey tries to sit through the hold by

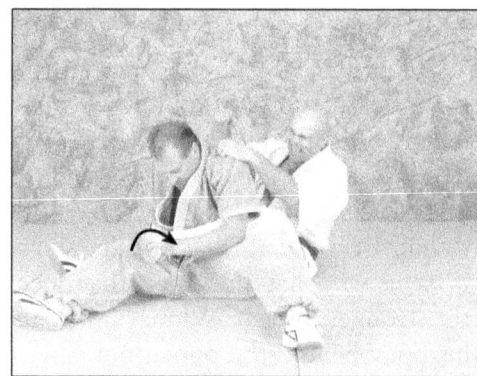

Figure 2-87

shooting his right leg under his own body and collapses onto his right hip (Figure 2-84). White reacts by pulling Grey backward into the seated position (Figure 2-85). This is a very difficult position for Grey to be in because White has his hands free to attack him (Figure 2-86). As White tries to choke Grey, Grey grabs White's left foot and twists it clockwise causing White to let go of his hold for fear of his knee dislocating (Figure 2-87). If you have someone in the reverse guard, one must be careful about your ankles. Your opponent can tie up both of your legs with one arm inserted

Chapter 2: The Science of Technique

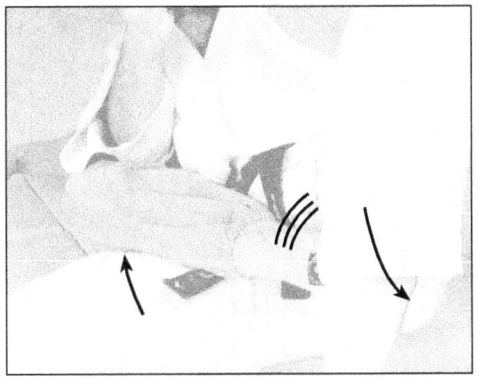

Figure 2-88

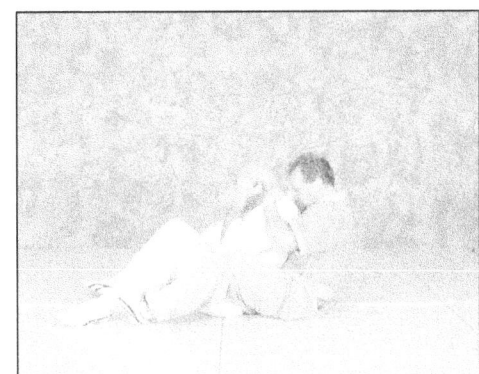

Figure 2-89

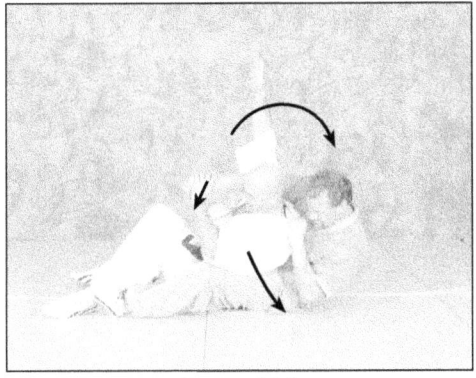

Figure 2-90

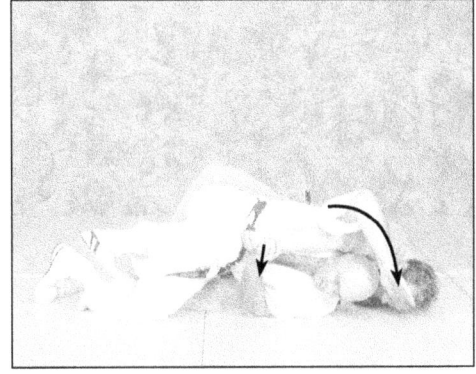

Figure 2-91

between crossed ankles or even an uncrossed ankle can be hyper-extended by your opponent's legs (Figure 2-88).

The best thing to do is to do a positional change. In Figure 2-89, Grey is seated behind White. As Grey tries to choke White with his right arm, White grabs Grey's right wrist and raises his own right arm above his head (Figure 2-90). As he does so, White rolls over onto his left side whole keeping Grey's right arm trapped between the right side of his head and his right arm that

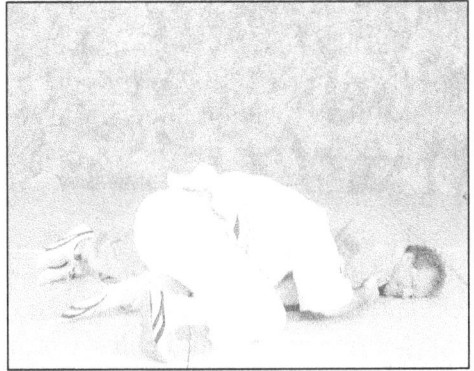

Figure 2-92

circles over to reach the mat (Figure 2-91). White assumes an all-fours position and continues to wrestle with Grey (Figure 2-92).

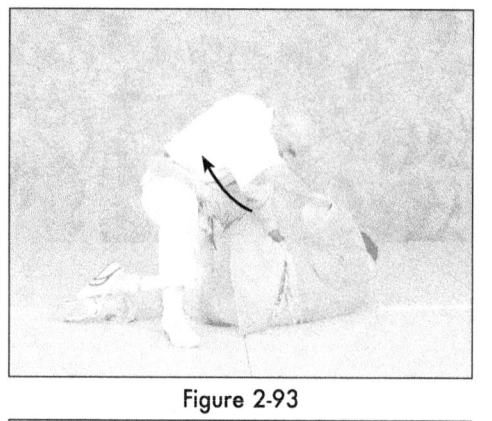

Figure 2-93

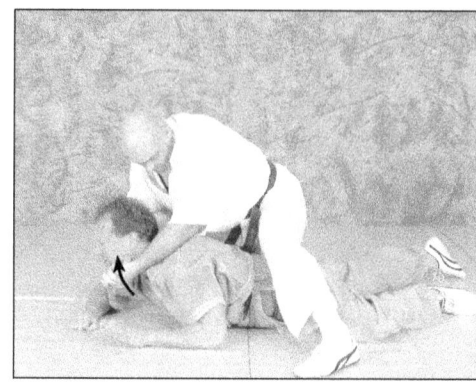

Figure 2-94

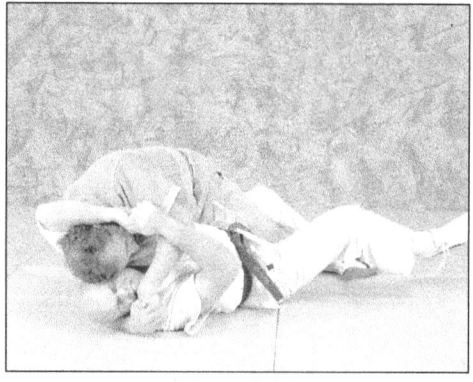

Figure 2-95

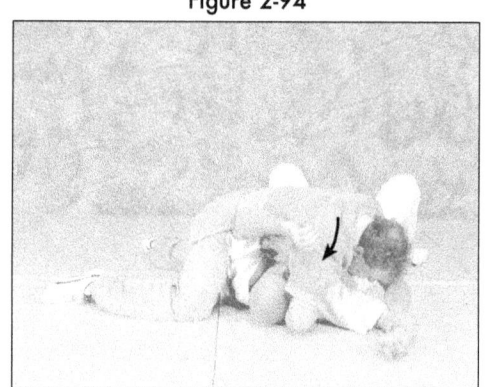

Figure 2-96

The Half Guard

The half guard is a transitional position as you move from the guard to other positions (Figure 2-93). As with the guard position, Grey can scissor White onto his back in order to mount him. If you are lying supine and someone rushes you, this is a good defensive posture to take, as it is more protective of the groin.

Prone

The prone position is the worst position to be in because you are completely defenseless (Figure 2-94). Never give your back to your opponent. This is a prime example of differentiating sport from the ugly reality of street fighting. In wrestling, this position makes it difficult for your opponent to 'pin' you, but on the street you are at his mercy. While on your back, you have all your limbs with which to defend and you can see your opponent (Figure 2-95).

The Cross Mount

The cross mount is often used as a transitional phase to the mounted position. The cross mount is achieved when your opponent is on his back and you are ninety degrees to him, basically facing him chest to chest (Figure 2-96). In this position, the person on top, Grey, has the advantage as he may strike, lock, or choke while

Chapter 2: The Science of Technique

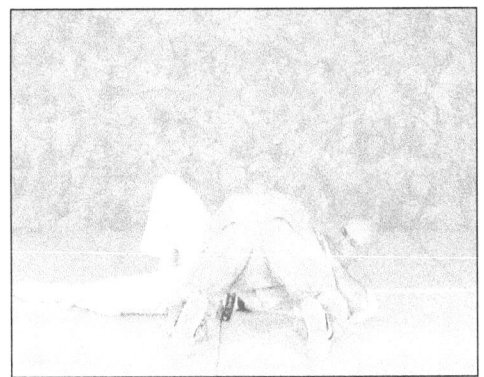

Figure 2-97

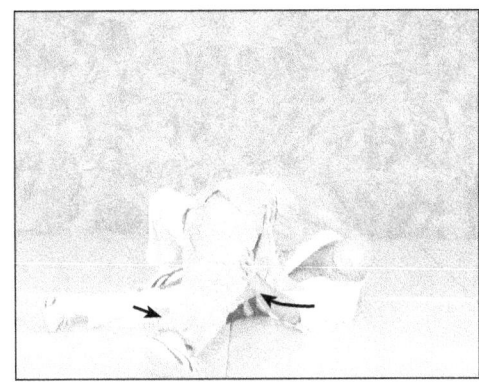

Figure 2-98

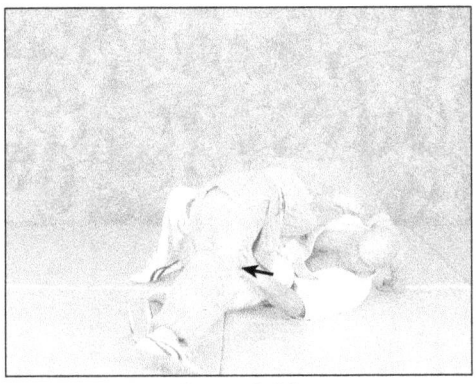

Figure 2-99

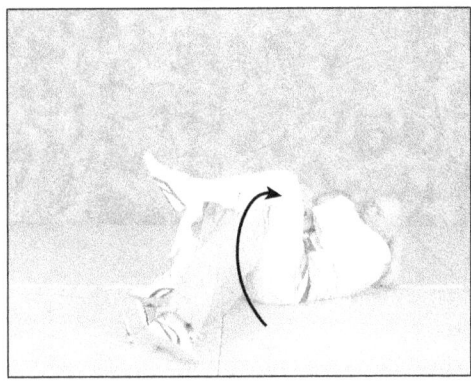

Figure 2-100

the person on the bottom, White, is limited to basically defending or trying to at least getting him into his guard position. Sometimes your opponent will move to an all-fours position before trying to mount you (Figure 2-97). White pushes Grey's right leg backwards at his knee while sliding his hips away from Grey (Figure 2-98). This gives White room to raise his left knee in front of Grey's left knee (Figure 2-99). White then forces his left leg straight, collapsing Grey's now semi-kneeling posture; he places it behind Grey's back (Figure 2-100) and completes the guard position (Figure 2-101).

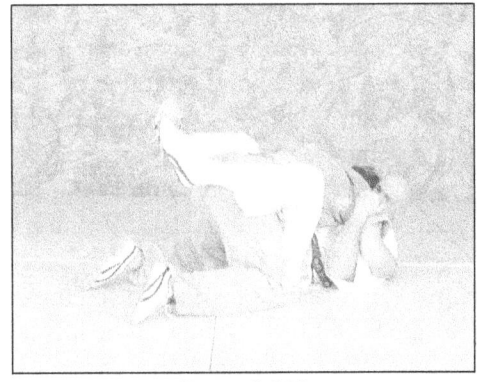

Figure 2-101

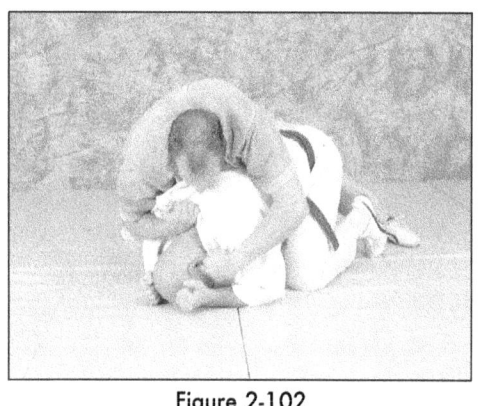

Figure 2-102

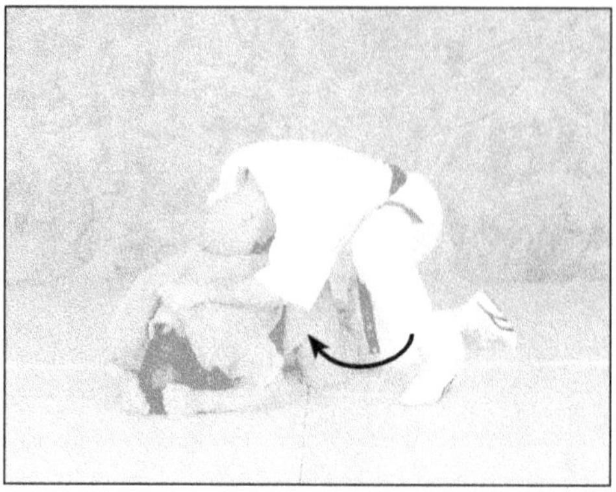

Figure 2-103

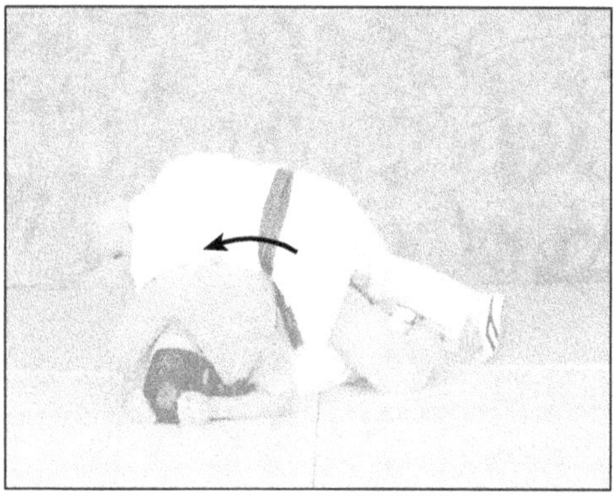

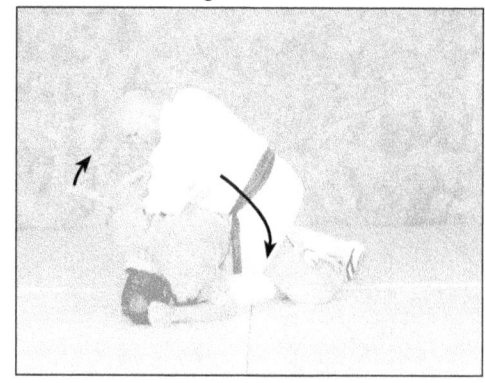

Figure 2-104

Figure 2-105

All Fours

This position of being on all fours is a common initial wrestling position. Although this is not a very good offensive position to be in, White can quickly 'turtle-up' into a tight ball (Figure 2-102) to keep a limb from being joint-locked, his anterior vitals from being exposed while protecting his neck. If your opponent does not launch striking and kicking attacks against you, he will try to insert an appendage to pry one of yours loose. In Figure 2-103, White has approached Grey who is on all fours. White inserts his left leg in between Grey's legs as he lays himself across Grey's back grabbing Grey's right arm as he does so (Figure 2-104). After White inserts his left forearm into the crook of Grey's right arm, he lifts it as he throws himself backward (Figure 2-105). White traps Grey's right arm under his left armpit while applying a headlock to Grey (Figure 2-106).

Kneeling

Kneeling positions are often used for transition purposes because when you are kneeling, your higher center of gravity makes you more mobile, but less stable (Grey is less stable than White in Figure 2-107) and you are unable to use your legs for offensive purposes unless delivering a knee strike (Figure 2-108). If your opponent assumes a kneeling position, it is better to attack him at this level than to allow him

Chapter 2: The Science of Technique

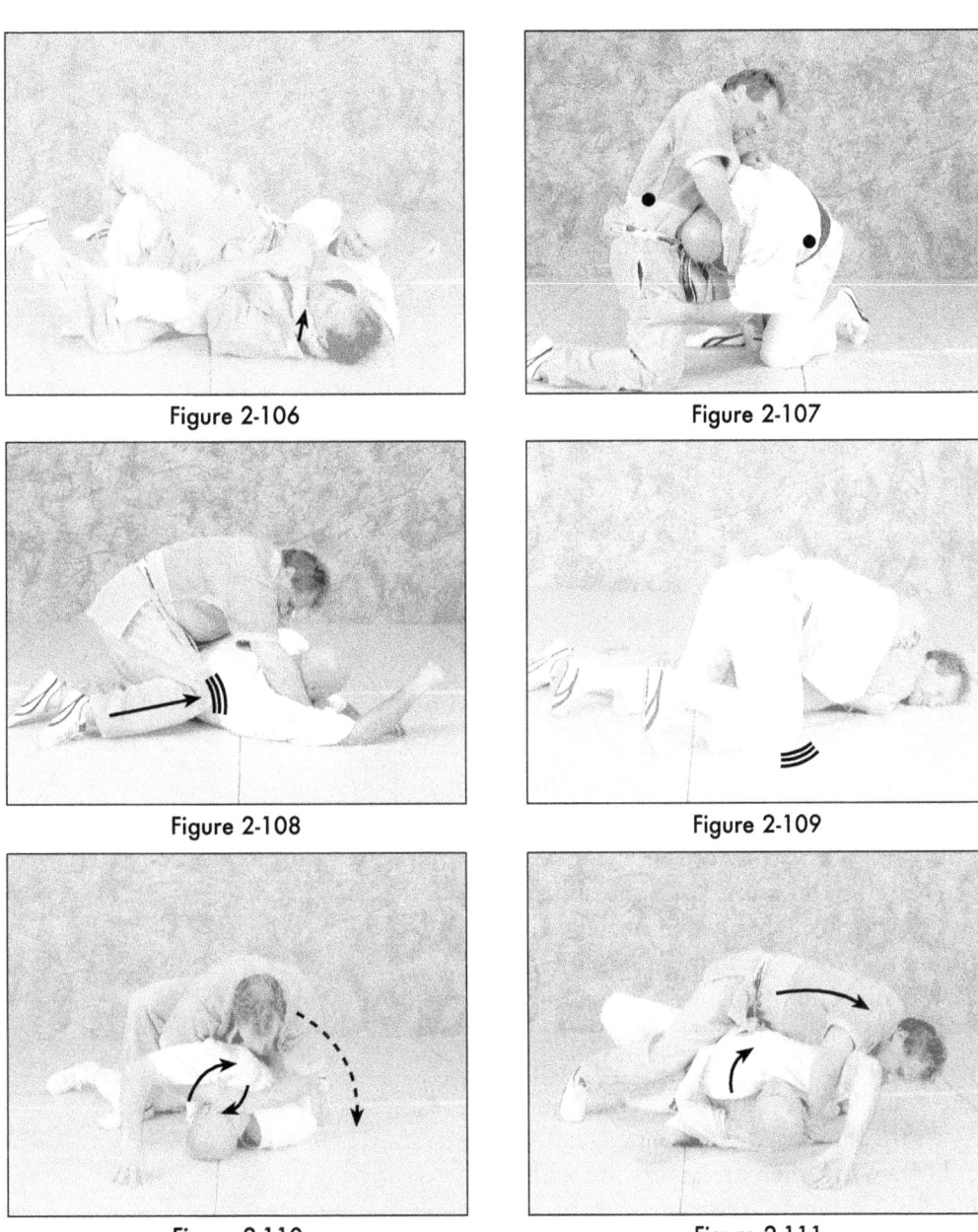

Figure 2-106

Figure 2-107

Figure 2-108

Figure 2-109

Figure 2-110

Figure 2-111

to climb on top of you. Kneeling gives you good mobility, but at a loss of some control over your opponent because some of your body weight is taken off of your opponent via knee contact with the mat (Figure 2-109). Figure 2-110 shows Grey kneeling with his left leg while straddling on top of White. Grey places him in a half Nelson while he rolls over onto his left side (Figure 2-111). Grey is now mounted

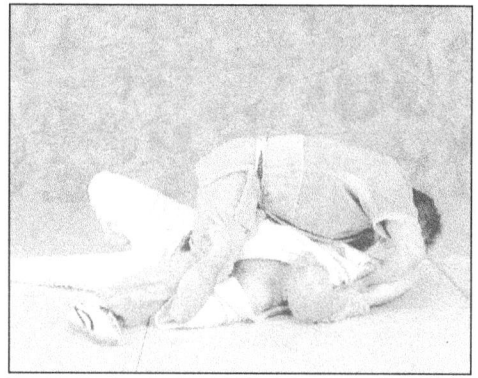

Figure 2-112

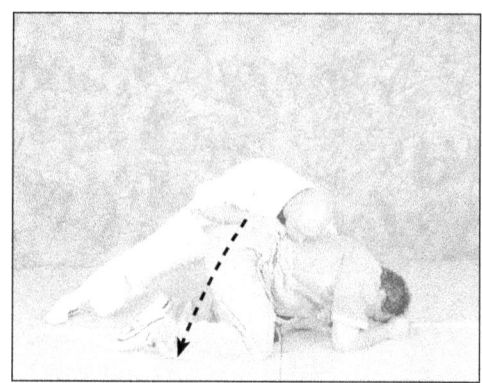

Figure 2-113

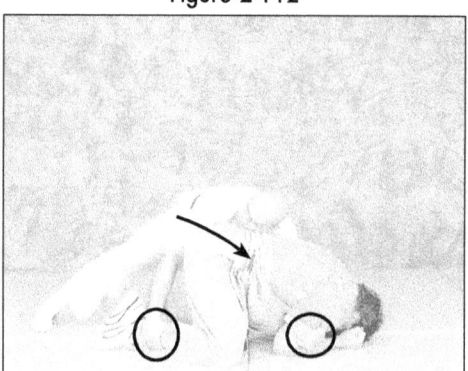

Figure 2-114

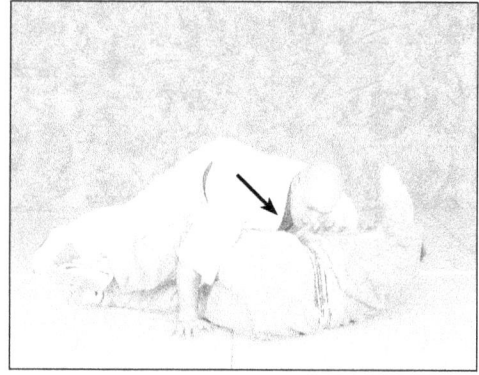

Figure 2-115

on top of White (Figure 2-112).

Kneeling does offer one the ability to drive with the legs when needed. In Figure 2-113, Grey has assumed an all-fours position while White assumes a semi-kneeling position. White then reaches under Grey with his left arm and grabs Grey's right upper arm while he also grabs Grey's right ankle (Figure 2-114). White then drives forward with his legs, rolling Grey onto his back (Figure 2-115). White then can wrestle with Grey in the cross-mounted position (Figure 2-116).

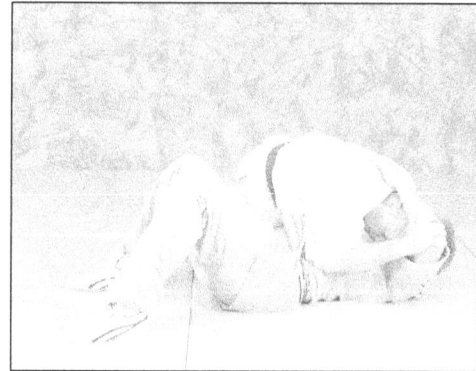

Figure 2-116

Chapter 2: The Science of Technique

Positioning

Now, there are many variations of all of these basic positions we have been talking about. Once you learn what techniques can be used from these different basic positions and which positions have limited possibilities for victory, you will want to start learning how to go from a position of disadvantage to a position of advantage. If the position is bad for us to defend from, obviously that is the position to have our opponents in. These transitions may not happen quickly in one smooth movement. It is a game of chess and you may have to work hard at getting to where you want to go, one small move at a time. We have shown some of the most basic positional changes to help get you started.

This topic lies outside the scope of this book and really should be learned from a qualified instructor because there are just too many different possibilities and variations. Otherwise, roll around on the mat and let your ingenuity fly. There is no substitute for mat work.

CHAPTER 3

Pressure Points of the Fourteen Meridians

3-1. INTRODUCTION

Pressure Points

One need not know the intricacies of acupuncture, meridian theory and acupuncture points that forms the basis of Traditional Chinese Medicine (T.C.M.) in order to apply Qin Na (Chin Na) technique to the numerous pressure points and cavities that exist in the human body. After all, there are 361 acupuncture points (670 points counting the bilateral ones) that lie on the 14 main meridians (see Figures 3-1 through 3-3). The meridians facilitate the flow of the life force *qi* throughout the human body according to T.C.M. theory.* These points were originally located and researched for healing purposes. Today T.C.M. and acupuncture is slowly gaining acceptance in the West as a viable alternative treatment. Indeed, it has been said that to know how to kill, one must know how to heal. We certainly do not claim any expertise in this field of study. This chapter includes a brief summary of the meridian theory gleaned from Li Ding's masterful book *Acupuncture, Meridian Theory and Acupuncture Points*. Others may wish to skip it and read the section about the location of the pressure points. Here again, we put in some detail about the nomenclature surrounding the naming of these points for those wishing to undertake a more academic study of these points.

Nomenclature

For those wishing to learn the names of the points, having an understanding of the rationale behind the nomenclature will help one to remember the point in question. For example, L.I. 4 Hegu means 'Converging Valley'. It is located in the web of the hand between the thumb and the index fingers. When these fingers are spread, the space between the first and second metacarpal bones is likened to that of a deep valley, so the (English) name and location should stick in your mind. There are many bases for labeling the points: some are named for an analogy to geography or topography (like L.I. 4 Hegu); astronomy (e.g., G. B. 24 Riyue-'Sun and Moon');

Acupuncture, Meridian Theory and Acupuncture Points by Li Ding, 1992, p. 35

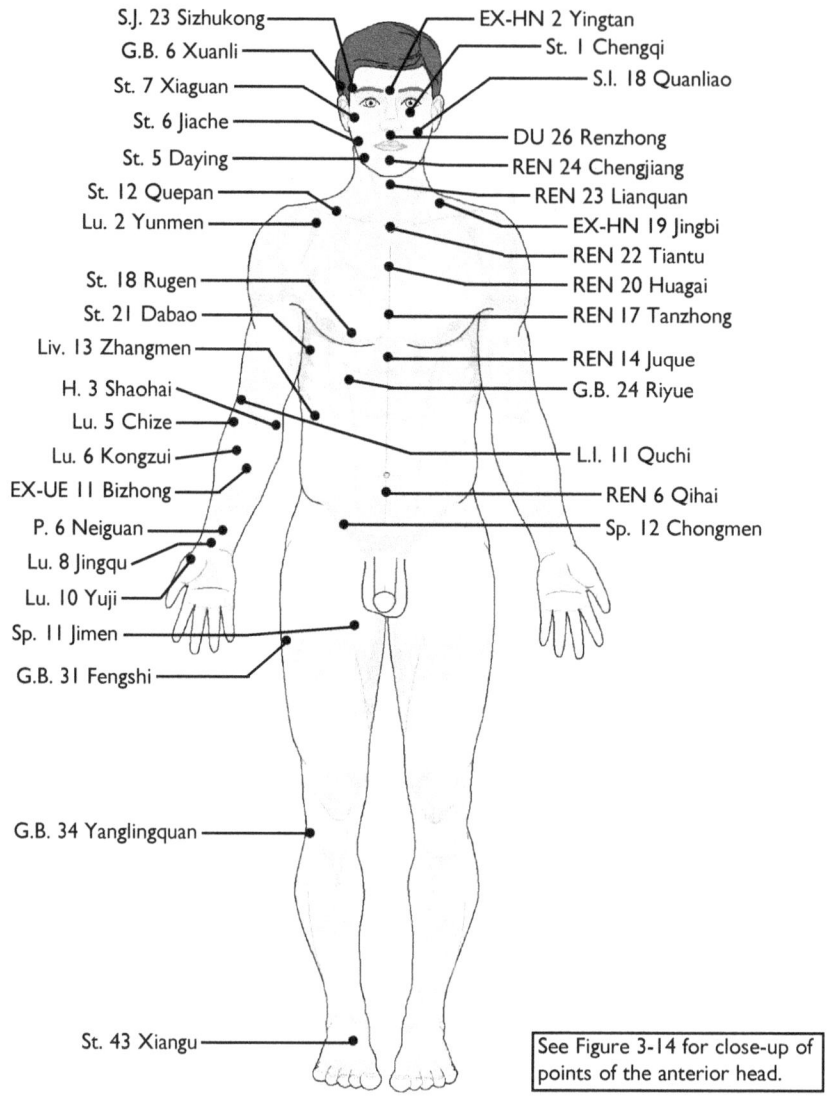

Selected Pressure Points of the Anterior Body.
Figure 3-1 More than half of 52 selected points can be accessed from the front. All points are bilateral (not shown) with the exception of those lying on the Conception Meridian (REN) which runs up the anterior mid-line of the body.

water flow (e.g., K.3 Taixi-'Big Stream'); names of animals were borrowed (e.g., St. 35 Dubai-'Ox Nose'); others relate to the physiological functions of proximal parts of the body (e.g., REN 17 Tanzhong–'Heart Palace'); or to realistic descriptions based on their locations and/or their indications (e.g., DU 15 Yamen-'Mute-saving Gate'). All acupuncture points were named for a reason; however, not all points have modern or easy to remember connotations.

Chapter 3: Pressure Points of the Fourteen Meridians

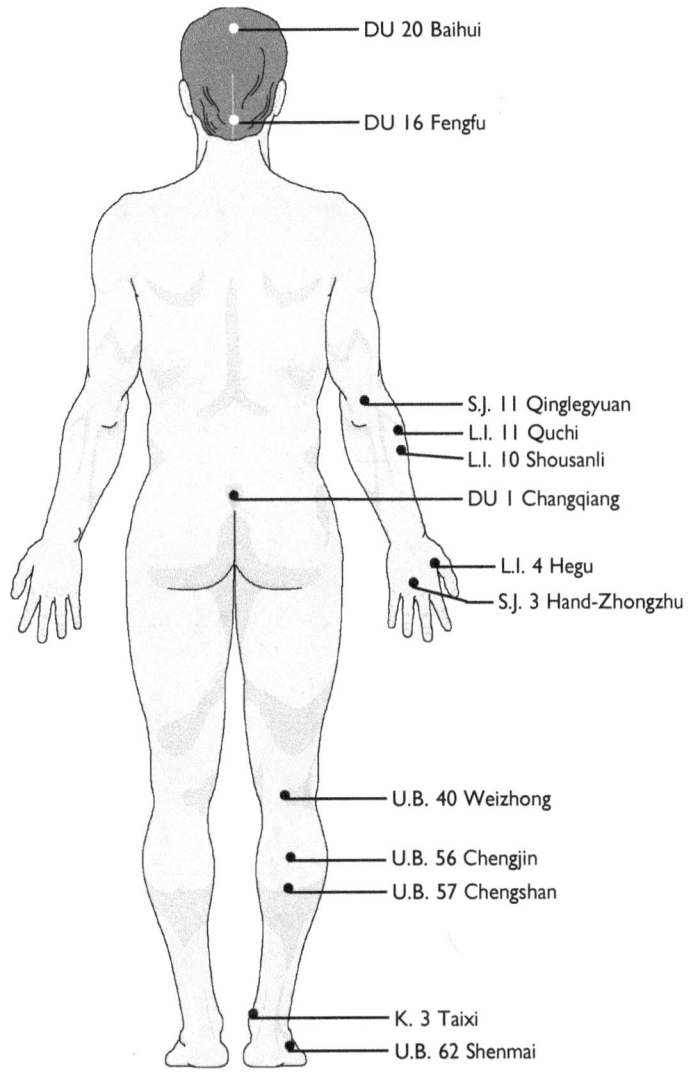

Selected Pressure Points of the Posterior Body.
Figure 3-2 Only a quarter of the 52 selected points can be accessed from the rear. An opponent in the prone position has limited attack and defense options, and is susceptible to choking techniques.

Pressure Point Locations

Having a rudimentary knowledge of the more common, practical pressure/vital points (*kyusho*) used in the martial arts for fighting purposes is a great asset, regardless of whether you can name them or not. Knowing where the motor nerves of the central nervous system (those voluntary nerves controlling body movement) run in the body is advantageous, particularly where they can be readily accessed. These nerves generally run along the bone contours under thick protective muscular covering. Where they emerge

Chin Na In Ground Fighting

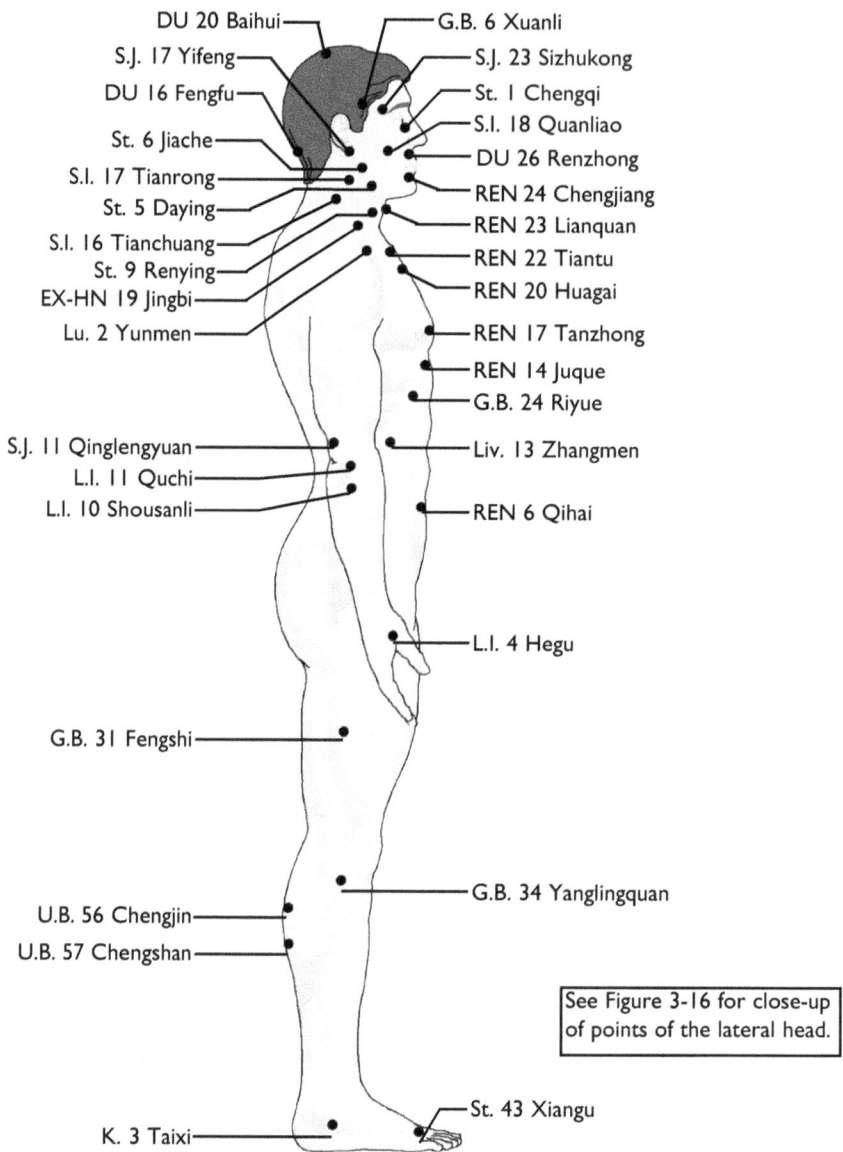

Selected Pressure Points of the Lateral Body.
Figure 3-3 About half of the 52 selected points can be readily accessed directly from the side. at the joints (and other locations), the muscular cover is greatly reduced, making them vulnerable to attack. Seizing and striking the relatively exposed nerve points will render the nerves (and corresponding innervated muscle) temporarily 'stunned'. The loss of muscle control, strength, numbness and pain associated with pressure point attacks can reduce your opponent's ability to fight with the affected limb. Take time and care to practice locating these points on yourself, at least the ones that you can reach (Figure

3-4) shows the author studying pressure points of the arm. Indelible ink was used to offer ample study time of these points). As these points are often located in the depressions at the ends of bone or muscle, they can be found relatively easily. Not only do these nerves lack protective muscular cover at these points, they are often lying across bony surfaces. As such, they are responsive to touch, making them ideal targets, for they are widely distributed around the body and strength does not play a major role in applying pressure. Of special interest are the 'Pressure Points and Control Tactics' nerve pressure points and nerve motor points that are used by police officers (See Table 3-2, p. 108). When applying pressure to pressure points, remember that a specific angle is needed to generate the best results. In many cases, it is just straight into the point, whereas others, an angled attack is required as to press a nerve against bone (e.g., Hegu L.I. 4). Counterpressure is required for maximum results, otherwise your opponent might just move away from the attack, unless that is your intention. This counterpressure may be provided by your other hand or more likely by another body part or by the ground itself because of your entwinement with your opponent.

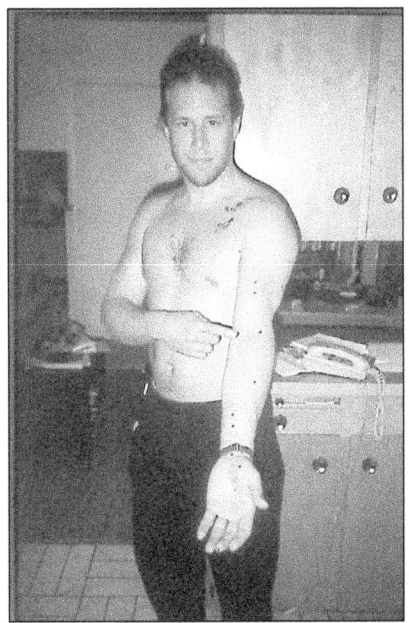

Figure 3-4 Author Al Arsenault researching pressure points (1993). Practice locating an accessing a few points at a time.

Indentations, in the body, such as behind the ear, the solar plexus and the shoulder well, are good places to access nerves which are thinly protected by muscle. There are 108 'cavities' that can be struck or pressed in order to affect the flow of *qi*. Attacking the cavities could lead to numbness or unconsciousness (72 points), or even death (36 points). Some of these points can be used as targets for distraction, setting up releases, joint lock manipulations and progressive strikes, while others cause injury or death.

Deadly Techniques

Attacking these various vital points is known as dim mak *(dian xue)* or *kyusho jitsu*. It appears that the earlier deadly forms of martial arts have been guarded family secrets by masters who handed down their deadly knowledge sparingly—sometimes to only a single trusted senior student—out of fear that their enemies might use their techniques against them. Life and death fighting were more common in the days of yore than they are now. Between this secretive attitude and the need to make the martial arts more civilian-friendly into the twentieth century, the 'softer' martial arts

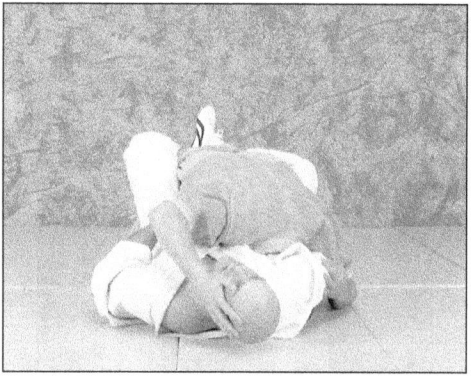
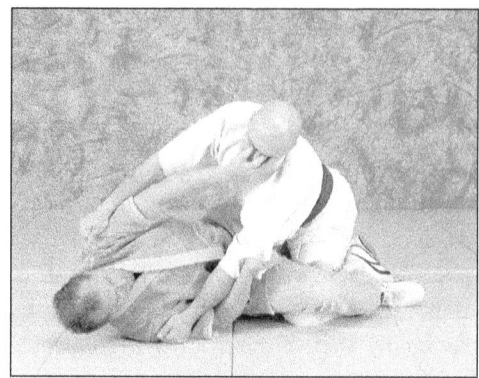

Figure 3-5   Figure 3-6

were created. The old bone-breaking 'Hell dojo' of the past have been greatly toned down. The deadlier and more risky techniques have been removed for the sake of propagation in the schools and our peaceful society in general. Today, the sports aspect of the martial arts is allowed to flourish because of these kinds of transformations. One must often look deeply into *kata bunkai* to understand the true meaning of the simplified techniques that had been made safer.

Value of Pressure Points

The more you have in your bag of tricks, the more likely you will be able to bail yourself out of a tight situation. Minimally, these pressure point attacks can be used to weaken your opponent's body, weaken his resolve to keep on fighting, or from applying a hold in a committed fashion. A crushing hold such as a headlock may be defeated with a single well-placed finger to your opponent's eye (Figure 3-5). Your opponent must free one of his own gripping hands in order to deal with the threat to his eye, thereby forcing him to partially relinquish his hold, otherwise he would suffer a debilitating injury. Often the eyes are vulnerable to attack even from relatively weak positions. Such attacks can be great equalizers (Figure 3-6). Distractions that force your opponent to change his body position or grip can be used to create openings for your own attacks.

A variety of body tools can be used to access these pressure points found all over the body. Do not limit yourself to just using your finger tips to this end (see Chapter Four). These pressure points can be struck, pressed, or gouged. This is makes using pressure points easy to access and difficult to defend against. Knowing that some points can be attacked to knock out (vascular neck restraint, Figure 3-7), stun (temple strike, Figure 3- 8), distract (hypoglossal gouge, Figure 3- 9) or merely annoy (sternal rub, Figure 3-10) your opponent could prove useful in your fighting strategy. Pain compliance techniques have limited utility when dealing with people high on drugs, mental incompetents, or who are extremely agitated or goal oriented persons. This makes techniques utilizing some pressure points, like those involved with vascular neck restraints, all the more valuable because submission is

Chapter 3: Pressure Points of the Fourteen Meridians

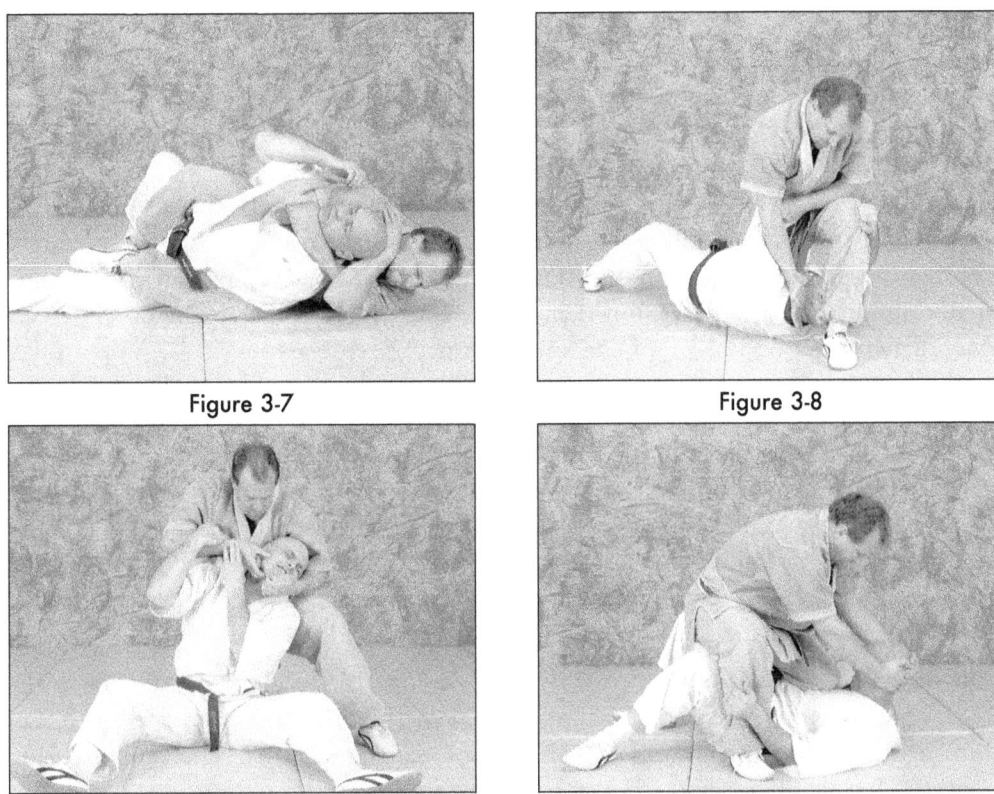

Figure 3-7

Figure 3-8

Figure 3-9

Figure 3-10

not dependent upon the feeling of pain, rather it is garnered from the rendering of your opponent unconscious.

3-2. MERIDIAN THEORY

Meridians and Acupuncture

In order to better understand pressure points, we will briefly outline the concept of the meridian theory, which is an important component of Traditional Chinese Medicine. Proponents of T.C.M. believe that the body is nourished and energized by an intangible life force or essence called *qi* (*chi* or *ki*) that is distributed throughout the body by a network of pathways or meridians. An essential function of the meridian systems is to transport blood and the *qi* to all cells within the body. Fourteen main meridians in all, these meridians are joined together in an endless pattern of circulation. A total of 361 superficial acupuncture points have been identified on these meridians to date. These superficial points, where blood and *qi* can be stimulated to affect the corresponding internal and external organs, are widely spread across the body. When disease affects the meridians and their collaterals (sub-branches), the flow of *qi* and blood is disturbed. These points are tender and reactive spots, hence the value of some for use in the martial arts. This organic relationship between acupuncture points and disease is the basis for the delayed death touch. Upset the flow of *qi* and disease occurs. A total cessation of *qi* means death.

Acupuncture, massage and *qigong* have utilized these meridians and their constituent points for thousands of years. It is hypothesized that as early the Stone Age, ancient man recognized that where there is pain, there is a point that can be used for healing local body tissues and even internal organs by pressing and puncturing these points. As each meridian has an organ pertaining to it, diseases can be cured through acupuncture (needling) to the various points. For example, angina pectoris may cause pain in the heart, but it may also extend down the course of the Heart Meridian (posterior border of the medial aspect of the upper arm). With much trial and error, it was learned that needling points along this part of the arm would affect the diseased condition of the heart. These points were mapped on the human body and they have been verified in modern times by differences in electrical skin resistance. It is not definitively known whether these meridians are related to the peripheral nerves and blood vessels, the central nervous system or are part of a yet undiscovered and unique organic structure. What is known is that acupuncture does work. China radically demonstrated this to the world by acupuncture anesthesia research released in the 1970s.

Yin and Yang Meridians

There are twelve pairs (bilateral) of regular meridians: three hand and three foot Yin meridians and three hand and three foot Yang meridians. The nomenclature suggests that the hands and feet were thought to be very important in the distribution of *qi* throughout the body. So was the concept of Yin and Yang, the polar generalizations of everything in the universe, being neither absolute nor independent. Yin and Yang are used to describe the relative functions of the parts within the body system. As the parts are interrelated, they are inseparable and mutually dependent. As such, the meridians are paired up, Yin and Yang, as shown in (Figure 3-11).

The hand and foot meridian triplets are ranked in descending orders of Yin (–) and Yang (+) *qi* and blood within them. The *zang* (Yin) organs stores *qi* but have no function of excretion; *fu* (Yang) organs transforms food into *qi* but have no storage capabilities, hence their polar and ranked pairings. Examination of the various meridian pathways will lead one to the following observations:

- Three of the **Yin** meridians of the hand run from the hand to the **chest**
- Three of the **Yang** meridians of the hand run from the hand to the **head**
- Three of the **Yin** meridians of the foot run from foot to the **abdomen**
- Three of the **Yang** meridians of the foot run from the head down to the **foot**

The meridians flow continuously to one another as follows:

Rank (i) Lung Meridian—Large Intestine Meridian—Stomach—Spleen Meridian—.

Rank (ii) Heart Meridian— Small Intestine Meridian—Urinary Bladder Meridian—Kidney Meridian—.

Rank (iii) Pericardium Meridian—Triple Burner Meridian—Gall Bladder Meridian—Liver Meridian—Lung Meridian (as shown in Figure 3-11).

The ranked meridians are distributed on the four limbs in a medial-lateral aspect symmetry as follows:

Rank (i) meridians are located on the anterior border of both the medial and lateral aspects of the four limbs.

Rank (ii) meridians are located on the midline of both the medial and lateral aspects of the four limbs.

Rank (iii) meridians are located on posterior border of both the medial and lateral aspects of the four limbs.

And so it can be seen that the Yang meridians all run either into or out from the head. The yin meridians of the hand (upper part) and foot (lower part) correspond to the chest (upper part) and abdomen (lower part), respectively. The Ren and Du Meridians for the most part, run vertically around the medial (sagittal) plane of the torso (and therefore do not have bilateral points like the twelve regular meridians) but of course have similar Yin and Yang aspects of the body, from being front and back meridians respectively. The meridian system is further composed of various collaterals (sub-branches) and other meridians. There are eight 'extra' meridians that store excess *qi* and blood when the twelve regular meridians are full. Of these, we will only deal with the Du and Ren Meridians.

3-3. PRESSURE POINTS

Martial Arts Pressure Points

Here are some of the more common pressure points for your consideration. These 52 points (see Figures 3-1, 3-2, and 3-3) have been chosen for their effectiveness, distribution on the body and popularity with martial arts scholars (Dillman, Mashiro, McCarthy, Siddle, Tedeschi). This latter issue is summarized in Table 3-1, but the readers may decide for themselves which points offer the best strategic and effective value in fighting.*

---

*The nomenclature of the points is that of the standard numbering system used in China. Variations of this system have been noted. The translations of the acupuncture point names have been subjectively interpreted by Dr. Li Ding and subsequently related by the authors. They have been rigidly and literally interpreted or they been given a loosely figurative interpretation by Dr. Ding, not all of which are clear. In any case, this text is highly recommended to those seeking to know more about acupuncture points. Note also Tedeschi's clear and informative work *Essential Anatomy* (2002) regarding the location of these points.

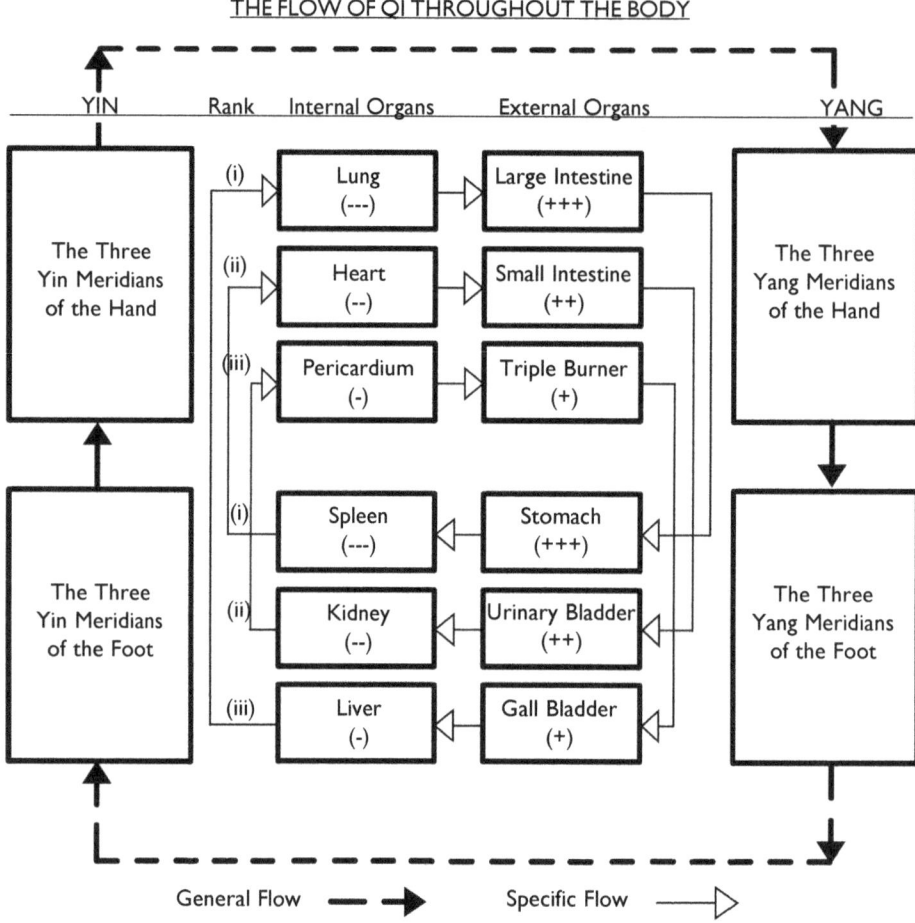

Figure 3-11 The regular meridians allows the bilateral flow of qi throughout the body in a 24 hour diurnal cycle starting in the Lung Meridian (Lu) and ending in the Liver Meridian (Liv).

Pressure Points and Control Tactics

The Pressure Point and Control Tactics pressure points outlined in this book were researched and developed by Bruce Siddle (P.P.C.T. Management Systems, Inc.). The pressure points highlighted (See Table 3-2) should be studied closely. The acupuncture points used to approximate these points, however, are of the author's own estimation and not those necessarily recognized by the P.P.C.T. system.

This extraordinary defensive tactics system is a leading source of self-defense training in the criminal justice system. The author was privileged to have been certified in this defensive tactics system in 1996. Having said that, the course must really be taken in order to understand the purpose and rationale behind the point selection

Chapter 3: Pressure Points of the Fourteen Meridians

Number (in this book)	Pressure Point	Dillman	Mashiro	McCarthy	Siddle	Tedeschi
1.	DU 1			•		•
2.	DU 16		•	•		•
3.	DU 20					•
4.	DU 26			•	•	•
5.	REN 6					•
6.	REN 14		•			
7.	REN 17	•				
8.	REN 20		•			
9.	REN 22		•	•	•	•
10.	REN 23		•			•
11.	REN 24			•		
12.	Lu. 2				•	
13.	Lu. 5	•	•			•
14.	Lu. 6	•				
15.	Lu. 8	•	•	•		
16.	Lu.10	•				
17.	H. 3					•
18.	P. 6	•	•			•
19.	L.I. 4	•	•	•		•
20.	L.I. 10	•	•	•	•	
21.	L.I. 11	•				•
22.	S.I. 16	•	•	•	•	
23.	S.I. 17					•
24.	S.I. 18	•				
25.	S.J. 3	•	•			•
26.	S.J. 11	•				
27.	S.J. 17	•	•	•		•
28.	S.J. 23	•	•			•
29.	St. 1		•	•		
30.	St. 5	•	•		•	•
31.	St. 6					
32.	St. 7	•				•
33.	St. 9	•	•	•		•
34.	St. 12			•	•	•
35.	St. 18		•			
36.	St. 43		•			
37.	U.B. 40		•	•		•
38.	U.B. 56		•		•	
39.	U.B. 57					•
40.	U.B. 62			•		
41.	G.B. 6		•	•		
42.	G.B. 24	•		•		•
43.	G.B. 31			•	•	•
44.	G.B. 34					
45.	Sp. 11	•			•	•
46.	Sp. 12	•	•			•
47.	Sp. 21	•				•
48.	K. 3		•			
49.	Liv. 13	•	•	•		•
50.	EX-HN 2		•			•
51.	EX-HN 19		•		•	
52.	EX-UE 11			•		
Total	52	23	27	19	13	31

Table 3-1 Selected Pressure Points of Interest to Martial Artists

Number (in this book)	Pressure Point	Pressure Point Name	PPCT Point
1.	DU 1	Changqiang (Long Strong)	
2.	DU 16	Fengfu (Wind Mansion)	
3.	DU 20	Baihui (Hundred Meeting)	
4.	DU 26	Renzhong (Person in Middle)	'infraorbital nerve pressure point'
5.	REN 6	Qihai (Energy Sea)	
6.	REN 14	Juque (Big Gateway)	
7.	REN 17	Tanzhong (Heart Palace)	
8.	REN 20	Huagai (Canopy)	
9.	REN 22	Tiantu (High Prominence)	'jugular notch pressure point'
10.	REN 23	Lianquan (Prism Spring)	
11.	REN 24	Chengjiang (Receiving Saliva)	
12.	Lu. 2	Yunmen (Door of Cloud)	'brachial plexus tie-in motor point'
13.	Lu. 5	Chize (One-foot Marsh)	
14.	Lu. 6	Kongzui (Supreme Passage)	
15.	Lu. 8	Jingqu (Passage of the Meridian Qi)	
16.	Lu.10	Yuji (Fish Border)	
17.	H. 3	Shaohai (Young Sea)	
18.	P. 6	Neiguan (Inner Pass)	
19.	L.I. 4	Hegu (Converging Valley)	
20.	L.I. 10	Shousanli (Three Li from Zhouliao)	'radial nerve motor point'
21.	L.I. 11	Quchi (Curved Pond)	
22.	S.I. 16	Tianchuang (Celestial Window)	'suprascapular motor nerve point'
23.	S.I. 17	Tianrong (Celestial Appearance)	
24.	S.I. 18	Quanliao (Zygomatic Crevice)	
25.	S.J. 3	Hand-Zhongzhu (Mid Islet)	
26.	S.J. 11	Qinglengyuan (Cooling Gulf)	
27.	S.J. 17	Yifeng (Ear-shielding Wind)	'mandibular angle pressure point'
28.	S.J. 23	Sizhukong (Bambooleaf Depression)	
29.	St. 1	Chengqi (Hold Tears)	
30.	St. 5	Daying (Great Meeting)	'hypoglossal nerve pressure point'
31.	St. 6	Jiache (Jaw Vehicle)	
32.	St. 7	Xiaguan (Lower Hinge)	
33.	St. 9	Renying (Man Pulse)	
34.	St. 12	Quepan (Broken Basin)	'brachial plexus clavicle notch p.p.'
35.	St. 18	Rugen (Breast Root)	
36.	St. 43	Xiangu (Sinking Valley)	
37.	U.B. 40	Weizhong (Popliteal Center)	
38.	U.B. 56	Chengjin (Supporting Tendon)	'tibial nerve motor point'
39.	U.B. 57	Chengshan (Supporting Hill)	
40.	U.B. 62	Shenmai (Relaxing Meridians)	
41.	G.B. 6	Xuanli (Correct Suspension)	
42.	G.B. 24	Riyue (Sun and Moon)	
43.	G.B. 31	Fengshi (Wind Market)	'lateral femoral nerve motor point'
44.	G.B. 34	Yanglingquan (Outer Mound Spring)	
45.	Sp. 11	Jimen (Basket Gate)	'femoral nerve motor point'
46.	Sp. 12	Chongmen (Pulsating Door)	
47.	Sp. 21	Dabao (General Control)	
48.	K. 3	Taixi (Big Stream)	
49.	Liv. 13	Zhangmen (Bight Door)	
50.	EX-HN 2	Yingtan (Decorating Hall)	
51.	EX-HN 19	Jingbi (Upper Arm)	'brachial plexus origin pressure point'
52.	EX-UE 11	Bizhong (Arm Center)	'meridian nerve motor center'

Table 3-2 Pressure Point Control Tactics

as well as the modes of applications of the techniques used to attack them. The tactical, medical and legal research that was put into this system is unparalleled in police training systems. All criminal justice workers who physically deal with criminals should undertake this training.

Dumai Meridian (Governor Vessel Meridian: G.V.)

Du means governor or controller, referring to the regulation of blood and *qi*, and *mai* means passages or meridians (Figure 3-12). It is called the governing vessel because it regulates or communicates with the *Yang Qi* (six Regular yang meridians) of the whole body through DU 4, DU 14, DU 15 and DU 16. DU 14 (Dazhui) for example, sees the convergence of the three meridians each of the hand and foot at the Du Meridian, like rivers flowing into the sea, hence this governing meridian is also called "the sea of Yang meridians". Also, this meridian has its distribution in the brain, the organ governing mentality, giving further reasoning for its name.

There are 28 single points on this meridian distributed along the head, face, neck, back and lower spine which are used to treat a wide variety of disorders ranging from fever, psychosis, epilepsy, impotence, to diarrhea.

Point 1: DU 1 Changqiang (Long Strong)

Chang means long, as in the case of the Du Meridian, which ascends along the spine over top of the head to the face. *Qiang* means strong, referring to the strong therapeutic effect that needling this point has. The entire spinal column atop this point is long and strong enough to bear the weight of the body, hence the name Long Strong.

It is located between the coccyx and the anus. The pudendal nerves are found here (inferior rectal, perineal, posterior scrotal, and dorsal nerves of the penis). A knee strike, kick with the top of the foot, or even an upward knife-edge strike can cause incontinence, painful urination, or unconsciousness.

Point 2: DU 16 Fengfu (Wind Mansion)

Feng refers to a pathogenic wind and *fu* means a mansion. This acupuncture point is used to treat any disorders caused by wind, hence the name Wind Mansion.

This cavity is located in the posterior hairline, in the depression between the trapezius muscles where the occipital bone meets the first cervical vertebrae at the base of the skull (Figure 3-13). The occipital nerves and a branch of the occipital artery can be affected here. A light blow from a fist or sword hand to this area could cause vertebral subluxation. A moderate blow can cause unconsciousness. A heavy blow can cause death due nerve damage and shock to the cerebellum. Cervical damage and disruption of the deeply underlying medulla oblongata can result in very serious injuries indeed.

Point 3: DU 20 Baihui (Hundred Meetings)

Bai means many in number and *hui* means to converge as in reference to the fact that all Yang meridians intersect at the body's vertex center (top of the head).

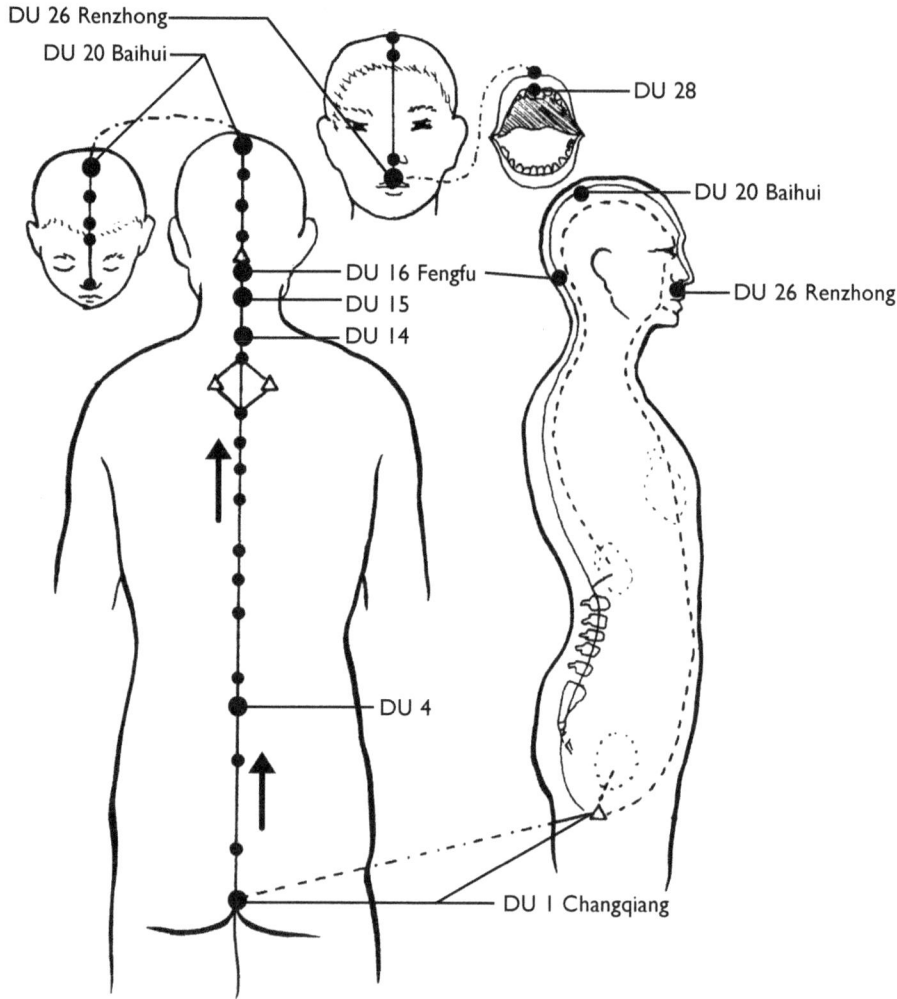

The Dumai (Governing) Meridian (DU)
Figure 3-12 The six regular Yang channels (of the hardened foot) converge at DU14. This "sea of yang meridians" is said to govern the brain, spine, and urogenital organs.

This cavity is located at the mid-point between the top of the nose and base of the skull, intersecting the line drawn between the ears, where a person's height is measured from (see Figure 3-13). Even when a light downward blow is struck at this weak point of the calvaria with the palm or hammer fist, dizziness or unconsciousness from the generation of a concussion may result. Cutting the scalp can lead to typically profuse, but non-life-threatening, bleeding from the superficial temporal and occipital arteries and veins that anastomose (cross-connect) freely across the scalp. A heavy blow can cause cranial swelling from internal bleeding from the mid-

Chapter 3: Pressure Points of the Fourteen Meridians

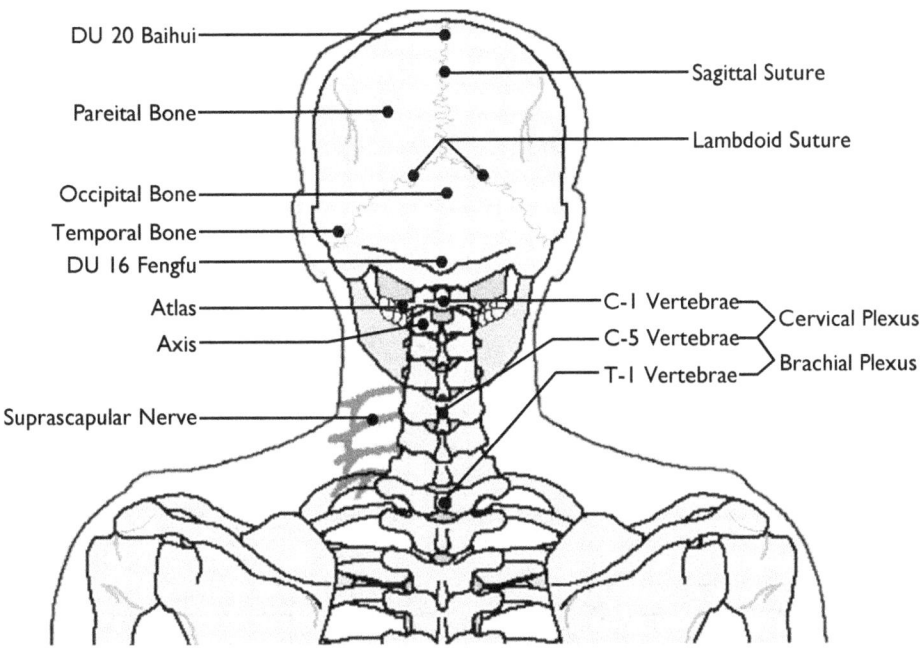

Bones of the Posterior Head and Neck
Figure 3-13 Note the location of DU16 at the juncture of the occipital bone and first cervical vertebrae (C-1). Note also the brachial plexus (C-5 to T-1).

dle meningeal artery and vein. As this is the coalescent point of the Du Meridian and the foot and hand Yang meridians, it is a major *qi* point. This area has the terminal points of the supraorbital nerves descending the front of the scalp as well as a branch of the great occipital nerve.

Point 4: DU 26 Renzhong (Person in Middle)

Ren means person and *zhong* means middle (between the nose and the mouth). As this point is located in between the intakes for the celestial and terrestrial *qi* respectively, its position is reminiscent of a standing person. A better name for this point is *shuigo* (ditch) as it lies in the nasalabial groove that resembles a trough or ditch.

This point is actually located on the medial plane (directly below the centerline of the nose) at the lower portion of the upper middle third of the philtrum (just below the gum line as shown in Figure 3-14). The loose protective skin of the philtrum can be stretched downward by using a pressing and rolling action with the knuckles or other attacking portions of the hand. This will reduce the thickness of this upper lip area (orbicularis oris muscle) and thereby allow maximal pressure penetration to this point (45 degrees upward towards the top of the head) on the infraorbital nerves lying on top of the maxilla bone of the skull. This is a popular police pressure point (infraorbital nerve pressure point) used for dealing with low levels of resistance. Easily

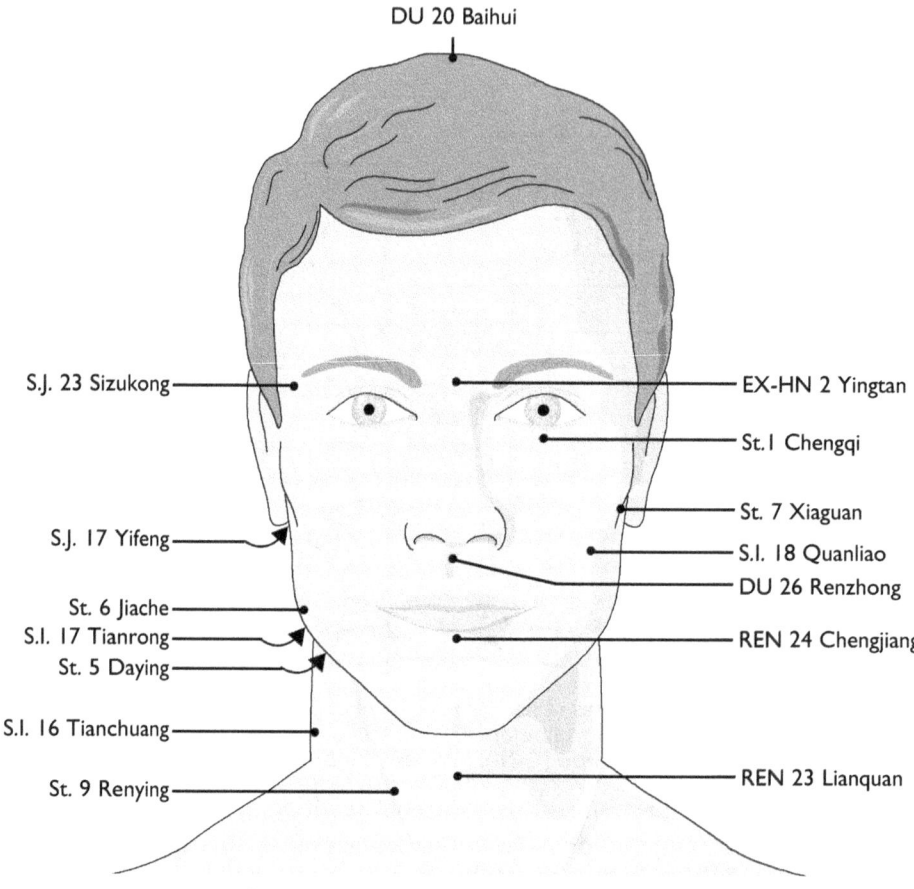

Selected Pressure Points of the Anterior Head
Figure 3-14 The face has some very accessible and easily located pressure points.

accessible and locatable as well as very reliable, pressure attacks to this point causes a painful watering of the eyes and even a mucous discharge from the nose due to the route that this nerve takes superficially in the face. It is painful enough to cause low level stunning, making it a good place to apply pressure as a means of creating distance or as a tool of distraction. It is therefore a useful pain compliance technique in order to get a person to relinquish their grip. Its proximity to the mouth (teeth) and position on a mobile base (head) make it a somewhat risky point to attack unless the head is immobilized. Heavier blows can cause fracturing of the maxilla, into which the upper teeth are affixed, at the intermaxillary suture (lying on the medial plane of the skull). As this bone is firmly fixed to the brain case, a concussion and concomitant knockout is likely to result if such an application of force is used.

Ren Meridian (Conception Vessel: C.V.)

Ren means responsibility or conception, as in becoming pregnant, and *mai* means meridian (Figure 3-15). This meridian links all of the hand and foot Yin meridians

Chapter 3: Pressure Points of the Fourteen Meridians

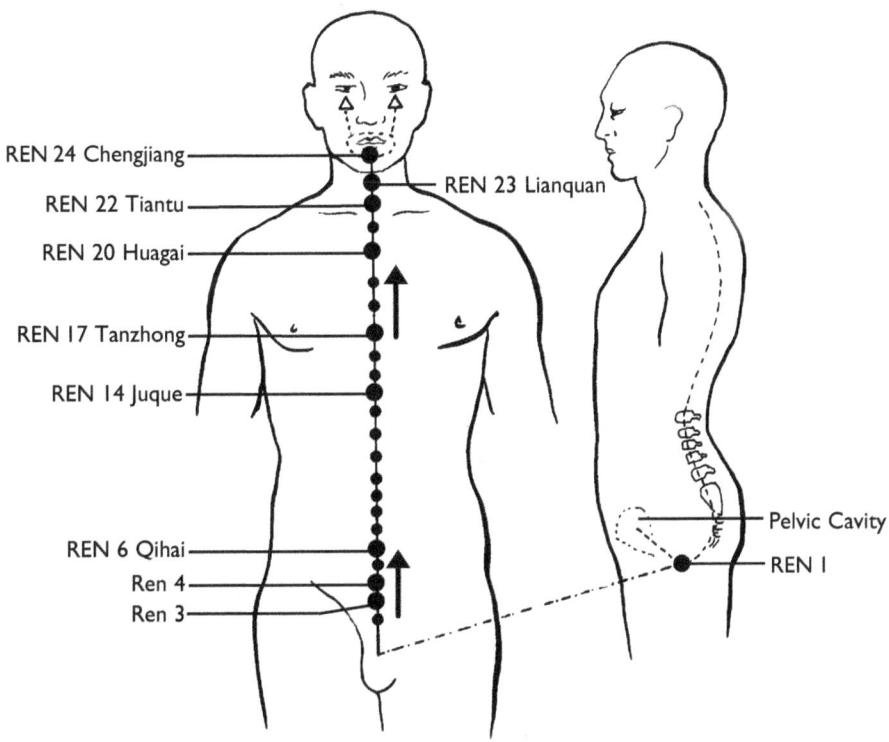

The Ren (Conception) Meridian (REN)
Figure 3-15 The six regular Yin channels (of the head and foot) are known collectively as the "sea of Yin meridians." It controls the reproductive and endocrinal systems.

of the body and is known as "the sea of Yin meridians". For example, the three Yin meridians of the foot converge at REN 3 (Zhongji) and REN 4 (Guanyuan). This meridian originates in the uterus and dominates this organ of conception, hence the name Conception Vessel Meridian.

There are 24 single points located in the facial region, neck, anterior midline of the chest and abdomen that are used to treat diseases of the endocrinal and reproductive systems as well as other disorders in the areas supplied by this meridian.

Point 5: REN 6 Qihai (Energy Sea)

Qi refers to vital energy and *hai* refers to a convergent place- the sea. This area is an abundant area for *qi*, hence the name Energy Sea.

It is located within the lower abdomen on the anterior midline of the body about one to one and a half inches below the umbilicus, the site of the lower of three *qi* reservoirs (*shiah dantien*). It is more commonly known as the *dantien* (field of elixir) or the *tanden*, in Japanese literature. This point is at the level of the L3 vertebrae. A penetrating blow directed straight inward could injure the small intestine and induce

113

unconsciousness due to the presence of the thoracoabdominal nerves. A kick or punch directed downward into this point can damage bladder, lower large intestine and reproductive system. Death may even ensue in some cases. Normally this area is well-muscled and therefore resistant to attack. According to acupuncture theory this area is the main reservoir for *qi* ('sea of *qi*'). Many types of martial arts consider this area to be the seat of power and it is close to the body's center of gravity.

Point 6: REN 14 Juque (Big Gateway)

Ju means big and *que* means gateway, implying *qi* may flow to the heart from this point.

It is located within the lower abdomen on the anterior midline of the body approximately one inch below the tip of the zyphoid process. It is also known as the Jong Dantien (Middle Dantien), the second of three major *qi* reservoirs (see EX-HN 2 and REN 6, the Upper and Lower Dantien respectively). A punch or kick directly into this point, unprotected by bone or muscle, will result in nausea and unconsciousness. This is a common martial arts target (solar or celiac plexus), because of the susceptibility of the diaphragm to being shocked via the affected phrenic nerves. Even light blows can cause the diaphragm to paralyze. This results in an inability to breathe easily, an uncomfortable albeit temporary condition. Heavier blows can affect the upper stomach and the lower portion of the liver (the liver is more exposed on full inspiration).

Point 7: REN 17 Tanzhong (Heart Palace)

Tan refers to the outer protective tissues of the heart and *zhong* means inside the plurae (enclosing membranes), hence the name Heart Palace. (Li Ding (p. 377) gives Shangzhong as the alternative spelling).

This point is located on the sternum, between the two nipples, at the level of the 4th intercostal space. A strike directly into this point will affect the medial anterior branch of the fourth intercostal nerve. An exceptionally heavy blow to this sternal shield might affect the underlying heart, lungs and thoracic nerves inducing unconsciousness and death if the circulatory and respiratory functions have been disrupted. Even pressing or rubbing pressure to this area is relatively painful.

Point 8: REN 20 Huagai (Canopy)

Huagai was the ancient umbrella protecting the emperor's carriage. The lung shields the other organs below it, including the imperial heart, hence its name Canopy.

It is located on the anterior midline of the chest at the level of the first intercostal space (between the first and second ribs. This point is slightly above the sternal angle, the juncture of the manubrium and the sternal body (two inches below the jugular notch). A heavy blow could break this weak point of the sternum and injure the underlying heart, lungs and thoracic nerves, shocking both the respiratory and circulatory systems. If a punch or kick is delivered straight into this point, high temperatures, coughing and unconsciousness and even death may occur.

Point 9: REN 22 Tiantu (High Prominence)

Tian means a high place as in the position on the body; *tu* means a prominence, referring to the Adam's apple, hence the name High Place.

It is found in the depression at the upper border of the suprasternal notch (manubrium sterni). An inward and downward press by one or two fingers into this jugular notch will affect the laryngeal nerves, carotid, and subclavian arteries. Even light finger pressure will cause discomfort and coughing because of the presence of the underlying trachea (windpipe), making it a favorite police pressure point (jugular notch pressure point) attack to push someone back away from you. Pushing straight inward or upward interferes with the trachea that could cause swelling and subsequent suffocation.*

Point 10: REN 23 Lianquan (Prism Spring)

Lian refers to the prism shape of the tongue and *quan* means spring as in the case of saliva emanating from the mouth, hence the name Prism Spring.

This point is located in the depression just above the Adam's apple, in the crease of the neck, in the recess of the upper edge of the hyoid bone (Figure 3-16). A downward application of force can injure the relatively brittle (to the cricoid cartilage of the trachea) thyroid cartilage (larynx). Inward pressure can fracture the hyoid bone, the floating base of attachment for the tongue (level with the third cervical vertebra). Any such breakage can result in a very painful (due to the presence of the internal branch of the superior laryngeal nerve), if not deadly injury due to suffocation resulting from swelling of the soft tissue surrounding these delicate throat structures. Speaking and swallowing would also be inhibited, along with an inability to breathe. Sealing the breath can easily terminate a fight (or a person's life). An opponent would, however, struggle violently from the intense pain and extreme panic of suffocation until the oxygen in his lungs is consumed and he passes out of consciousness.

Point 11: REN 24 Chengjiang (Receiving Saliva)

Cheng means to receive and *jiang* means river, referring here to saliva. Since saliva will flow onto the chin if it flows out of the mouth, this point is called Receiving Saliva.

This point is located in the center of the depression under the lower lip (labiomental groove) as shown in (Figure 3-14). Pressure to this point is somewhat painful due the presence of the inferior labial branches of the mental nerves that innervate the lower lip. Heavy pressure or a forceful blow can dislocate the jaw and/or fracture the mandible, although this bone is resistant to fracture.

---

*The trachea is a cartilaginous and membranous airway that consists of 16-20 imperfect cricoid rings. Contrary to popular belief, this structure is highly elastic, becoming calcified and therefore brittle only in advanced stages of life. Also, this 4.5 inch long pipe is only 3/4 of an inch in outside diameter, making it smaller in diameter then your baby finger. At the upper extreme of the trachea is the larynx voice box). This cartilaginous structure begins to calcify from age 25 years and is a larger and more brittle structure than the trachea. See the author's autopsy photo (Figure 7-4).

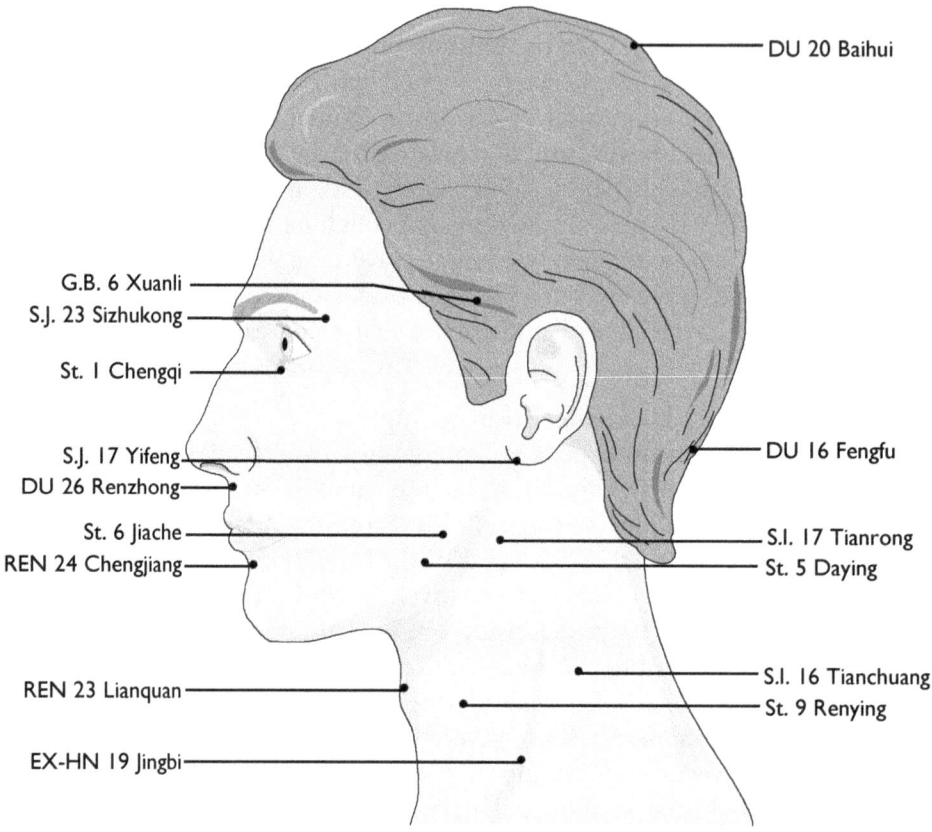

Selected Pressure Points of the Lateral Head and Neck
Figure 3-16 Many of these pressure points can be attacked fairly easily in a ground fighting situation.

Lung Meridian

There are 11 bilateral points on this Yin meridian starting from the stomach and ending at the medial side of the tip of the thumb. Nine of these points are found on the medial side of the arm. These points are used to treat disorders of the respiratory system, hence the name Lung Meridian (Figure 3-17). The host organ (lung) is paired internally with the large intestine.

Point 12: Lu. 2 Yunmen (Door of Cloud)

Yun means cloud and *men* means gate or door. If *qi* and blood are likened to a lofty cloud as it nourishes everything below, then this highest point of the Lung Meridian gives its name Door of Cloud.

This point is in the recess (when the arms are held akimbo) below the lateral end of the clavicle (Figure 3-17). A heavy downward blow can break the collarbone and affect functioning of the arm and hand. The axillary vein and axillary artery run beneath the collar bone at this point at a 45-degree angle from the neck to the armpit, so they can be torn by the breakage of the collar bone to cause internal bleeding. The

Chapter 3: Pressure Points of the Fourteen Meridians

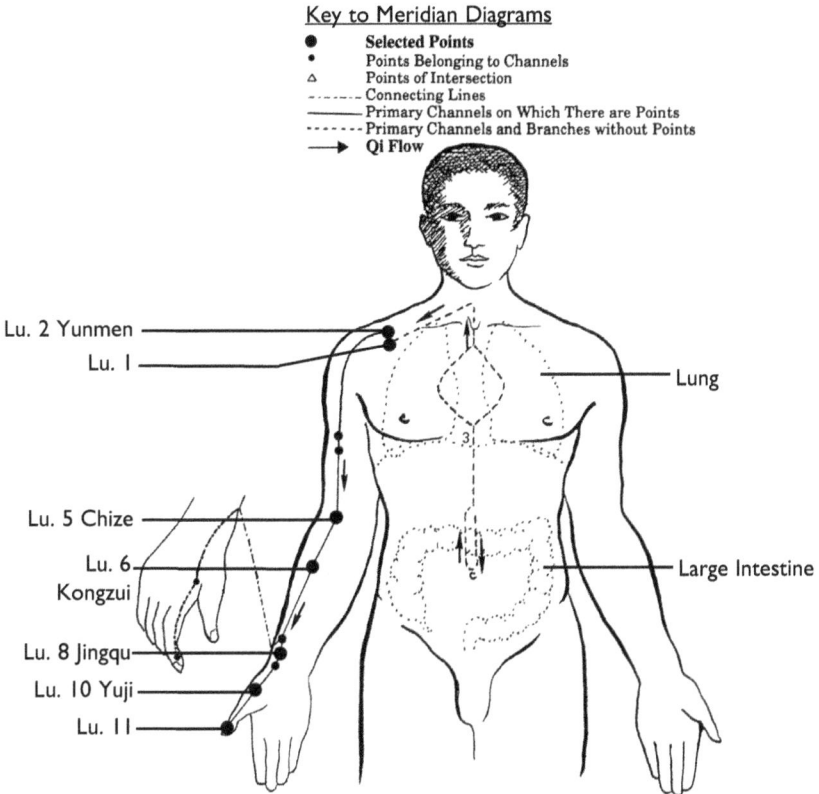

The Lung Meridian (Lu.)
Figure 3-17 There are eleven bilateral points on this Yin meridian. The host organ (lung) is paired internally with the large intestine.

brachial plexus also runs superior to these vessels down the arm, innervating the arm and hand. Gouging downward and inward from this point can access this plexus. The deltoid, pectoralis major muscles and at a deeper level (and slightly laterally), the biceps and pectoralis minor muscles, attach to the clavicle and coracoid process of the scapula respectively. Even a punch directed straight into this spot could cause numbness and even severely impair the use of the arm and hand. This makes it a popular police motor nerve point target (brachial plexus tie-in motor point).

Point 13: Lu. 5 Chize (One-foot Marsh)

Chi refers to the forearm section of an ancient Chinese system of measurement that used the distance from the wrist to the elbow crease (one chi). *Ze* means marsh or pond referring to the fact that this point is a *He-sea point* of the meridian, where *qi* pools like waters merging into the sea, hence the name One-foot Marsh.

This point is located at the midpoint of the transverse cubital crease of the arm, on the radial side of the biceps brachii tendon, at the origin of the brachioradialis muscle (Figure 3-18). Digital penetration here can affect the lateral cutaneous nerve

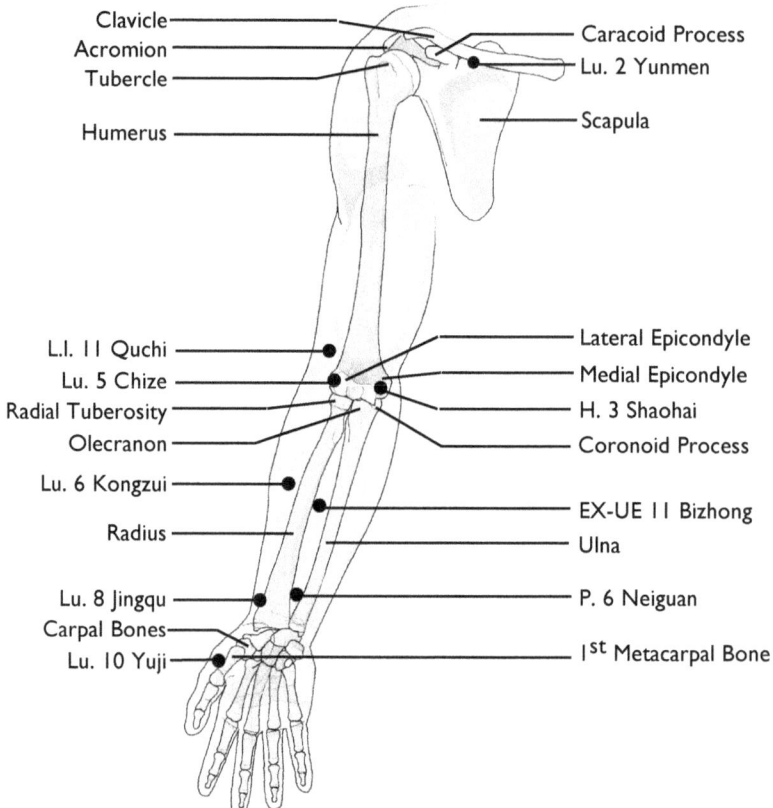

Selected Pressure Points of the Anterior Arm (and Underlying Bones)
Figure 3-18 Notice that the pressure points are found close to the bones.

and more deeply, the radial nerve. A well-focused penetrative strike to this point can affect the functioning of the radial part of the forearm and the thumb and first two fingers of the hand.

Point 14: Lu. 6 Kongzui (Supreme Passage)

Kong means a passage and *zui* means most superior or supreme. Used in ancient times as the best point to treat febrile (fever) disease, this Supreme Passage point could also help the lung disperse *qi* and control the opening and closing of the pores.

This point is located on the radial side of the arm slightly above the midpoint between the wrist and the elbow (Figure 3-18). Digital or percussive blows to this point can affect the lateral branch of the cutaneous nerve and the superficial branch of the radial nerve. This will affect the functioning of the radial part of the forearm and the thumb and first two fingers of the hand.

Point 15: Lu. 8 Jingqu (Passage of Meridian Qi)

Jing-river points are one of the five *shu* points where the *qi* of the Lung Meridian increases in abundance, hence the name Passage of the Meridian Qi.

It is located on the medial aspect of the top of the styloid process of the radius, about an inch above the transverse crease of the wrist (Figure 3-18). It is in this recess on the radial side of the radial artery where the pulse is taken. As with Lu. 6, the lateral branch of the cutaneous nerve and the superficial branch of the radial nerve can be affected by digital or percussive blows to this point. This will affect the functioning the thumb and first two fingers of the hand (See Figure 2-42).

Point 16: Lu. 10 Yuji (Fish Border)

Yu means fish and *ji* means border or margin. This point is located at the juncture of the red palmar skin and white skin from the back of the hand in the ball of muscle of the thumb (thenar eminence). As this is much like the meeting of the red and white skin of a fish belly, this point is called Fish Border.

This point is located on the middle of the first metacarpal bone on the thenar eminence (Figure 3-18). Gouging or one-knuckle striking straight into this point affects the superficial branch of the radial nerve and is useful in loosening a person's grip.

(Figure 3-18) shows the pressure points in the arms which are also found close to the bones.

Heart Meridian

There are 9 bilateral points on this Yin meridian, beginning in the heart with a string of eight medially oriented posterior arm points terminating at the inside tip of the little finger. Cardiovascular problems (and some mental disorders) are treated with these points, hence the name Heart Meridian (Figure 3-19).

Point 17: H. 3 Shaohai (Young Sea)

Shao refers to the Heart Meridian of the Hand-*Shaoyin* (lesser or young yin meridian) and *hai* means sea. This is the *He-sea* point of the Heart Meridian. As the heart dominates the flow of *qi* through blood circulation, *qi* is most abundant here, like waters converging into the sea, hence the name Young Sea.

This point is located at the medial end of the transverse cubital crease of the flexed elbow, in the anterior recess of the medial epicondyle of the humerus (Figure 3-19). Gouging into this point presses the medial antebrachial cutaneous nerve against this bone to affect the functioning of the ulnar portion of the forearm.

Pericardium Meridian

There are nine points on this Yin meridian, originating from the chest (the pertaining organ, the pericardium), hence the name Pericardium Meridian (Figure 3-20). All but one point of the meridian are found along the central line of the palmar aspect of the arms. It terminates at the center tip of the middle finger nail. These points are used to treat disorders of the cardiovascular system, nausea, etc.

Point 18: P. 6 Neiguan (Inner Pass)

Nei means interior and *guan* refers to the passage where *qi* enters and exits, hence the name Inner Pass.

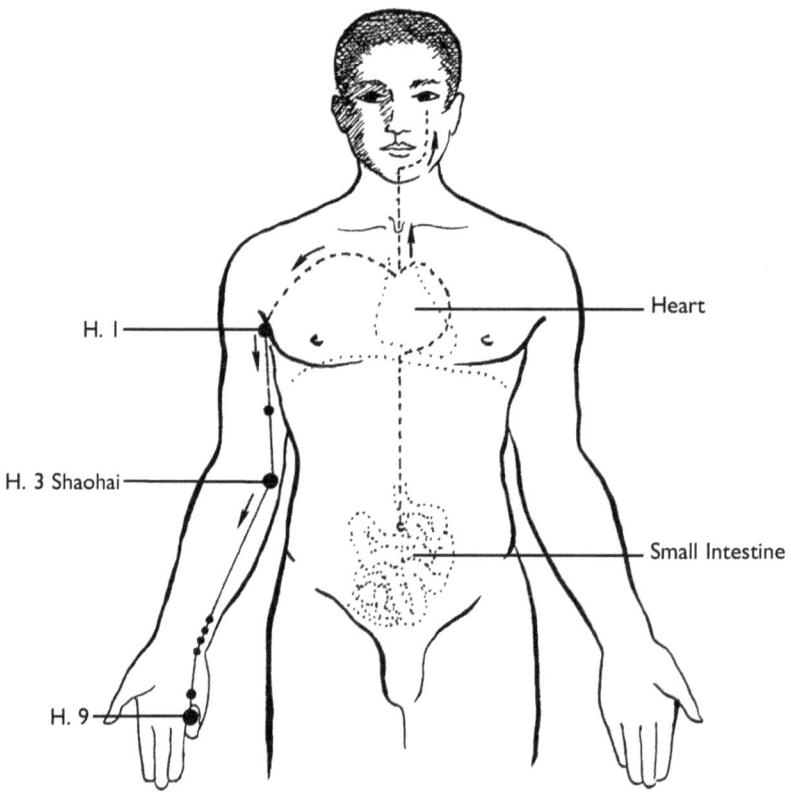

The Heart Meridian (H.)
Figure 3-19 There are nine bilateral points on this Yin meridian. The host organ (heart) is paired internally to the small intestine.

This point is located about two inches above the midpoint of the transverse crease of the wrist, in the soft spot between the tendons of the palmaris longus and the flexor carpi radialis muscles (Figure 3-18). This point can be digitally accessed by pressing inward towards the wrist to affect the anterior branch of the medial cutaneous nerve and the palmar cutaneous branch of the medial nerve, which will impair the use of thumb and first two fingers. Such digital penetration can cause nausea as well as intense pain to this area and is helpful in grip releases.

Large Intestine Meridian

There are 20 bilateral points on this Yang meridian, 15 of which are located along the inside of the arms, starting with the tip of the index finger, with five more points located on the face and neck. Though these points are used to treat disorders of the face and throat, the five sense organs and the lateral aspects of the arms, this meridian enters into the large intestine, its pertaining organ, hence the name Large Intestine Meridian (Figure 3-21).

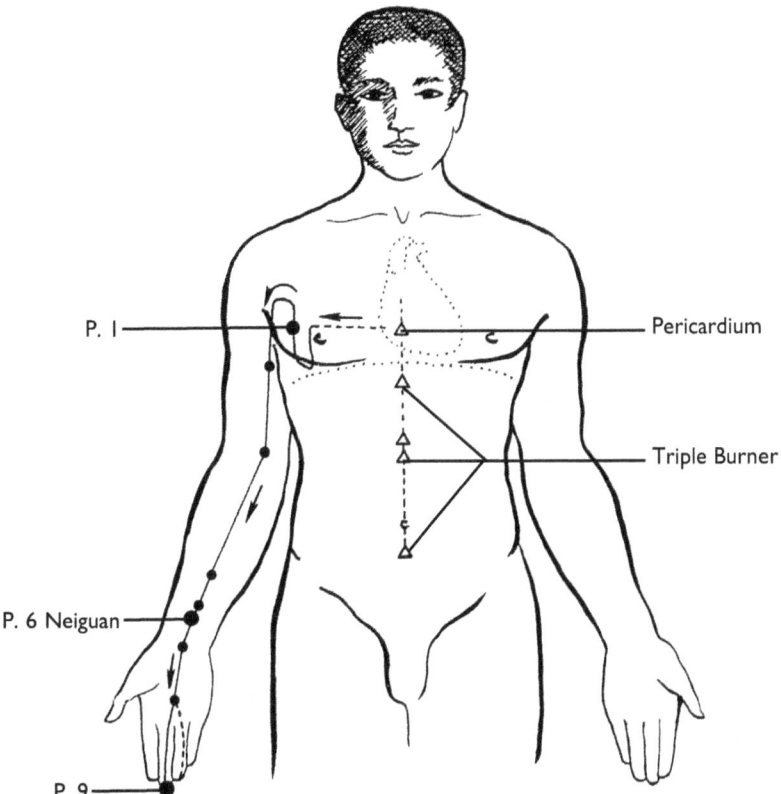

The Pericardium Meridian (P.)
Figure 3-20 There are nine points on this Yin meridian. The host organ (pericardium) is paired internally to the triple burner.

Point 19: L.I. 4 Hegu (Converging Valley)

He means to converge and *gu* refers to a valley from which a spring emanates to join a stream. When the thumb and index finger are separated, the web area is like a valley, hence the name Converging Valley.

This point is located in the 'valley' created by the first and second metacarpal bones (Figure 3-22). When the thumb and index fingers are pressed together (in the plane of the palm) a medial crease appears between the muscular process on top of the hand and the thumb. At the high point of this mound, level with the tip of the crease, lies this point. Pressure should be directed 45 degrees into the plane of the hand against the mid-point of the second metacarpal bone. A one-knuckle punch or a finger gouge to this readily accessible point can cause a lot of pain due to the presence of a superficial branch of the radial nerve. This makes it a good release point against grabs.

Point 20: L.I. 10 Shousanli (Three Li From Zhouliao)

Li refers to an ancient measuring unit; *san* means three, referring to the fact that

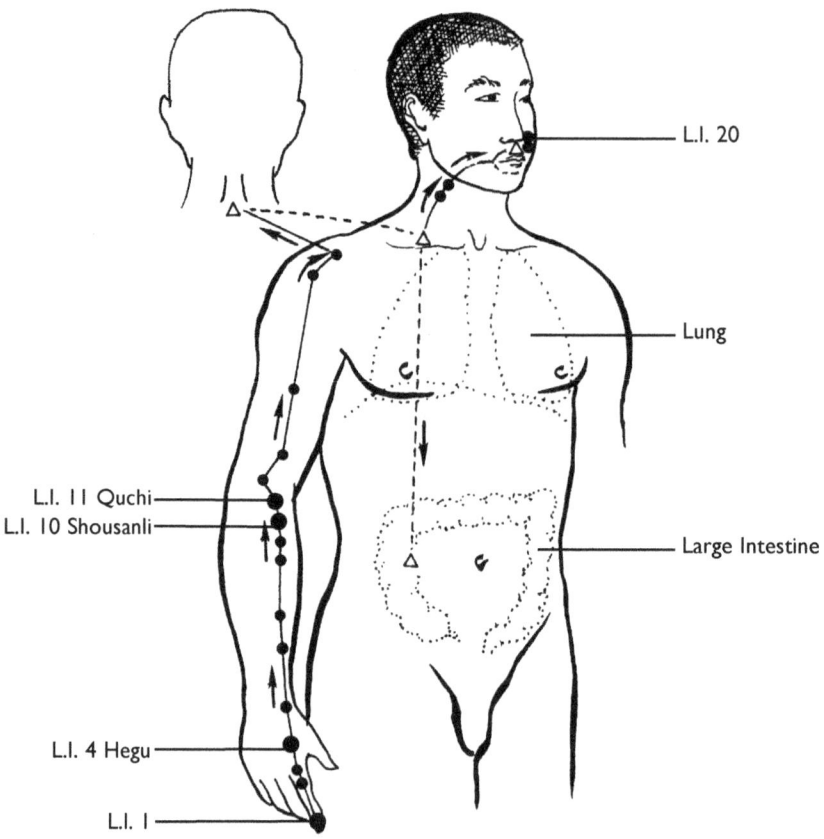

The Large Intestine Meridian (L.I.)
Figure 3-21 There are twenty bilateral points on this Yang meridian. The home organ (large intestine) is paired internally with the lung.

this point is three *cun* (thumb widths) from Zhouliao (Elbow Crevice), hence the name Three Li From Zhouliao.

This point is located about two inches distal to L.I. 11, on the lateral side of the radius, between the supinator longus (brachioradialis) muscle and the extensor carpi radialis longus muscle (Figure 3-23). Gouging or striking into this spot will affect the posterior antebrachial cutaneous nerve; a deep branch of the radial nerve that will result in numbness of the radial edge of the forearm and hand. This is a good spot to attack in order to break loose from a hold such as a rear chokehold or to release a grip on a weapon, making this point a popular police control tactics target (radial nerve motor point).

Point 21: L.I. 11 Quchi (Curved Pond)

Qu refers to the flexion of the elbow the crease created makes a curved depression likened to a *chi* (pond), hence the name Curved Pond.

This point is located in the recess of the lateral epicondyle of the humerus, at

Chapter 3: Pressure Points of the Fourteen Meridians

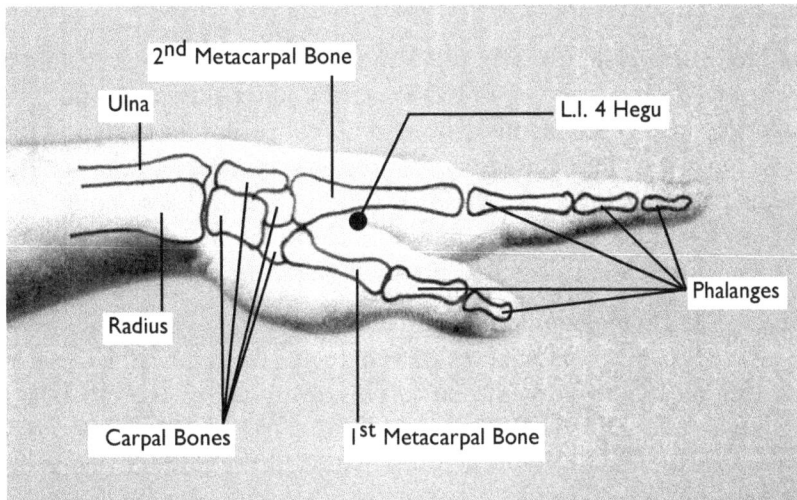

Bones of the Radial Edge of the Hand
Figure 3-22 Hegu (L.I. 4) is a useful point in the 'convergent valley' between the first and second metacarpal bones of the hand (at the tip of the medial curve).

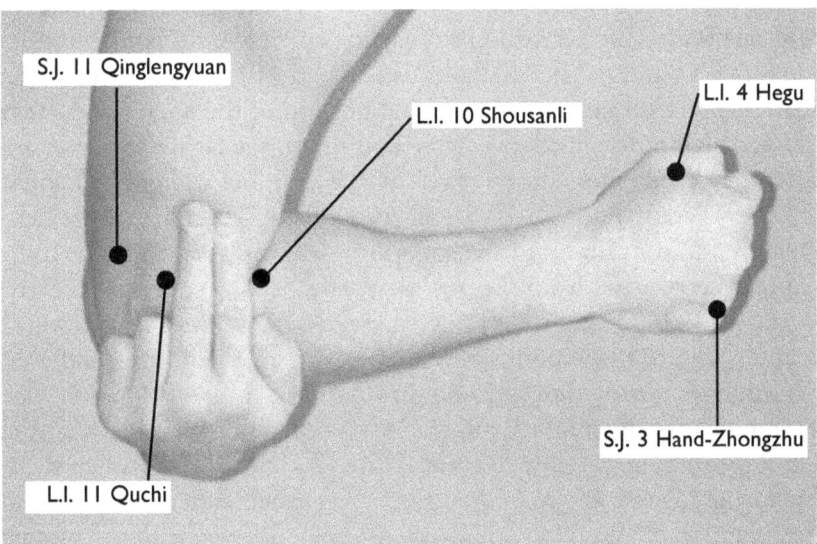

Selected Points of the Posterior Arm
Figure 3-23 Here are several important pressure points on the back of the arm and hand.

the lateral end of the transverse cubital crease of the elbow in the bulge between the extensor carpi radialis and brachioradialis muscles (Figure 3-23). As with L.I. 10, gouging or striking into this spot will affect the posterior antebrachial cutaneous nerve and the deep branch of the radial nerve. This will result in numbness of the radial edge of the forearm and hand.

Small Intestine Meridian

There are 19 bilateral points on this Yang meridian, starting at the outside tip of the little finger. Eight points are found along the ulnar side of the posterior aspect of the forearms, with the remaining eleven points distributed in the shoulder, neck and facial areas. This meridian enters the torso to terminate in the small intestine, hence the name Small Intestine Meridian (Figure 3-24). These points are used to treat head, neck and back disorders as well as along the ulnar side of the arms. The host organ (small meridian) is paired internally with the heart.

Point 22: S.I. 16 Tianchuang (Celestial Window)

Tian means heaven or celestial region in reference to the head and neck. *Chuang* means an opening (referring to the ears). This point can be used to treat deafness, hence the name Celestial Window.

This point is located on the side of the neck, on the posterior edge of the sternocleidomastoid muscle at the level of the top of the Adam's apple (Figure 3-24), in the posterior triangle of the neck (the triangle formed between the sternocleidomastoid, the trapezius muscles and the collar bone). A knife-edge blow or squeeze into this point at about a 30-degree angle from back to front can cause unconsciousness. This point central to the cervical plexus, being the nerve roots three upper cervical vertebrae (C2-C4) and the brachial plexus (C5–C7, T1) as shown in (Figure 3-13). The transverse cervical nerve, the emerging portion of the great auricular nerve and the lesser occipital nerve, accessory nerve and the supraclavicular nerves are affected (this latter nerve emerges under cover of the sternocleidomastoid muscle). The accessory nerve (cranial nerve XI) may also be affected. It is the motor nerve for the sternocleidomastoid muscle and the superior portion of the trapezius muscles. The suprascapular nerve arises from the posterior aspect of the superior trunk of the brachial plexus (C4-C6). This spot is targeted as a primary motor nerve point by police (suprascapular motor nerve point) because of the mental stunning and concomitant motor dysfunction of the shoulder and arm muscles.

A rare but always fatal injury can ensue if a heavy sideward blow is directed into the neck, rupturing the vertebral (cervical) artery as it ascends between the transverse foramina of the first six cervical vertebrae, through which it passes. This important artery feeds much of the outer brain (meninges) and cerebellum. Internal hemorrhage could not be controlled without doing irreparable damage to the brain.

Point 23 S.I. 17 Tianrong (Celestial Appearance)

Tian means heaven or celestial region in reference to the head. *Rong* means appearance. Ancient Chinese women wore ear rings that touched this spot and needling here was used to treat cosmetic problems affecting the neck and face, hence the name Celestial Appearance.

It is located on the side of the neck, posterior to the angle of the mandible, in the depression at the anterior border of the sternocleidomastoid muscle (Figure 3-24). A knife edge blow or squeeze to this point can cause unconsciousness. This spot is

Chapter 3: Pressure Points of the Fourteen Meridians

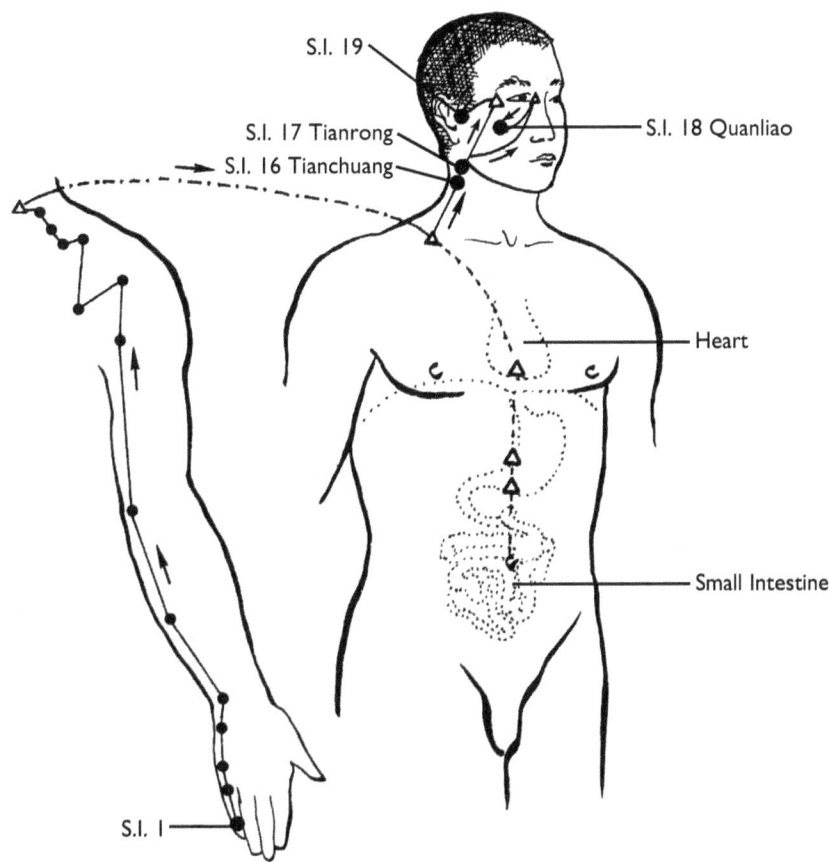

The Small Intestine Meridian (S.I.)
Figure 3-24 There are nineteen bilateral points on this Yang meridian. The host organ (small intestine) is paired internally with the heart).

very susceptible to a painful pressure point attack due to the presence of a branch of the great auricular nerve, a cervical branch of the facial nerve, and a superior cervical ganglion of the sympathetic trunk that lies along side the internal carotid artery and the internal jugular vein.

Point 24: S.I. 18 Quanliao (Zygomatic Crevice)

Quan refers to the zygoma (cheek bone) and *liao* means a crevice in a bone. This point is in the depression under the highest point of the cheekbone, hence the name Zygomatic Crevice.

This point is located directly below the outer canthus (corner of the eye), in the depression below the cheekbone (Figure 3-24). Gouging this point inward and upward against the zygomatic arch creates a relatively intense pain from the facial and infraorbital nerves being stimulated. A single knuckle press, thumb gouge or radial bone squeeze from an actual 'head' lock can cause considerable pain should you require a distraction or a release technique.

Sanjiao Meridian (Triple Heater/Warmer/Burner Meridian)

This Yang meridian has 23 bilateral points on either side of the body, 13 of which lie on the midline of the posterior aspect of the upper arms, originating from the tip of the ring finger. This meridian enters the torso and connects the upper, middle and lower *Jiao* (referring to the chest, stomach and lower abdomen respectively) known collectively as *Sanjiao*, its pertaining 'organ'. *San* means three and *jiao* means junction or crossroad, hence the name Sanjiao Meridian (the triple heater / warmer/burner – Figure 3-25). The remaining 10 points are located on the neck or head, terminating in the infraorbital area (lateral side of the eye).

Point 25: S.J. 3 Hand Zhongzhu (Mid Islet)

Zhong means middle and *zhu* means a small island or an islet. As this point is located between the fourth and fifth metacarpal bones 'downstream' from S.J. 2 (Fluid Gate) so it gets its name.

It is located on the dorsum (back) of the hand one quarter of the way along and in between these two metacarpal bones (Figure 3-25). This point is accessible to painful finger pressure when directed 45 degrees into the hand. This presses a dorsal cutaneous branch of the ulnar nerve against the fourth metacarpal bone, numbing the hand. Punching the hand at this point can reduce its ability to grasp.

Point 26: S.J. 11 Qinglengyuan (Cooling Gulf)

Qing means cool; *leng* means cold; and *yuan* means a gulf. This point is indicated in diseases relating to the accumulation or retention of heat and it is used to cool the blood, hence the name Cooling Gulf.

This point is located on the back of the upper arm (Figure 3-25) about two inches above the olecranon (tip of the elbow). The nerves affected by grinding or striking this point are the posterior brachial cutaneous nerve and the muscular branch of the radial nerve. Stimulating these nerves weakens the lower arm. This point is useful for attacking the elbow in order to straighten it during the application of a straight arm bar.

Point 27: S.J. 17 Yifeng (Ear-Shielding Wind)

Yi refers to a fan (shaped like an ear) and *feng* means wind. Its name is derived from the position of this point, which is shielded behind the ear lobe (Figure 3-16).

This point is found in the depression under the ear lobe between the mandible and the mastoid process (Figure 3-25). This pressure point can be accessed by finger/knuckle strikes, although it is a popular police pressure point (mandibular angle pressure point), because of the great pain that can be generated without causing injury. Pressure attacks directed inward and forward towards the nose will cause low level stunning and extreme pain due to the presence of the great auricular nerve and the emergence of the facial (seventh cranial) nerve, which feeds the muscles of facial expression. A punch in this same direction could dislocate the jaw and result in unconsciousness or even death.

Chapter 3: Pressure Points of the Fourteen Meridians

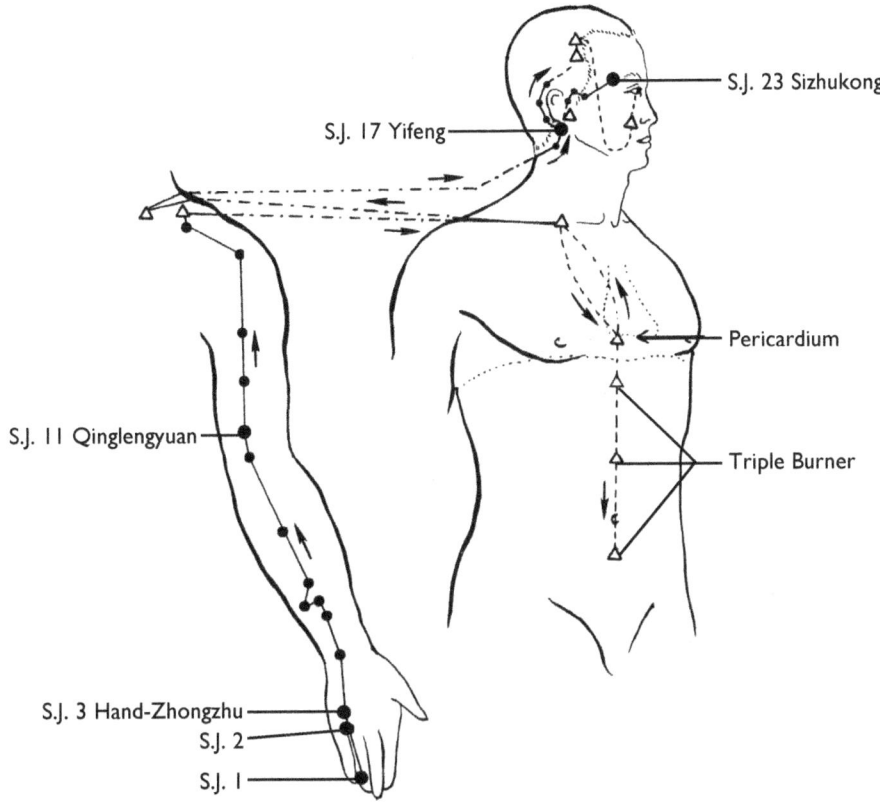

The Triple Burner Meridian (S.J.)
Figure 3-25 There are 23 bilateral points on this Yang meridian. The home organ (upper, middle, and lower burners) is paired internally to the pericardium.

Finger pressure can be applied in a variety of ways such as: c-clamping this point and the nose; pinching the ear lobe with the thumb and index finger to stabilize the penetrating middle finger; grasping the back of the neck with the fingers so that the thumb(s) can press inward; and even just using the middle knuckle to drill into this cavity.

Point 28: S.J. 23 Sizhukong (Bamboo Leaf Depression)

Sizhu means a tiny bamboo leaf (referring to the eyebrow); *kong* means a depression, as found at the lateral end of the eyebrow, hence the name Bamboo Leaf Depression.

This point's location is just posterior to the zygomatic process (upper side portion of the eye socket) in the beginning of the temple, the depression formed by the sphenoid bone (Figure 3-16). As the sphenoid bone is the smallest and only concave bone of the calvaria (skull cap), it is susceptible to injury. A blow directed directly into this area can fracture this relatively weak bone and rupture internal (deep temporal) arteries causing a fatal hematoma (pooled blood pressure on underlying cerebral cortex) within hours of the injury. The superficiality of the zygmaticotemporalis nerve makes it an easy target as well for a pressure point attack using a knuckle or fingertip.

Stomach Meridian

There are forty-five bilateral points on this Yang meridian, beginning under the eyes and terminating at the lateral tip of the second toe. Fifteen points lie on the anterior border of the lateral aspect of the legs, while the rest are found on the abdomen, chest, face and head. The meridian passes through the stomach, hence the name Stomach Meridian (Figure 3-26). These points are used to treat diseases of the stomach, intestines, head and front of the legs. The home organ (stomach) is paired internally with the spleen.

Point 29: St. 1 Chengqi (Hold Tears)

Cheng means to hold and *qi* refers to tears. Tears flow down to collect at this point of the eye, hence the name Hold Tears.

This point is located directly below the pupil just above the midpoint of the infraorbital ridge (Figure 3-26). Here lie branches of the infraorbital and oculomotor nerves, as well as the muscular branch of the facial nerve. This point can be used to approximate any attack to the eyeball. Any minor finger poke be very distracting and cause the eyes to water profusely and temporary blindness. Increasing pressure and penetration leads to the displacement of the eyeball causing extreme pain and blindness. Primarily the paper-thin ethmoid bone, making access to the brain via a finger or weapon attack a possibility, forms the medial wall of the eye socket. Any such attack to the eyes should be reserved for life-threatening situations. In these situations, attacks should be directed to your opponent's "vision, wind (airway), and limbs", in that order.

Point 30: St. 5 Daying (Great Meeting)

Da means big or great and *ying* means mandible as well as referring to the meeting at this point of branches from St. 8 and St. 1 before descending to St. 9, hence the name Great Meeting.

This point is found about an inch anterior to the angle of the jaw (in the notch along the bottom of the jaw as shown in (Figure 3-26). One can hook fingers up under the jaw line or poke a thumb inward and upward at a 45-degree angle to access the hypoglossal nerve and the buccal nerve (hypoglossal nerve pressure point). This can cause excruciating pain making it a popular police hold for distracting passive resistors and for assisting people unto their feet. The shape and size of the mandible makes it one of the more resistant bones of the body. An upward blow can cause dental damage and or lingual lacerations (if the tongue is extended past the teeth) and even cause a concussion or whiplash. Sideward blows can dislocate the jaw but this is more readily done if the bone can be attacked from a 45-degree angle to the front of the face at the jaw hinge (see St. 6).

Chapter 3: Pressure Points of the Fourteen Meridians

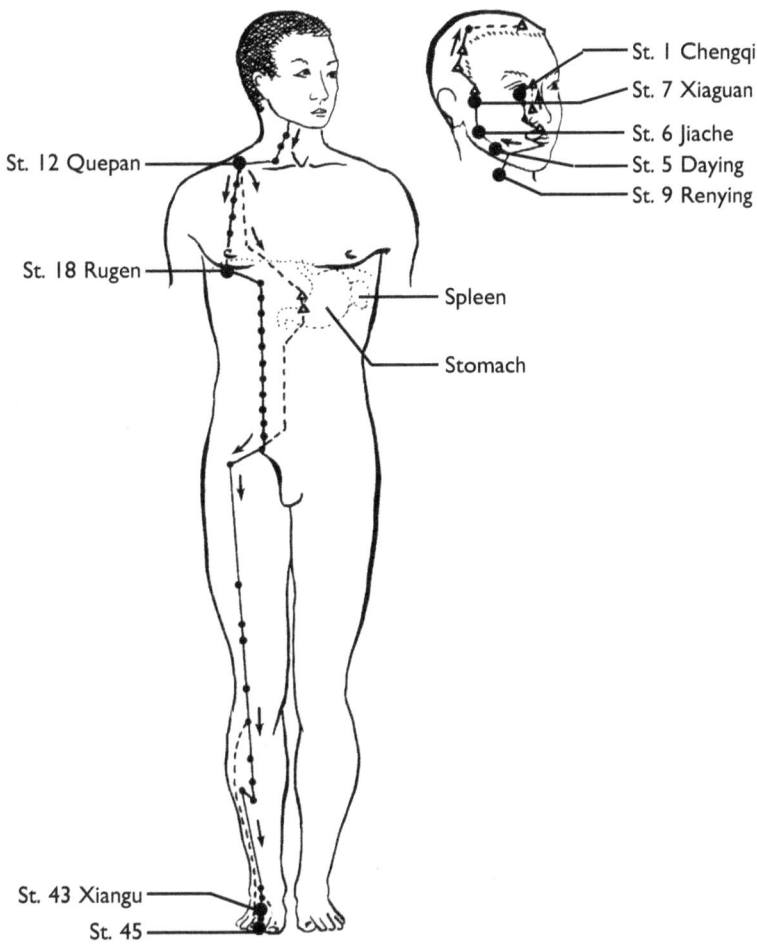

The Stomach Meridian (St.)
Figure 3-26 There are 45 bilateral points on this Yang meridian. The home organ (stomach) is paired internally to the spleen.

Point 31: St. 6 Jiache (Jaw Vehicle)

Jia means the lateral aspect of the jaw. The mandible's ancient name was *Jiachegu* or Vehicle Jaw Bone, as this bone moves the lower teeth during eating. Since this point is on the jaw near the mandibular angle, it is called Jaw Vehicle in deference to its old name.

It can be located about a half inch above the mandibular angle below the prominence of the muscle formed by the clenched teeth (Figure 3-26). This point can be assaulted by pressure point attack using a knuckle press (affecting the great auricular, facial and masseteric nerves) or by a jaw-dislocating blow directed from the back to front at a 45-degree angle inward. A sideward blow can twist the head to cause a concussion or whiplash.

Point 32: St. 7 Xiaguan (Lower Hinge)

Xia means the lower part; *guan* means the joint or hinge. As this point is located on the lower part of the junction of the jawbone and the mandible, which acts as a hinge to allow movement of the mandible, the point is called Lower Hinge.

It is located in front of the mid-ear, in the depression at the lower border of the zygomatic (upper mandible) arch (in the temporomandibular joint at the origin of the masseter muscle-the muscle that flexes which the jaw is clenched as shown in (Figure 3-26). As with St. 6, this point can be assaulted by pressure point attack (to the underlying branch of the facial nerve and a branch of the auriculotemporal nerve) or by a jaw-dislocating blow directed 45 degrees downwards.

Point 33: St. 9 Renying (Man Pulse)

Ying means palpitation, as with the throbbing of an artery where a pulse can be taken; *ren* refers to the middle (man) mode (the others being the upper heaven and lower earth modes) of the upper region of the bodies three-pulse regions, hence the name Man Pulse.

It is located at the level of the tip of the larynx (Adam's apple) on the posterior side of the carotid artery (where it splits into the internal and external carotid arteries) in front of the sternocleidomastoid muscle (Figure 3-26). A punch, slap or pressure point attack here can cause unconsciousness due to the presence of the vagus nerve and the carotid body (carotid sinus). This reaction reduces blood flow to the brain because the body interprets the externally applied pressure as high blood pressure (see the section 'Sealing the Vein' in Chapter Seven for the physiological reasons for this response).

Point 34: St. 12 Quepan (Broken Basin)

Que means broken and *pan* means a depression or basin. Since ancient times, this point has been referred to as Broken Basin as it is along the midpoint of the curved bone, the supraclavicular fossa.

This cavity is also known in police circles as the brachial plexus clavicle notch pressure point, because it is located in the hole or notch behind the mid-clavicle vertically aligned with the nipple (Figure 3-26). A hard downward penetration of the fingers here can lead to paralysis of the arm, mental stunning and possibly unconsciousness because of the stimulation of the (superficially) intermediate supraclavicular nerve and (deeper) the brachial plexus. If the clavicle breaks, the subclavian artery can be torn causing death quickly through massive hemorrhaging.

Point 35: St. 18 Rugen (Breast Root)

Ru means breast and *gen* means the root or base of something. Since this point is in the lower part of the breast, it is called Breast Root.

This point is located in the fifth intercostal space, directly below the nipple (Figure 3-26), in the 'root of the breast' (below the pectoralis muscle). A punch, kick, elbow or knee directly into this point can break the ribs relatively easily as the fifth and sixth ribs articulate with the costal cartilages at the bony tip of the ribs, affording maximal leverage against the ribs. This could cause injury to the lungs and affect the fifth intercostal nerve.

Point 36: St. 43 Xiangu (Sinking Valley)

Xian means sinking as with a depression and *gu* means valley. This point lies in a depression between two bones that is akin to a valley. It is used to treat the deficiency or sinking of stomach qi, hence the name Sinking Valley.

This point is located in a recess between the second and third metatarsal bones of the top of the foot (Figure 3-26). Gouging into this point affects the medial dorsal digital nerves and causes considerable pain. Striking this area can greatly reduce your opponent's ability to use the affected foot. Gouging in between the long bones of the foot (like the hands) can serve as distractions and can cause your opponent to release a leg lock.

Urinary Bladder Meridian

This Yang meridian consists of sixty-seven bilateral points starting at the medial corners of the eyes and running down the posterior length of the body beside the Du Meridian as bifurcated branches. It continues down the posterior aspect of the lower limbs (eighteen points) terminating at the lateral aspect of the little toe. It derives its name from the fact that it passes through the urinary bladder, hence the name Urinary Bladder Meridian (Figure 3-27). These points are used to treat eye, neck and back illnesses as well as disorders of the backs of the legs. The home organ (urinary bladder) is paried internally with the kidney.

Point 37: U.B. 40 Weizhong (Popliteal Center)

Wei refers to the popliteal fossa, behind the knee, and *zhong* means center, hence the name Popliteal Center.

This point is located on the midpoint of the transverse crease of the popliteal fossa (the diamond-shaped depression behind the knee) between the tendons of the biceps femoris and the semitendinosus muscles (Figure 3-27). Here the tibial nerve lies shallow and relatively unprotected by muscle, but the posterior muscle tendons of the knee and hamstrings offer considerable resistance to applications of pressure, particularly when the leg is extended. A blow to this area may drop your opponent by buckling the leg (with a sympathetic reaction by the other leg). If a heavy blow is rendered, the posterior cutaneous femoral and the tibial nerves will be affected, thereby partially disabling the lower leg and foot.

Point 38: U.B. 56 Chengjin (Supporting Tendon)

Cheng means to support or hold; *jin* means tendons. This point is used in acupuncture to treat tendon spasms in the legs that support the body, hence the name Supporting Tendons.

This point is located mid-calf between the two heads of the gastrocnemius muscle (Figure 3-27). A strike directly into this area affects the medial sural cutaneous nerve

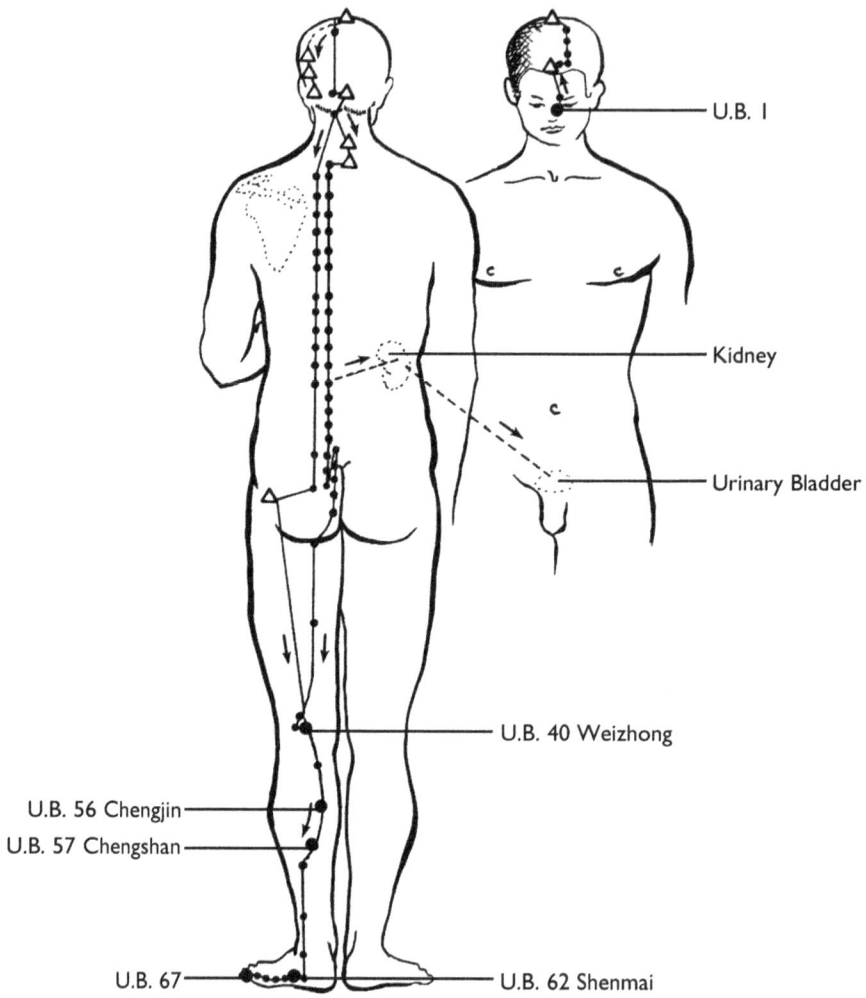

The Urinary Bladder Meridian (U.B.)
Figure 3-27 There are 67 bilateral points on this Yang meridian. The home organ (urinary bladder) is paired internally to the kidney.

and more deeply, the tibial nerve, the latter nerve innervating in part, the flexor muscles in the leg. A painful but temporary paralysis of the foot (inability to plantarflex the foot) will result if this area is targeted. Due to the presence of the protective muscle mass, applied pressure should be directed inward with an elbow or other pointed tool, or stuck with considerable force for penetrative effects. This point is a common police pressure control point for baton strikes (tibial nerve motor point).

Point 39: U.B. 57 Chengshan (Supporting Hill)

Cheng means to support or hold; *shan* means hill. As this point lies at the highest part of the hill of supporting calf muscle, it is called Supporting Hill.

This point is located in the depression at the lower border of, and between the two heads, of the gastrocnemius muscle (Figure 3-27). As with UB 56, the tibial nerve will be affected, although there is less muscle mass protecting the tibial nerve at this point. It is therefore more susceptible to painful pressure point attacks directed straight into the underlying superior border of the calcaneal (Achilles) tendon.

Point 40: U.B. 62 Shenmai (Relaxing Meridians)

Shen means to relax or stretch and *mai* refers to the blood vessels and meridians. Since this point is used to assist in relaxing the tendons and muscles of the lumbar area as well as promote blood circulation, it is called Relaxing Meridians.

This point lies in the recess directly under the lower extremity of the external malleolus (outside anklebone) as shown in (Figure 3-28). Gouging or striking directly into this point will affect the sural nerve (branches of the tibial and common fibular nerves) that innervates the lateral aspect of the foot and part of the heel.

Gall Bladder Meridian

This Yang meridian consists of forty-four bilateral points starting at the lateral side of the eye and moving down along the chest, hip and the lateral aspect of the leg (fifteen points). Since it passes through the gall bladder, it takes its name as the Gall Bladder Meridian (Figure 3-29). These points are used to treat diseases of the head, liver, gall bladder, chest and lateral extremities of the legs. The home organ (gall bladder) is paired internally with the liver.

Point 41: G.B. 6 Xuanli (Correct Suspension)

Xuan means suspending and *li* means correct or straight. This point derives its name, Correct Suspension, because of the potential to correct headache, dizziness, and blurred vision from points that are suspended on either side of the head.

This point is located in the slight depression at eyebrow level, midway between the eye socket and the anterior edge of the ear (Figure 3-29). Underlying this point is the pterion, the juncture of the sphenoid, temporal, frontal and parietal bones. Underlying the pterion, in grooves within the inner surface of the skull, are the anterior branches of the middle meningeal vessels. A blow directed directly into this area of the temple can fracture these thin bones (1/16 inch thick compared to the average thickness of 3/16 inch and a maximum of 3/8 inch) and rupture this artery causing a fatal hematoma (pooled blood pressure on underlying cerebral cortex) within hours of the injury. A moderate strike to the temple can cause blurred vision, dizziness, and unconsciousness, all symptoms indicative of a concussion. Apart from the weakness caused by these bones meeting in such close proximity, is the fact that they all join to the much smaller sphenoid bone, which has the dubious distinction of being the only skull bone to be concave inward, making it even further structurally weaker. A heavy blow can actually splinter the inner side of the calvaria without externally breaking the skull, thereby causing the above-mentioned, life-threatening hematoma. The superficiality of the auriculotemporal nerve makes it an easy target as well for a pressure point attack using a knuckle or fingertip.

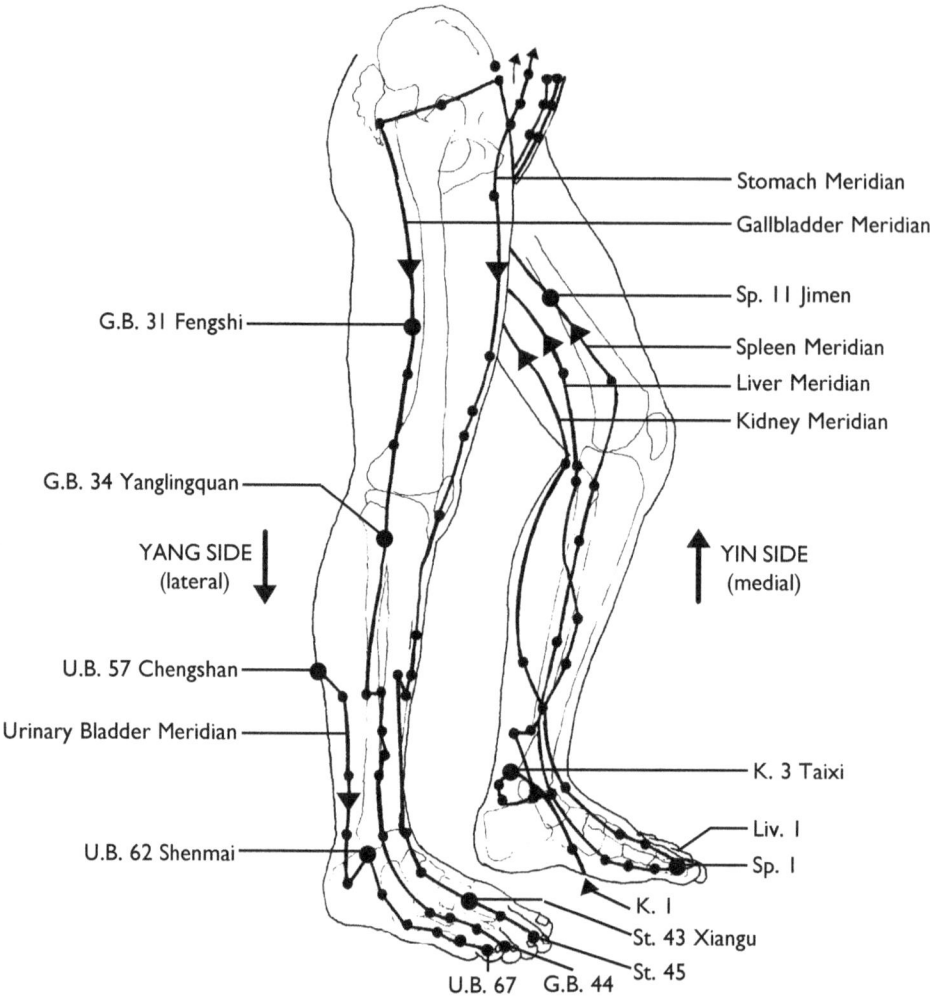

Selected Points of the Lateral and Medial Leg
Figure 3-28 The three meridians on the outside of the leg flow downward (Yang meridians). The three meridians on the inside of the leg flow upward (Yin meridians).

Point 42: G.B. 24 Riyue (Sun and Moon)

Ri means the sun and *yue* means the moon. The characters for these two celestial bodies combine to form *ming* meaning clear and distinct. Since the gall bladder is considered to be the organ dominating decision-making, as with a clear and distinct mind, this point is called Sun and Moon.

This point is located below the nipple, between the seventh and eighth ribs (seventh intercostal space as shown in (Figure 3-29). Striking this point will affect the seventh intercostal nerve. A heavy blow delivered to this spot can cause unconsciousness or death by internal bleeding, especially if the liver (right side) or the stomach/spleen (left side) is injured. The diaphragm may also be injured causing a difficulty in breathing.

Chapter 3: Pressure Points of the Fourteen Meridians

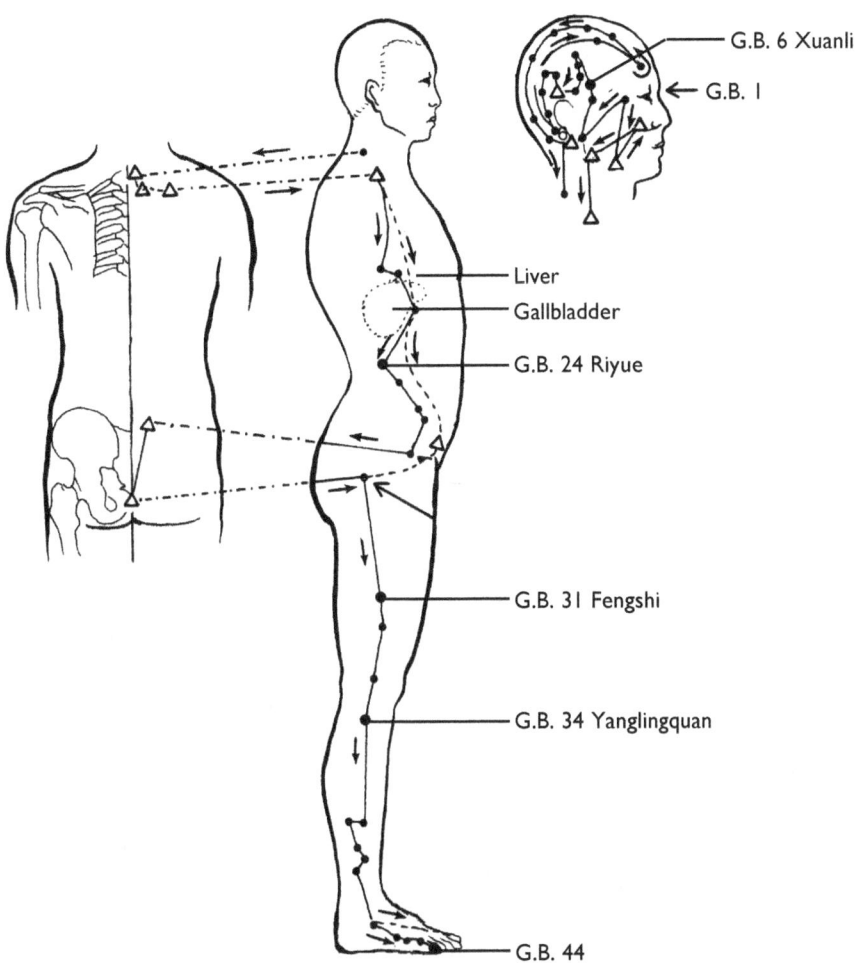

The Gall Bladder Meridian (G.B.)
Figure 3-29 There are 44 bilateral points on this Yang meridian. The home organ (gall bladder) is paired internally to the liver.

Point 43: G.B. 31 Fengshi (Wind Market)

Feng means wind and *shi* means a market (convergent) place. In Traditional Chinese Medicine, this is the most important point for eliminating wind from the lower extremities of the body, hence the name Wind Market.

It is easily located by where the tip of the middle finger touches the outside of the leg by the fully down-stretched arm (Figure 3-28). This is a very popular police control tactics spot (lateral femoral nerve motor point) for inducing a 'Charley horse' to temporarily paralyze the leg (vastus lateralis muscle) with a knee strike, kick, or baton strike, as it affects the lateral femoral cutaneous nerve and muscular branch of the femoral nerve.

Point 44: G.B. 34 Yanglingquan (Outer Mound Spring)

Yang in this case refers to the lateral (outside) aspect of the leg; *ling* means a high place or a mound (the head of the fibula); *quan* refers to a spring in a depression (below the head of the fibula), hence the name Outer Mound Spring.

This point is located in the recess on the lateral (outside) portion of the leg below the knee between the fibula and tibia (Figure 3-29). It is painful to touch due to the presence of the common peroneal nerve, which branches into the superficial and deep peroneal nerves. Striking this point can immobilize the lower leg.

Spleen Meridian

There are twenty-one bilateral points on this Yin meridian beginning at the tip of the big toe and terminating at the tongue. Eleven points lie on the anterior aspect of the medial sides of the legs with the rest being distributed on the abdomen and chest, having passed through its pertaining organ, the spleen, hence the name Spleen Meridian (Figure 3-30). These points are used to treat disorders of the abdomen, spleen, stomach, genitals, etc. The home organ (spleen) is paired internally with the stomach.

Point 45: Sp. 11 Jimen (Basket Gate)

Ji refers to the abducted position of the legs, like holding a basket between the knees, when this point is being located. *Men* means gate, hence the name Basket Gate.

This point is located on the medial side of the sartorius muscle of the middle inner thigh (Figure 3-30). The anterior femoral cutaneous nerve and more deeply, the saphenous nerve may be accessed by gouging with the elbow inward and upward toward the front of the thigh or by striking with hand or foot. This will affect the functioning of the anterior and medial side of the leg. This loss of motor control in the leg makes this femoral nerve motor point a prime target for police control tactics.

Point 46: Sp. 12 Chongmen (Pulsating Door)

Chong means rushing or pulsating and *men* means gate. This point is close to a palpation point of the femoral artery and this Spleen Meridian enters the abdominal cavity as if through a door, hence the name Pulsating Door.

This point is located in the inguinal crease just lateral to the femoral artery at the level of the pubic symphysis (Figure 3-30). Gouging this point with the thumbs or elbow can affect the femoral and ilioinguinal nerves as well as the anterior branch of the obturator nerve. The femoral nerve, for example, innervates the anterior muscles of the thigh, and hip and knee joints, hence the functioning of the leg will be hampered.

Point 47: Sp. 21 Dabao (General Control)

Da means big or general. *Bao* means totally controlling something. Since this point is the main governing point for all of the Yin and Yang meridians, and the spleen feeds *qi* to all of the *zangfu* organs as well as the four limbs, it is called the General Control point.

Chapter 3: Pressure Points of the Fourteen Meridians

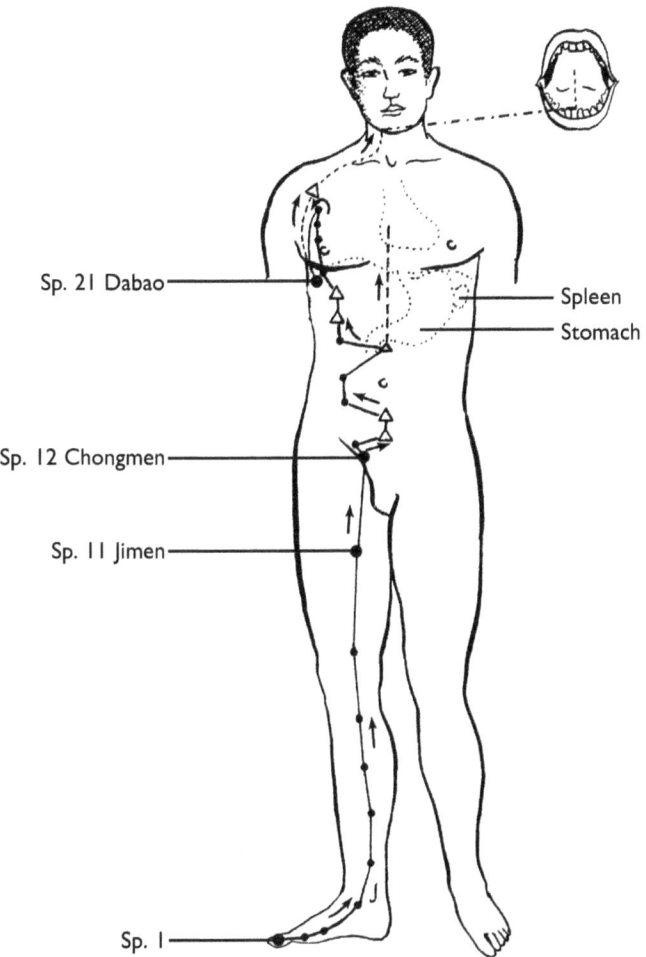

The Spleen Meridian (Sp.)
Figure 3-30 There are 21 bilateral points on this Yin meridian. The home organ (spleen) is paired internally to the stomach.

A punch or kick directed straight into this point, located midway down the ribs (level with the solar plexus between the seventh and eighth ribs) on the lateral plane of the body, can injure the liver (right side), or the stomach/spleen (left side) and cause unconsciousness or death by internal bleeding (Figure 3-30). The diaphragm will also be temporarily paralyzed due to the presence of the seventh intercostal nerve.

Kidney Meridian

This Yin meridian consists of twenty-seven bilateral points beginning from the base of the small toe, through the sole of the foot, up the posterior aspect of the lower legs (ten points) and along the anterior mid-line of the torso, and terminating in the root of the tongue. As this meridian passes through its pertaining organ, the kidney, it

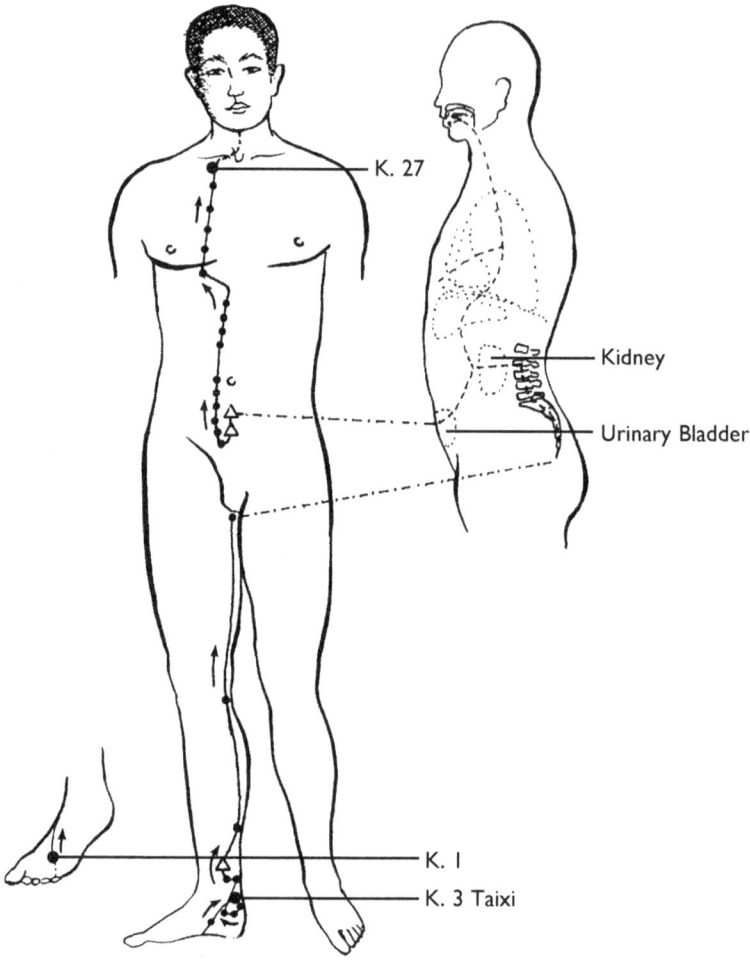

The Kidney Meridian (K.)
Figure 3-31 There are 27 bilateral points on this Yin meridian. The home organ (kidney) is paired internally to the urinary bladder.

derives its name as the Kidney Meridian (Figure 3-31). These points are used to treat diseases of the urinary and reproductive systems, as well as head and throat ailments. The home organ (kidney) is paired internally with the urinary bladder.

Point 48: K. 3 Taixi (Big Stream)

Tai means big and *xi* means stream. Since the *qi* of the kidney meridian pours out of K.1 through this point after converging and strengthening at this point, it is called Big Stream.

This point is located in the recess of the inner ankle midway between the tip of the medial malleolus (anklebone) and the tendo calcaneus (Achilles tendon) as shown in (Figure 3-31). The medial crural cutaneous nerve can be gouged with the thumb or elbow to effect a release from a leg lock.

Chapter 3: Pressure Points of the Fourteen Meridians

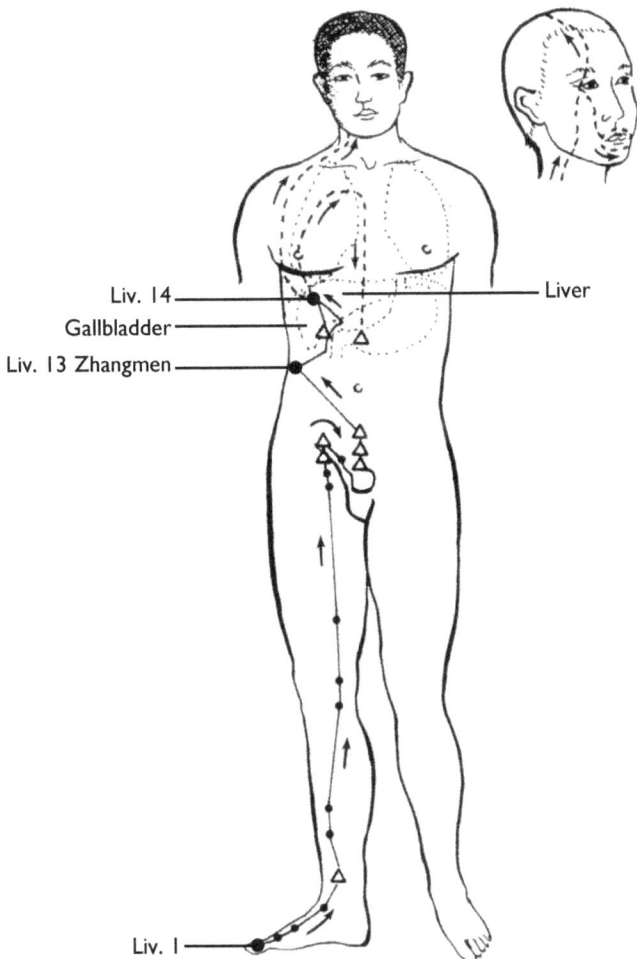

The Liver Meridian (Liv.)
Figure 3-32 There are 14 bilateral points on this Yin meridian. The home organ (liver) is paired internally to the gall bladder.

Liver Meridian

This Yin meridian consists of fourteen bilateral points, twelve of which lie on the medial aspect of the legs, with the remainder being located on the abdomen and chest. It begins near the medial end of the big toe and runs up the inner side of the leg entering the abdomen, passing through its pertaining organ, the liver (hence the name Liver Meridian- (Figure 3-32), and ending in the chest cavity. These points are used to treat a wide array of head, chest and genital disorders.

Point 49: Liv. 13 Zhangmen (Bright Door)

Zhang means bright, in reference to the brightness that the spring color green and *men* means door, hence the name Bright Door.

This point can be located at the lateral sides of the body where the tip of the

139

elbow touches the torso, below the free end of the eleventh 'floating' rib in the internal and external oblique muscles (Figure 3-32). A gouge or blow to this area will affect the tenth intercostal nerve. These floating ribs are so named because they are not connected to the sternum by costal cartilages. As such, these ribs can be easily broken, and damage to the liver, spleen and stomach can occur. Death can ensue from internal bleeding, if an attack is directed diagonally upward at this point to damage these organs.

Extra Points

Extra points are those not indicated on the 14 regular meridians, although they may lie on them. They vary in number from 20 to 1,500, depending on the source; however, 30-60 are in common use. Some have a history of traditional use in acupuncture whereas others have been recently discovered.

Point 50: EX-HN 2 Yingtan (Decorating Hall)

Yin means to dye or stain and *tan* means a place or hall. This point used to be dyed with red ink for cosmetic purposes, hence the name Decorating Hall. Also known as Shang Dantien (Upper Dantien), this is the uppermost of the three main *qi* reservoirs (see Ren 14 and Ren 6).

This point is located in the smooth hairless spot between the eyebrows at the top of the nasal bone (Figures 3-14). Known as the glabella, a heavy blow to this area can be fatal due to the concussive impact to the frontal lobes of the brain. Lighter blows can cause unconsciousness and concussion. Breakage of the nasal bone slightly below this point will rupture the vein that enters into the nasal cavity (angular vein), causing significant bleeding that could interfere with breathing. Although this is a painful injury (from the stimulation of the external and internal nasal nerves and the anterior ethmoidal nerves), which temporarily causes blurred vision, it is not a life-threatening one.

Point 51: EX-HN 19 Jingbi (Upper Arm)

Jing means neck and *bi* means upper arm. This point is located on the brachial plexus that runs from the neck (C5- C7, T1) to the arm, hence the name Upper Arm.

This point is located in the lower neck (one inch above the junction of the medial 1/3 and the lateral 2/3 of the clavicle) in the recess at the posterior border of the sternocleidomastoid muscle (Figure 3-1). The brachial plexus origin pressure point is a useful police pressure control point that may be painfully gouged by digitally penetrating directly into the center of the neck. The brachial plexus root and the anterior branch of the supraclavicular nerves can impair motor functioning of the affected shoulder, arm and hand. Branches of the superficial carotid and transverse cervical arteries and veins can also be affected.

Point 52: EX-UE 11 Bizhong (Arm Center)

Bi means forearm and *zhong* means middle or center. As this point is located mid-arm between the bones of the arm, it derives its name Arm Center.

This point is located halfway between the transverse creases of the wrist and elbow, between the radius and ulna bones (see Figure 3-18). This point lies directly on the median nerve and a strike or gouge can also affect the anterior and posterior interosseous nerves. This will interfere with the functioning of the hand making it a prime target in police control tactics median nerve motor point).

CHAPTER 4

Body Tools and Vulnerable Points

4-1. INTRODUCTION

The Body as a Weapon

Anyone studying the martial arts has heard various body parts referred to as being weapons ("my hand is my sword", "my whole body is a weapon", "his hands and feet have to be registered as deadly weapons with the police", etc.). Some parts are used as tools for setting up attacks or for defensive purposes. There is a clear advantage of applying your hard, bony body parts to your opponent's weaker or softer body parts. Indeed, pressure point attacks are directed at your opponent's weaker, nerve rich areas along the acupuncture meridians via gouging techniques and well-placed strikes. Always use your weapons/tools in an effective manner. Many combatants have done themselves damage by misapplying their weapons (or by applying their weapons to inappropriate parts of their opponent's body) or have wasted their efforts by using techniques that are ineffective to the targeted area of the body. Some examples of this would be:

1. To apply a head butt using your own temple area against the front top section of your opponent's head (your temple is the weaker area).
2. To head butt your opponent's buttock (though a strong weapon, this technique is ineffectual to such a well muscled part of the body).
3. Fingertip punching a well-muscled chest (your fingers may only get injured).
4. A bear hug is applied to a large torso (not enough strength to be effective).

All parts of the body, your hands, arms, legs, head and even the torso can be utilized to achieve your goal. Sometimes tools not normally considered in fighting, such as the torso and teeth, can be used with an element of surprise, both defensively and offensively respectively.

Learn the Principle

For example, the straight arm bar can be applied in many ways (see Chapter Two). One needn't try to remember all the ways as being separate techniques. If you understand the biomechanical principle behind bending the arm past its full range of extension, using a fulcrum at the elbow, then it is left to your own creativity to discover and apply all the ways of applying this technique and its variations. Consider applying the arm bar using your body tools like the torso (or your head, arms, legs, pelvis, shoulder, etc.). By having a total awareness of body parts of both yourself and your opponent, you could have the advantage in a fight. Look at the damage a head butt to the face or a bite to the nose or ear can do to distract or otherwise put your opponent out of commission.

Know the Body

Having an intimate knowledge of the anatomical strengths and weaknesses of the human body and a kinesthetic sense of how to apply your body tools to your opponent's exposed weak points and vital areas such as pressure points, muscles/tendons, joints, veins/arteries, and so on, is crucial for the effective fighter. Although there are over 200 joints in the human body, one need only concentrate on the 15 major joints that we can manipulate or attack, namely those of the head, neck, torso, upper arm, lower arm, hand, upper leg, lower leg and foot (Figure 4-1).

4-2. Body Tools

Breaking the Machine

The body may be regarded functionally from a martial arts perspective as being a collection of organic tools, capable of exerting force on an opponent by pressing, striking or by gripping his weak points or otherwise neutralizing his tools. This fighting machine can be immobilized or controlled through the strategic biomechanical application of force (pain compliance/pinning). When pain compliance does not work, or such low level uses of force are ineffective or inappropriate, the human machine may be rendered temporarily inoperative (veins/arteries and/or breath can be sealed to yield unconsciousness) or it may be physically damaged to prevent further aggression (joint breakage), or it may even be permanently destroyed (death). Simply put, a wide variety of your body parts may be applied to conquer your opponent's body. We can divide the groups of body tools (arms, legs, neck/head, torso) in accordance to their utility (pressing, striking, and gripping).

Hand Tools

The human hand is comprised of 27 bones (eight wrist bones, five hand bones, fourteen finger bones) and numerous muscles, tendons and ligaments. Each of the four fingers has three joints accompanied by and a two-jointed thumb. The hand is attached to the lower arm via the wrist joint. The unsurpassed manual dexterity of the hand makes hand tools the most versatile means by which to attack your opponent through pressing, striking, and gripping techniques. These kinds of

Chapter 4: Body Tools and Vulnerable Points

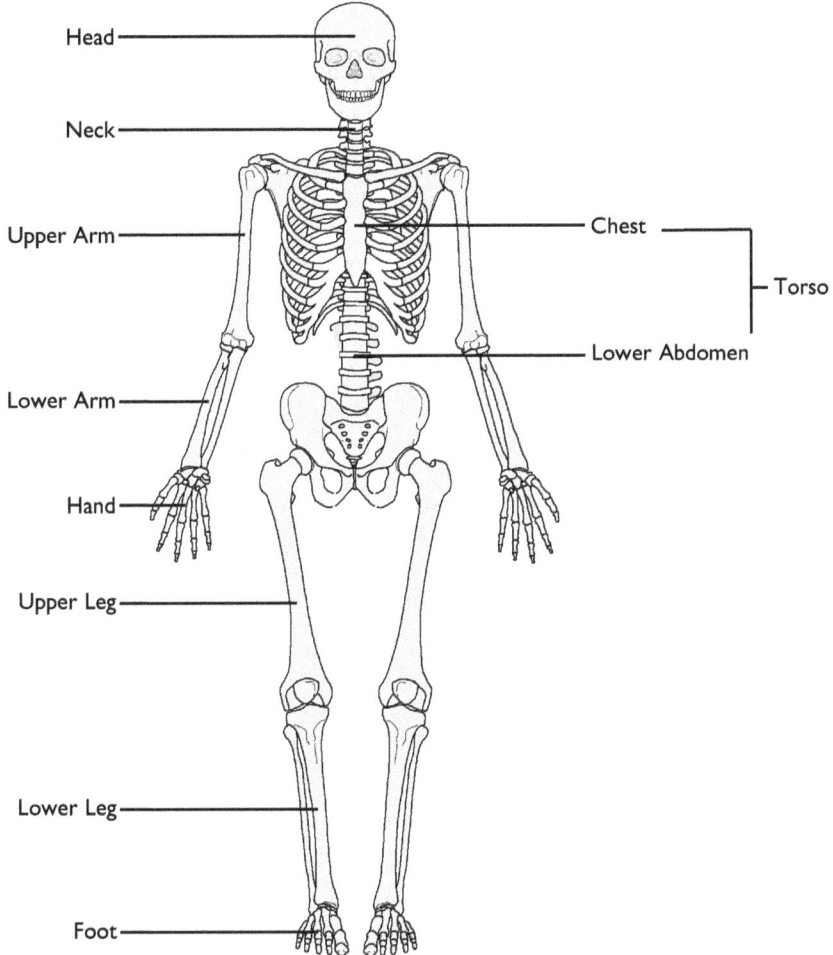

Skeletal Segments
Figure 4-1 There are 206 bones in the human body, forming over 200 joints. We need only concentrate on those few joints between body segments for fighting.

force applications are essential in both Qin Na and ground fighting. Several force-related considerations are: 1) the use of the minimum surface area of the tool, 2) the duration of force application (over time: slow = pressing; fast = striking), 3) the practical application of your soft/hard tools against the weaker anatomical points of your opponent. Striking hand tools can be applied in conjunction with both Qin Na and ground fighting applications in order to incapacitate, distract or otherwise weaken your opponent's grip on you or his resistance towards you in both offensive and defensive capacities. Pressing hand tools can be also used against pressure points or other body tools for leverage and immobilization purposes.

Let's look at the many types of hand tools available for combative use and look at how and where they can be applied to the body.

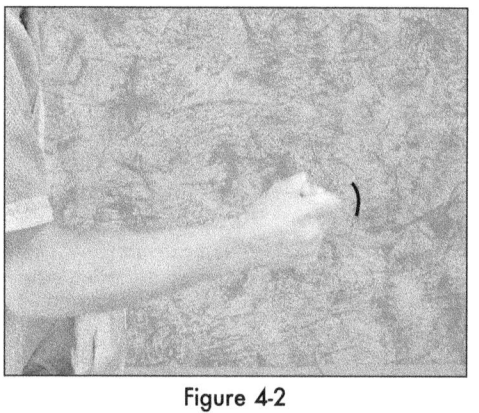

Figure 4-2

Figure 4-3

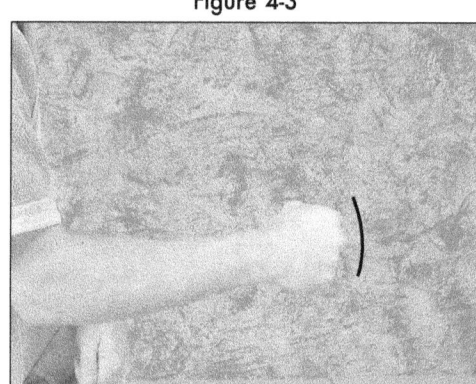

Figure 4-4

Figure 4-5

(i) **Pressing Hand Tools:**

   a) Finger Tools

   Knuckle Presses and Their Applications
   - One knuckle press (Figure 4-2) to sternum, temple, ear.
   - Thumb knuckle press (Figure 4-3) to ribs, temple.
   - Fore knuckle press (Figure 4-4) to triceps tendon.
   - Fist press (Figure 4-5) to leg, neck.

Figure 4-6: Grey attacks White's ear (S.J. 17) with a single knuckle press. Note the counterpressure on White's head with Grey's other hand.

Figure 4-7: Grey attacks White's ribs (Liv. 13) with a thumb gouge. Note the augmentation and the anchoring of the gouging hand with the other hand.

Figure 4-8: Grey attacks White's triceps tendons (S.J. 11). Note the use of Grey's grabbing of the clothing to anchor his knuckles to the target. Grey grabs White's clothing at the elbow so that the tip of White's elbow rests in the space between Grey's fingertips and palm heel. When Grey's knuckles are rolled forward while gripping the clothing, his fore knuckles will be in the correct position on the back of the arm to affect the triceps tendons.

Chapter 4: Body Tools and Vulnerable Points

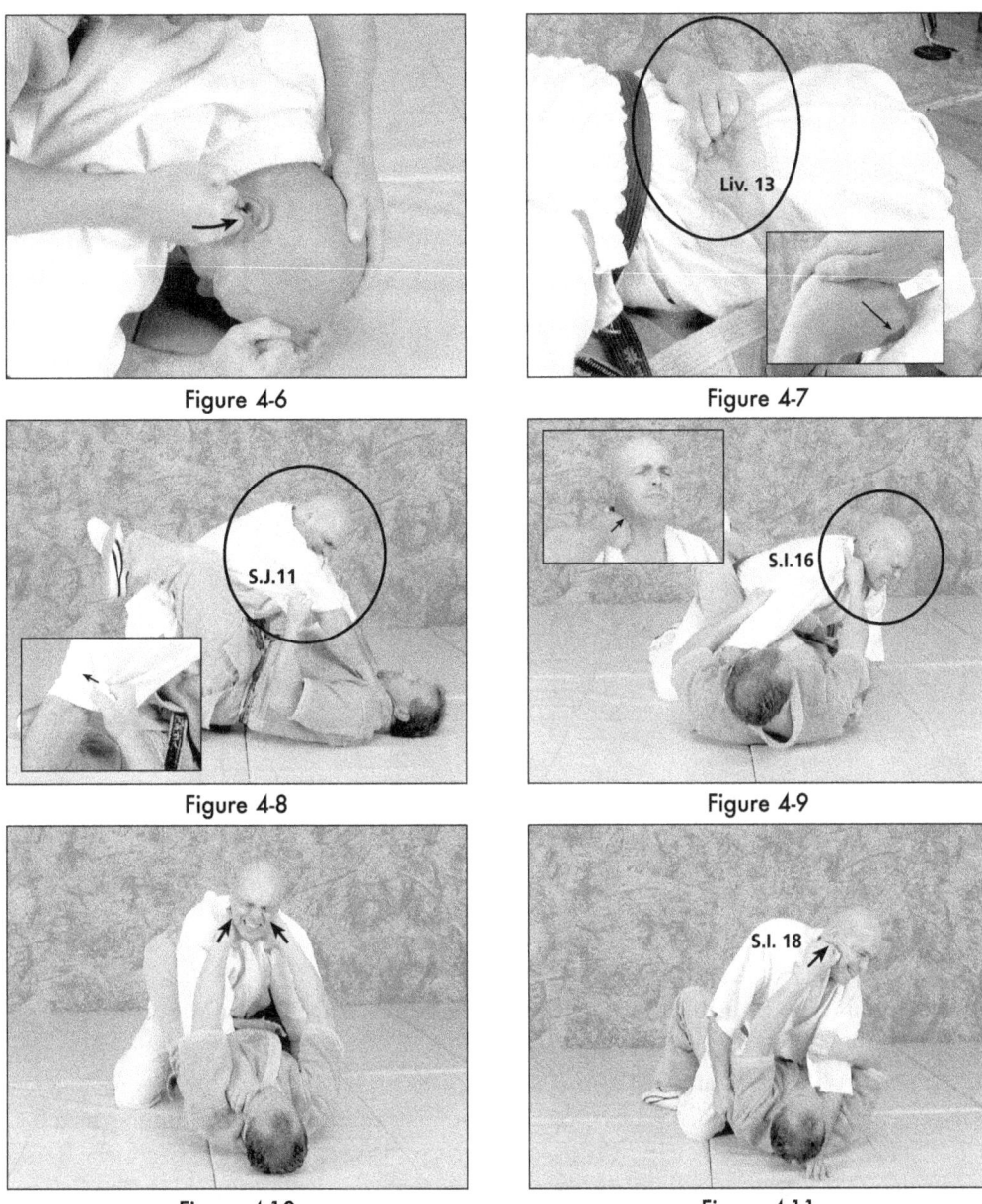

Figure 4-6

Figure 4-7

Figure 4-8

Figure 4-9

Figure 4-10

Figure 4-11

Figure 4-9: Grey attacks White's neck (S.I. 16) with a one-handed fist press while anchoring his hand to White's gi top.

Figure 4-10: Grey attacks the sides of White's neck (L.I. 17) with both hands. Grey grips White's collars and turns his fists inwards to choke White.

Figure 4-11: Grey applies a fore knuckle press to White's cheekbone (S.I. 18) while holding onto his gi top.

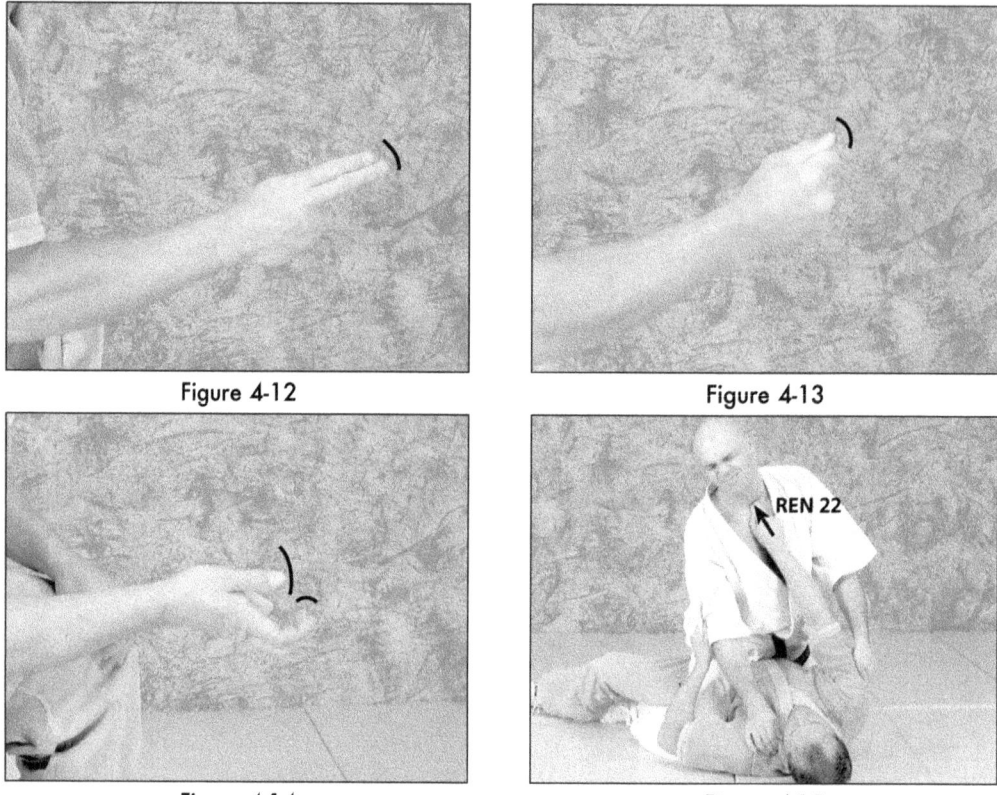

Figure 4-12   Figure 4-13

Figure 4-14   Figure 4-15

Finger Tip Presses and Their Applications
- One/two finger presses (Figure 4-12) to jugular and clavicle notches, eyes.
- Thumb tip press (Figure 4-13) to eyes, mandibular angle, under cheek bone.
- Finger(s)-thumb squeeze (Figure 4-14) to throat, brachial plexus, hypoglossal nerve.

Figure 4-15: Grey attacks White's throat (REN 22) with his fingertips. Balance displacement can be achieved by pressing with the fingers into this jugular notch.

Figure 4-16: Grey attacks Whites jaw line (St. 5) with his fingertips. Grey hooks his fingertips under White's jaw to affect the hypoglossal nerve. Note how Grey stabilizes White's head by holding it like a football tucked in to his left arm.

Figure 4-17: Grey attacks White's shoulder (St. 12) with his fingertips. Grey accesses White's brachial plexus at the clavicle notch by hooking his fingers deeply into this 'shoulder well'.

Chapter 4: Body Tools and Vulnerable Points

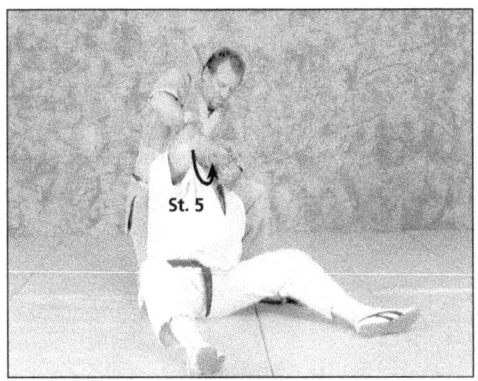

Figure 4-16

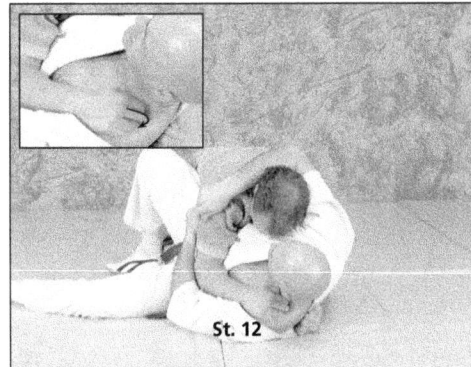

Figure 4-17

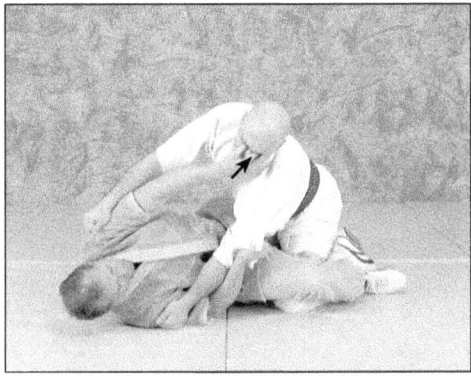

Figure 4-18

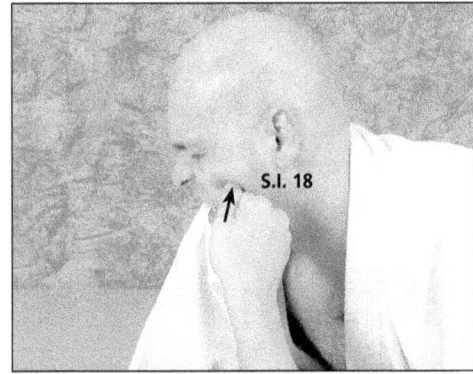

Figure 4-19

Figure 4-18: Grey attacks White's eyes (St. 1) with his fingertips. Grey need not penetrate White's eye sockets fully to effect balance displacement.

Figure 4-19: Grey attacks White's cheekbone (S.I. 18) using the tip of his thumb. Grey stabilizes his right thumb by pressing the pad of his last thumb segment onto the side of his own pointer finger (this is stronger than the loose 'hitch-hiker's' thumb).

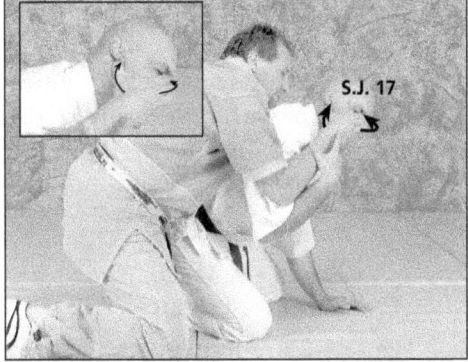

Figure 4-20

Figure 4-20: Grey attacks White's nose and ear (S.J. 17) with a c-clamp. Grey anchors his right fingers across White's nose and uses his opposing thumb to gouge into White's mandibular angle pressure point.

149

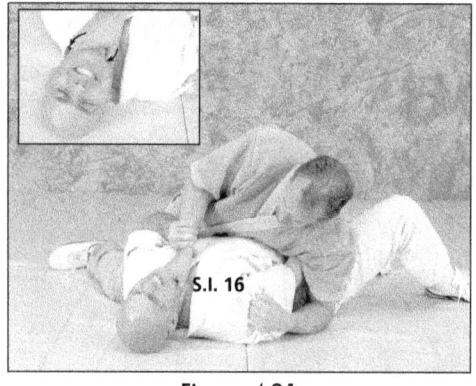

Figure 4-21   Figure 4-22

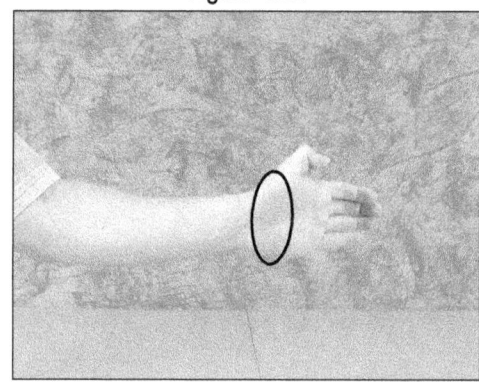

Figure 4-23   Figure 4-24

Figure 4-21: Grey applies a c-clamp (finger scissors) to White's throat (S.I. 16) to effect major structural damage to the front of White's neck.

Figure 4-22: Grey attacks White's brachial plexus tie-in point (Lu. 2) from the front and from within the armpit using a finger grab.

Figure 4-23: Grey grabs White's groin with a hand grab. White will feel excruciating pain when Grey grabs, twists and pulls on White's testicles.

b) Base of Hand Tools

Palm Press and Its Applications
- Palm press (Figure 4-24) to chin, neck, arm, wrist.

Figure 4-25: White applies a hand press to the back of Grey's neck (DU 16) using a lock (White has captured Grey's right arm with his left arm to help stabilize this move).

Figure 4-26: White peels Grey off of him using a combined chin twist/hair pull. Notice how White maximizes the hair pulling torque by reaching around with his left arm to grab the hair on the far (left) side of Grey's head.

Edge of Hand Presses and Their Applications
- Sword hand (baby finger side) edge (Figure 4-27) to triceps, throat.
- Ridge hand (thumb side) edge (Figure 4-28) to infraorbital ridge: under the nose.

Chapter 4: Body Tools and Vulnerable Points

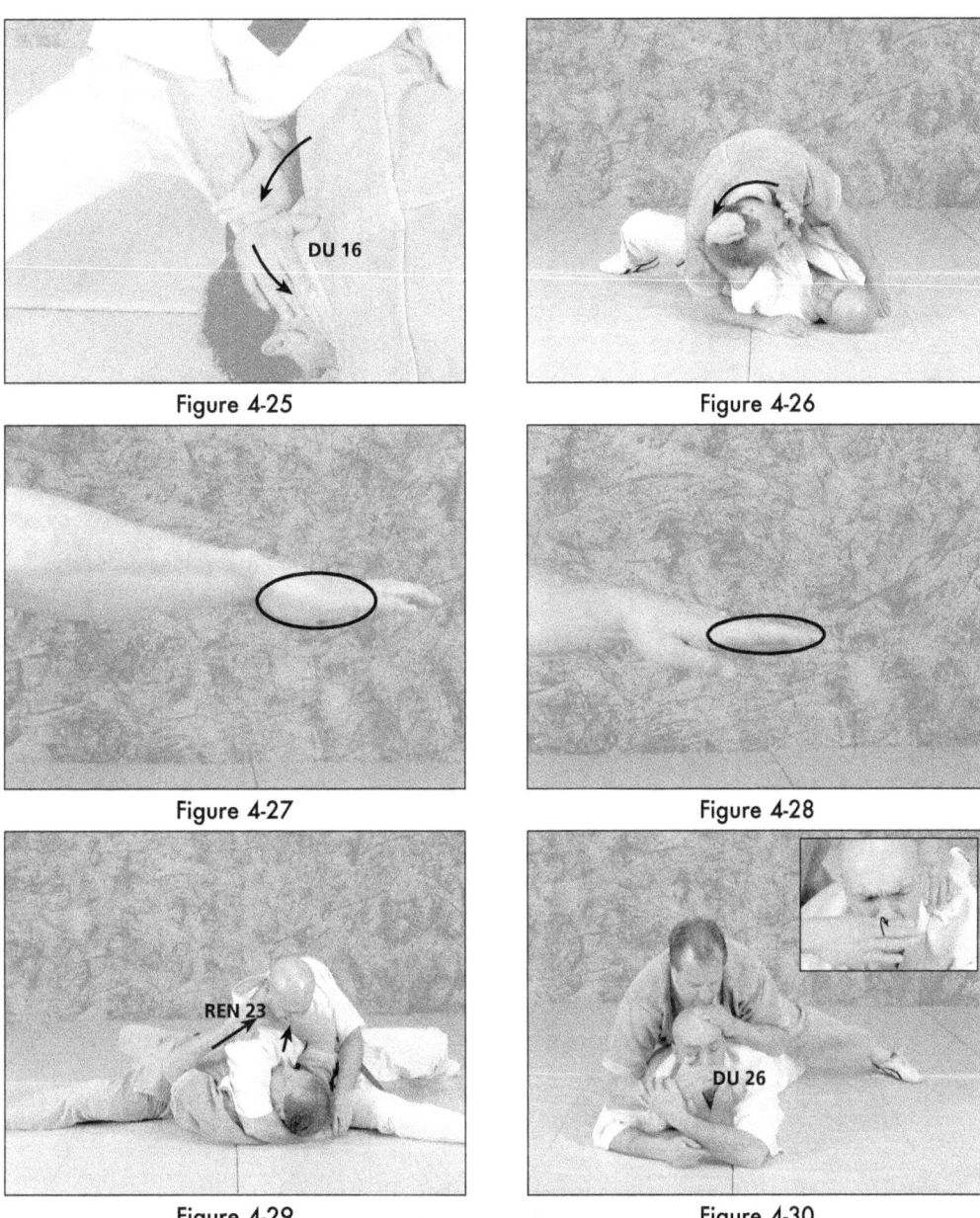

Figure 4-25

Figure 4-26

Figure 4-27

Figure 4-28

Figure 4-29

Figure 4-30

Figure 4-29: Grey frames White's neck (REN 23) with his right wrist. The harder White squeezes, the more pressure he puts on his own neck.

Figure 4-30: Grey presses the mid-knuckle of his right hand under White's nose (DU 26) then turns his hand inwards (as to level it out). This action stretches White's upper lip downward to reduce the thickness of it over the philtrum to effect maximal pain on the infraorbital nerve.

Chin Na In Ground Fighting

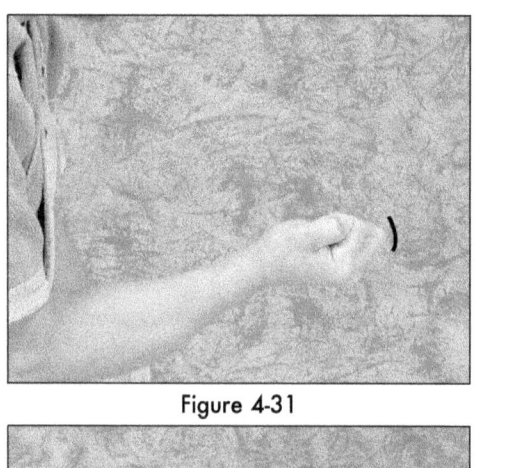

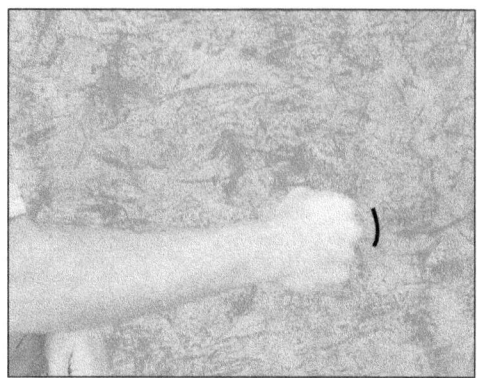

Figure 4-31 Figure 4-32

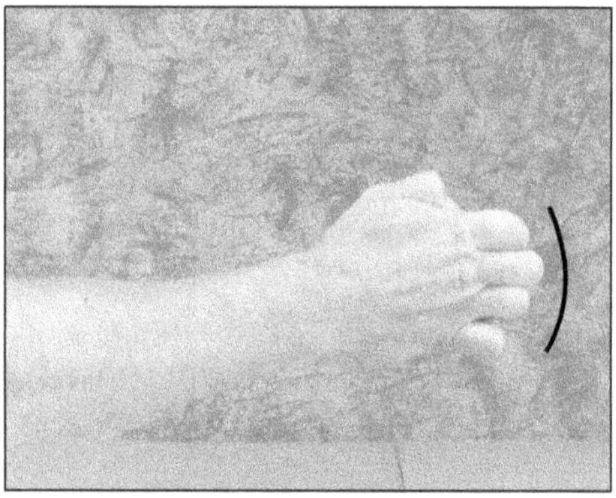

Figure 4-33 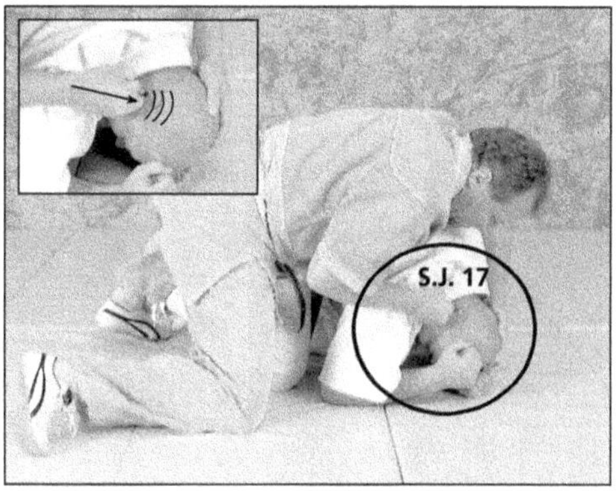 Figure 4-34

(ii) Striking Hand Tools:

a) Finger Tools

Knuckle Punches and Their Applications
- One finger (dragon fist) punch (Figure 4-31) to eye, ear, throat.
- Root knuckle (first two knuckles) punch (Figure 4-32) to nose, chin.
- Fore knuckle strike (Figure 4-33) to throat.

Figure 4-34: Grey uses a single knuckle punch to White's ear (S.J. 17).
Figure 4-35: Grey punches White's chin (REN 24) with a root knuckle punch.

Finger Tip Strikes and Their Applications
One, two, four finger strikes (to throat, eyes, Figure 4-36)
Figure 4-37: Grey punches White's throat (REN 22) with a double finger poke.

Chapter 4: Body Tools and Vulnerable Points

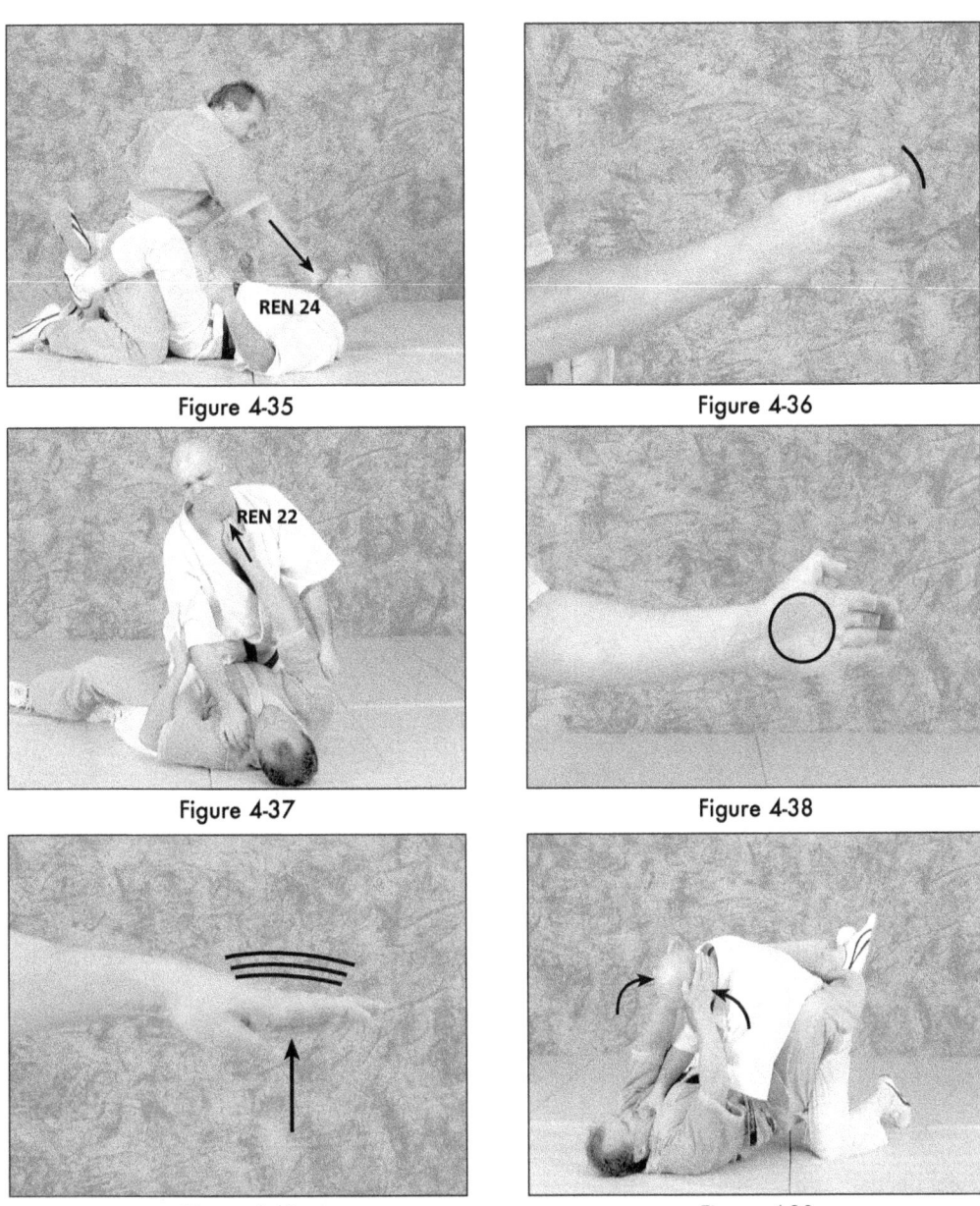

Figure 4-35

Figure 4-36

Figure 4-37

Figure 4-38

Figure 4-40

Figure 4-39

b) Flat of Hand Tools

Hand Palm Slap and Its Applications
• Palm slap (Figure 4-38) to ears, side of neck.

Figure 4-39: Grey slaps White's ears from both sides. The painful percussive effect of this will be to break White's eardrums and severely impair his balance and will to fight.

153

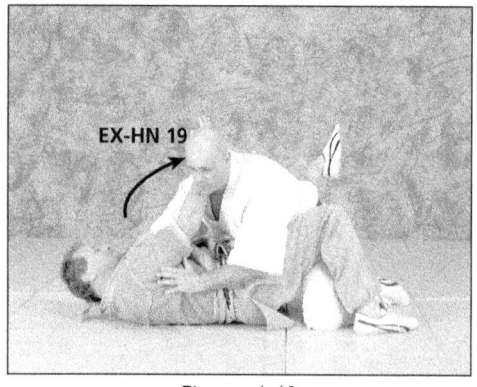

Figure 4-41

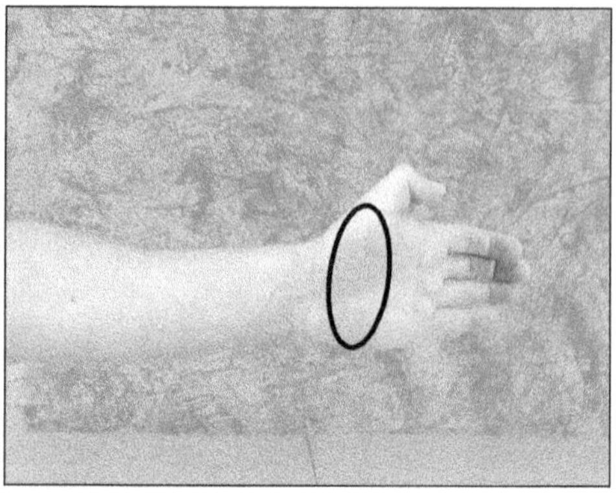

Figure 4-42

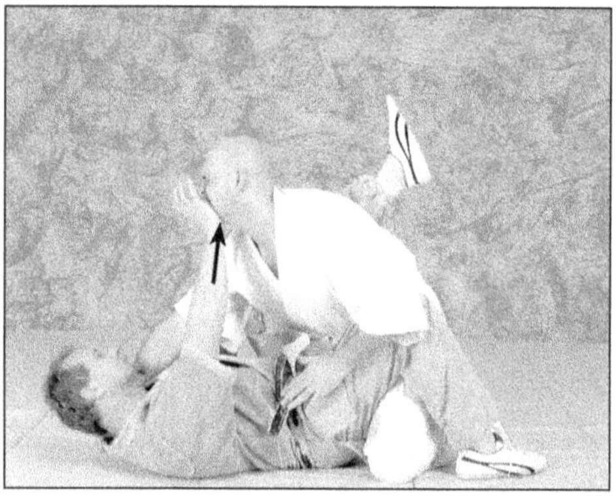

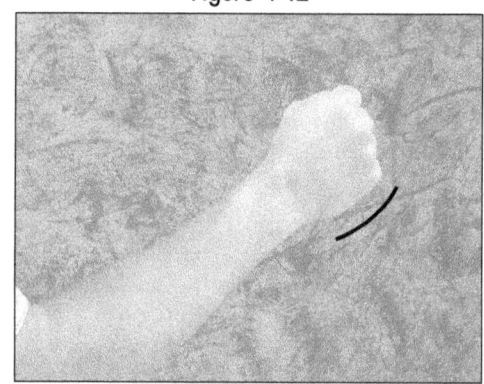

Figure 4-43

Figure 4-44

Back of Hand Slap and Its Applications
- Back of hand slap (Figure 4-40) to ears, nose, neck.

Figure 4-41: Grey applies a back of hand/forearm strike to the side of White's neck (EX-HN 19). This brachial plexus stunning technique will serve to weaken his resolve.

c) Base of Hand Tools

Palm Heel Strike and Its Applications
- Palm heel strike (Figure 4-42) to solar plexus, brachial plexus, nose.

Figure 4-43: Grey punches upward against White's exposed chin with the palm heel of his hand.

Top of Wrist Strikes and Their Applications
- Back fist strike (Figure 4-44) to temple, nose.
- Top of wrist (Figure 4-44) to throat, solar plexus.

Figure 4-45. Grey attacks White's neck with a back fist strike.

Edge of Hand Strikes and Their Applications
- Knife hand strike (baby finger side, open hand) edge (Figure 4-46) to clavicle, back of neck.

Chapter 4: Body Tools and Vulnerable Points

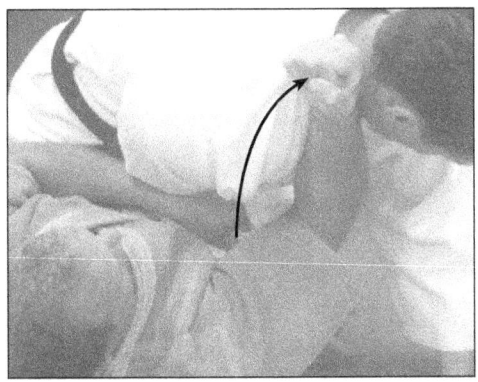

Figure 4-45

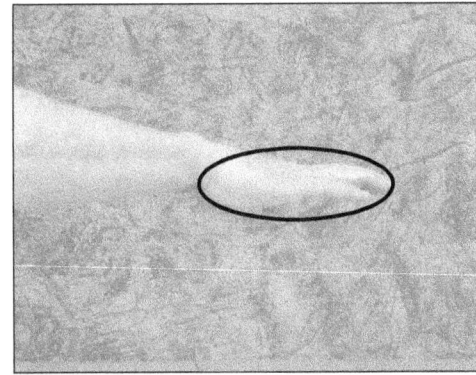

Figure 4-46

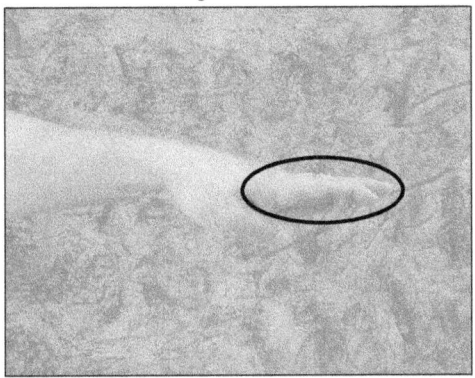

Figure 4-47

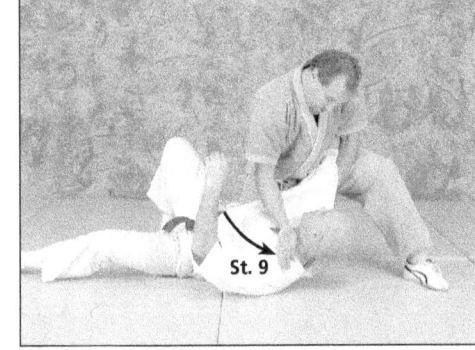

Figure 4-48

- Ridge hand strike (thumb side, open hand) edge (Figure 4-47) to nose, testicles.
- Hammer fist strike (baby finger side, closed fist) (Figure 4-44) to jaw, floating ribs, kidneys, top of head.

Figure 4-48: Grey attacks White's neck (St. 9) with a knife hand strike.

Figure 4-49: Grey applies a hammer fist strike to the top of White's head (DU 20).

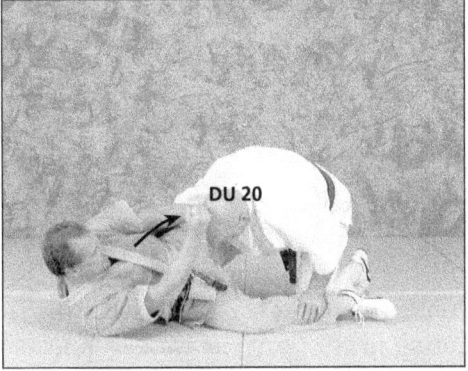

Figure 4-49

Arm Tools:

The arm is comprised of the lower forearm (radius and ulnar bones) and the upper arm (humerus bone), connected at the elbow joint. The upper arm is in turn connected to the torso at the shoulder joint. There are six arm muscles and fifteen smaller muscles that work the fingers, all with their concomitant tendons and ligaments. The arm tools are often used in conjunction with the gripping hands, but they may also be powered by other muscles or through the use of body weight.

155

Chin Na In Ground Fighting

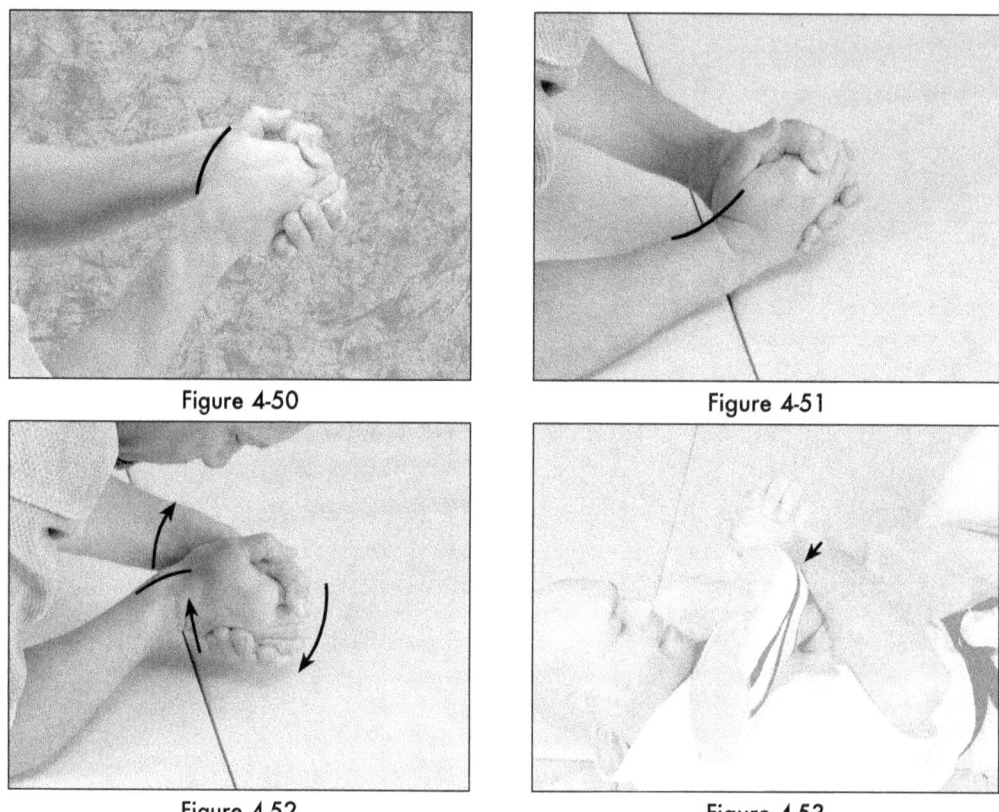

Figure 4-50
Figure 4-51
Figure 4-52
Figure 4-53

(i) Pressing Arm Tools:

   a) Wrist Tools

      Inner Wrist Press and Its Applications
- Radial edge wrist lever (Figure 4-50) to side of neck, mid-calf, Achilles tendon.

Figures 4-51 to 4-52. Grey demonstrates how the wrist lever works. When applying a two-handed gripping technique involving the application of pressure by the radial edge of the wrist, firstly cinch up the hold with the arms with the wrists unflexed (wrists bent away from the target as shown in Figure 4-51). After the arms bring in the wrists as close as possible to the target, then apply the wrist lever by flexing the wrists inwards to the target, thereby applying tremendous pressure into the target (Figure 4-52). This technique has many applications such as with neck restraint, heel locks, etc. Notice how Grey's right wrist moves from a concave to a convex shape upon application. Both the left hand and the mat anchors the right hand in place while the right hand twists clockwise in the palmar plane. The left hand also augments this twisting action. Although the wrist only moves a matter of a

Chapter 4: Body Tools and Vulnerable Points

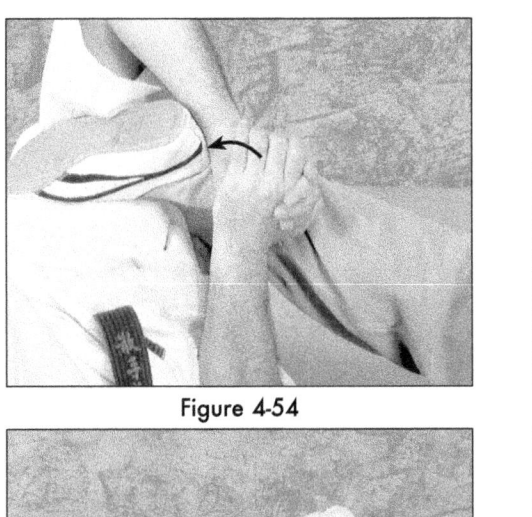

Figure 4-54

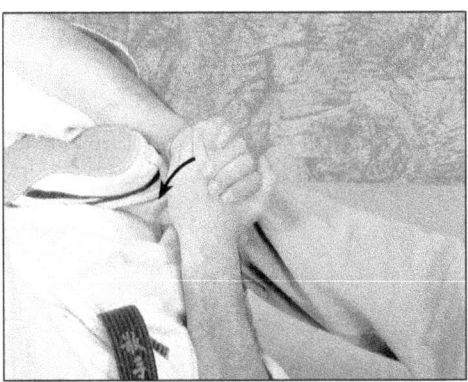

Figure 4-55

Figure 4-56

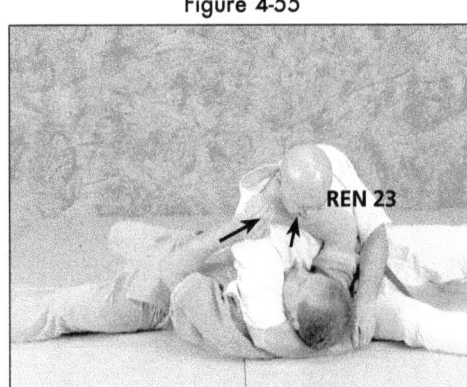

Figure 4-57

few inches at most, this slight movement of the wrist inward translates into extreme pressure when all the slack of the technique has been removed by arm pressure prior to its application.

Figure 4-53: White bridges the top of Grey's foot on his shoulder and applies the radial edge of his wrist to Grey's Achilles tendon using a heel hook technique. This bony edge gouges into Grey's tendon causing significant pain, particularly when the wrist lever is applied.

Figures 4-54 to 4-55: In a similar move, White has hooked Grey's heel and traps Grey's foot in his armpit. He applies a scooping action inward and upward to apply pressure on Grey's Achilles tendon.

Outer Wrist Press and its Applications
• Ulnar edge scissors (Figure 4-56) press to sides of neck.

Figure 4-57: Grey uses a framing technique to keep White from effectively headlocking him, by placing his right wrist/forearm across White's throat (REN 23), Grey can apply pressure to White's neck by White's own squeezing.

157

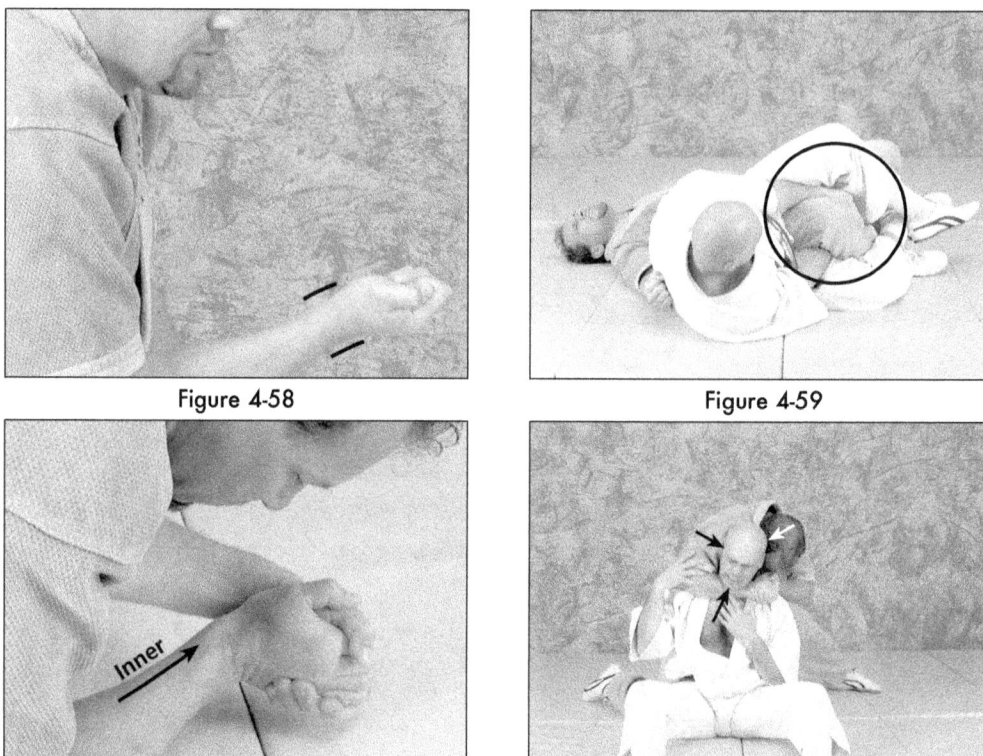

Figure 4-58

Figure 4-59

Figure 4-60

Figure 4-61

Top/Bottom Wrist Press and Its Applications
- Top and bottom wrist pressing (Figure 4-58) across the throat, to knee joints passively.

Figure 4-59: White has Grey's right leg in a leg scissors and he has inserted his own right wrist into the crook of Grey's knee in order to apply a knee block. When White flexes Grey's knee, the block will cause great pressure on the knee joint, dislocating it in the process.

b) Forearm Tools

Inner Forearm Press and Its Applications
- Radial edge press (Figure 4-60) all sides of neck, mid-calf.

Figure 4-61: Grey uses the radial edge of his forearm to apply excruciatingly painful choking pressure to White's throat (REN 23). Notice how Grey presses his head and shoulder into the back of White's head/neck in order to stabilize the head and to defeat rear head butts.

Figure 4-62: White uses the radial edge of his forearm to apply pressure to Grey's Achilles tendon, having figure-foured Grey's left leg to also effect a leg lock.

Outer Forearm Press and Its Applications
- Ulnar edge press (Figure 4-63) to throat, all sides of neck.

Chapter 4: Body Tools and Vulnerable Points

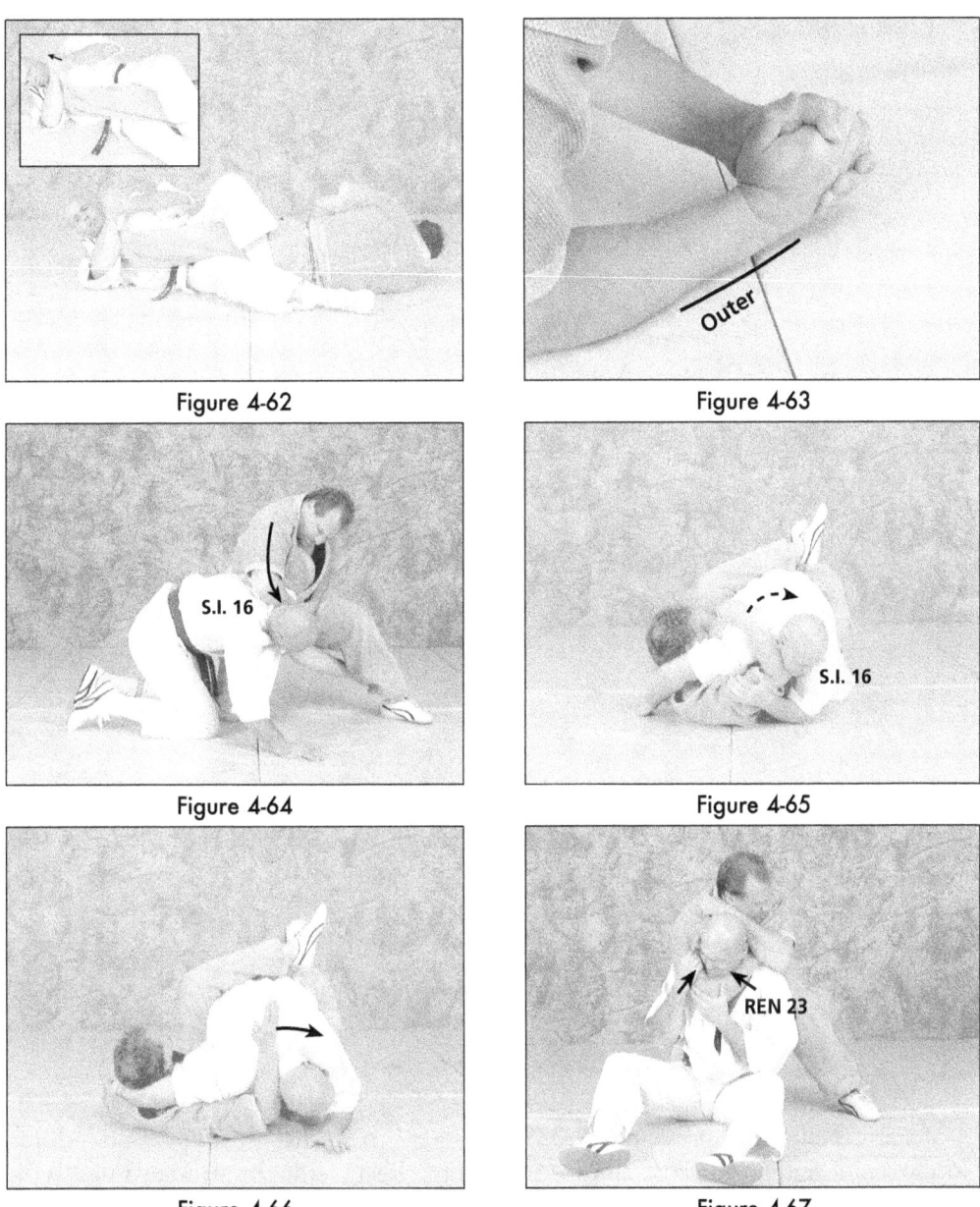

Figure 4-62

Figure 4-63

Figure 4-64

Figure 4-65

Figure 4-66

Figure 4-67

Figure 4-64: Grey is pulling on White's right collar to increase the pressure exerted on the left side of White's neck (S.I. 16) with his right ulnar edge of his forearm. Grey may be able to render White unconscious by sealing the vein using this technique.

Figures 4-65 to 4-66: Grey uses the ulnar edge of his right arm to the right side of White's neck (S.I. 16) in order to prevent White's attack on him.

Figure 4-67: Grey uses neck restraint with chancery in order to both seal the vein and seal the breath. Notice how the ulnar edge of Grey's left arm presses against the

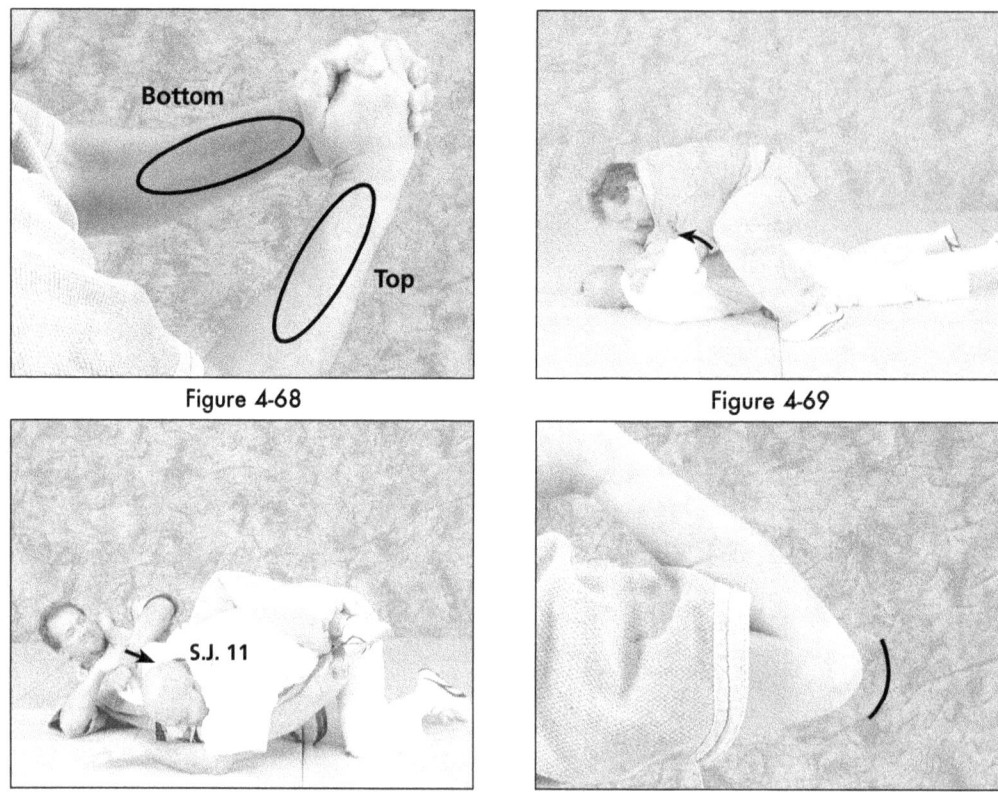

Figure 4-68

Figure 4-69

Figure 4-70

Figure 4-71

back of White's neck (DU 16) forcing White's throat (REN 23) into the crook of Grey's right arm.

Top of Upper Arm Press and Their Applications
• Top arm press (Figure 4-68) arm locks, leg locks.

Figure 4-69: Grey uses the top of his left upper arm to press White's forearm toward his own head in a bent arm lock.

Bottom of Upper Arm Locks and Their Applications
• Bottom arm press (Figure 4-68) arm locks, leg locks.

Figure 4-70: Grey uses the bottom of his left forearm to press down on White's straightened right arm at the elbow (S.J. 11) to effect a straight arm bar hug.

c) Elbow Tools

Elbow Joint Press and Its Applications
• Elbow press (Figure 4-71) to sternum, ribs, spine.

Figure 4-72: Grey uses his right elbow to grind into White's spine as he levers White's right arm upward.

Chapter 4: Body Tools and Vulnerable Points

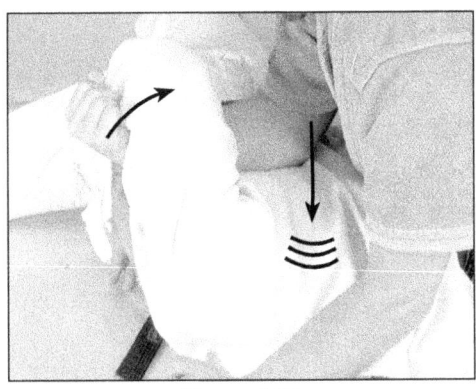

Figure 4-72

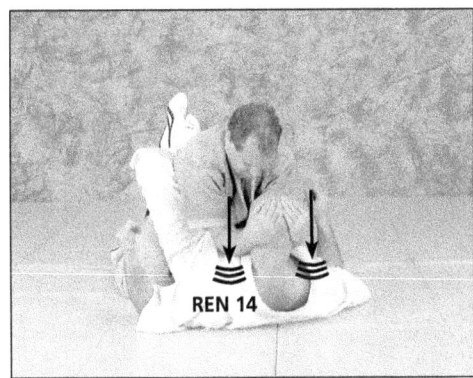

Figure 4-73

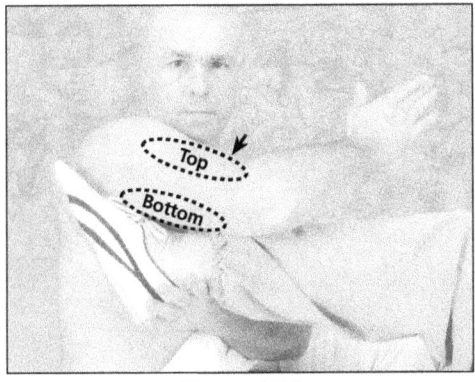

Figure 4-74

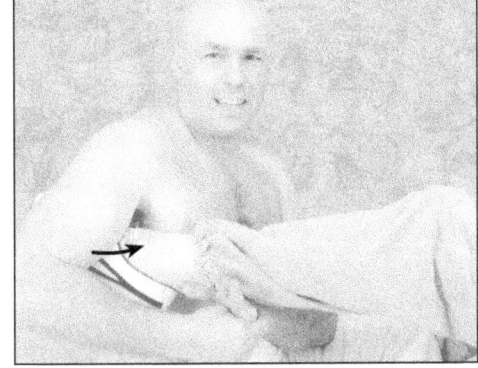

Figure 4-75

Figure 4-73: Grey digs both of his elbows into White's chest (REN 14) as he levers White's head forward.

d) Upper Arm Tools

Bottom of Upper Arm Press and Its Applications
- Arm Press (Figure 4-74) to arm, to sides of foot.

Figure 4-75: White uses the bottom of his right arm to squeeze Grey's foot in order to apply an ankle lock.

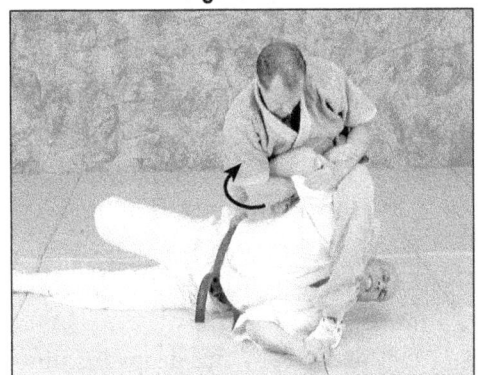

Figure 4-76

Figure 4-76: Grey uses the bottom of his right inner arm to press White's lower right arm clockwise in order to effect a shoulder crank.

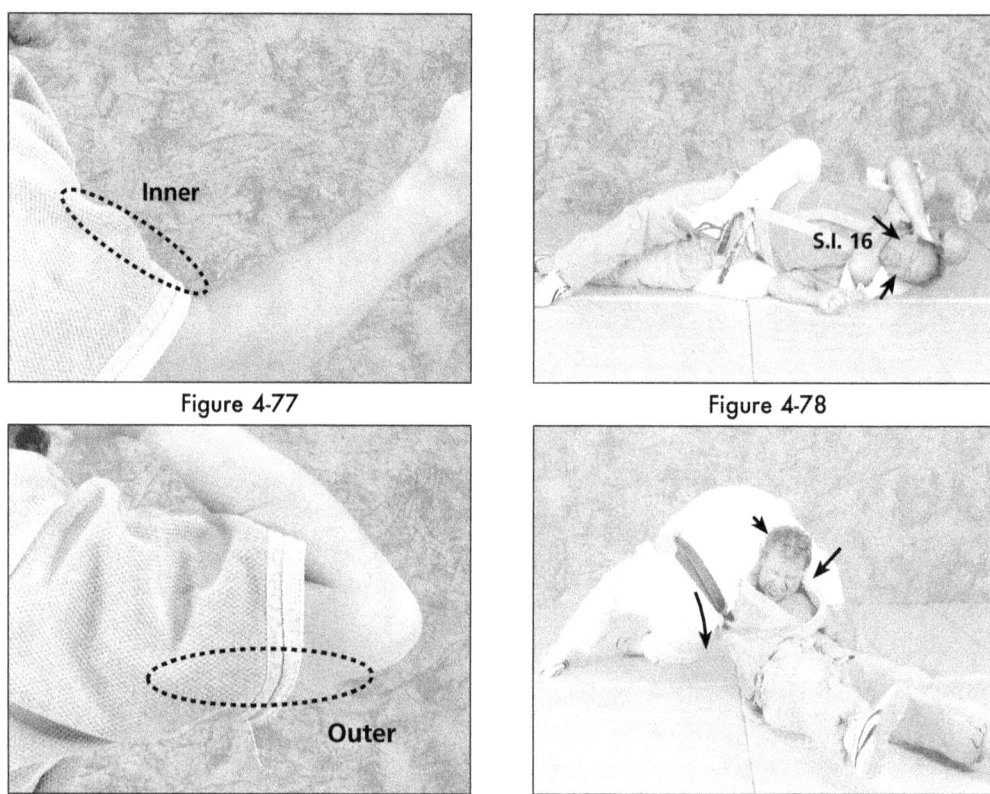

Figure 4-77
Figure 4-78
Figure 4-79
Figure 4-80

Inner Upper Arm Press and Its Application
• Biceps press (Figure 4-77) neck restraint to sides of neck.

Figure 4-78: White uses his left inner arm to press into the right side of Grey's neck (S.I. 16) in order to effect neck restraint on him.

Outer Upper Arm Press and Its Applications
• Upper arm press (Figure 4-79) to neck.

Figure 4-80: White uses his ribs and right outer upper arm to press backward against the back of Grey's neck while effecting a death lock on him. Use extreme caution.

Figure 4-81: White drops his outer upper arm downward against Grey's throat (REN 23) while effecting a straight arm bar on him.

e) Shoulder Tools

Shoulder Joint Press and Its Applications
• Armpit press (Figure 4-79) to upper arm, leg, back of neck.

Figure 4-82: Grey uses his right shoulder joint to press against White's left upper back/shoulder in order to effect an armpit hold.

Figure 4-83: Grey uses his armpits to press White's ankles downward as he presses upward with his forearms in order to effect the Boston Crab on him.

Chapter 4: Body Tools and Vulnerable Points

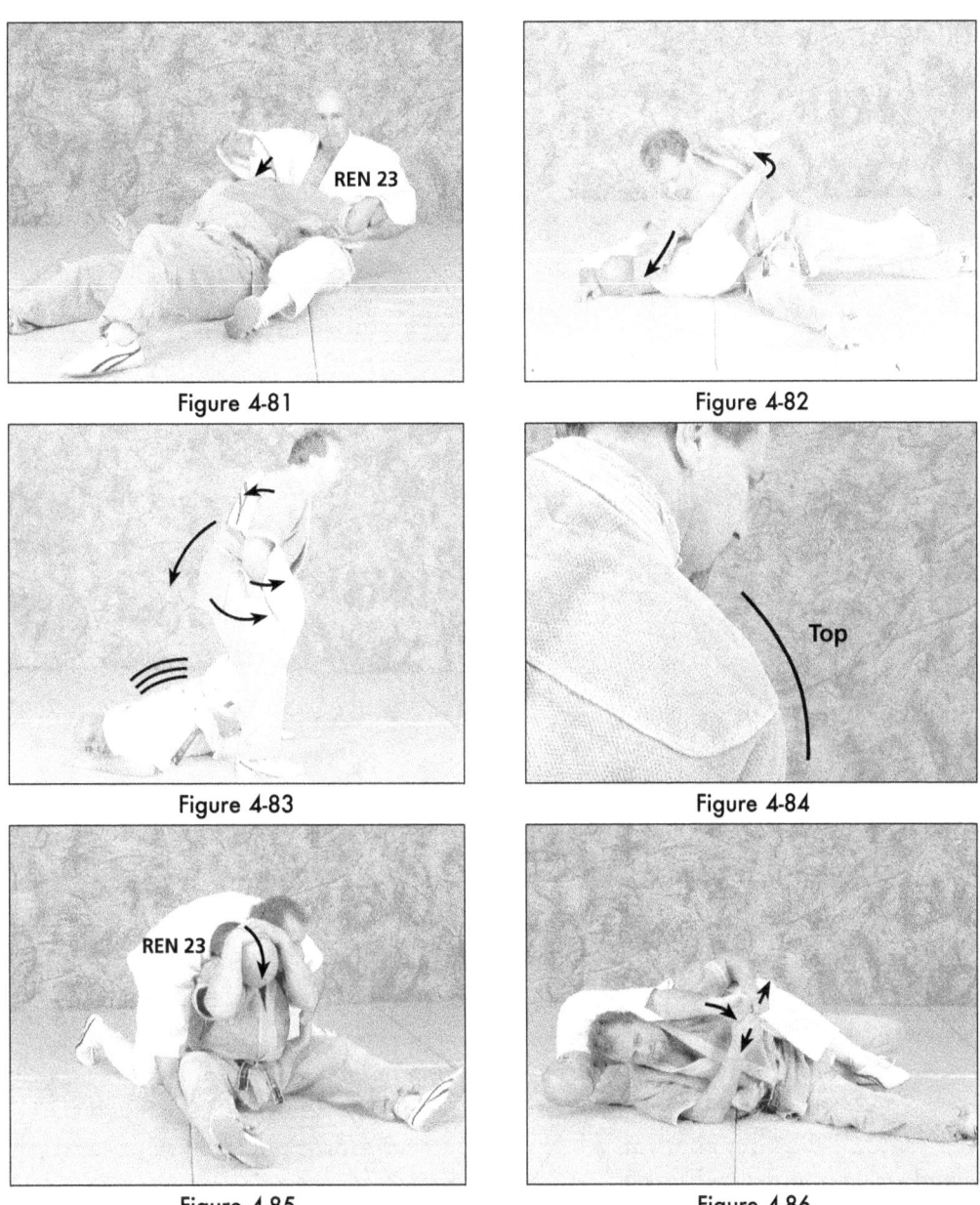

Figure 4-81

Figure 4-82

Figure 4-83

Figure 4-84

Figure 4-85

Figure 4-86

Top of Shoulder Press and Its Applications
• Shoulder press (Figure 4-84) to throat, arm.

Figure 4-85: Grey chokes White by pulling his head down. Grey forces White's throat (REN 23) down onto the top of Grey's shoulder.

Figure 4-86: Grey uses the top of his left shoulder as a fulcrum in order to effect a straight arm lock on White by pulling his left arm down. Note the use of finger-splitting Qin Na while doing so.

Chin Na In Ground Fighting

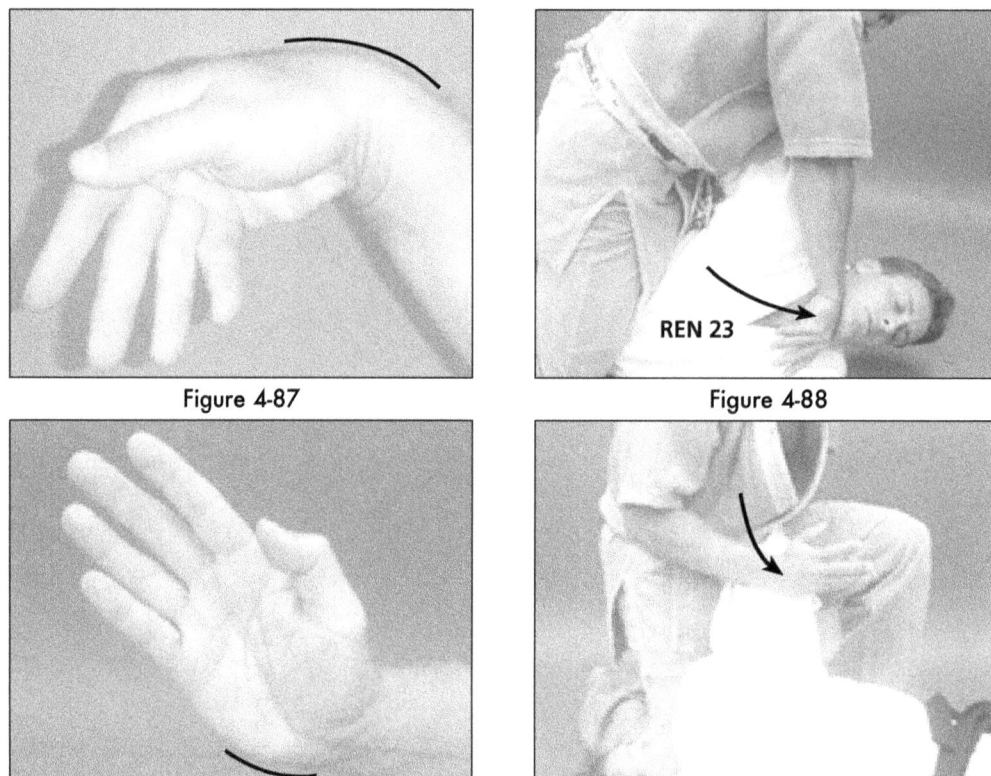

Figure 4-87 Figure 4-88

Figure 4-89 Figure 4-90

(ii) Striking Arm Tools

a) Wrist Joint Tools

Inside of Wrist Joint Strike and Its Applications
- Chicken head wrist strike (Figure 4-87) to throat.

Figure 4-88: Grey kneels over White and strikes his vulnerable throat area with a chicken head wrist strike.

Outside of Wrist Joint Strike and Its Applications
- Ox jaw hand strike (Figure 4-89) to the clavicle, sides of neck.

Figure 4-90: Grey chops at White's straightened arm at the elbow with an ox jaw hand strike in order to break it.

Top of Wrist Joint Strike and Its Application
- Crane head strike (Figure 4-91) to the chin, solar plexus.

Figure 4-92: Grey strikes at the side of White's jaw with a crane head strike as he tries to pass his guard.

Bottom of Wrist Joint Strike and Its Applications
- Palm heel strike (Figure 4-93) to the solar plexus, temple, ear.

Chapter 4: Body Tools and Vulnerable Points

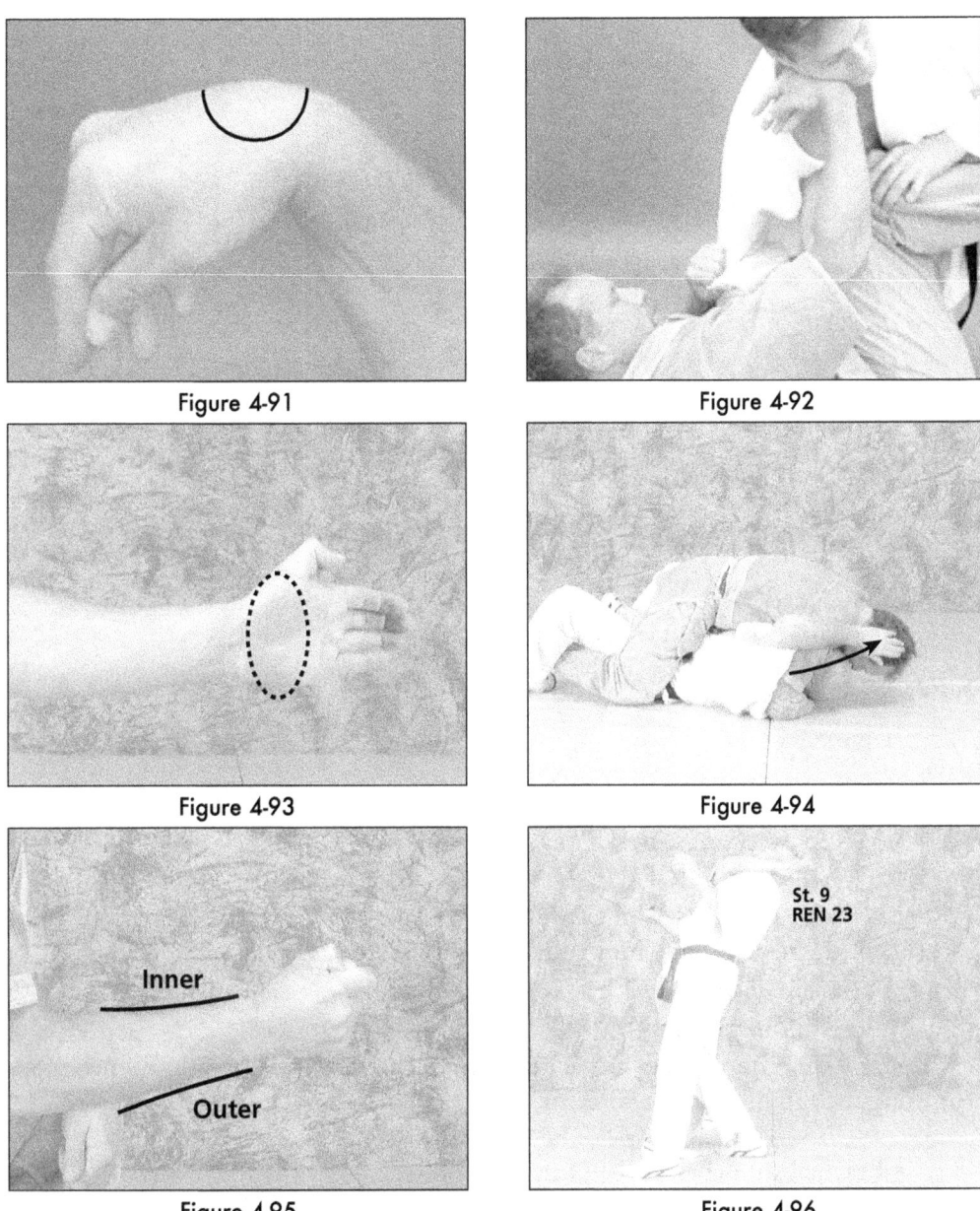

Figure 4-91

Figure 4-92

Figure 4-93

Figure 4-94

Figure 4-95

Figure 4-96

Figure 4-94: White applies a palm heel strike to Grey's right ear in order to escape a painful neck hold.

b) Forearm Tools

Inner Forearm Strike and Its Applications
• Clothesline strike (Figure 4-95) to throat.

Figure 4-96: Grey applies a clothesline strike to White's throat (St. 9, REN 23) in order to effect a takedown.

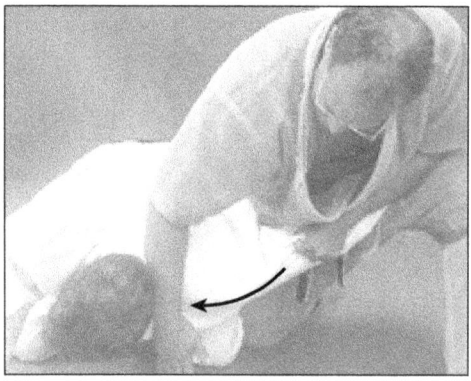

Figure 4-97 Figure 4-98

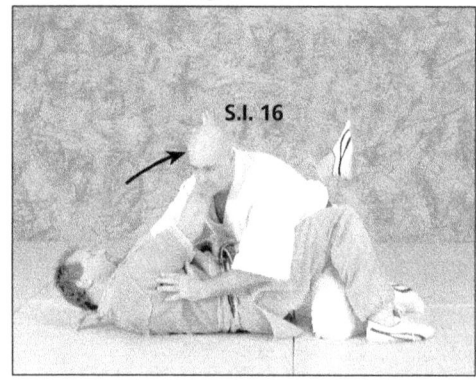
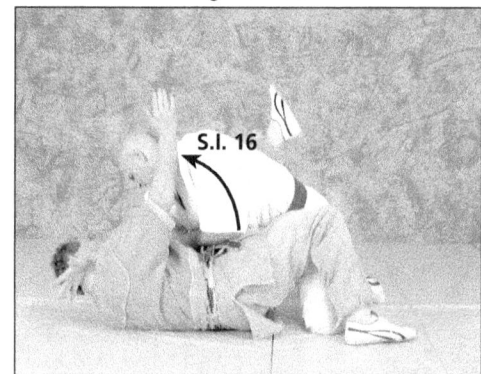

Figure 4-99 Figure 4-100

Outer Forearm Strike and Its Applications
- Forearm chop (Figure 4-95) to throat.

Figure 4-97: Grey has White in an arm bar and he uses a forearm chop to the backside of the neck to stun him before moving into *waki gatame*.

Top of Forearm Strike and Its Applications
- Brachial stun (Figure 4-98) to sides of neck.

Figure 4-99: Grey applies a brachial stun to the right side of White's neck (S.I. 16) using the top of his right forearm.

Bottom of Forearm Strike and its Applications
- Brachial stun (Figure 4-98) to sides of neck.

Figure 4-100: Grey applies a brachial stun to the left side of White's neck (S.I. 16) using the bottom of his right forearm.

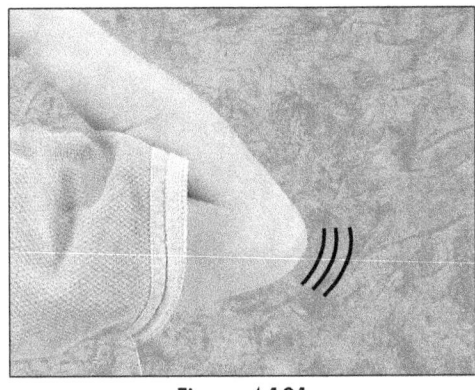

Figure 4-101

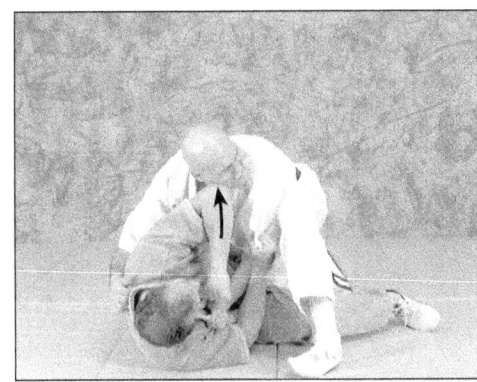

Figure 4-102

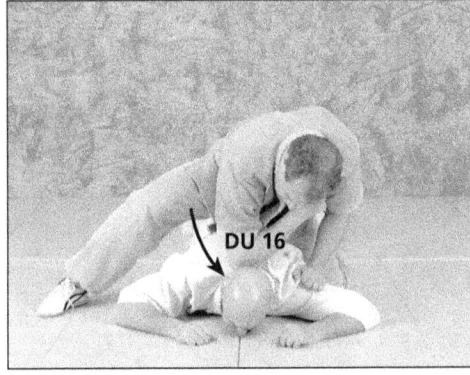

Figure 4-103

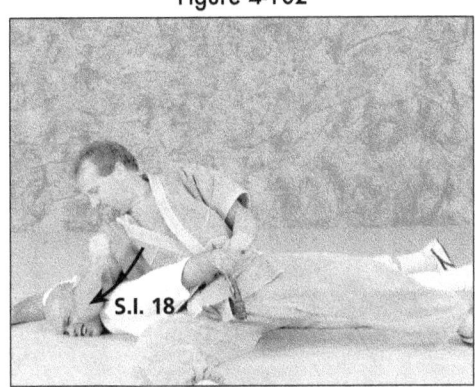

Figure 4-104

c) Elbow Tools

Elbow Joint Strikes and Their Applications
- Elbow strikes (Figure 4-101) in all directions and to most parts of the body.

Figure 4-102: Grey uses an elbow strike into White's right cheekbone (S.I. 18) from a bottom position as White advances upon him.

Figure 4-103: Grey applies a downward elbow strike to the back of White's neck (DU 16) as he lies prostate on the ground.

Figure 4-104: Grey strikes the left side of White's head (S.I. 18) with a reclining right elbow.

Chin Na In Ground Fighting

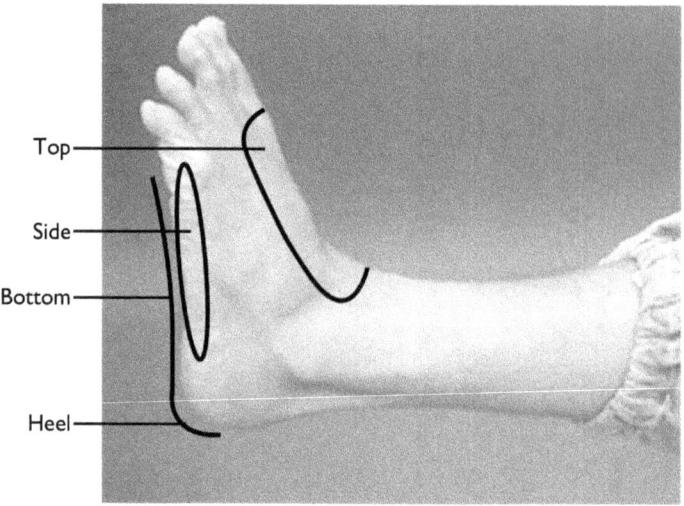

Figure 4-105

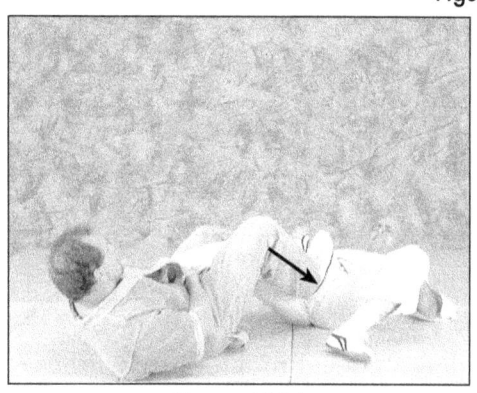

Figure 4-106

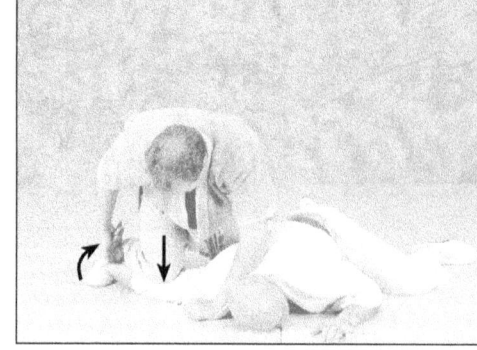

Figure 4-107

Leg Tools

The various parts of the legs can also be used to press or strike your opponent. Ground fighters will be far more familiar with using these tools than the Qin Na practitioner. With practice, these tools can be added to your fighting arsenal.

(i) Pressing Leg Tools

a) Foot Tools

Outside of Foot Press and Its Application
- Press (Figure 4-105) to groin.

Figure 4-106: Grey uses the outside edge of his right foot to press against White's groin during the execution of an ankle lock.

Top of Foot Press and Its Application
- Press (Figure 4-105) top of wrist onto foot.

168

Chapter 4: Body Tools and Vulnerable Points

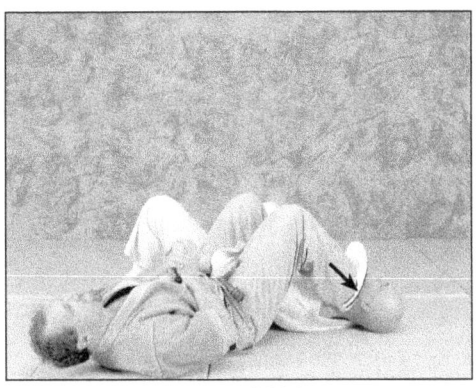

Figure 4-108

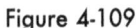

Figure 4-109

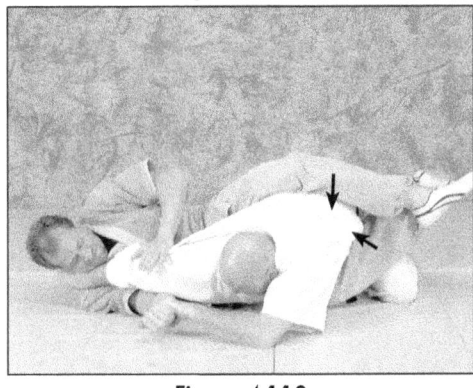

Figure 4-110

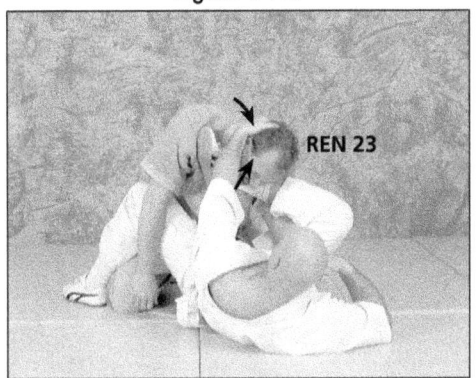

Figure 4-111

Figure 4-107: Grey wedges his right foot under White's right wrist to create a bridge so that his knee pressure on this arm will hyperextend White's right arm.

Bottom of Foot Press and Its Application
- Press (Figure 4-105) to sides of neck.

Figure 4-108: Grey uses the bottom of his right foot to press against the left side of White's neck while applying an arm bar to White's left arm.

b) Lower Leg Tools

Inside of Lower Leg Press and Its Application
- Leg scissors (Figure 4-109) around torso, neck.

Figure 4-110: Grey applies leg scissors to White's torso while trying to put on a straight arm bar on White's right arm.

Top of Lower Leg Press and Its Applications
- Shin press (Figure 109) to throat, calf.

Figure 4-111: White presses Grey's throat into his right shin press (REN 23) by grabbing the back of Grey's head.

169

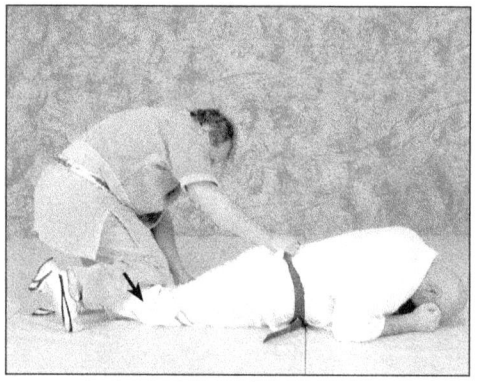

Figure 4-112

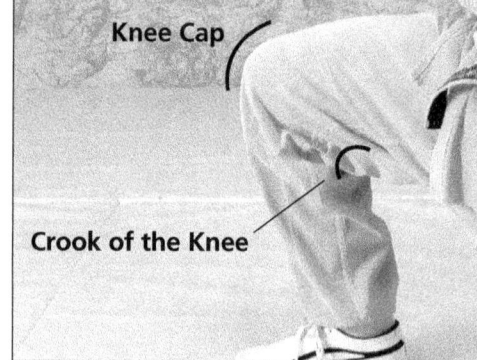

Figure 4-113

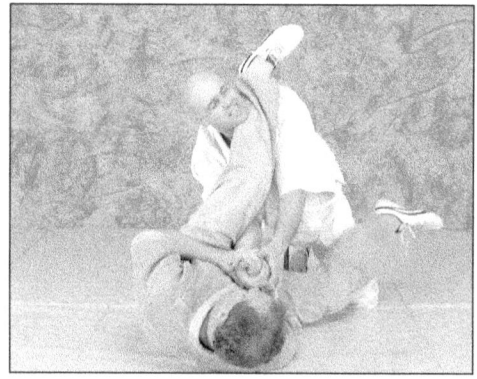

Figure 4-114

Figure 4-115

Figure 4-112: Grey uses his right shin to press against White's right calf (U.B. 56, U.B. 57).

Bottom of Lower Leg Press and Its Applications
• Triangle choke (Figure 4-109) to back of neck.

Figure 4-113: Grey has White in a triangle choke. Grey's bottom right lower leg presses against the back of White's neck. Grey can flex his calf muscle to increase the pressure on White's neck.

Figure 4-114: Grey uses the bottom of his left lower leg to hook White's neck and draw him over onto his back in order to effect an arm bar on White's right arm.

c) Knee Tools

Knee Cap Press and Its Applications
• Press (Figure 4-115) to torso.

Figure 4-116: White uses his right kneecap to press on Grey's right rib cage (G.B. 24). White can intensify this pressure by transferring his weight onto Grey and by pulling his own body down onto Grey by cupping the back of Grey's head and grabbing Grey's right lower leg.

Chapter 4: Body Tools and Vulnerable Points

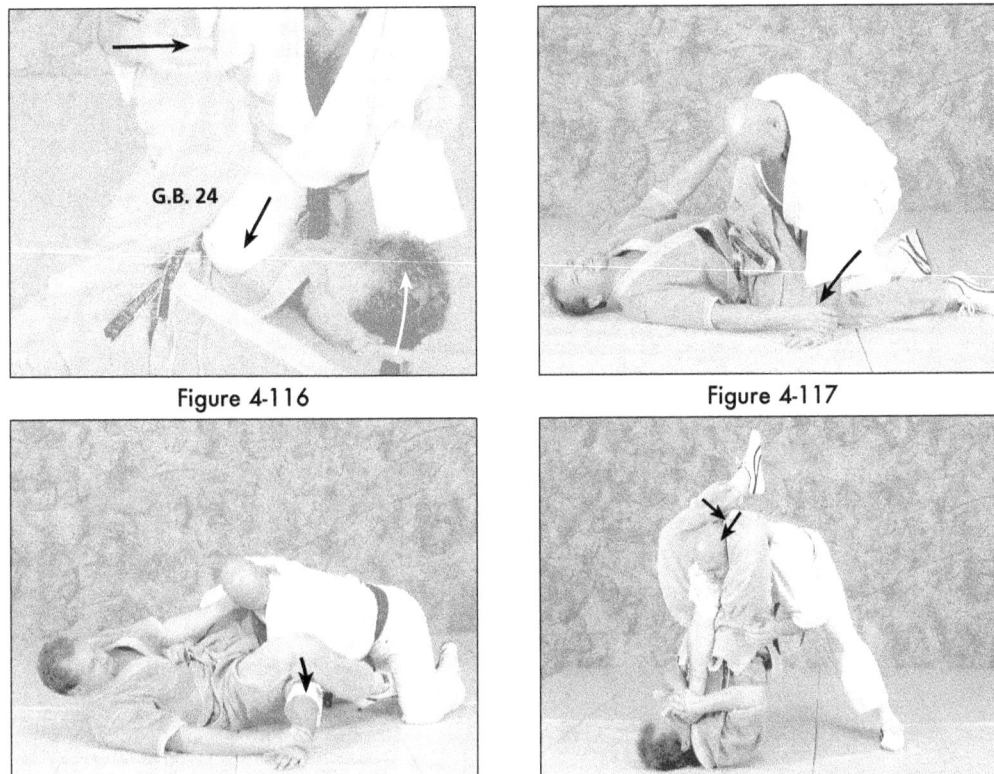

Figure 4-116

Figure 4-117

Figure 4-118

Figure 4-119

Figure 4-117: White knees on Grey's right inner thigh (Sp. 11) while making a positional change.

Crook of Knee Press and Its Applications

Press (Figure 4-115) arm lock and to back of neck in triangular choke.

Figure 4-118: Grey uses the crook of his right knee to press down onto White's straightened arm in order to effect a straight arm lock. Notice how Grey anchors his right foot under White's left thigh. He merely has to straighten this leg to break Grey's arm at the elbow.

Figure 4-119: Grey applies a triangle choke to White using the bottom of his right leg to press against the back of Grey's neck and using the bottom of his left leg to lock his own right leg in place. Grey also simultaneously tries to effect a straight arm bar to White's right arm.

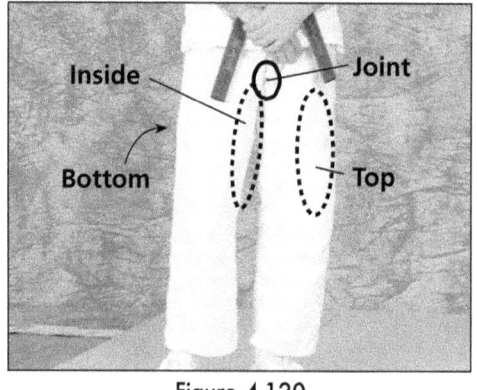

Figure 4-120

Figure 4-121

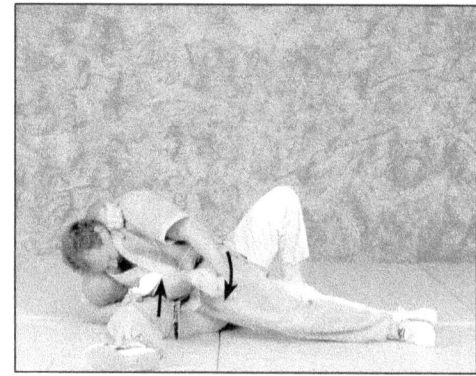

Figure 4-122

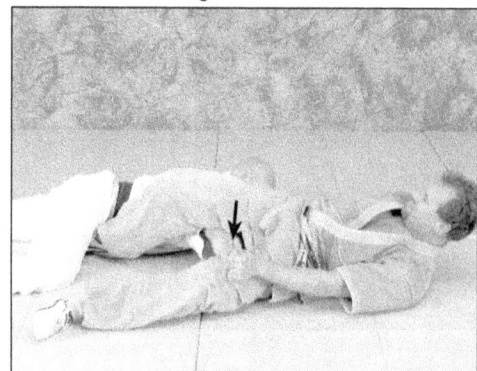

Figure 4-123

d) Upper Leg Tools

Inside of Upper Leg Press and Its Application
- Pressing fists (Figure 4-120) into sides of neck as a counter to a choke.

Figure 4-121 White scissors Grey's torso to control his movement.

Top of Upper Leg Press and Its Application
- Press down (Figure 4-120) with arm as with the scarf hold.

Figure 4-122: Grey uses the top of his right thigh as a fulcrum in order to effect a straight arm bar on White while he has him in a scarf hold. Notice Grey's use of finger Qin Na to enhance his control over White's right arm.

Bottom of Upper Leg Press and Its Application
- Press (Figure 4-120) to leg in leg lock.

Figure 4-123: Grey applies a straight arm bar to White's right arm using the bottom of his right thigh. Grey has anchored his right foot under White's right thigh. Grey need only to straighten his leg in order to break White's arm at the elbow.

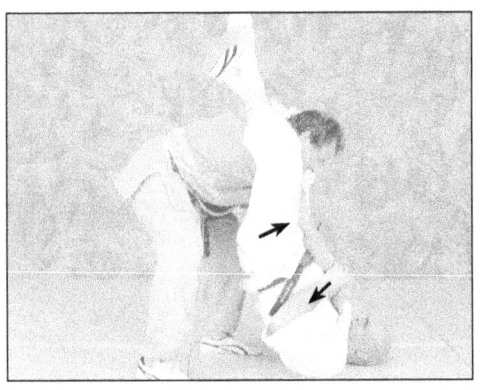

Figure 4-124 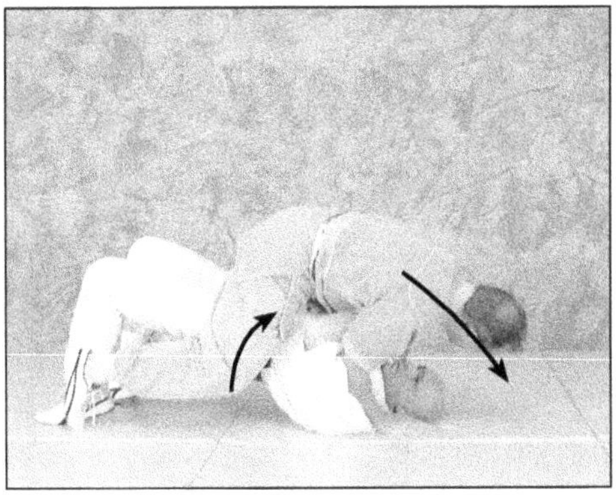   Figure 4-125

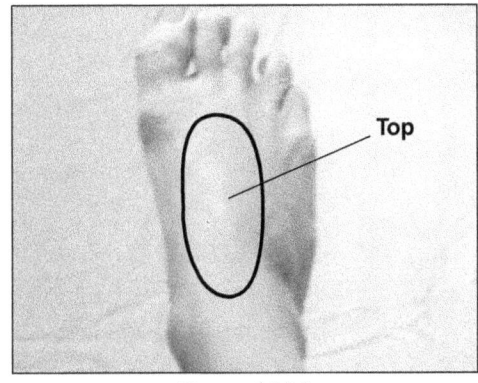

Figure 4-126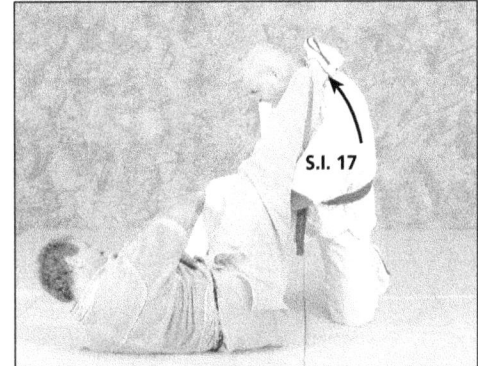

Figure 4-127

e) Hip Tools

Hip Joint Press and Its Application
- Press (Figure 4-120) to back of elbow in inverted arm bar.

Figure 4-124: White uses his pelvic joint to press against the back of Grey's right elbow during the application of an inverted straight arm bar.

Figure 4-125: White bucks Grey off of him by bridging his body, thrusting his hips upward to displace Grey's center of gravity away from his own.

ii) Striking Leg Tools

a) Foot Tools

Top of Foot Strike and Its Application
- Roundhouse kick (Figure 4-126) to face, sides of neck.

Figure 4-127: Grey kicks White on the left side of his neck (S.I. 17) with a right roundhouse kick using the top of the foot/shin in order to repel White's advance.

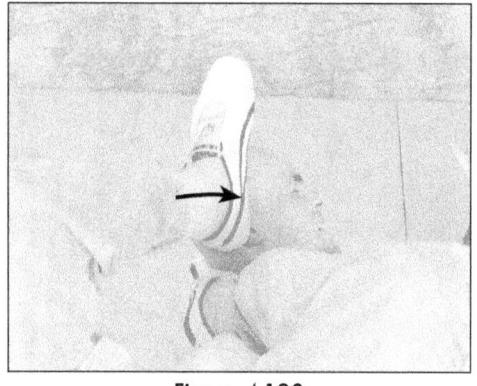

Figure 4-128   Figure 4-129

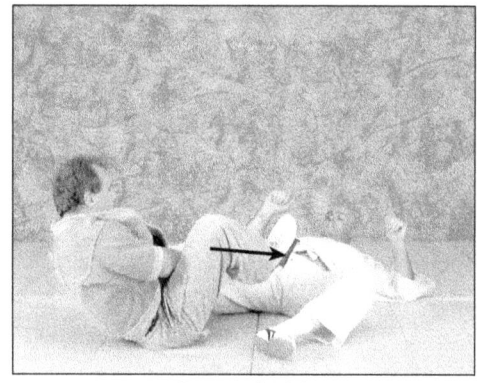

Figure 4-130   Figure 4-131

Bottom of Foot Strike and Its Application
• Stomp (Figure 4-105) to sides of neck.

Figure 4-128: Grey stomps the right side of White's head (S.J 17) with the bottom of his left foot.

Heel of Foot Strikes and Their Applications
• Stomp or thrust (Figure 4-105) to neck, groin, ribs, kidneys.

Figure 4-129: Grey applies a downward heel kick to White's face (DU 26, St. 1) while effecting a straight arm bar on White's left arm.

Figure 4-130: Grey stomps White's exposed groin while applying an ankle lock to White's right ankle.

Figures 4-131 and 4-132: Grey applies a heel kick to White's solar plexus (REN 14) while effecting a straight arm bar to White's left arm. Note the application of finger Qin Na to White's right hand.

Figure 4-133: Grey attacks White's throat (REN 23) with a distracting backward heel kick as he steps over White's head in order to apply a shoulder crank to White's right arm.

Chapter 4: Body Tools and Vulnerable Points

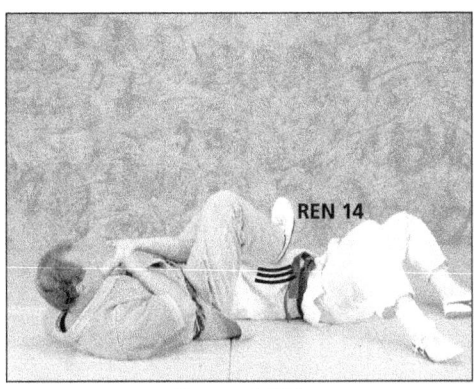

Figure 4-132

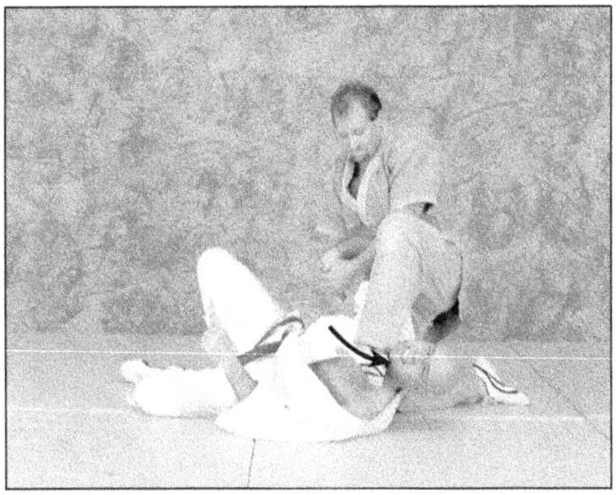

Figure 4-133

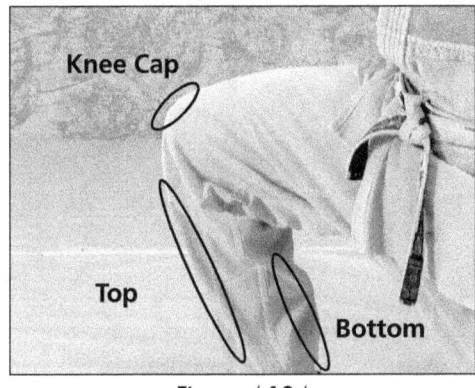

Figure 4-134

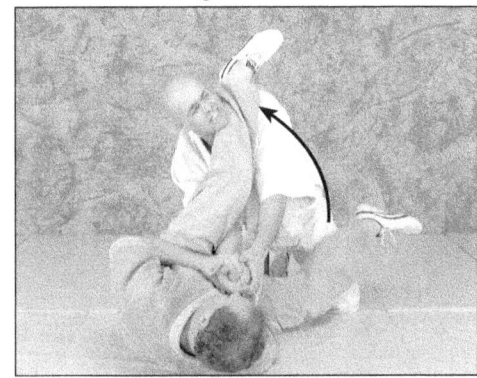

Figure 4-135

b) Lower Leg Tools

Top of Leg Strikes and Its Application
• Shin kick (Figure 4-134) to throat.

Figure 4-127: Grey kicks White in the head/neck with his shin.

Bottom of Leg Strike and Its Application
• Stomp (Figure 4-134) to throat.

Figure 4-135: Grey uses the bottom of his left lower left to apply a hook kick to White's neck to drop him over onto his back in order to effect an arm bar on White's right arm.

175

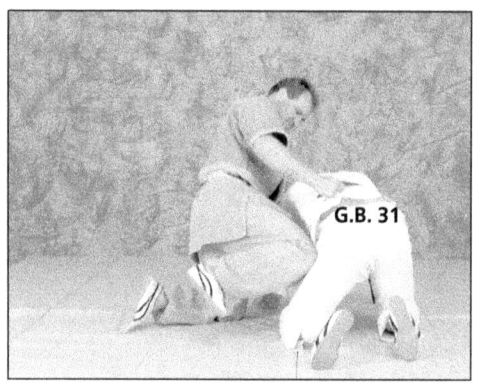
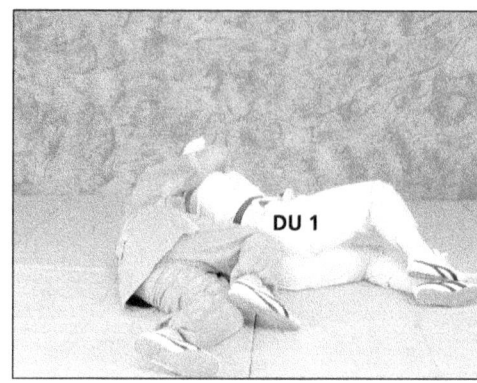

Figure 4-136   Figure 4-137

c) Knee Tools

Kneecap Strikes and Their Applications
- Knee strikes (Figure 4-134) to tail bone, ribs, face.

Figure 4-136: Grey drives a right knee strike into White's left outer thigh (G.B. 31) in order to reduce his mobility.

Figure 4-137: Grey drives a right knee strike into White's tailbone (DU 1) while lying on his left side.

Head Tools

To the Qin Na practitioner, the use of head tools may be unfamiliar. Ground fighters often use their heads for bridging, grinding, pushing, striking, and so on because their other limbs are often tied up.

(i) Pressing Head Tools

Any part of the skull and the point of the jaw (Figure 4-138) may be used to press on your opponent (grind the pressure points). The head is a useful tool in bridging the body, pushing (bulldozing) your opponent, levering, striking, holding, etc.

Head Press and Its Applications

Figure 4-139: Grey uses the front top of his head to push White over.

Figure 4-140: Grey uses the rear of his head to effect a body bridge while uprooting White.

Figure 4-141: Grey buries the right side of his head against the rear of White's head in order to prevent a reverse head butt while applying neck restraint. This pressing action of the head also stabilizes White's head during the execution of this technique.

Chapter 4: Body Tools and Vulnerable Points

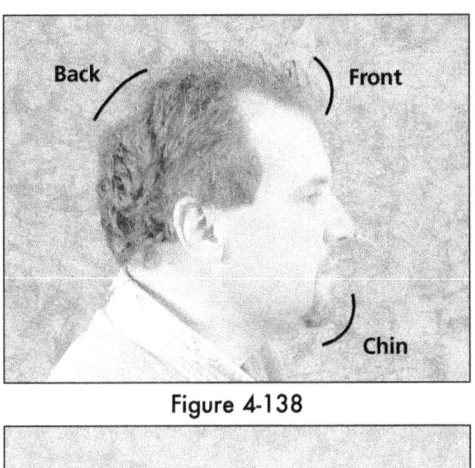

Figure 4-138

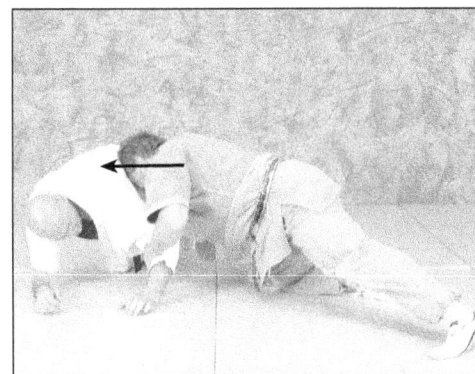

Figure 4-139

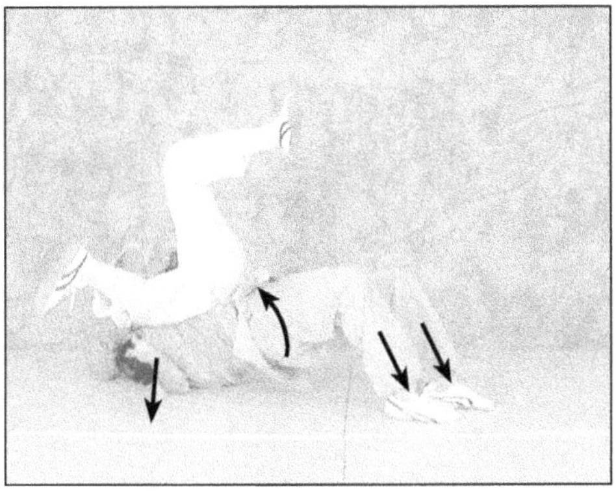

Figure 4-140

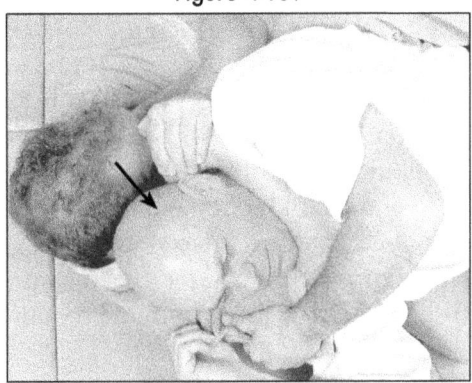

Figure 4-141

(ii) Striking Head Tools

The head can move 360 degrees about the spinal axis and swivel 180 degrees in the horizontal plane as well, making it a short range but versatile tool. Well-developed neck muscles enable powerful striking abilities. The head is a much overlooked and neglected tool that can have devastating and vicious in-fighting consequences. The head butt is affectionately known in some cultures as 'the Scottish handshake' or 'nutting' and it is often used as a 'sucker blow'. Indeed, the unwary can pay a brutal price for their ignorance about this deceptively innocuous and powerful tool.

If you literally go head to head with an opponent (as in a clinching situation), press your head against his to keep from being head butted. If your opponent is giving you the space to move your head freely, then attack his jaw, teeth (be careful of cuts and blood born pathogens!), temple, bridge of nose, eye socket, etc. The best place to deliver a head strike with is the thicker frontal area of the forehead but the back of the head can be used to deliver a reverse head strike as well. The face is a good target-rich area. Bear in mind that the skull is thinnest at the temple should serious incapacitation be required.

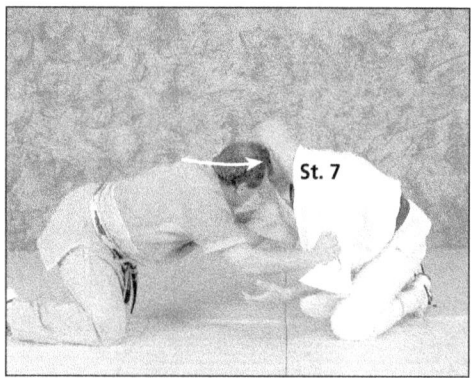

Figure 4-142

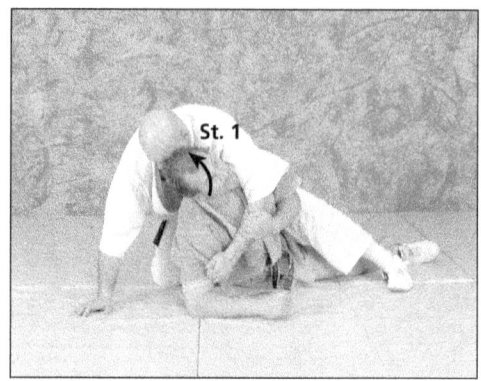

Figure 4-143

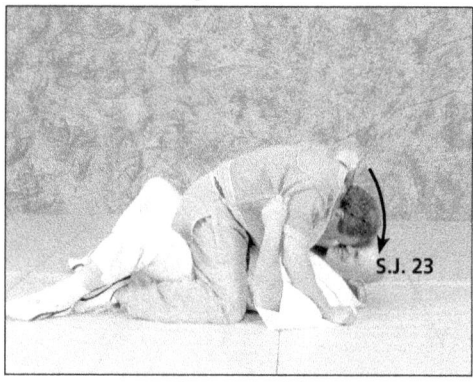

Figure 4-144

Head Strikes and Their Applications

Figure 4-142: Grey applies a head butt to the side of White's head (St. 7) from kneeling position.

Figure 4-143: Grey applies a reverse head butt to White's face (St.1).

Figure 4-144: Grey head butts White's head (S.J. 23) from the mounted position.

Torso Tools

The torso is the heaviest yet the softest of all the available categories of body tools. It is however, used as a power base for all of the other tools. The torso is reliant on the appendages for mobility and stability. Use your body weight to help control your opponent.

(i) Pressing Torso Tools

Your torso will often provide you the fulcrum necessary to complete a technique and/or the dead weight that is needed to help pin your opponent. For example, the straight arm bar can be delivered across your chest, over the shoulders, over the pelvis, etc. The constant pressing of the body into your opponent will help to wear him down, reduce his mobility, and make it difficult for him to breathe.

Torso Presses and Their Applications
• Presses (Figure 4-145) all sides.

Figure 4-146: Grey leans onto White's back while applying a hold down technique on him. Grey also applies a wristlock to White's straightened right arm.

Figure 4-147: Grey applies his body weight via his torso onto White's chest/head thereby placing pressure onto the back of White's neck (DU 16) due to the placement of Grey's arms behind White's neck.

Chapter 4: Body Tools and Vulnerable Points

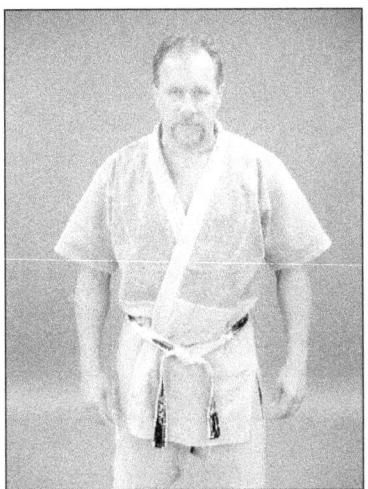

Figure 4-145

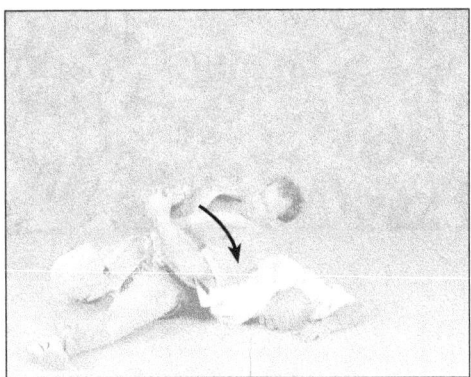

Figure 4-146

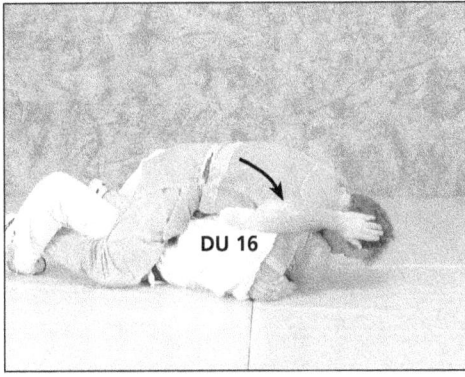

Figure 4-147

(ii) Striking Torso Tools

Apart from the dropping of a weight upon a take down, there is little ability for the torso to effect striking blows in a ground fighting situation (unlike from the body slamming possible in the throwing situation).

4-3. OTHER VULNERABLE AREAS AND MISCELLANEOUS TOOLS

Applying Other Tools

Apart from the vulnerable areas and tools already discussed, it is necessary to mention other body parts. Consider the types of application and the relative ease of applying these tools (and your own vulnerabilities) when you review these.

Hands

Clearly, the human hand is not the

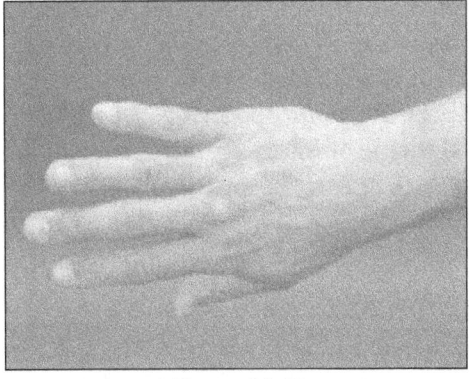

Figure 4-148

ideal weapon, given that there are five fingers and twenty-seven bones that can be broken when punching, being punched or grabbed (Figure 4-148). The number of applications for the hand in combat is too numerous to list. Always consider grabbing and bending or breaking a finger or two in order to break loose from a hold or to partially incapacitate an aggressor. Indeed the ancient Greeks used finger and arm twisting (along with punching) in the beginning stages of their pankration matches

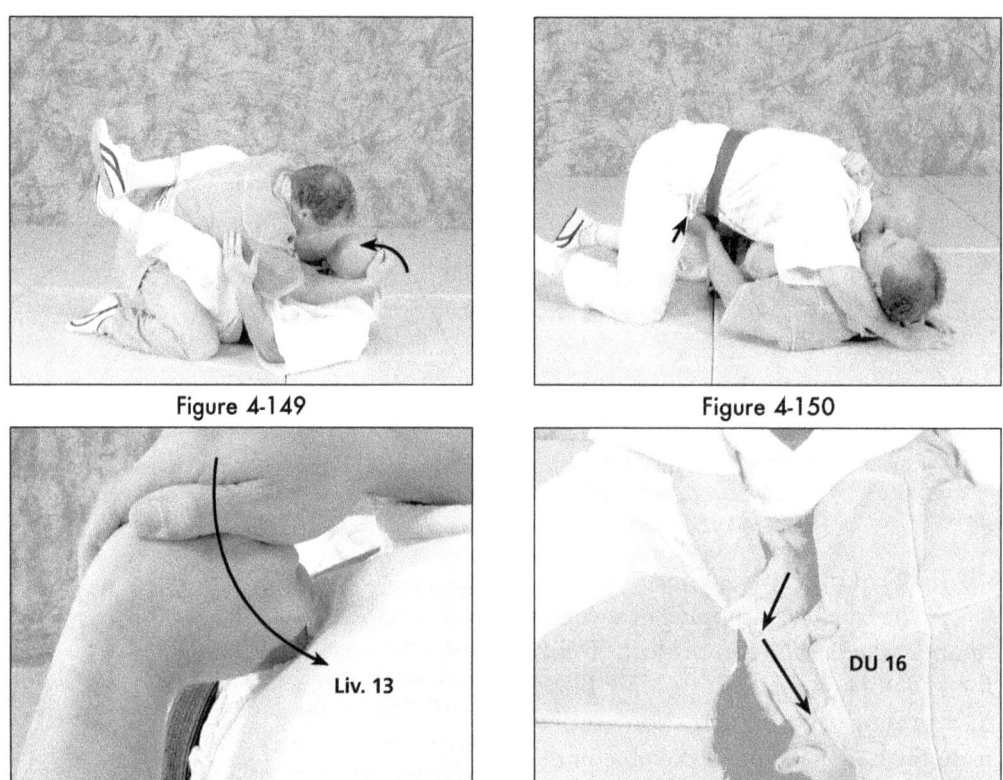

Figure 4-149

Figure 4-150

Figure 4-151

Figure 4-152

at the Olympic games (see Chapter One). It is difficult to fight on the ground if one's hands are broken because of the reliance on being able to make a strong grip. However, many fights have been waged despite having suffered minor broken bones. Breaking your opponent's hands is a good, safe (liability-wise) strategy. Inflicting this type of injury on the dominant hand would also restrict your opponent's ability to access and use a weapon against you.

Hands as Tools and Their Applications

Figure 4-149: Grey uses his hands to hyperflex the neck by pulling the head forward.

Figure 4-150: Grey grips White's testicles in order to prevent his advance. If your opponent's pants are stretched taut, you may find it difficult to apply a squeezing attack. Results of attacking this target are varied.

Figure 4-151: Grey grips his own hands and inflicts pain upon his opponent (grinding his knuckles into his opponent). For example, this technique can be applied to the floating ribs (Liv. 13).

Figure 4-152: White uses a figure-four grip to apply pressure onto the back of Grey's neck (DU 16).

Figure 4-153: White grabs Grey's right wrist to control a limb directly.

Chapter 4: Body Tools and Vulnerable Points

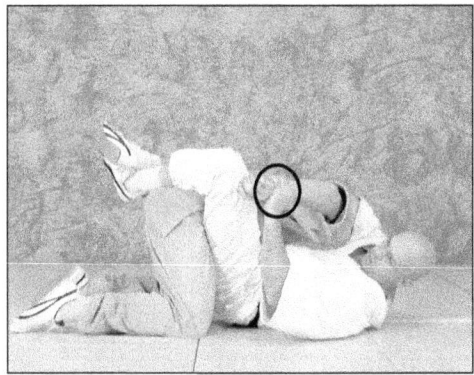

Figure 4-153

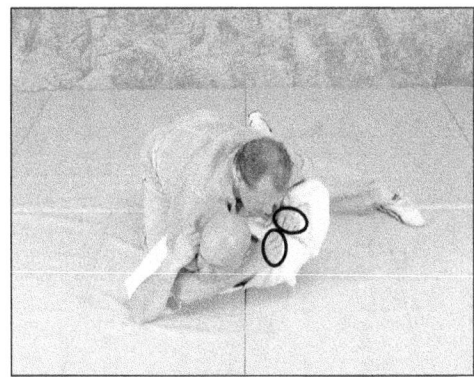

Figure 4-154

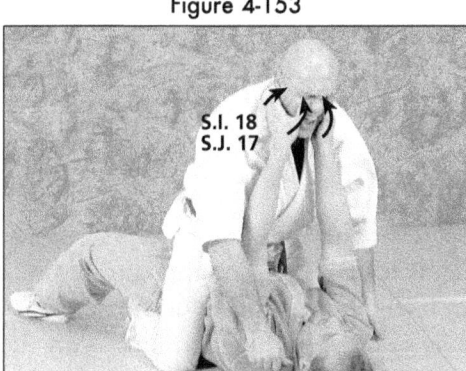

Figure 4-155

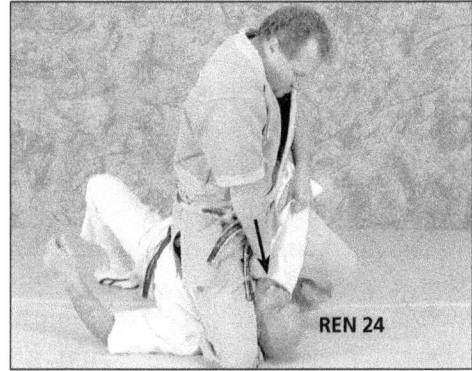

Figure 4-156

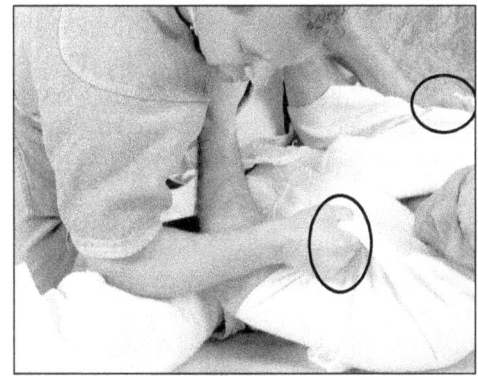

Figure 4-157

Figure 4-154: Grey grabs White's clothing in order to anchor himself and thereby strengthen his holding techniques. If your opponent is very strong and you do not wish to relinquish a hold, use a clothing grip to fix his appendage where it is.

Figure 4-155: Grey gouges under White's cheekbones (S.I. 18) with his thumbs. Grey can also simultaneously hook into the depression under the ear and behind the jaw (S.J 17) with his pointer fingers to effect a c-clamp onto these pressure points.

Figure 4-156: Grey uses his right fist to punch White's face (REN 24) while kneeling on top of him. Punches landed from this position can have great impact because the head is resting against the floor.

Figure 4-157: Grey and White clinch each other's clothing. Though not always available, the grasping of clothing can be advantageous in grappling situations, because you can create handles where one may not exist naturally.

181

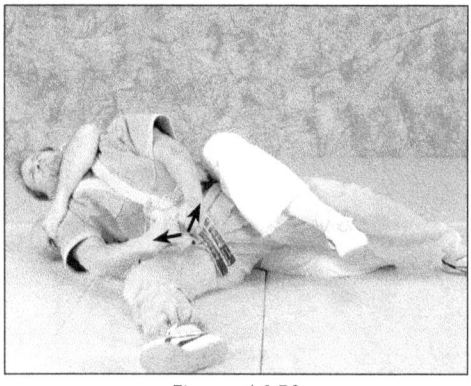 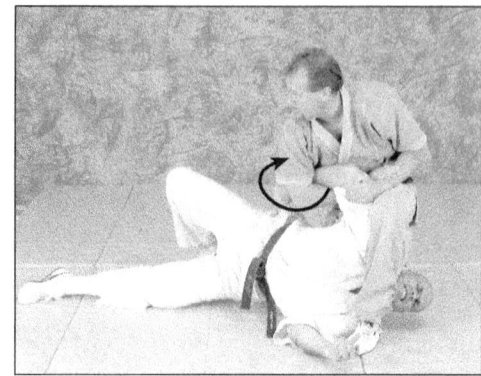

Figure 4-158   Figure 4-159

Figure 4-158: Grey uses finger Qin Na to break White's fingers in order to escape from a very disadvantageous position. Such techniques may not end a fight but they can serve as serious distracters and can weaken your opponent's ability to grip, strike or hold a weapon.

Arms

Structurally, the elbow is the weakest part of the arm, so never sacrifice a straightened arm to your opponent lest he bends it in another, more painful direction. Consider bending the arm at 90 degrees to the normal plane of movement as well as the standard hyperextension break. For in-close fighting, striking with the elbows can yield devastating results. Your opponent can only present his arm to you either bent or straight. Use what ever he gives you. Arms allow the hands to do their work and to ensnare your opponent into you, but they may also be used offensively. Well-placed piercing strikes to the nerves and muscles (motor nerve points) of the arm can render the arm and hand temporarily functionless. The bones in the arms are relatively resilient but are susceptible to breakage under the right conditions.

Arms as Tools and Their Applications

Figure 4-159: Grey applies a painful shoulder crank to White's right shoulder as a means of controlling his right arm. This is a great holding technique because: this hold can be maintained relatively strain-free for a long period of time, dislocation of the shoulder can be easily accomplished with little muscular strength, the vertical posture allows you to readily scout for additional threats, and you are free to disengage quickly from it into the standing position if necessary.

Figure 4-160: Grey uses his arms to clinch to prevent White from attacking him effectively and while he bridges out of White's hold down.

Figure 4-161: White uses his left arm as a basis for support. It is preferable not to tie up an arm for balance when ground fighting, but sometimes it is unavoidable.

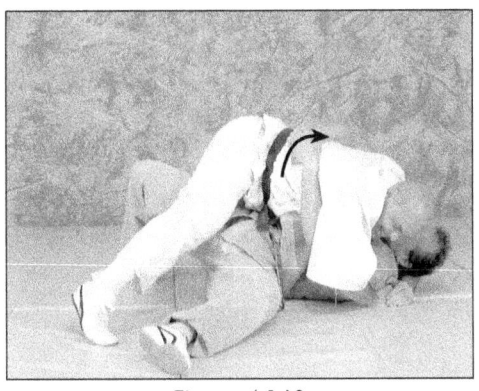

Figure 4-160

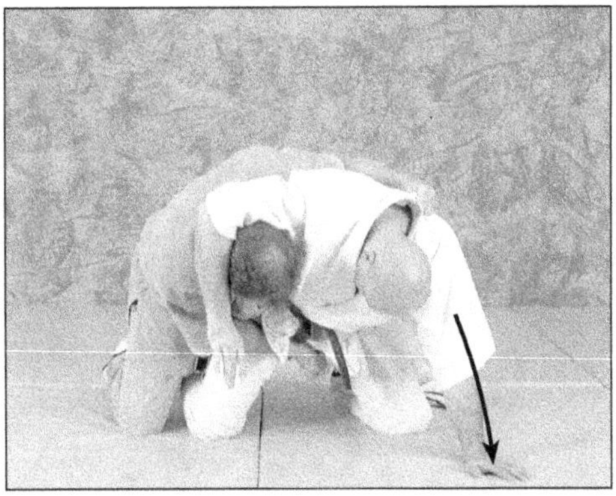

Figure 4-161

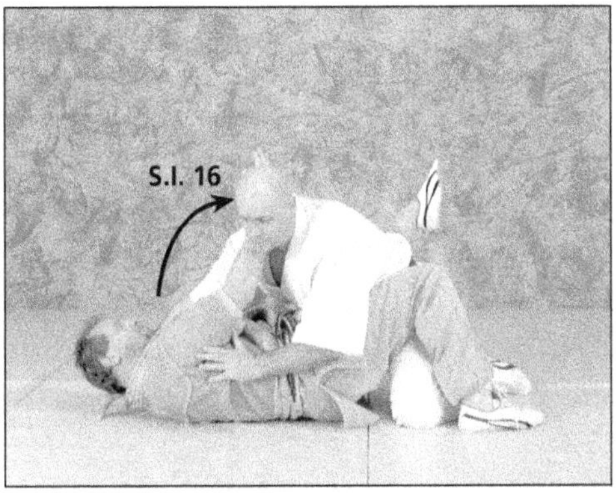

Figure 4-162

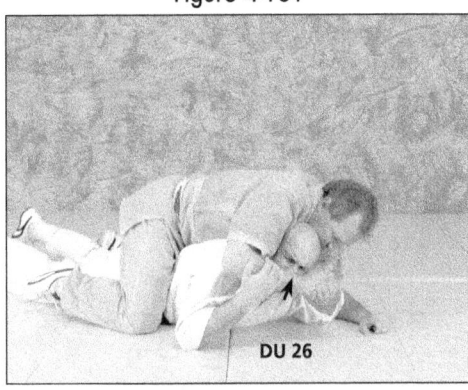

Figure 4-163

This is another good reason for not getting into a prone-oriented position.

Figure 4-162: Grey uses the top of his right arm as a means of striking White's brachial plexus (S.I. 16) in a back-handed motion.

Figure 4-163: Grey uses the radial edge of his right wrist, augmented by his left hand grip, to apply pressure to the pressure point under White's nose (DU 26).

Legs

Like the elbows are to the arms, the knees are the structural weak points of the legs. Special consideration should be given to sideward pressure to facilitate breakage of the knee joint when doing leg locks, given the overall strength of the oppositional leg muscles. Special care should be given to joint lock attempts as your opponent's free leg can deliver powerful and punishing blows. The kneecap is a vulnerable spot on the leg that may be accessed on the ground via a heel kick. Ancient Greek pankrationists were allowed to use leg and foot holds in concert with both upright and ground wrestling. Whenever possible, use your legs for kicking, blocking, clinching, bridging and levering when ground fighting.

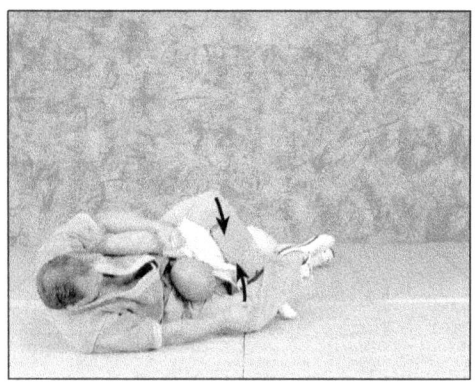
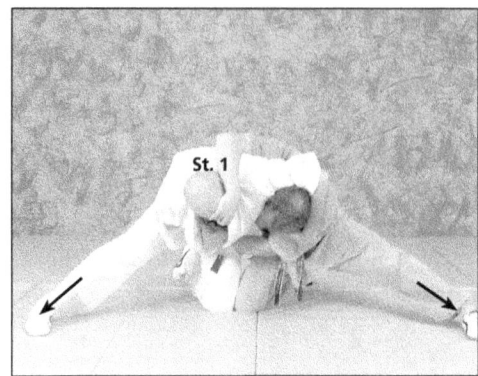

Figure 4-164   Figure 4-165

Legs as Tools and Their Applications

Figure 4-164: Grey uses his legs to clinch White. The leg scissors can be used more effectively to apply pressure to your opponent's body than the arms, given the relative strength potential of these sets of limbs.

Figure 4-165: Both Grey and White are dependent upon a leg as a means of support as they initiate the grappling phase. Grey reaches with his right arm to gouge White's eyes (St. 1).

Figure 4-166: Grey uses a downward heel strike to attack White's exposed groin.

Figure 4-167: Grey uses his leg as a means of applying pressure to the back of White's outstretched left arm.

Figure 4-168: White uses his legs in a figure-four lock as a means of controlling a limb, in this case Grey's straightened left leg.

Head/Neck

Protecting the head and neck is critical during a fight. This is not a surprising revelation, considering that the important organs of the senses of sight and hearing are contained in the head. By far the most vital organ, that which controls all bodily functions, is the brain. Lose consciousness in battle and all is lost. One can be struck at the 'sweet spot' (point of the chin) or at any point on the skull hard enough to produce a percussive blackout. One can also be 'choked out' into unconsciousness by starving the brain of oxygen in a wide variety of ways, be it by sealing the breath or sealing the vein (See Chapter 7).

Being adept at defending against the choke and neck restraints (and conversely knowing how to choke your opponent out) is paramount in ground fighting. Your spinal column attaches to the base of the skull via the cervical vertebrae. If your neck gets broken in a fight, you are minimally quadriplegic and you could easily die from such an injury.

The pulling of the hair is a much over-looked aspect of ground fighting, given its association to 'dirty fighting' or 'fighting like a girl'. The ancient Greek wrestlers were turned out with short hair to keep their opponents from gaining advantage over them

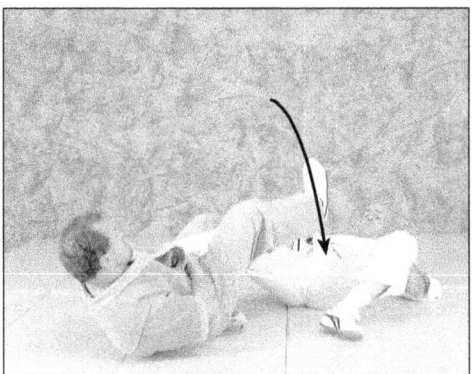

Figure 4-166

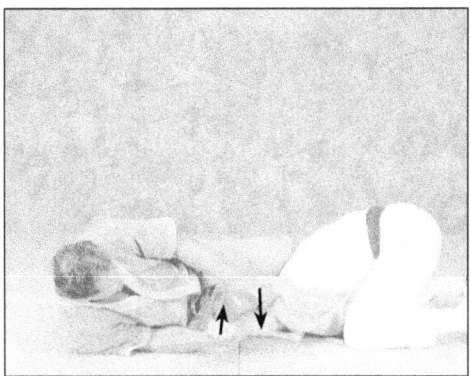

Figure 4-167

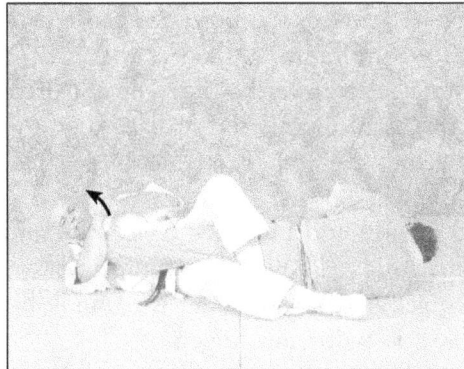

Figure 4-168

in this manner (but on the other hand, at one period in history, they wrestled each other nude). Hair pulling can be a useful means to access the throat or otherwise control the head. If you want to pull the chin off the chest from behind in order to apply a choke, grasp the hair in a twisting motion towards the front of the scalp (not the rear) in order to get more leverage from the pull. So having a closely cropped head of hair can be a distinct advantage in a ground fight.

The eyes are relatively vulnerable to poking attacks in particular, with evasive head and defensive hand movements being the remedy against painful blinding. Moderate pressure on the eyes reduces the resolve of most people and they are forced to deal with this impending threat of blindness. Even ancient Greek *pankration*, arguably the most punishing of the ancient combative sports, short of boxing with the *caestus* (forerunners of the knuckle dusters), banned the practice of eye gouging and biting, although pottery scenes depict that these were dirty tricks that contestants tried to get away with. Those caught trying such unsportsmanlike fouls were beaten by a stick-wielding referee.

The ears too are susceptible to attack from many angles. A blow to the exterior of the ear can be painful and can cause the recipient to lose his balance or even black out. A cupped hand slapped over one or both ears can cause a painful puncture to the eardrum. Unlike stand up fighting situations, the absence of both sight and hearing is not critical to winning on the ground, but the pain of losing them during the fight would probably be a big determining factor.

The skull is the 'Stone Age bone cage' that protects the all-important brain and houses the sensory organs of the eyes and ears. Remember that the skull is thickest at the front central part of the skull and weakest at the temporal regions.

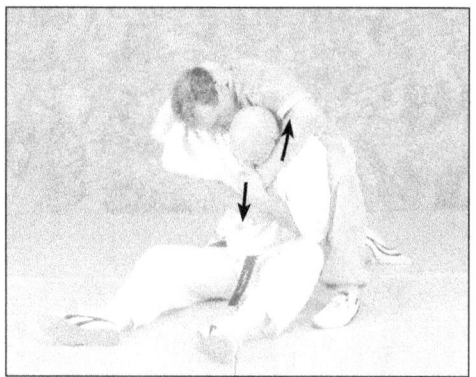

Figure 4-169

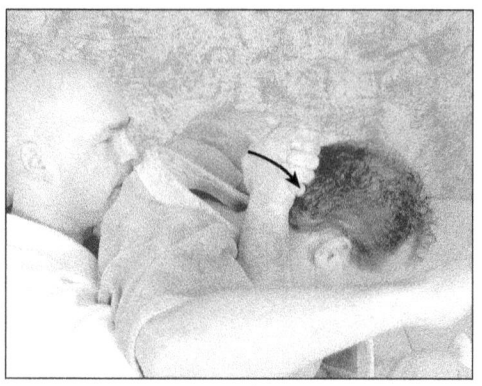

Figure 4-170

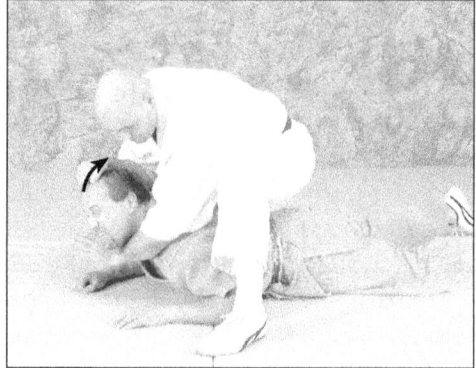

Figure 4-171

A blow to the nose can cause it to bleed profusely and cause the eyes to water. An upward strike will not drive the nasal bone (it is cartilage anyway) up into the brain cavity, as some street lore will have it. The blow can serve as a painful and bloody distracter should the situation call for it. A creative way to get at your opponent is to hook his nostrils with your fingers.

The mouth can be attacked by smashing the teeth (and cutting the lips) as well as by hooking the lips and insides of the cheeks with your fingers. A punch to the chin against an extended tongue is a bonus. One must be very careful in this day of extreme diseases (blood-born pathogens) that you do not cut yourself on your opponent's teeth, nor are you bitten. The exchange of blood (or any bodily fluids for that matter) can have serious medical consequences (infections), long after the fight is over.

As mentioned earlier, a strike upwards and into to the point of the chin can knock a person out cold. The brain is a very sensitive organ and if starved of oxygen, subjected to high internal (blood) pressure or treated to a concussive shock, it may shut your whole system down. A sideways blow to the jaw can dislocate it, as can backward pressure exerted from behind by a pair of choking arms (when you drop your chin to defend against such a choke).

The throat has several weak areas within it, most notably the Adam's apple. A blow to this area is painful and dangerous because of the swelling that can accompany it's breakage (and that of the lower hyoid bone). People have been known to die from asphyxiation as the result of blows to the throat or from being choked out improperly. A blow to the brachial plexus along the sides of the neck can cause mental and physical stunning of the brain (and body) and can result in unconsciousness.

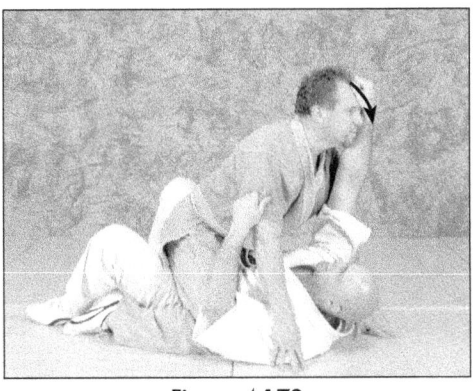

Figure 4-172

Figure 4-173

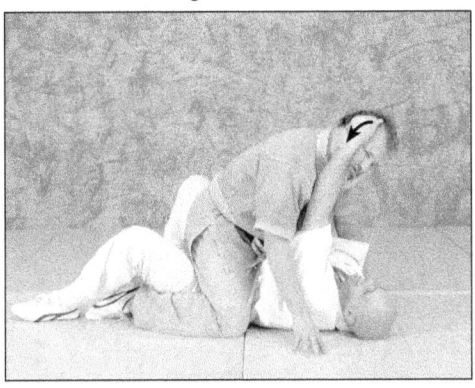

Figure 4-174

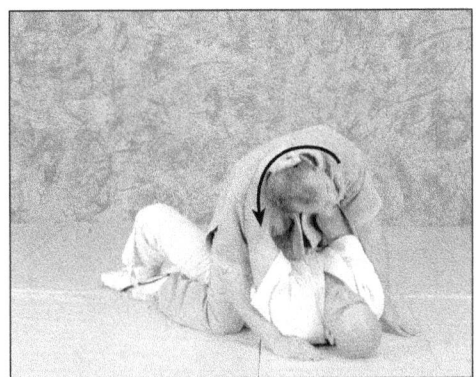

Figure 4-175

Head and Neck Tools and Their Applications

Figure 4-169: Grey attacks White's neck with a choke using White's collar. White protects himself by dropping his chin to his chest and by grabbing Grey's choking left hand with his own left hand and pulling downwards to relieve the pressure on his throat.

Figure 4-170: White attacks Grey's neck with a forward neck crank using a Full Nelson hold.

Figure 4-171: White grabs Grey's frontal hair in order to expose his neck for a choke.

Figure 4-172: White ineffectively grabs Grey's frontal hair while in the mounted position.

Figure 4-173: White applying a more effective hair pull on Grey's hair, by reaching further behind Grey's head to gain an increased mechanical advantage.

Figure 4-174: White grabs Grey's front-side portion of his hair for an ineffective hair pull.

Figure 4-175: White demonstrates a proper hair pull by reaching to the other side of Grey's head to get more pulling purchase.

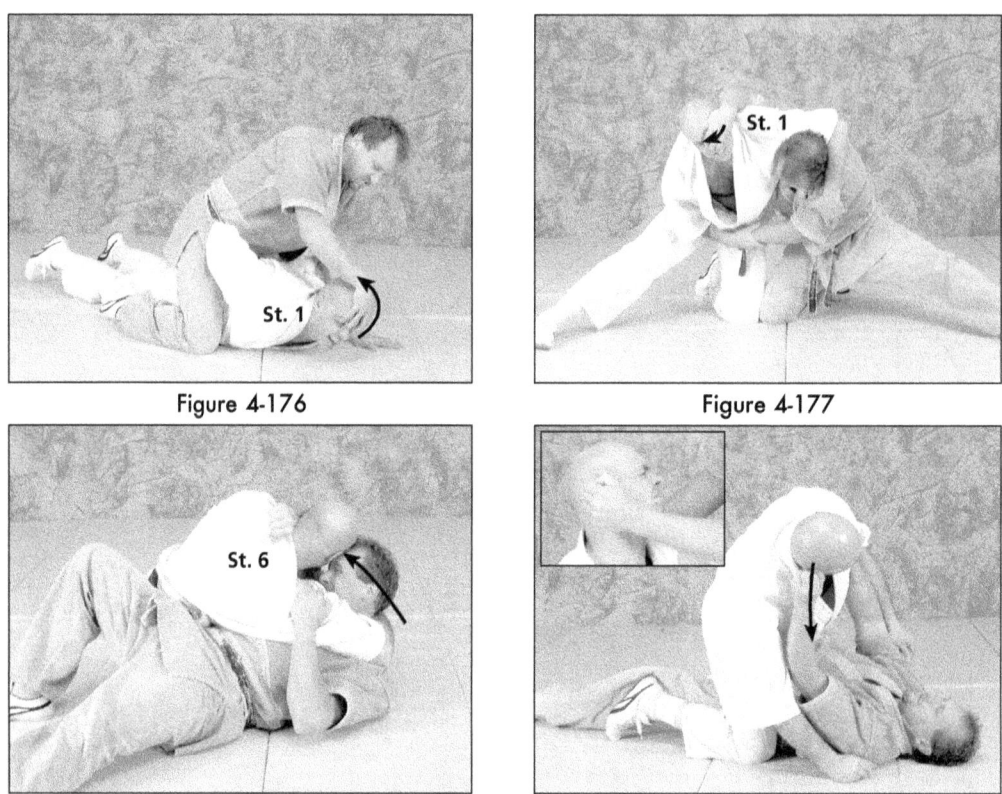

Figure 4-176

Figure 4-177

Figure 4-178

Figure 4-179

Figure 4-176: Grey attacks White's eyes and hooks the eye sockets (St. 1) to hyperextend the neck.

Figure 4-177: Grey gouges White's eyes (St. 1) in order to effect a release from White's headlock.

Figure 4-178: Grey attacks White's temporal region (G.B. 6) with a head butt from the bottom position. Head butts are also very effective in breaking the thin nasal bones at the base of the nose to produce massive bleeding and tearing of the eyes.

Figure 4-179: Grey rips White's right ear in order to unbalance him.

Figure 4-180: Grey attacks Whites temporal area (G.B. 6) with a back knuckle strike.

Figure 4-181: Grey palm heels White's nose from the mounted position.

Figure 4-182: Grey rips (fish-hooking) White's right cheek.

Figure 4-183: Grey punches the point of White's jaw (the 'sweet spot' in boxing) in an attempt to knock him out.

Figure 4-184: Grey uses his teeth as a weapon to bite White's left ear as a technique to distract the opponent.

Figure 4-185: Grey attacks the left side of White's neck with a ridge hand strike immediately upon taking him down (S.I. 16).

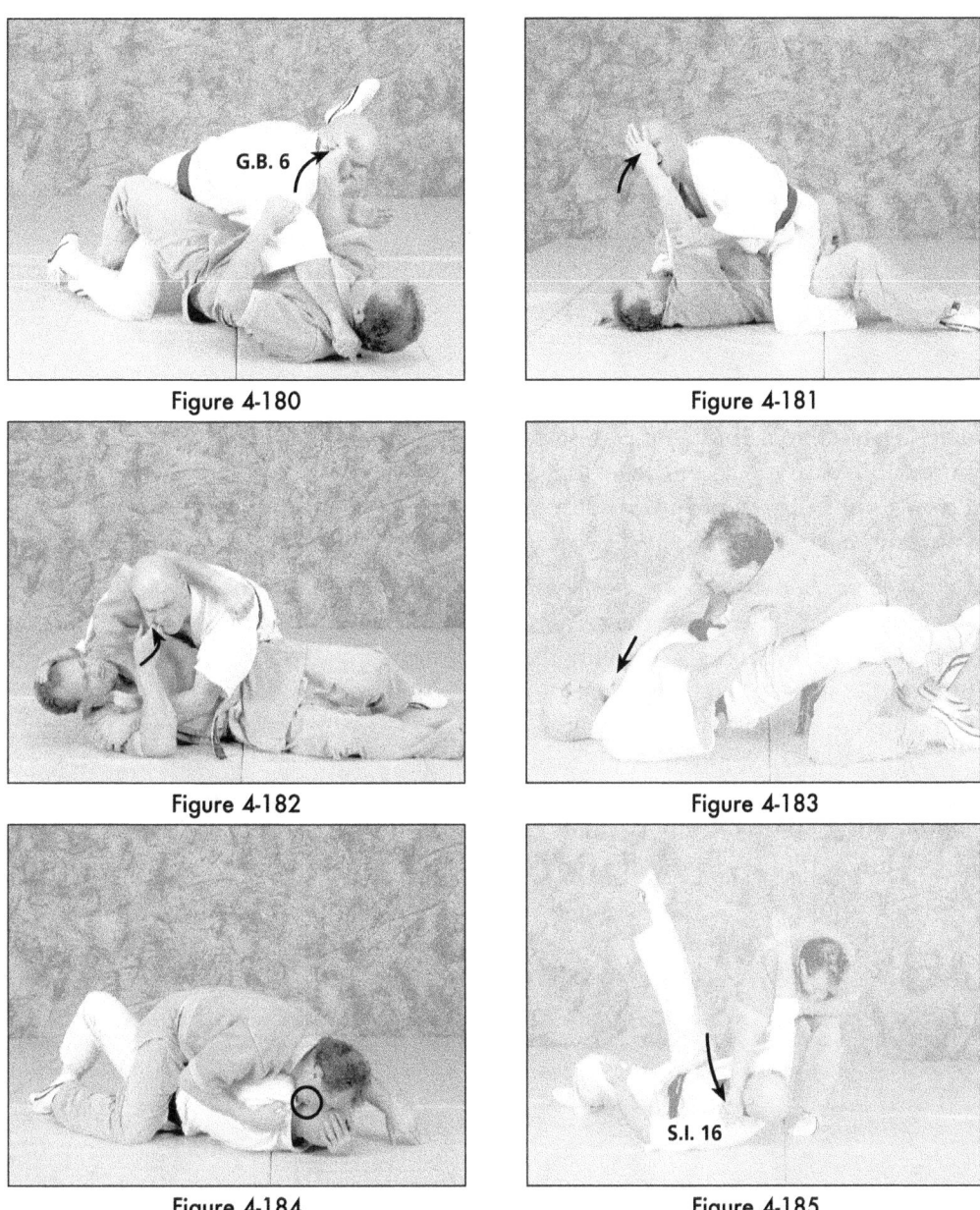

Figure 4-180

Figure 4-181

Figure 4-182

Figure 4-183

Figure 4-184

Figure 4-185

Torso

Much damage can be done if the torso is struck with heavy blows such as stomping heel kicks and elbow strikes, particularly if the spine, groin and kidneys are targeted. Vital organs such as the heart and lungs are fairly well protected by the rib cage but ribs can be broken to perforate these organs. Heavy abdominal conditioning can minimize damage to this area. Apart from doing body conditioning exercises (such as *Da Peng Qigong*–Iron Shirt training) and using your arms and legs

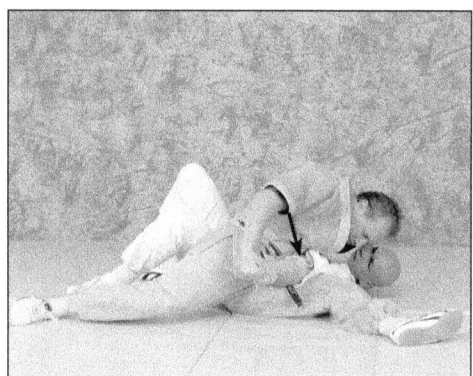

Figure 4-186

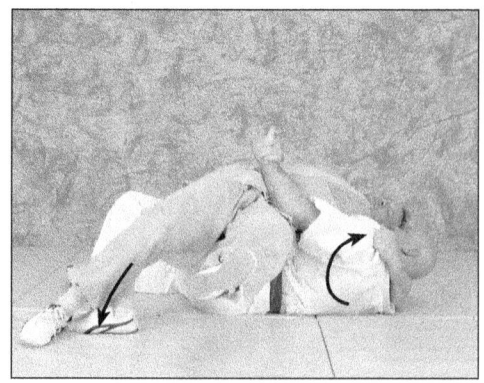

Figure 4-187

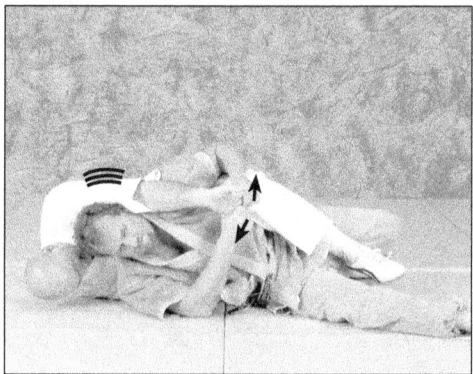

Figure 4-188

defensively there is little you can do to protect all parts of the torso at once. Forcing your opponent into defense is a good strategy.

Torso Tool and Its Applications

Figure 4-186: Grey uses his torso to weigh down White's body. Keeping the butt off the floor is helpful in achieving this 'spiking' feeling.

Figure 4-187: White uses his torso (powered by the legs) to roll Grey over onto his back.

Figure 4-188: Grey uses his shoulders as a fulcrum for applying a straight arm bar.

PART TWO

Joint Locks

CHAPTER 5

Controlling the Arm

5-1. INTRODUCTION

The Arms as Tools

The Qin Na (Chin Na) practitioner excels in arm/wrist locking techniques because the arm is the primary target of control. This is not surprising given that the hands are most people's main attacking and controlling tools that are readily available in a stand up fighting situation, which is where many martial artists prefer to remain. There is more of a tendency for the untrained fighter to use his hands for hitting and grabbing and to use the feet solely for moving the body (unless the opponent has fallen down then kicking seems to be a more natural mode of attack). The legs gain increased importance as a controlling (and controllable) tool in the ground fighting situation, as their primary function for mobility is reduced and the legs become more functional and accessible for grappling purposes.

The Qin Na practitioner's ability to use his techniques is hampered on the ground because of the lack of mobility and concomitant shifting of his center of gravity that is so important to the effective implementation of these techniques. Some Qin Na techniques do not require a lot of mobility to be effective so these techniques can be successfully used on the ground. The other techniques will have to rely on a good degree of improvisation to work; others simply cannot be done from the ground. We will leave it to the readers to sort out what Qin Na techniques are workable from the ground. Get on the mat and practice pure Qin Na technique with your partner to get a feeling of what it is like not to be able to use your legs for mobility and how this effects the overall dynamics of your techniques. Discover also the possibilities for controlling your opponent using your legs. The same biomechanical principles used to gain control over the arms can be adapted to the legs.

The ground fighter can learn a lot about controlling the arm from a good Qin Na practitioner even though his techniques are somewhat limited from the ground. Cross training would be beneficial to him, both in the standing and ground fighting situations, as most ground fighters have learned their art through a sport-based martial art such as judo or jiu jitsu. Remember, there are no rules in a street fight (other than legal/moral ones concerning use of force issues) other than those concerning survival. The use of illegal or 'dirty fighting' techniques could determine success or defeat on the street.

There has been much written on the art of Qin Na, particularly by Dr. Yang Jwing-Ming, so the authors defer to his written works (we highly recommend his most recent book titled *Comprehensive Applications of Shaolin Chin Na*). As such, we will not go into detail about Qin Na technique, rather we will look at the basic principles that underlie the techniques and highlight these various techniques as moves of augmentation or distraction, particularly for fingers and to a lesser degree, wrist Qin Na, as they occur throughout the text.

Anatomy of the Arm

There are a total of 64 bones of the upper extremities as follows (from the shoulders to the finger tips):

2 collar bones (clavicles)	2 scapula (shoulder blades)
2 humerus (upper arm bones)	2 radius (inside forearm bones)
2 ulna (outside forearm bones)	16 carpals (wrist bones)
10 metacarpals (hand bones)	28 phalanges (finger bones)

Not only are the arms and hands the most agile parts of the body, they also have the greatest ranges in motion. The upper and lower arms form an angle of about 165-170 degrees, but the elbow can only flex and extend about 140 degrees. The brachial plexus feeds nerves from the lower neck, under the mid-collar bone, through the armpit after which they split into the radial, median and ulnar nerves, which can be readily accessed at the elbow and wrist.

The shoulder joint, formed by the ball and socket joining of the humerus into the scapula, is the largest joint of the upper body. The head of the joint is much larger than its socket, hence only about one third of it is contained in the socket and it is held in place by few and relatively weak ligaments. This allows significant mobility about three axes, but these same factors causes this joint to be very weak and unstable. The lower front area of the joint is particularly susceptible to dislocation due to minimal ligament support there.

The elbow joint is actually three joints of the humerus, radial and ulna bones contained in a single joint capsule that are mutually dependent and supportive. All rotational movement of the elbow is done by the shoulder joint. The inward and outward rotation of the lower arm involves the bones of the forearm as well as the shoulder joint. The radius and ulna bones cross on inward rotation (to a maximum of 140 degrees); an outward rotation of 15-25 degrees is possible. The combined rotational capabilities of the lower arm that uses the shoulder joint is 360 degrees (if the arm is bent, the wrist can only be twisted 270 degrees). Locking the wrist will lock the elbow, which in turn will lock the shoulder, hence the importance of controlling the elbow and locking the shoulder when applying wrist locks. Locking a joint in isolation may allow your opponent to retaliate. Conversely, the combined locking of the joints can immobilize the entire body.

The wrist is made up of eight bones (two rows of four bones) joined by ligaments, but only a few of these bones are connected at the wrist joint to the radius. This allows the wrist to flex, extend, rotate in and out as well as move in a circle. As with the elbow joint, the radial, ulnar and median nerves are accessible here by pressure point attacks.

The hand consists of five fingers containing fourteen joints (three per finger and two for the thumb). The five palmar bones in the body of the hand itself connect the wrist to the fingers. The hand is capable of sophisticated movement including the ability to form a multitude of hand tools and to grip. The lateral range of motion and strength of the fingers however is relatively very small, hence grabbing a few fingers can damage ligaments, cause dislocation or breakage, all of which are painful. Locking fingers can lead into wrist, elbow, and shoulder locking, as well as cause weakening of the hand and low effort pain compliance. Additionally, nerves in the hand can be readily accessed and compressed against the bones of the hand by pressure point attacks due to a paucity of thick protective musculature. The fingers/wrist will be dealt with as a secondary augmenting means of control, deferring to the more reliable joint lock manipulations of the arm and shoulder.

Locking the Arm

The larger the joint, the more serious the consequences that your opponent faces should it be broken. There is simply no comparison to breaking a finger versus breaking an arm in a fight. Breaking a finger in combat is therefore not a reliable means to end a street encounter. Conversely, the larger the joint, the more difficult it will be to control it and to break it. We will concentrate on the arm as a whole, emphasizing the elbow joint, as it is a very reliable joint to lock.

Remember that every lock requires some counterpressure, be it from the opponent's own body weight, your body or from a fixed object such as the mat, otherwise your opponent will move in the direction of the locking force to escape.

There are only two ways your opponent can present his arm to you: straight or in a bent position. When at either extreme ranges of motion, the arm is at its weakest. The fingers and wrists offer secondary targets for attack in order to assist in gaining control over a person or to weaken their resolve when you are in a defensive situation requiring an escape.

5-2. STRAIGHT ARM BARS

Applying Straight Arm Bars

The straight arm bar is the most basic and practical type of arm lock. One of the most common ground fighting techniques in judo is *juji gatame* (cross-mark hold). It is simply a transverse arm bar that has many applications. The arm bar itself can be applied from a wide variety of angles and relative body positions. It is ideal if your opponent offers you a straight arm as you don't have to try and forcefully straighten it. If you do, use the weight of your body and the principle of leverage (see Chapter One.) to do the work for you.

The underlying principle behind the straight arm bar is to bend or hyper-extend the arm beyond its normal range of movement so that the structural integrity of the elbow is compromised. The wrist area of the lower arm is the lever handle (force point) where the most mechanical advantage can be utilized. Basic physics tells us that the shorter the lever (force arm), the less mechanical advantage there is to do the work. Although the hand is a very mobile handle, it may be manipulated to create additional pain or to set yourself up for a more substantial lock. The fulcrum (axis of rotation) should be located just above the elbow joint, preferably on the triceps tendon (about two inches above the tip of the elbow – S.J. 11). If the fulcrum is below the elbow joint, then the force becomes directed towards the forearm rather than the elbow. If you are levering against a hard, bony fulcrum here, you will inflict more pain, making you seem stronger than you are. The extra pain is always a valuable asset when trying to gain submission. Judoka turn the hand of the arm being pried such that the thumb points in the arm's plane of movement in order to diminish the strength of the biceps over that of the weaker triceps muscles.

Straight Arm Bar from a Single Leg Takedown

White has taken down Grey with a single leg take down of his left leg (Figure 5-1). White foolishly reaches across the belt line in an attempt to grab Grey's left arm as he picks up Grey's left leg (Figure 5-2). Grey seizes White's outstretched arm initially with his left hand then his right hand as he rolls onto his back, scissor-kicking backwards at White to unbalance him as he does so. This takes White with him onto their backs. Grey quickly secures White's right arm in a 'figure four' lock with his legs (Figure 5-3). Grey cinches up the hold by pulling White's arm upward along his body. He then pulls White's arm towards the mat to apply the pressure on the elbow at the correct angle. Grey can twist his right hip upwards to further stress Grey's elbow joint. Grey may also apply a finger lock or wrist lock of his choice to ensure that submission is gained (Figure 5-4).

Chapter 5: Controlling the Arm

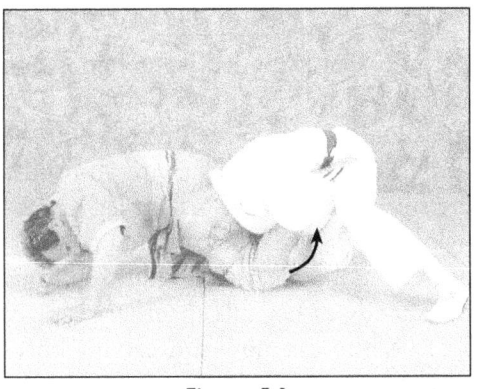

Figure 5-1

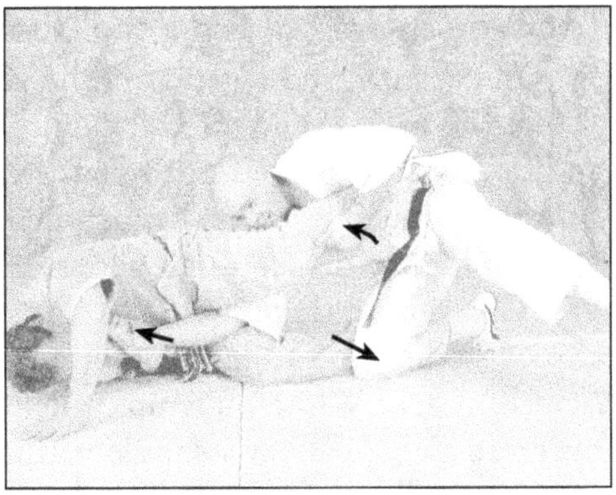

Figure 5-2

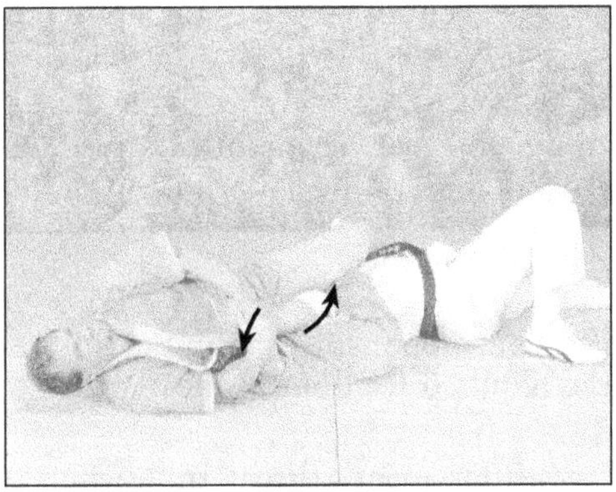

Figure 5-3

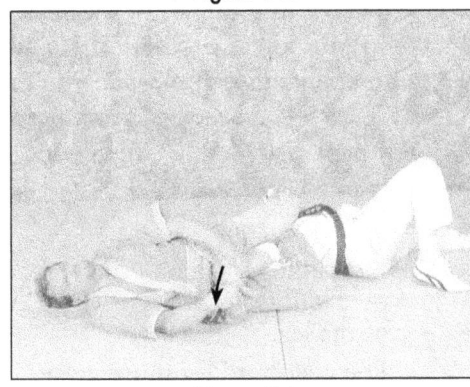

Figure 5-4

Key Points

1. Pull your pelvis as close to your opponent as needed to ensure that this fulcrum is above the elbow joint or else much of the mechanical advantage is diminished.
2. Also, if the elbow is below the pelvis, escape by your opponent is possible if he were to drop his elbow to the mat.
3. If your opponent is very strong and you need some additional control, finger and wrist Qin Na can give you that additional help.
4. In order to make the application of this type of hold less painful (for the men) do not pry against your groin for obvious reasons. Use the hip joint or upper thigh to achieve the same purpose. Depending on the angle that your opponent is lying relative to you, you may have to push or rotate your hips in the opposite direction of the prying or even use other body parts in order to maintain the correct and pure angle of attack.

Transverse Arm Bar From the Guard

Grey is in White's guard and he attempts to do a two-handed frontal choke on White (Figure 5-5). White seizes Grey's hands to reduce the pressure on his neck and to ensure that he is not struck in the face should Grey suddenly abandon the choke. White pulls Grey's hands to his right side as he unlocks his guard and slides his own hips to the left. This allows White the freedom to swing his left leg up and over Grey's head (Figure 5-6). White now kicks Grey's head sideways in a counter-clockwise direction using his right leg as a power base. This action will drop Grey onto his back. White pulls upwards on Grey's hands as he rolls in order to place his groin tight to Grey's shoulder (Figure 5-7). White can now squeeze his knees together, pull Grey's hands downwards to his chest, and raise his hips to effect the elbow lock. White can also lock his ankles together to further secure the arm. The final end position is a variation of judo's *juji gatame,* which has the near-head leg over the opponent's throat and the other leg bent against the near-side of the rib cage (Figure 5-8 shows this classical hold from the opposite viewpoint). In this case, White's bent right leg at Grey's rib cage prevents Grey from rolling into White in an effort to escape.

Key Points

1. The sliding of the hips at right angles to your opponent is an important preparatory move in order to create the required freedom of movement of the leg.
2. The near-head leg must always be over your opponent's throat; otherwise the opponent could easily escape by merely sitting up. Be mindful of your opponent's ability to bite your calf (respond with a heel kick to the face or to the solar plexus or groin with the other leg if you cannot extract your leg).
3. The leg that is placed against the rib cage prevents your opponent from rolling into you and dropping his elbow, allowing him to escape.
4. Squeeze your knees together to further fold his arm in order to making more difficult for your opponent to escape.
5. If your opponent twists his arm, you must change the angle of your hip pressure by raising and/or twisting the hips in the corresponding direction (opposite to the direction of the controlling force).

Chapter 5: Controlling the Arm

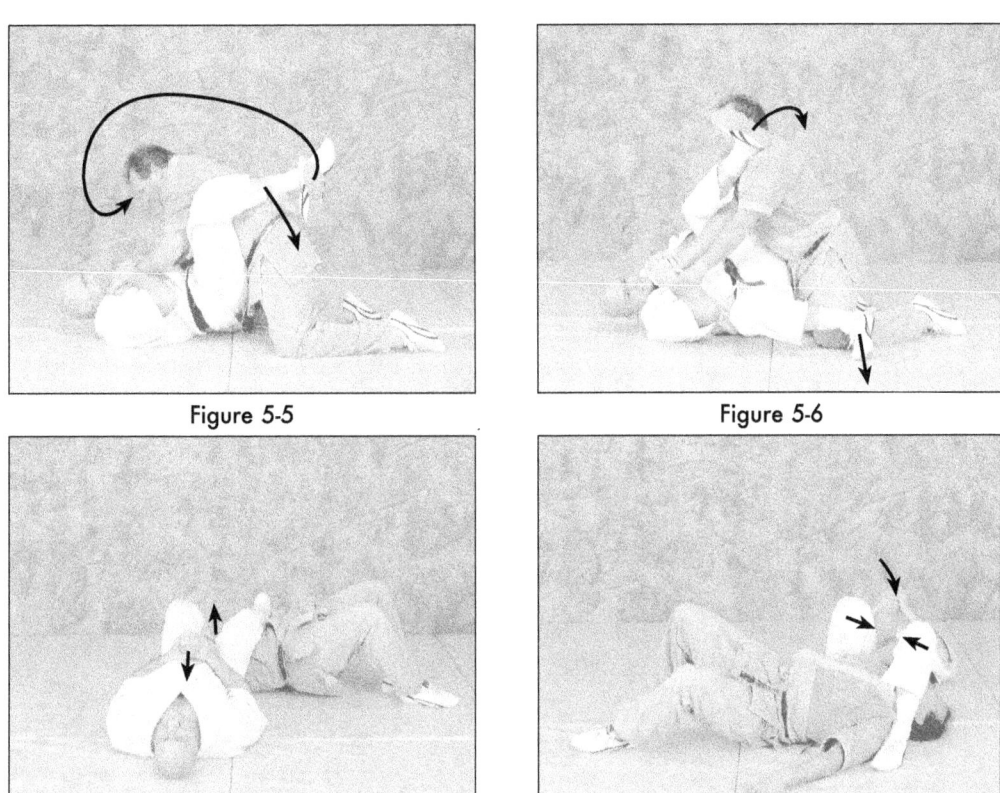

Figure 5-5

Figure 5-6

Figure 5-7

Figure 5-8

199

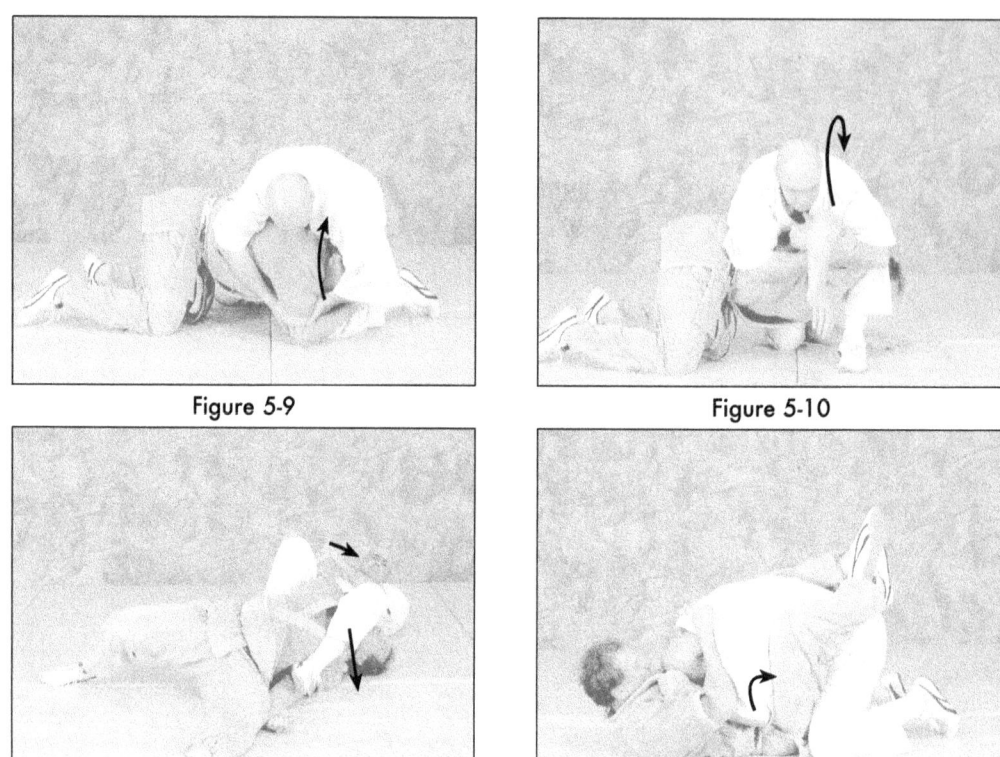

Figure 5-9

Figure 5-10

Figure 5-11

Figure 5-12

Transverse Arm Bar From a Roll Over

Grey has attempted to take White down by shooting for his legs, but White steps back and presses his chest onto Grey's back (Figure 5-9). White places both of his hands under Grey's right arm and pulls up as he shifts 90 degrees to the Grey's left side in a semi-kneeling position, placing his left leg on the right side of Grey's neck (Figure 5-10). White lays backward to roll Grey over while levering on Grey's right arm. As White lies back, his left kneeling knee comes off the mat to be positioned against Grey's right ribs and his other leg remains pressed against Grey's neck (Figure 5-11). White now peels Grey's arm to his chest by transferring his grip to Grey's wrist and raises his hips to effect the arm lock.

Key Points

1. Let your body weight and momentum do the work in rolling over your opponent.
2. Use your opponent's arm as a lever to effect this positional change on him.
3. Do not be too concerned if you do not land in the perfect position. Go for the lock while you are in transition if possible and apply it immediately.

Chapter 5: Controlling the Arm

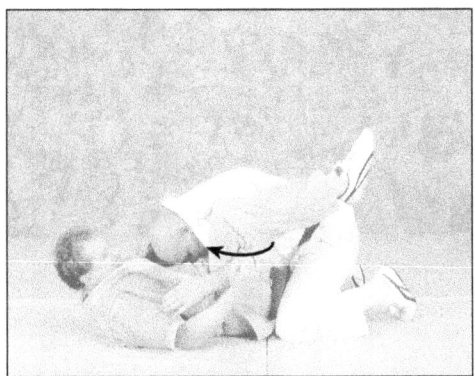

Figure 5-13

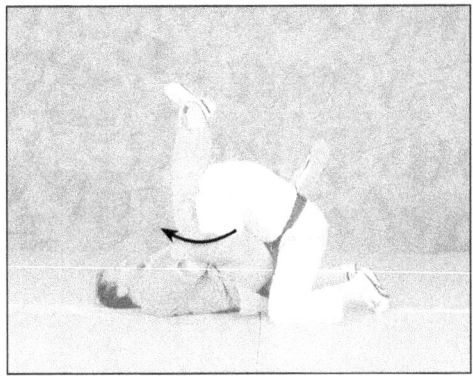

Figure 5-14

Inverted Straight Arm Bar

White is in Grey's guard and White begins to insert his left forearm against the inside of Grey's right thigh (Figure 5-12). White presses his elbow into Grey's thigh to break the guard and he hooks his left arm around the crook of Grey's right knee (Figure 5-13). White then attempts to pass completely out of Grey's guard by trying to pass Grey's right leg up and over White's head (Figure 5-14). Grey grabs White's right

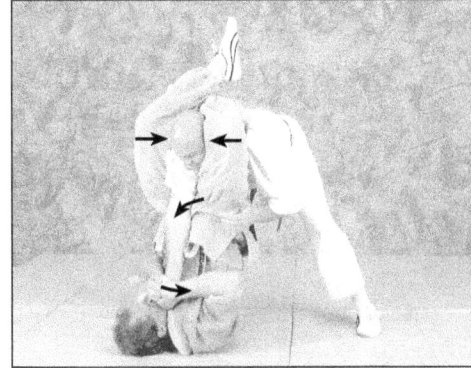

Figure 5-15

arm as he does this and pushes his leg down against White's left shoulder in order to prevent the pass. Grey then swings his other leg up to figure four his legs as he pulls White's arm to his chest. White tries to stand up out of the technique, but Grey holds on and presses his hips forwards to lock out the elbow (Figure 5-15). Grey is also in a position to apply the triangle choke should he be able to work his right inside into the crook of his own left knee.

Key Points
1. Passing the guard by throwing a leg up and over your opponent's own head is a good time for you to look at doing the triangle choke and/or the straight arm bar.
2. Do not be too concerned if your opponent's body position changes while attempting an arm lock. You can win from any position (although your opponent may elect to apply his body weight onto your neck).

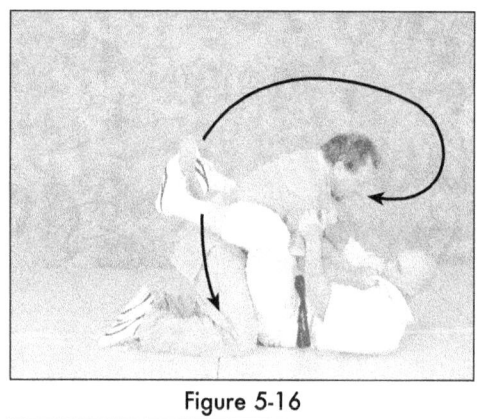

Figure 5-16

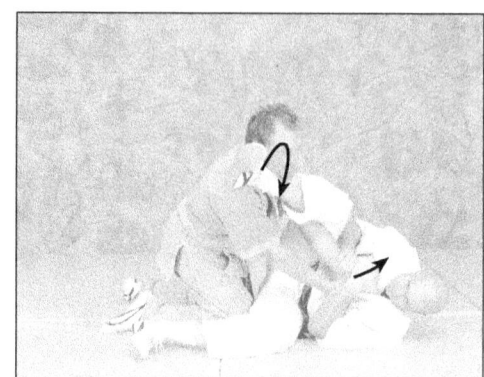

Figure 5-17

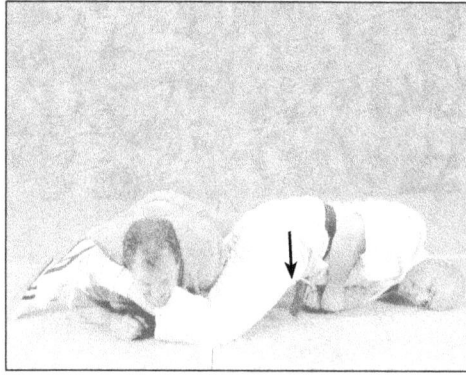

Figure 5-18

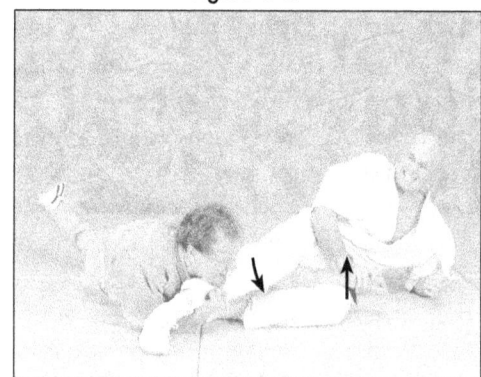

Figure 5-19

Straight Arm Lock

Grey is in White's guard and Grey tries to do a two-handed frontal choke on White (Figure 5-16). White tries to peel Grey's fingers off his clothing and he tries a kick over with his right leg, intending to scissor Grey over onto Grey's left side (Figure 5-17). White is unable to complete the kick over so he quickly reverses his hip rotation in the other direction while gripping Grey's right wrist so that he can use this arm as a lever to roll Grey over onto his stomach (Figure 5-18). Both combatants are now prone. White can easily put pressure on Grey's elbow and hyperextend it merely by letting his weight drop through his hips towards the mat. A variation of this technique may be gained during the roll over transition (Figure 5-19). If the roll over is unsuccessful and you still retain Grey's left arm, you may scissor your legs to effect an arm bar, without having to use your arms. White need only press his right knee down (using Grey's neck as an anchor) above the elbow joint while simultaneously raising the left knee up (if necessary).

Chapter 5: Controlling the Arm

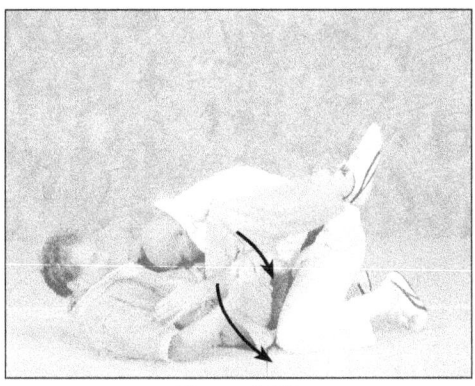

Figure 5-20

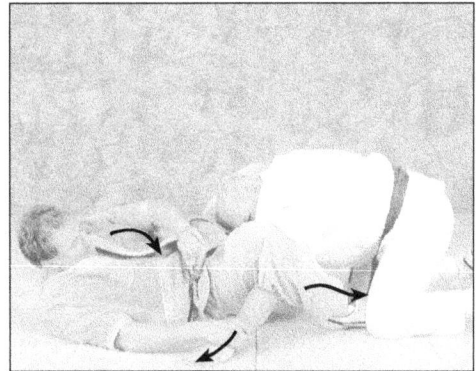

Figure 5-21

Key Points

1. If you cannot move in one direction, look for an opportunity for a quick reversal.
2. Be careful when practicing this technique because it is very easy to hyperextend your partner's elbow.
3. The placement of the knees is important in this leg scissors variation. Remember to keep the knees apart so that leverage can work for you. If your knees

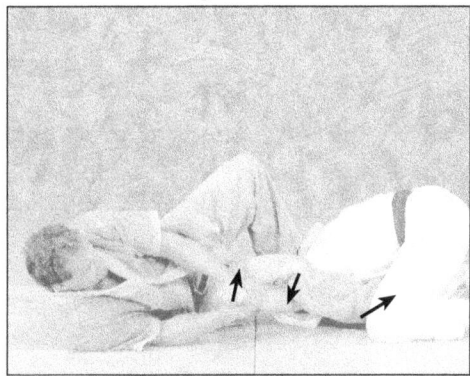

Figure 5-22

are stacked on top of each other, no pressure will be generated on the elbow.
4. There are numerous possibilities for applying the straight arm bar in many ground fighting situations. Try not to give your opponent that opportunity.

Straight Arm Bar Using a Leg Lever

White is attempting to pass Grey's guard by passing over Grey's right leg with his left arm (Figure 5-20). Grey thwarts this by seizing White's left wrist and forcing it to the mat with the help of his right leg as he rolls towards his right side. Grey also inserts his right foot inside White's left thigh (Figure 5-21). Grey then pulls up on White's left arm as he straightens his right leg that is well-anchored under White's pelvis to put pressure on White's elbow joint (Figure 5-22).

Key Points

1. Bring your opponent's straightened arm away from his body so that your leg can work on the elbow.
2. This technique allows Grey's left leg to be free should he need to kick White.

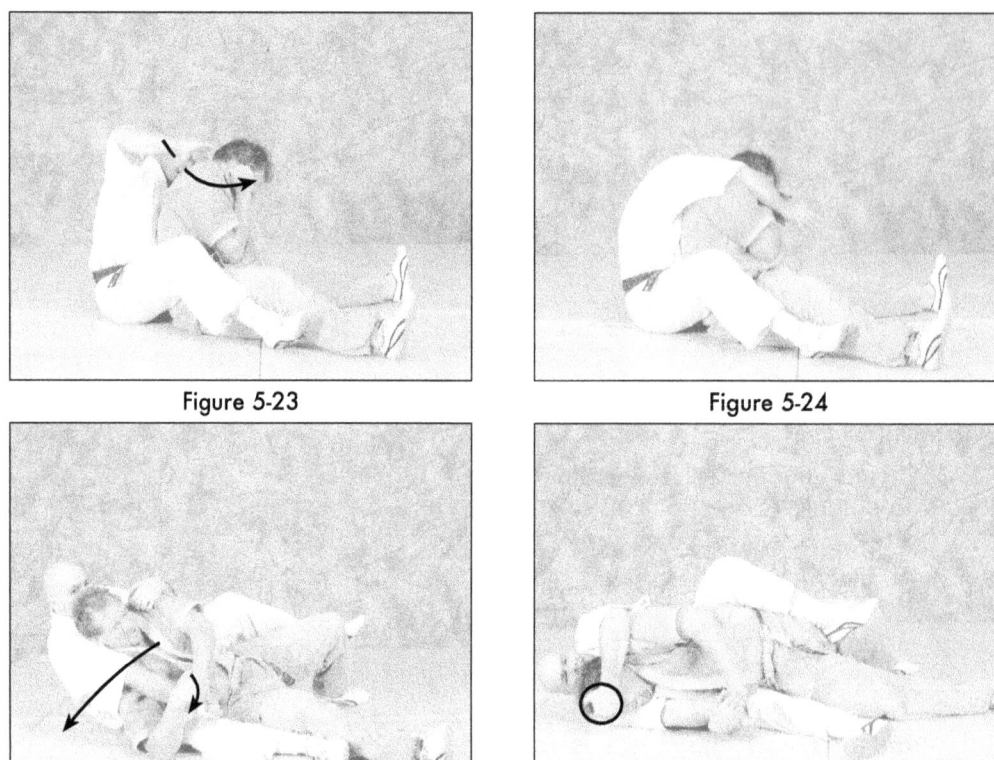

Figure 5-23

Figure 5-24

Figure 5-25

Figure 5-26

Straight Arm Bar From the Reverse Guard

White is behind Grey, both being in the seated position (Figure 5-23). White tries to choke Grey, but Grey covers up (Figure 5-24). Grey grabs White's right wrist and pulls down on this arm using his own shoulder as a fulcrum. As he does this, Grey also pushes backwards and rolls towards his right shoulder (Figure 5-25). Grey can now exert full pressure on White's arm, locking it out (Figure 5-26). Unless Grey can gain submission and break White's arm quickly, White will be in a position to gouge his face.

Key Points

1. Having an opponent directly behind you is very disadvantageous in ground fighting as you have few opportunities to attack and you are vulnerable many kinds of attack including the choke. Even if you do manage to get a hold, you are still at risk of attack from the free arm.
2. By rolling over onto his shoulder, Grey prevents White from sliding his arm off of his shoulder because it is tight against the mat.
3. It is always a good strategy to trap limbs beneath your body so that your arms can concentrate solely on offensive maneuvers (Figure 5-27).

Chapter 5: Controlling the Arm

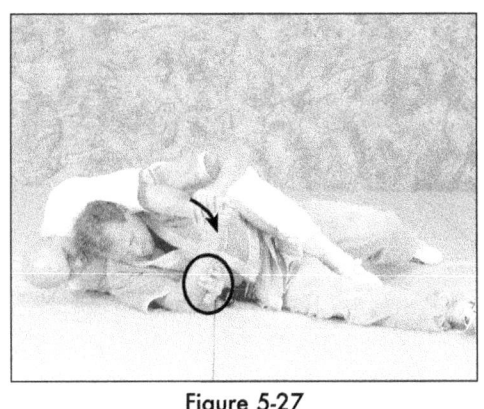

Figure 5-27

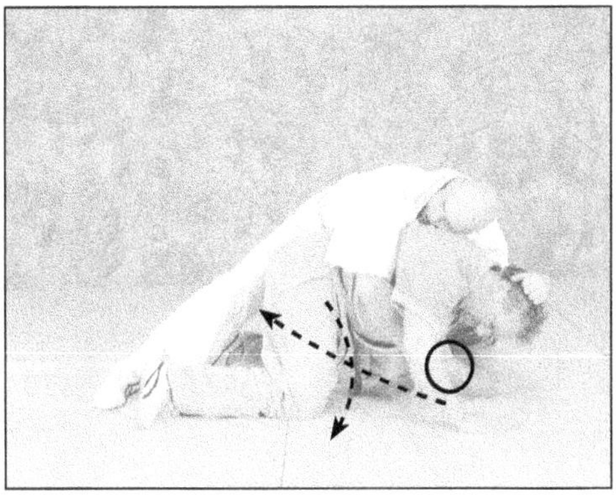

Figure 5-28

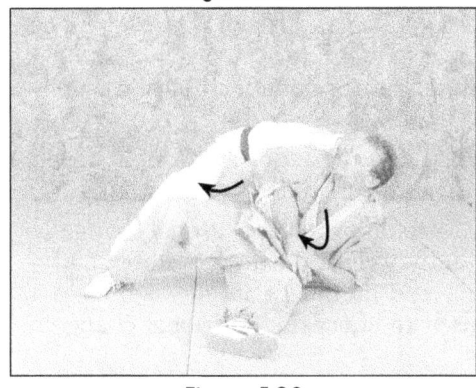

Figure 5-29

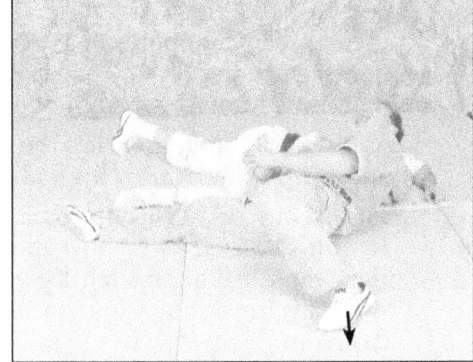

Figure 5-30

Straight Arm Bar From a Sit Out

White has taken down Grey onto all fours and he attempts to gain control over him while in a semi-kneeling position with his right arm in a semi-bear hug around Grey's stomach (Figure 5-28). Grey grabs White's right wrist with his left hand and Grey then shoots his left leg underneath his own body between his weight-bearing appendages and 'sits out'. Grey places his free right arm behind White's right knee as he does his sit out (Figure 5-29). As Grey sits through onto his right buttock, he presses White's right shoulder to the mat (Figure 5-30). Grey leans backwards onto White's right upper arm/shoulder to complete the technique (as shown from the reverse angle in Figure 5-31). Grey may also put on any finger lock or wrist lock of his choice, in this case a bent wrist lock to create additional pain and control (Figure 5-32).

Key Points

1. This technique is a variation on judo's *waki gatame* (armpit hold) which would put the person doing the hold down on the other side of his opponent's arm (i.e., lying more on his torso than his shoulder). This latter hold is more reliable in terms of your ability to pin your adversary because of your ability to maintain torso-to-torso contact.

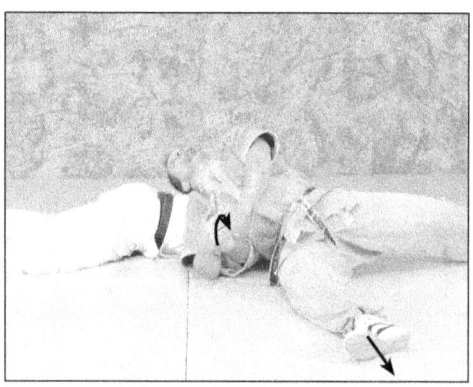
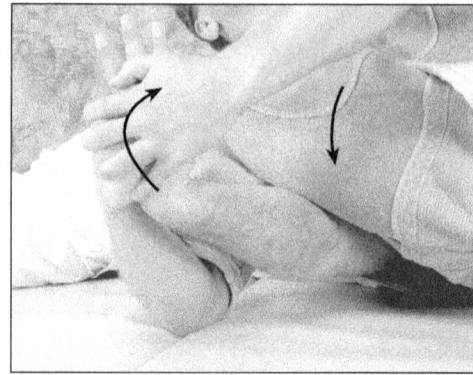

Figure 5-31   Figure 5-32

2. Grey uses his right arm to lever against White's right leg. White's leg is used as an anchor point or as a power base so that Grey can generate some levering action. Try to think about using your opponent's body to your physical advantage whenever you can.

3. As Grey sits through, he lets the combined levering action of his right arm and the dead weight of his body press White's shoulder to the mat.

4. The 'sit out' or 'sit through' is a good way to do a quick positional change. It works because Grey puts all of his body weight on his left elbow and right foot, making his left leg very light and mobile. This allows him to shoot his leg through underneath himself to effect the positional change desired.

5. Grey may increase the pressure on White's elbow by transferring his weight from White's shoulder to White's upper arm. Grey chose an augmenting wrist lock whose direction is consistent with the direction of the main arm lock. This keeps the opponent pinned in place and aligns the offensive pressures exerted by Grey.

Chapter 5: Controlling the Arm

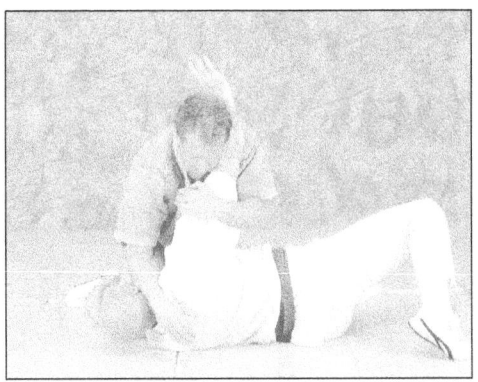

Figure 5-33

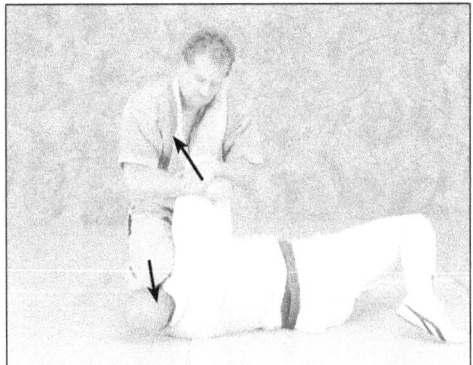

Figure 5-34

Kneeling Straight Arm Hold

Grey has taken down White onto his back and kneels over him from his left side. Grey immediately reaches up with his right arm to try and encircle Grey's neck. Grey gathers White's arm just above his elbow (Figure 5-33). Grey then elects to place his right knee on the right side of White's head (as opposed to kneeing him in the face) and hugs White's arm towards Grey's abdomen to achieve an arm bar that is bridging off of Grey's left shoulder (Figure 5-34).

Key Points

1. This technique is a classical judo move called *ude garumi* (arm hold). It can also be applied by bridging the lower forearm off of the chest or side of the rib cage as well depending upon your relative body configurations.
2. The bridging of the arm, off the shoulder in this case, is crucial to the success of this technique. Then you load the bridging arm with your squeezing arm pressure until the 'bridge' collapses mid span (at the elbow).
3. You may obtain additional control over his arm by pinching his wrist between your shoulder and neck.
4. Your knee across his head/neck will ensure that your opponent will not rise up to escape and will provide additional painful impetus to submit.
5. You may choose to grind the bony part of the radial side of your wrist into his triceps tendon until you find that tender spot (S.J. 11), so that your pressure achieves maximum results. Be mindful though that when you move from palm control to wrist edge control, you lose some ability to keep your opponent from rotating his arm away from the locking pressure.

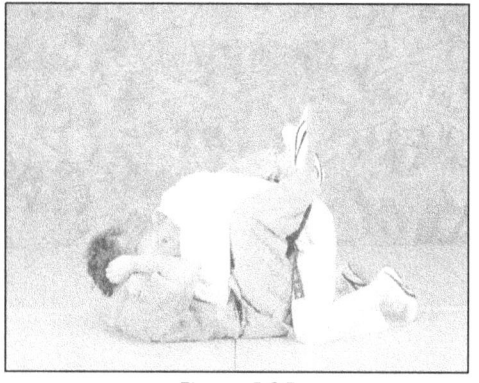

Figure 5-35

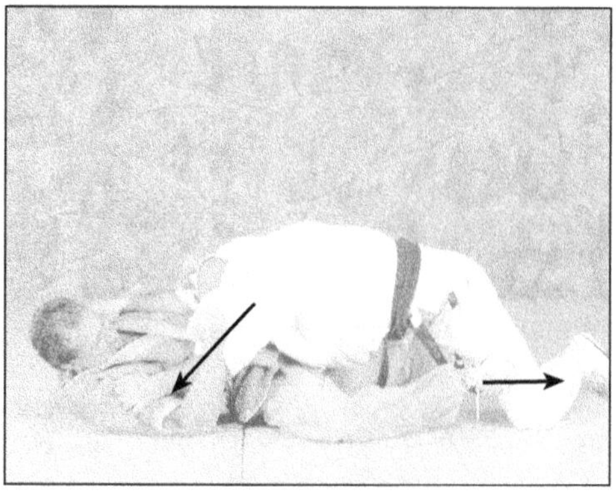

Figure 5-36

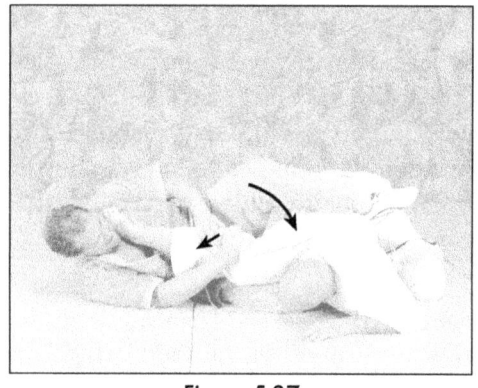

Figure 5-37

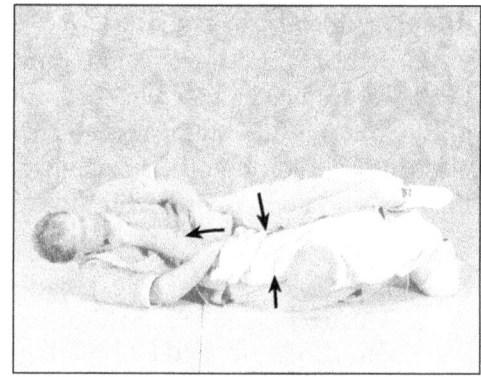

Figure 5-38

Reclining Straight Arm Hold

White is in Grey's guard and he chooses to pull himself in very tight to Grey (Figure 5-35). Grey unlocks his guard and kicks out White's left leg with his right foot while pulling sideways and forwards on White's left shoulder to help unbalance him (Figure 5-36). Grey slides out to his left and grabs White's right arm as he swings his free left leg over the top of White's shoulders (Figure 5-37). Grey squeezes his knees together and applies his right wrist, powered by a cross grab with his other hand, in towards his own body (Figure 5-38).

Key Points

1. Use your leg to take away a point of his balance, and your arm to take another away, both in the direction you want to take him, so that you can escape from under him.

2. Squeeze your knees together for additional arm control.

3. You may elect to initially hold his wrist to your chest as you kick him out flat, before working on his elbow.

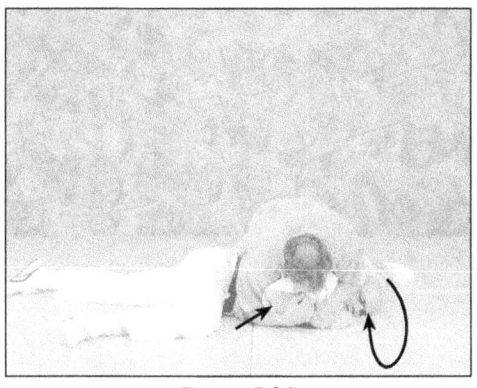
Figure 5-39

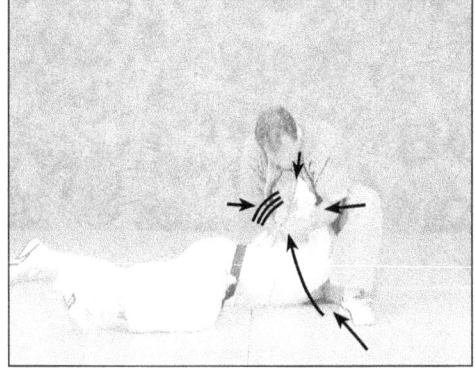
Figure 5-40

5-3. BENT ARM LOCKS

Applying Bent Arm Locks

As mentioned in the previous section, there are only two arm configurations that you have to deal with. The arm is either straight or bent. Any appendage at the extreme end of its range of movement is at its weakest position, biomechanically speaking. There are a number of bent arm locks that do not take the limb to its hyper-flexive state, rather the arm is bent at 90 degrees for the purposes of torquing the arm lateral to the arm's plane of movement. As such, the arm is in a position to offer resistance more readily than if it was at either end of its range of motion. For this reason, these locks can be more problematic to apply. You also need to move a lot closer to your opponent's upper body to effect these locks and this may not always be desirable. Bent arm locks though are a valuable class of holds to have in your repertoire. Unlike the massive hip joint of the leg, the comparable shoulder joint can be manipulated beyond its breaking point.

Sometimes your opponent takes on a defensive posture by covering up his head with his arms or by bending his arm to thwart your attempt to get him in a straight arm bar. Rather than trying to physically out-muscle him, go with what he gives you and try to snap on a bent arm lock.

As with the straight arm locks, take note that you can supplement your bent arm locks with finger and wrist Qin Na techniques to give your opponent maximum pain.

Prone Bent Arm Lock

Grey has taken down White into the supine position and pins him in a cross body mount, and then he takes control over White's right wrist with his left hand while he slides his right forearm under White's right elbow (Figure 5-39). Grey then steps over White's head with his left knee, adopting a semi-kneeling position, squeezing his opponent's torso between his legs to keep him from turning (Figure 5-40). Grey also bends White's right wrist toward his own body and augments the hold with his other hand. Grey scoops White's arm up between his forearms and

Chin Na In Ground Fighting

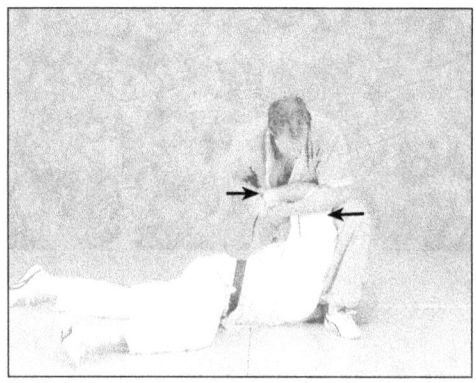

Figure 5-41

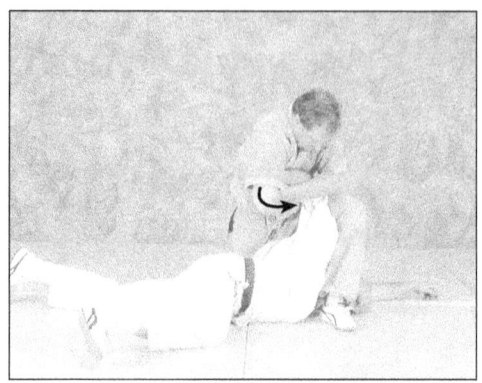

Figure 5-42

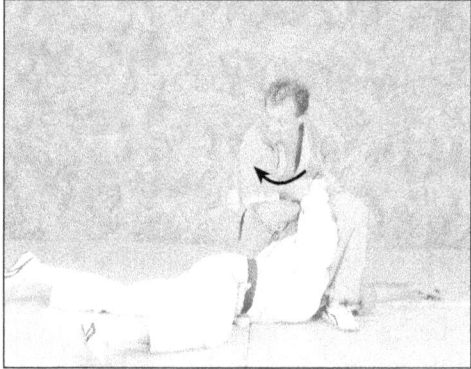

Figure 5-43

lifts his hands upwards against White's wrist, bracing White's elbow against Grey's chest to effect the lock.

Key Points

1. Be sure that when you are pinning your opponent, rest as little weight as possible on your knees and feet so that there is a maximum transfer of your body weight into your opponent.
2. Notice that Grey braces White's elbow against his chest for a more immediate and stronger locking counterpressure.
3. Grey may kick White in the face as he steps over his head to soften him up if required.
4. Grey can pull White's bent arm into himself, locking the elbow and even the shoulder joint as all the slack is taken out of the arm.

Shoulder Crank

As a continuation from the previous technique, prone bent arm lock, Grey could rotate White's right forearm clockwise (Figure 5-41). Grey maintains the bent wrist lock with his left hand while threading his right arm under his own left arm (and White's right arm) as deep as it will go (Figure 5-42). Grey can let go of the wrist lock and extract his left arm and clasp his other arm that is entwined with White's right arm (Figure 5-43).

Key Points

1. It is important to maintain the wrist lock through the transition with the arm crank, otherwise your opponent will sense the loss of control and try to escape.

Chapter 5: Controlling the Arm

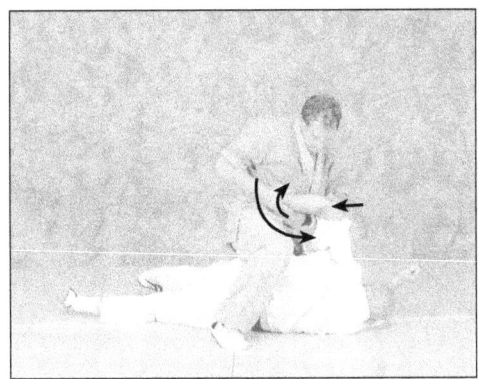

Figure 5-44

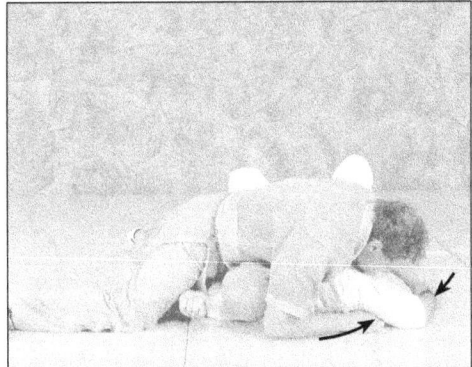

Figure 5-45

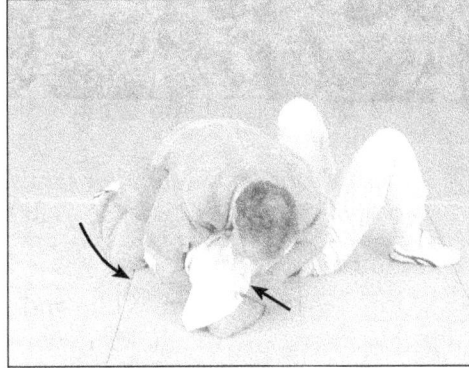

Figure 5-46

2. You may figure four your own wrist or adopt a power grip to secure this final hold.
3. The shoulder is highly inflexible beyond the frontal plane so little torque is needed to cause excruciating pain to your opponent (and you have plenty of potential torque to deliver).
4. Be wary of your opponent biting your ankle. Place your heel tightly against his throat. Posting your heel at his throat will also deter him from trying to rotate his body in the direction of the arm torque.
5. This technique can be delivered while facing your opponent in the opposite direction as well. Step over your opponent's lower back and apply a wrist lock, crank his left arm away from you by pulling his elbow towards you and simultaneously pushing his wrist away from you (Figure 5-44). You may also figure four his arm by threading your left arm under his forearm from the outside and grab your own wrist (not shown).

Transverse Arm Wrap

Grey has White in the cross mounted position and he grabs White's right wrist with his left hand while he begins to slide his right arm under White's right armpit (Figure 5-45). Grey then grabs White's right lower forearm and pulls this wrist toward White's armpit in order to hyperflex the elbow (Figure 5-46).

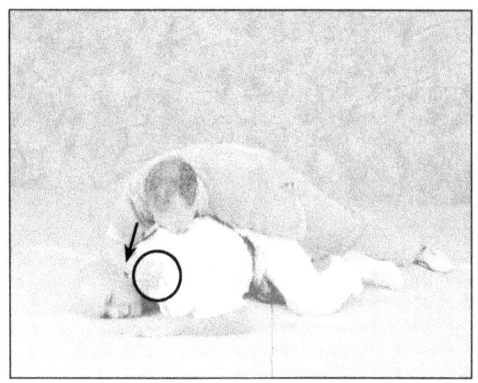
Figure 5-47

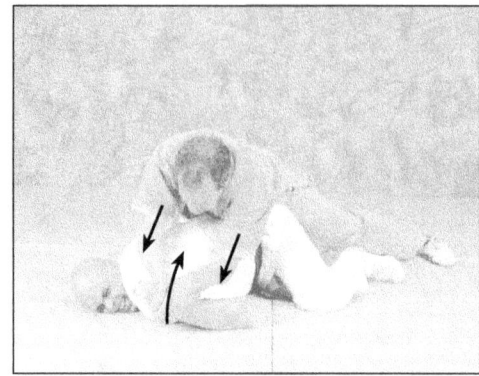
Figure 5-48

Key Points
1. The presence of the mat prohibits Grey from cranking White's arm down to lock it and cranking it upwards is too far to go in this situation, so Grey draws the hand into White's own armpit, as there is little mobility in this direction.
2. Grey can pin White's left arm with his right knee or knee White's head/neck should White try to grab his groin.

Double Lever Lock

Grey has taken down White and they are in the prone position with Grey on top (Figure 5-47). Grey holds down White by grabbing his left rear shoulder and levering the ulnar edge of his forearm against the back of White's neck. Grey may also attack his groin from this position. Grey then secures White's left wrist with both hands keeping both forearms on his opponent and he levers upwards to break the elbow joint (Figure 5-48).

Key Points
1. Notice how Grey uses White's own clothing to create an anchored power base for his right elbow.
2. By keeping the forearms or elbows on White, Grey can apply his arm strength and body weight into the levers as well as help pin his opponent.
3. The bent arm has very limited mobility in both the elbow and shoulder past the frontal plane of the body. When your opponent is prone, his arm is nearly at the end of its range of motion, making it an ideal target for a lock from this position.

Chapter 5: Controlling the Arm

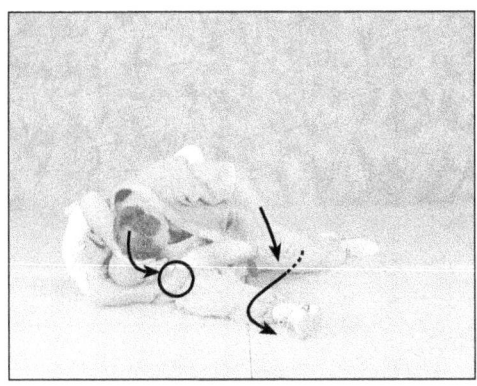

Figure 5-49

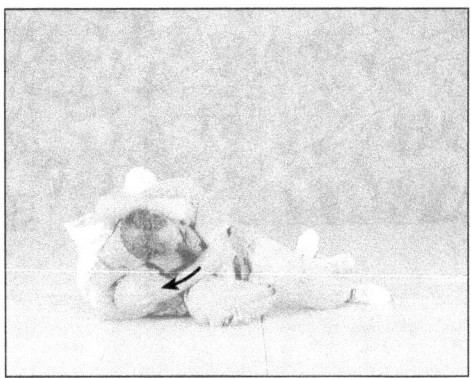

Figure 5-50

Bent Arm Lock from a Scarf Hold

Grey has taken down White and they land on their sides. Grey immediately puts on a scarf hold around White's neck, buries his head to protect it and bends White's straightened right arm across White's right upper thigh (Figure 5-49). Grey is being attacked by White's free left arm so Grey places White's right wrist under his right knee. Grey secures this arm by bending this leg and crossing his ankles (Figure 5-50). Gray can now gouge White's face or he can secure White's left arm with a finger lock and punch him in the face (Figure 5-51).

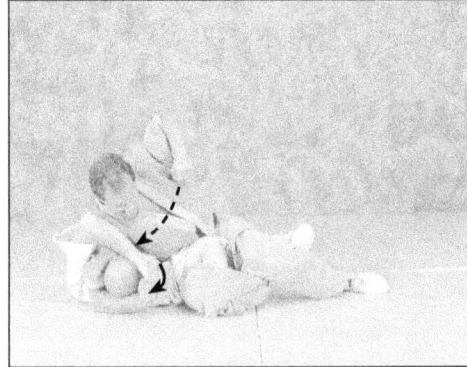

Figure 5-51

Key Points

1. This technique is a variation of judo's *kesa gatame* (scarf hold). It is an excellent way to pin an opponent.
2. Do not let your weight ride too high up onto your opponent's torso or he may pull you over backward.
3. Notice how Grey has grabbed his own pant leg with his encircling right hand anchoring it in order to free up his other hand.
4. Some instability to Grey's front quarter will be created when the opponent's arm is secured with his forward leg.
5. You may do a straight arm bar on your opponent if you have the clearance from the mat.
6. Grey can create additional torque on the bent arm by raising his hips upwards and/or sliding the right retaining leg backwards to lock the shoulder as well.

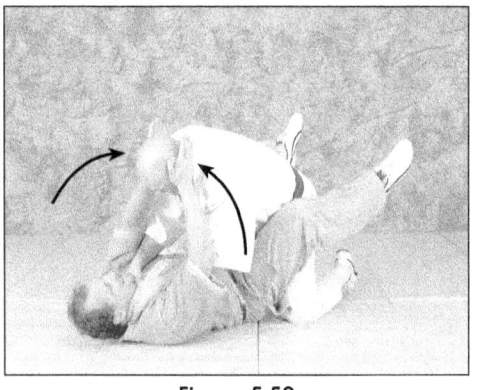

Figure 5-52

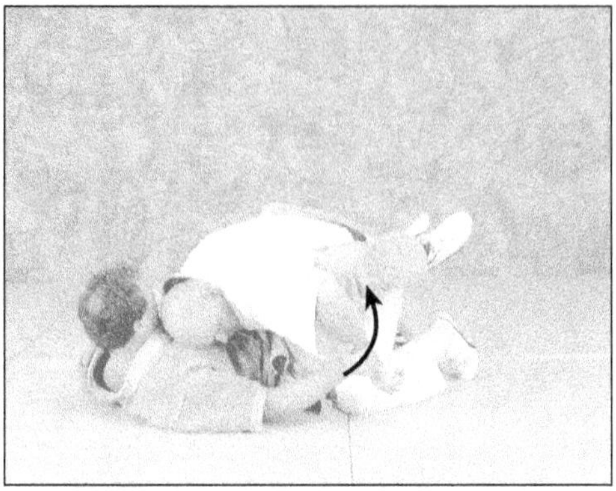

Figure 5-53

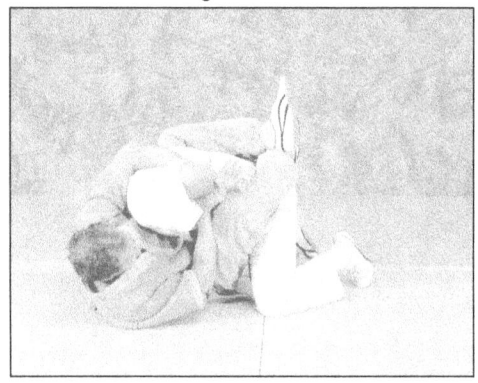

Figure 5-54

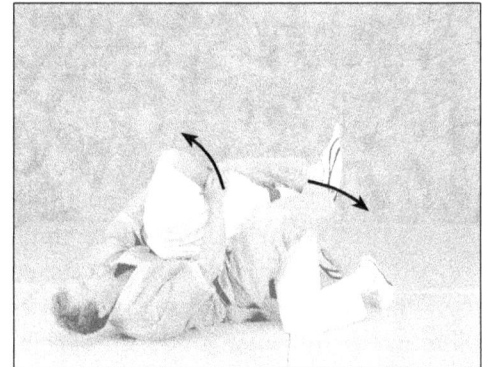

Figure 5-55

Rear Bent Arm Lock from the Guard

White has bowled Grey over and tries to choke him while in his guard. Grey immediately slaps both of White's ears in response to this threat (Figure 5-52). Grey grabs White's left wrist with his right hand, pushing it backward while he unlocks his legs and shifts his hips to the left (Figure 5-53). Grey now reaches over Grey's head and left shoulder to grab White's left wrist with his left hand, re-locking his legs as he does so (Figure 5-54). Grey now has a firm hold on White's left bent arm and he pulls it up White's back by leaning backward and pushing White's hips in the opposite direction by straightening his leg (Figure 5-55).

Key Points

1. The key to this technique is to get the arm bent past the frontal plane of the body, where it becomes weak and loses mobility. Using any distraction technique is beneficial to setting up your main technique.
2. By scooting your hips to one side, you can more easily reach over White's left shoulder.
3. Think of stretching your opponent's spine as you pull up the body with your arms and down with the legs.
4. If your opponent is very flexible in the arms push his arm upward (away from the back) to lock the arm.

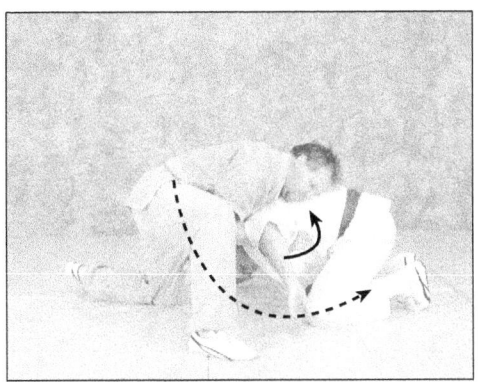

Figure 5-56

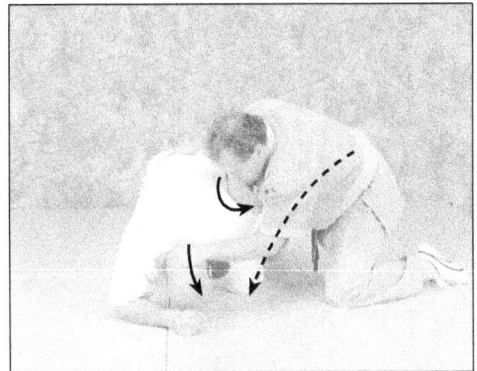

Figure 5-57

Hammer Lock

Grey approaches White who is on all fours and places his torso on top of White's back as he kneels on his left knee and underhooks White's left arm (Figure 5-56). Grey scoots counterclockwise around White's body while maintaining his body pressure on him, bending White's arm to the rear in the process. Grey pulls White's neck toward himself to keep White from sliding away from him to escape the

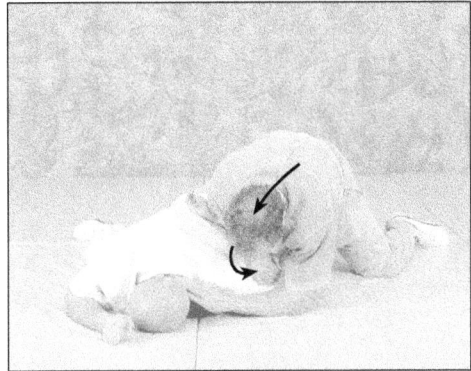

Figure 5-58

forming lock (Figure 5-57). Grey then drives forward with his legs in order to flatten out White and further reduce his chances of escaping (Figure 5-58).

Key Points

1. Use your legs, other muscles and body weight to defeat resistance encountered from a seized limb.
2. Make use of mechanical advantage by levering his arm with the crook of your elbow closer to his lower forearm (as opposed to his elbow).
3. You may grab your own top at the right biceps to firmly lock the hold in place.
4. Keep your body weight on your opponent to prevent him from rolling away from you to escape.

CHAPTER 6

Controlling the Leg

6-1. Introduction

Practicality of Leg Locks

When we talk about controlling the leg in ground fighting, it can be likened to knee and ankle Qin Na (Chin Na). These are two joints of the leg that can be attacked and controlled more easily than the hip, although the massive leg musculature and larger joint sizes pose significant control problems. As such, it is usually more difficult to control the leg than the arm because of these differences. The leg locking techniques generally require more power than an elbow or wrist technique. The principles involved in controlling these limbs, however, are identical given that their structures are similar. The ankle is similar to the wrist; the knee is similar to the elbow; toes are similar to the fingers; the hip is similar to the shoulder. When we attack the ankle, we are using the Qin Na principle of dividing the muscle/tendon. When we are attacking the knee, we are using the principle of misplacing the bone. The hip is seldom attacked given its size.

Qin Na practitioners do not have the experience that a seasoned ground fighter has when dealing with leg locks, because they seldom go to the ground to effect their techniques. The legs become more susceptible to these locks when your opponent has his weight off of them such as when he's on the ground. Many schools disregard ankle locks in particular because of the presence of footwear. Toe Qin Na is virtually unheard of partly because of this factor and due to the fact that toe injuries are not nearly as debilitating in a fight as finger injuries are (compare the effect on a ground fight that three broken fingers have versus three broken toes). Some of the ankle locks will work with shoes or boots on nonetheless. The reader can explore these possibilities on his own and see what will and will not work with regards to the presence of footwear.

Anatomy of the Leg

There are a total of 62 bones of the lower extremities (from the hip to the tips of the toes):

2 innominate bones (hip bones)	2 femur (thigh)
2 patella (knee caps)	2 fibula (minor lower leg bones)
2 tibia (major lower leg bones)	14 tarsals (ankle bones)
10 metatarsals (foot bones)	28 phalanges (toe bones)

The legs are a more critical target in stand up fighting than on the ground because of their requirement to support the body, providing the requisite balance and mobility to the fighting machine. They also serve as powerful tools for attack and defense. Like the arm, the leg has an upper bone connecting two lower bones at a joint. The knee joint has a protective free-floating kneecap over the joint though. The hip joint is a ball and socket joint that is somewhat susceptible to dislocation because of a relative lack of strong ligamentation and muscularity toward the rear of the joint. This joint is large and well muscled, making manipulation difficult. It is capable of rotation around three axes with movement possible through flexion (114 degrees with leg bent, knee towards chest, and 80 degrees with the leg straight), backward extension (32 degrees), expansion outward (45 degrees away from mid-line), inward rotation (15 degrees) and outward rotation (35 degrees) as well as circular movement (360 degrees).

The knee is a complicated and fairly large joint of the femur and tibia that is overlaid frontally by the patella. Four major ligaments stabilize the knee. The large sciatic nerve which runs down the back of the leg from the hip, splits into the fibular and tibial nerves and passes around the outside of the knee and behind the knee respectively. A branch of the femoral nerve runs through the knee itself.

The ankle joint can only move along one axis (26 degrees of movement) with limited inward and outward movement. It is comprised of the tibia and fibula that sits on top of the talus bones of the foot. It is held in place by several major ligaments. Many nerves pass through the ankle into the foot making it an opportune place to do pressure point attacks.

Leg Blocks

One thing that we can do with the legs that is not normally done with the arms, given that they are larger, longer and stronger than the arms, is to 'block' them. This means to place a physical block on the inside of the knee joint to act as a fulcrum so that the lower leg can lever the knee apart. The relative shortness of the two main segments of the arm compared to that of the leg plus the proximity of your upper body to his upper body with his main weapons, leaves little opportunity to effectively and safely apply a block to the elbow joint.

6-2. Ankle Locks

Learning the Lock

Ankle locks are difficult to learn safely from a book. It is for this reason that we will have a close look at two of the basic positions for attacking the ankle. Once you are able to do these locks correctly, you will have a foundation to work from. Play with variations in the technique bearing in mind the pertinent Qin Na principles. If your partner does not feel pain or experiences it up the calf as opposed to the ankle, take corrective measures in setting up your technique properly. Take care in practicing these techniques, as knee and ankle injuries are serious and debilitating injuries. Many schools do not teach them for this reason.

Chapter 6: Controlling the Leg

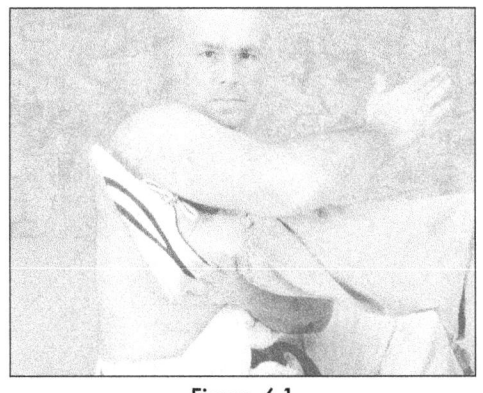

Figure 6-1

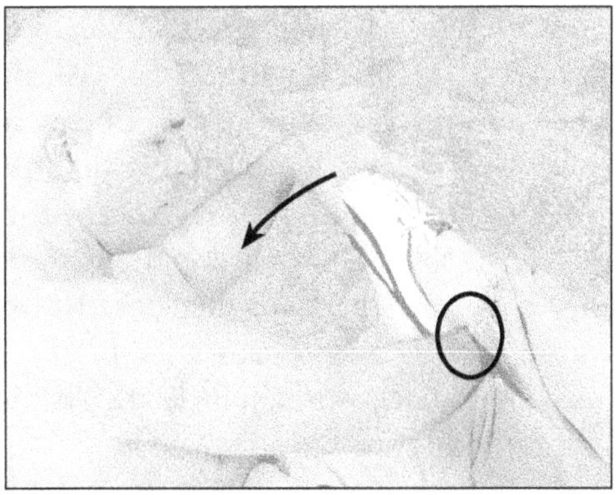

Figure 6-2

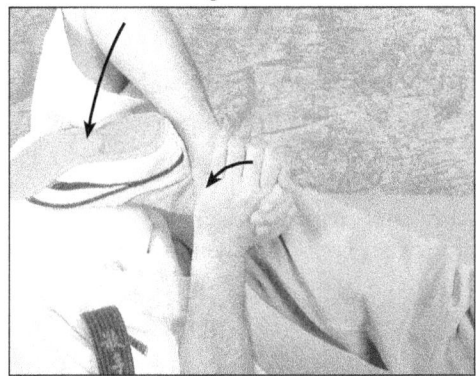

Figure 6-3

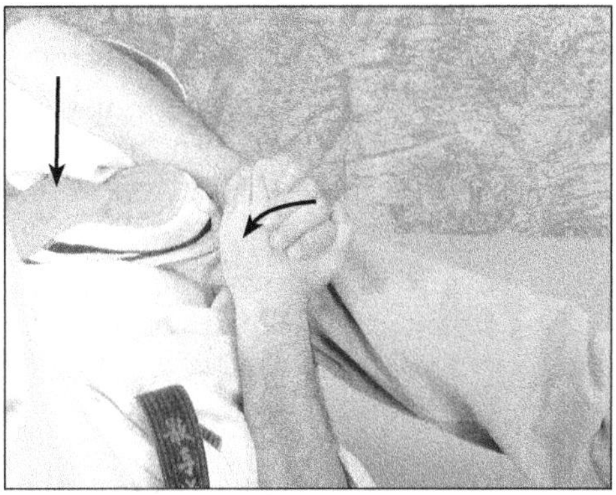

Figure 6-4

Basic Ankle Lock #1

White places Grey's left instep under and behind his right armpit (Figure 6-1) so that the inside of Grey's instep is in direct contact with White's latissimus dorsi / triceps muscles.

The exact placement of the narrow bony radial edge of the wrist is directly behind the ankle and under Grey's Achilles tendon (Figure 6-2) to ensure that there is a maximum, and painful, transfer of force into this tendon. Using the power grip, clasp both hands

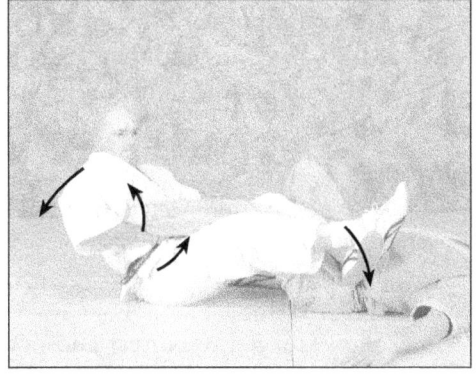

Figure 6-5

together and bring your elbow to your hip (Figure 6-3) while flexing your latissimus dorsi muscles and squeezing the foot in the arm pit. Be sure to do an inward and upward grinding movement with your wrist in order to maximize the pain and control potential (Figure 6-4).

White now places his left leg over his opponent's outstretched and tightly cap-

219

tured left leg with his left ankle over Grey's left hip (Figure 6-5). White then crosses his own ankle effectively scissoring Grey's leg. White can now effectively control Grey's leg and he can use his crossed ankles as a base to push down on as he leans backwards for more torque. White can raise his hips as he reefs backwards in order to get his entire body into action.

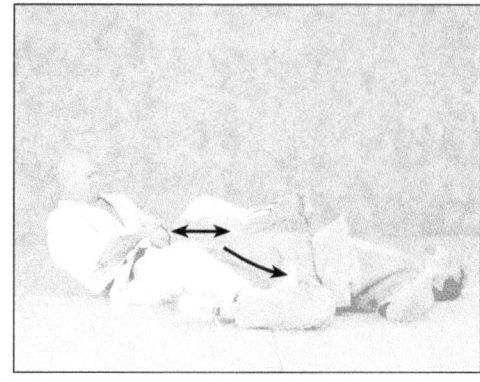

Figure 6-6

Key Points
1. The exact placement of the foot in your armpit is crucial for a good ankle lock.
2. The squeezing of the foot between the upper arm and your lat muscles can cause excruciating pain in the phalanges and metatarsal knuckles of the feet in itself, and further lock in the foot, preventing an escape.
3. This crunching of the foot knuckles would be difficult to do if your opponent had foot wear on. If that is the case, then concentrate solely on the attack of the Achilles tendon. Low cut footwear is not problematic for this type of ankle attack.

Basic Ankle Lock #2

Instead of White merely crossing his legs over Grey's leg as in the previous technique, White will apply a leg lock (Figure 6-6 shows the opposite configuration for clarity). If your opponent insists on trying to kick with his non-captured leg, White unlocks his figure four and the near side leg can kick back or push more directly into Grey's leg which assists in his backward push for power. This helps to effect control over both legs.

Key Points
1. The only difference between this lock and the previous one is the placement of the legs.
2. This method of pushing against your opponent's other leg also facilitates the stretching of his held leg thereby removing the slack from it. This allows for a more direct and positive response to your locking pressure.

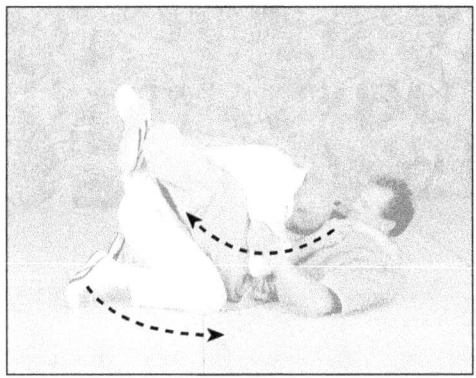

Figure 6-7

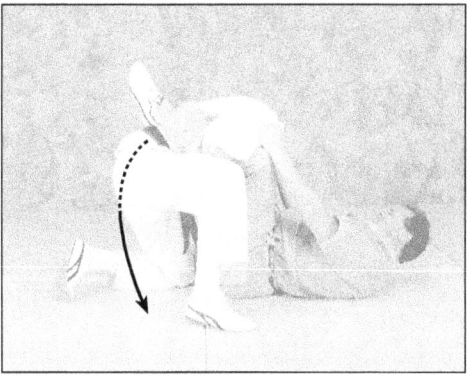

Figure 6-8

Basic Ankle Lock from the Guard

Starting in Grey's guard, White breaks free by pressing with his elbows against the inside of Grey's thighs (Figure 6-7). White then overhooks Grey's left leg while he comes up on his right leg to a semi-kneeling position (Figure 6-8). White pins Grey's other leg to the mat with his left hand. White then sits back and slides his right arm into the basic ankle lock position behind Grey's Achilles tendon while

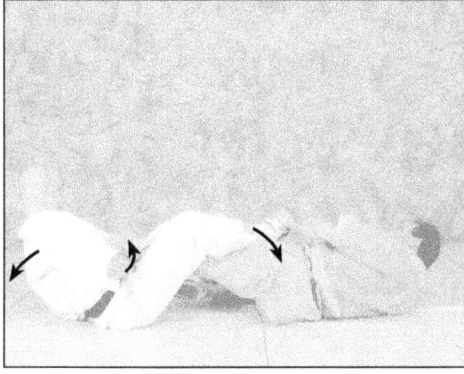

Figure 6-9

clasping his hands together in a power grip and inserting his left leg between Grey's legs (Figure 6-9). White may either use his left leg to push against his opponent's aggressive right leg or cross his ankles applying a lock to Grey's leg, securing the ankle lock.

Key Points

1. There are many ways to get to the basic ankle lock. We will show you two ways to effect this hold. Using your legs to control his legs and provide torquing power on the ankle is important.
2. Be sure to grind the bony part of the radial side of your wrist into your opponent's Achilles tendon.

Chin Na In Ground Fighting

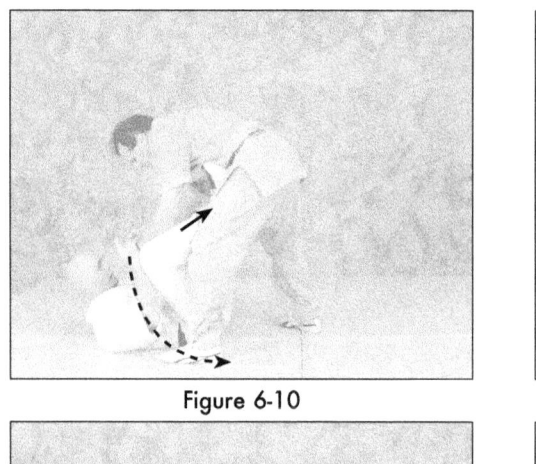

Figure 6-10

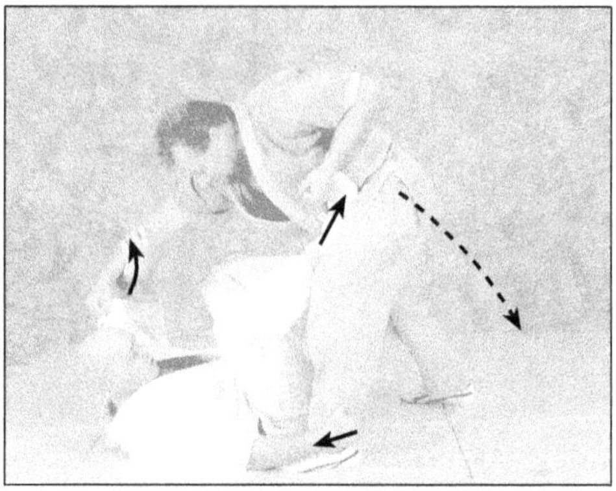

Figure 6-11

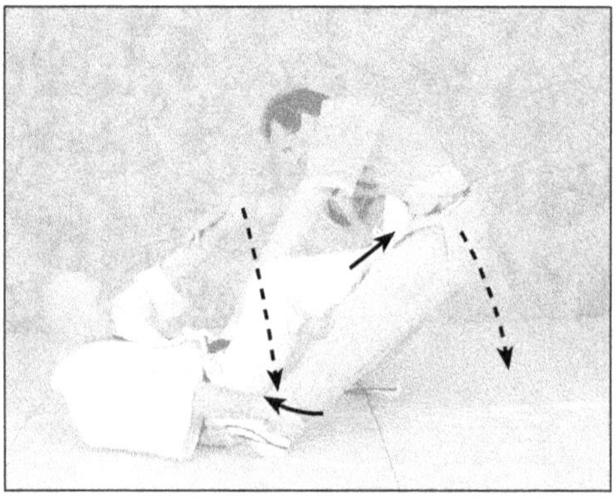

Figure 6-12

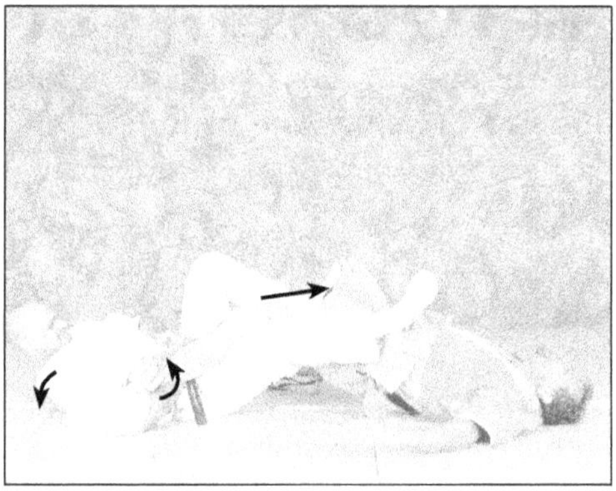

Figure 6-13

Basic Ankle Lock from a Defensive Position

Grey has knocked White to the mat and is attempting to finish him off. White places his legs against Grey's hips while controlling Grey's hands (Figure 6-10). White grabs Grey's left heel when he finds an opening to do so (Figure 6-11). White then thrusts at Grey's left hip with his right leg while pulling Grey's foot towards himself causing Grey to fall backwards (Figure 6-12). As Grey falls, White lets his right leg slide down over Grey's left leg as he scoops up his ankle with his right arm (Figure 6-13). White is now set up for the basic ankle lock and he may adopt the final leg placement of his choosing.

Key Points

1. Use your legs on your opponent's hips to control the distance.
2. In this case, White pushes on Grey's right thigh with his left foot to give him counterpressure for his ankle lock and to control his opponent's free leg.
3. White has tremendous mechanical advantage using Grey's entire leg as a lever with power for the take down supplied by his legs.
4. Try to keep your opponent's lower back on the mat by pushing down with your feet or by spreading his free leg to keep him from bridging upwards and thereby reducing the pressure on the lock.

Chapter 6: Controlling the Leg

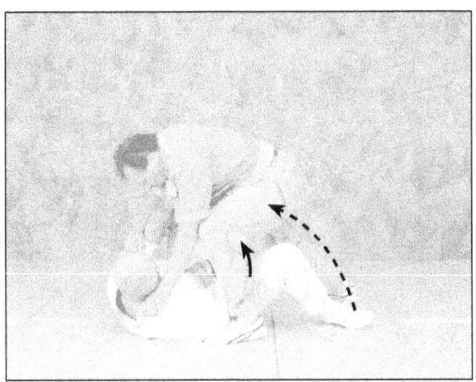

Figure 6-14

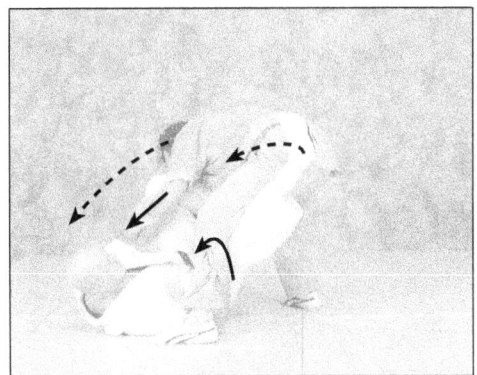

Figure 6-15

Heel Hook

In this case, Grey has taken down White and is attempting to mount him (Figure 6-14). White grabs Grey's left leg with his right hand under and behind Grey's left knee in order to try and buckle the leg and to use it to help spin himself counterclockwise. White simultaneously grabs Grey's left shoulder/arm with his left hand. White then kicks in a circular motion (similar to a crescent kick) with his right leg up and

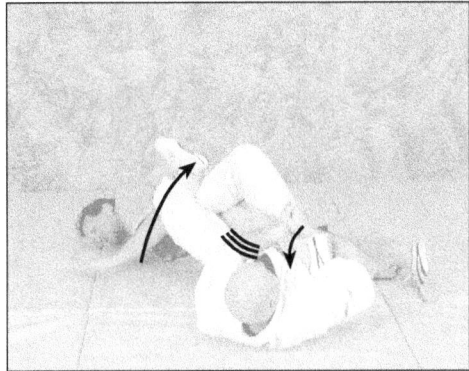

Figure 6-16

over Grey's left leg (Figure 6-15) while pulling crossways on Grey's left shoulder/arm to further unbalance him. Grey falls forward landing face down on the mat as White continues to snake his right leg around Grey's left leg and he secures it by crossing his ankles or figure-fouring it (Figure 6-16). White also secures White's left ankle by hooking Grey's heel with his right wrist held in a power grip. White further traps Grey's lower leg between his right lat muscle and right inner forearm such that the top of the instep lies across White's lat muscle (90 degrees to the basic ankle lock). White can then raise his hips up while bringing his hands to his chest, causing pain in both the ankle joint and the inside of the knee.

Key Points
1. This heel hook is a devastating technique because you are attacking the ligaments of the knee as well as the ankle itself. Exercise caution when practicing this technique. Note that it can be adopted from a variety of positions.

Chin Na In Ground Fighting

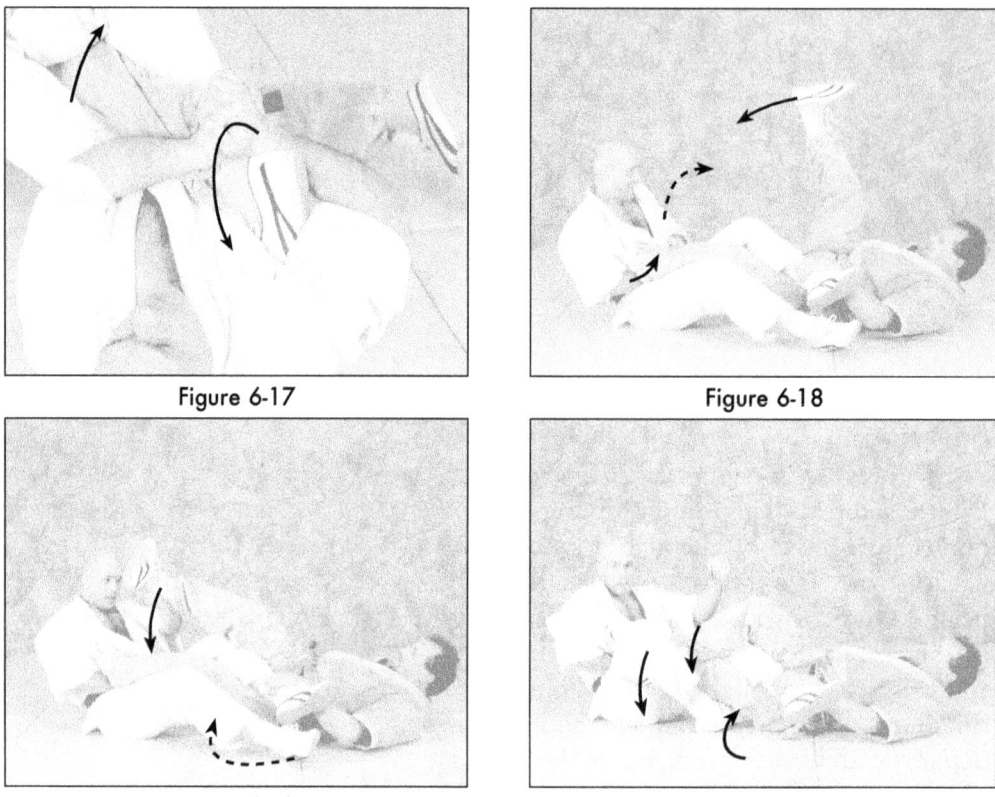

Figure 6-17

Figure 6-18

Figure 6-19

Figure 6-20

2. The main difference between this technique and the basic ankle lock is the placement of the hands relative to the ankle (Figure 6-17). White has placed his right wrist to the inside of Grey's left ankle. The exerted inward pressure works the ankle outward sideways (and the knee joint is pressured in the opposite direction).

3. The ankle has a very limited range of motion sideways, making this an opportune angle for attack.

Double Leg Lock

White is just in the process of applying the basic ankle lock when Grey attempts to deliver an axe kick to White's stomach (Figure 6-18). White parries the kick to his right side with his left hand while starting to swing his own right leg outwards and upward over Grey's deflected leg (Figure 6-19). White then traps Grey's kicking leg by swinging the crook of his right knee over Grey's right ankle that he places under Grey's own left thigh (Figure 6-20). White now can proceed with his original basic ankle lock by taking a power grip on Grey's left ankle. Alternatively, White may choose to secure a one-handed clothing assisted grip on this same ankle, freeing up his left hand to pull downwards on Grey's right knee to lock it as well (Figure 6-21). White now has Grey's left ankle and his right knee locked.

Chapter 6: Controlling the Leg

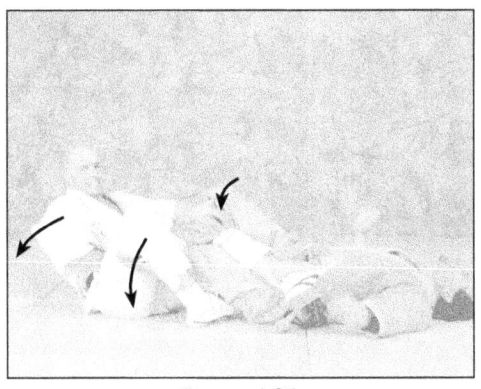

Figure 6-21

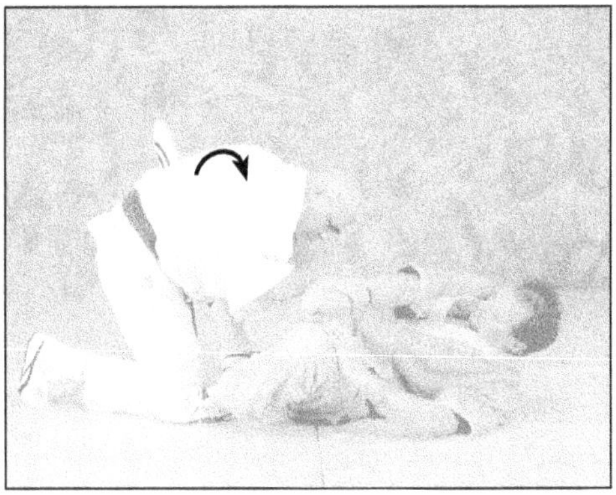

Figure 6-22

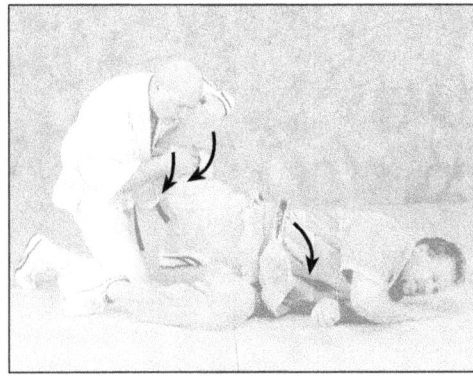

Figure 6-23

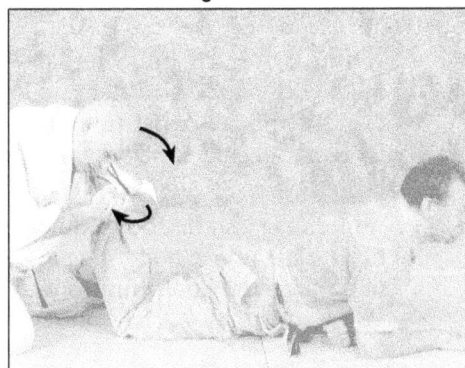

Figure 6-24

Key Points

1. Like with any martial arts technique, if you do not execute it with speed and precision, your opponent may counter the technique. The most natural way to try to counter an ankle lock is to kick your way out of it. If this happens, try this double leg lock.
2. Note that White secured this lock by placing his own right foot under the back of Grey's left upper thigh. Use your opponent's body to your advantage whenever possible.

Reverse Ankle Lock From the Guard

White finds himself in Grey's guard so he breaks out of it and under-hooks Grey's right leg with his left arm while stepping up with his left leg into a semi-kneeling position (Figure 6-22). White then turns Grey onto his stomach by levering against Grey's right lower leg with both of his hands behind Grey's knee and using his left arm/shoulder for additional torque (Figure 6-23). White immediately slides the left radial edge of his wrist to the Achilles tendon just below the rear of Grey's right heel making sure to secure this ankle with a power grip (Figure 6-24). Notice the placement of Grey's right instep on White's left shoulder.

Chin Na In Ground Fighting

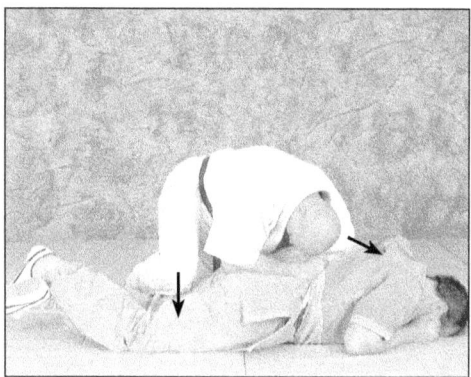

Figure 6-25

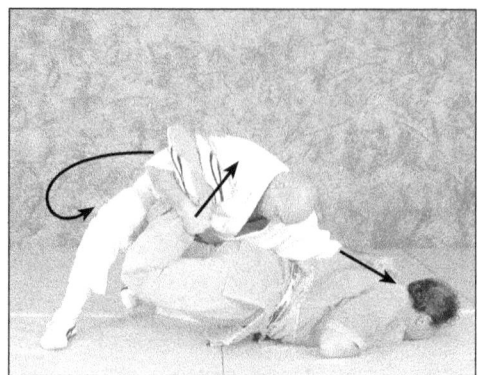

Figure 6-26

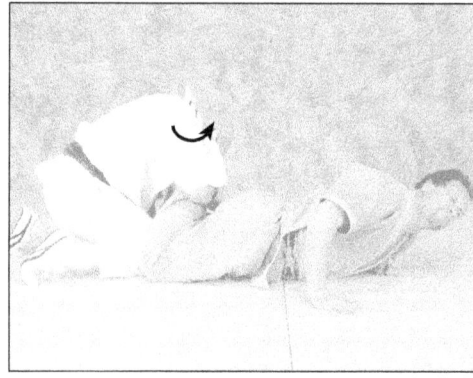

Figure 6-27

Key Points
1. White is free to press forwards with his left shoulder while grinding his left wrist in a circular fishhook-like motion towards himself.
2. White may also decide to quickly torque his upper body clockwise to damage the knee joint as well.

Double Ankle Lock

White has taken down Grey into the prone position. Grey adopts a defensive position by crossing his legs and protecting his neck with his hands. White immediately grabs Grey's clothing between Grey's shoulder blades for control and kneels on the back of Grey's left upper leg with his right knee to cause pain that distracts and to help immobilize him (Figure 6-25). White underhooks both of Grey's ankles with his right arm and lifts Grey's lower body off the mat, pressing his weight onto Grey's back to keep him in place and help thwart a counterattack (Figure 6-26). White then spins around directly behind Grey as he places Grey's crossed ankles on his right shoulder taking care to place the radial edge of his right wrist against Grey's Achilles tendon as he exerts inward pressure using both hands powered by his torso (Figure 6-27).

Key Points
1. It is usually not a good idea to cross your ankles defensively when your opponent can access them because both legs can be easily tied up and put into a painful lock as well.
2. Secure your hands with a power grip and grind this tendon with a circular inwards and upwards motion of this bony part of your wrist.
3. Simultaneously, apply counterpressure by pressing forward with your right shoulder. Because both ankles are crossed, pain will be experienced in both of your opponent's ankles.

Chapter 6: Controlling the Leg

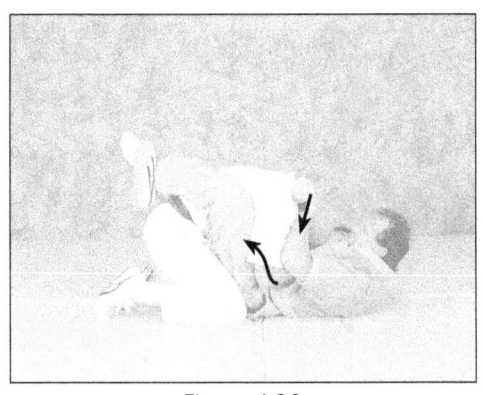

Figure 6-28

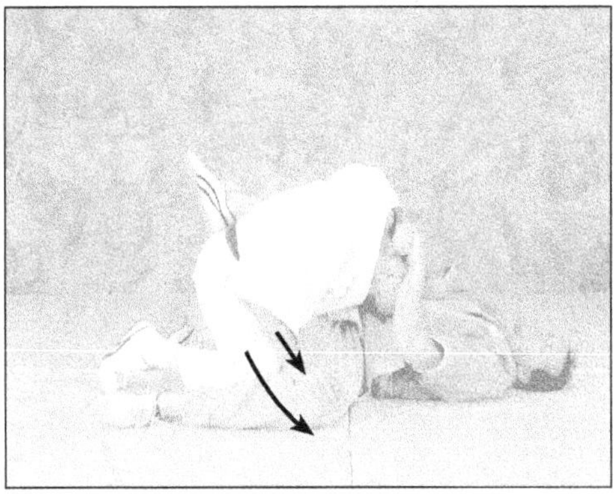

Figure 6-29

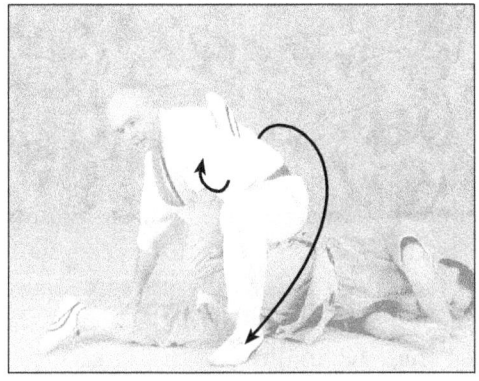

Figure 6-30

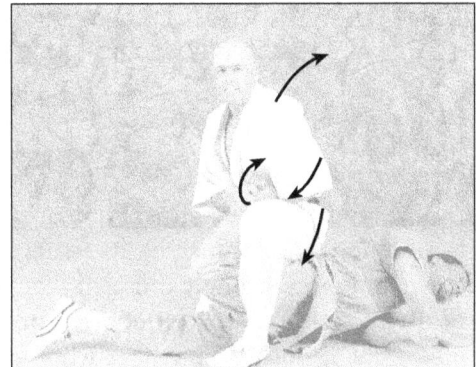

Figure 6-31

Kneeling Ankle Lock

White finds himself in Grey's guard (Figure 6-28). White breaks open Grey's guard by applying his right elbow to Grey's left inner thigh. As he does so, White overhooks Grey's right leg with his left arm, continues to open up the guard, and pins Grey's left leg by pressing down on his thigh, with his right hand (Figure 6-29). White then steps over Grey with his left leg clockwise, using Grey's right leg as a lever to turn him over onto his front in the process (Figure 6-30). Now White sits on Grey's buttock as he secures the ankle with a power grip and by bringing his left elbow towards his left hip (Figure 6-31).

Key Points
1. Notice the placement of Grey's left foot and White's left wrist (under Grey's Achilles tendon). This is exactly the same position as the basic ankle lock, only Grey is in the prone position.
2. Notice how White used Grey's right leg as a lever in order to turn him over onto his front. The knee is easily susceptible to lateral injury, hence your opponent can offer little resistance for fear of a knee injury.
3. The circular pressure of the wrist upward and inward is done in conjunction with White moving his hips forward as he arches backwards.

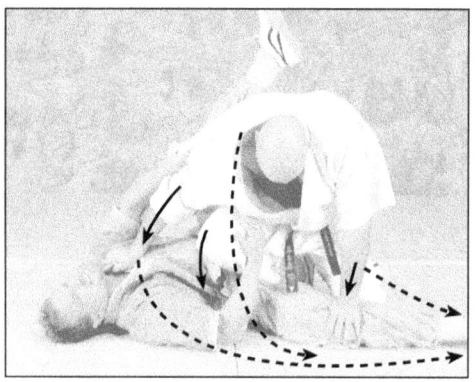 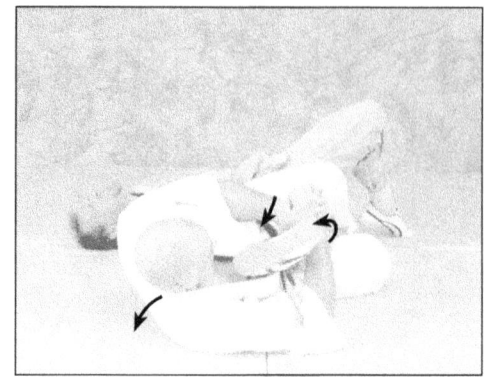

Figure 6-32   Figure 6-33

4. White also lets his body weight work for him as he sinks down onto Grey, keeping him pinned and diminishing the joint angles of the leg.

6.3. Knee Locks

Applying Knee Locks

We know that the knee is similar to the elbow and hyperextension of both joints is a prime way of damaging its structural integrity. We also know that the legs are larger and more strongly muscled than that of the arms, so more physical force must be used to effect these techniques. Applying the movement of your whole body is an important factor to remember when effecting these techniques on this large joint. Ankle locks may also be used in conjunction with knee locks.

Basic Knee Lock

White breaks free of Grey's guard and pins Grey's right leg to the mat with his right hand while bringing his right knee on top of Grey's right hip and thigh area (Figure 6-32). White also uses his left arm against Grey's chest to help control him. White then pulls Grey's right leg up with his left hand as Grey drops his right knee to the mat and rolls over onto his right side with his back to Grey. White scoops Grey's right heel with his right hand as he does so. White's right foot stays in Grey's right hip joint and his pelvis remains in direct contact with Grey's right knee creating a fulcrum that can be used to hyper-extend the knee. White pushes his hips forwards while pulling back on Grey's leg to effect the technique (Figure 6-33). Notice that White has also secured Grey's right ankle with a power grip to effect an ankle lock.

Key Points

1. You may often combine ankle and knee locks for a synergistic effect. In this case, White can also grab Grey's foot with both hands and torque it counterclockwise to take any slack out of it and put additional stress on the knee joint (Figure 6-34).

Chapter 6: Controlling the Leg

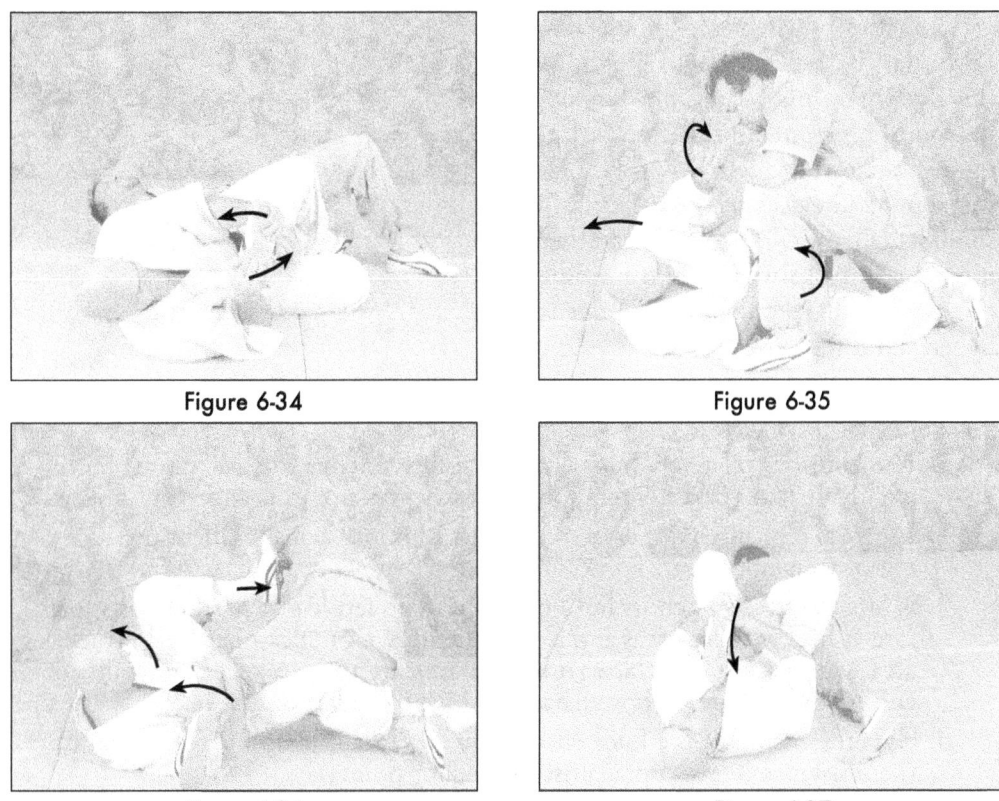

Figure 6-34

Figure 6-35

Figure 6-36

Figure 6-37

2. This basic knee lock position is using the same principle as the transverse straight arm bar (cross-mark hold); using the pelvis as a fulcrum just above the mid-appendage joint in order to hyper-extend it.

Knee Lock from the Half Guard

Grey has taken down White who has landed in the half guard position (Figure 6-35). Grey, in a semi-kneeling position, lords over White. White controls Grey's left arm with his left hand to keep from being punched. White pulls Grey's left arm to White's left side as he hooks Grey's left knee from behind with his right arm and rolls onto his back, levering Grey forward onto his front (Figure 6-36). White also kicks at Grey's left side to assist in turning him around. White continues to roll completely onto his back with Grey's left leg now securely between White's legs (Figure 6-37). White can now pull down on Grey's left heel with both hands (applying the basic ankle lock if he wants to) while crossing his ankles (or apply a figure four) so that the hips may be raised to hyperextend the knee joint.

Sometimes when making a kick down (as in the previous situation), the opponent may land on his side instead of his front. In this case, White figure fours Grey's left leg and places the top of Grey's instep on his right shoulder (Figure 6-38). White can then move his hips forward while he pulls backwards on Grey's ankle in order to hyperextend the knee.

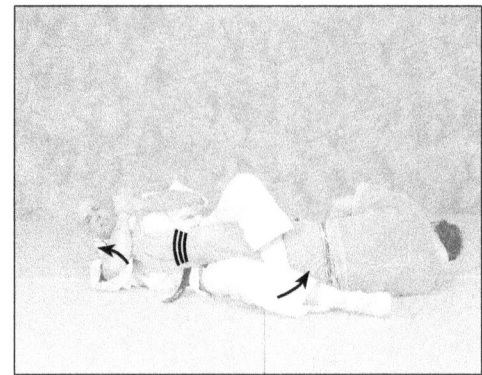

Figure 6-38

Key Points
1. The knee has relatively poor lateral stability. Hence, the leg can be more readily de-stabilized if you apply sideways pressure to it with your arms.
2. Use your legs in conjunction with your hips and arms to effect the turning of your opponent.
3. White effectively anchors both ends of Grey's left leg by pulling down on Grey's heel with his arms and by pushing down on his upper leg/buttocks area with his feet. The latter move is necessary to help keep Grey pinned and to give a stronger power base for his pull down on the heel.
4. Hyperextension of the knee ensues when White lifts up his pelvis against the resistance he sets up against his anchor points.
5. White may combine an ankle lock with the knee lock by gouging the Achilles tendon with the radial edge of his forearm or by simply twisting the foot.

Chapter 6: Controlling the Leg

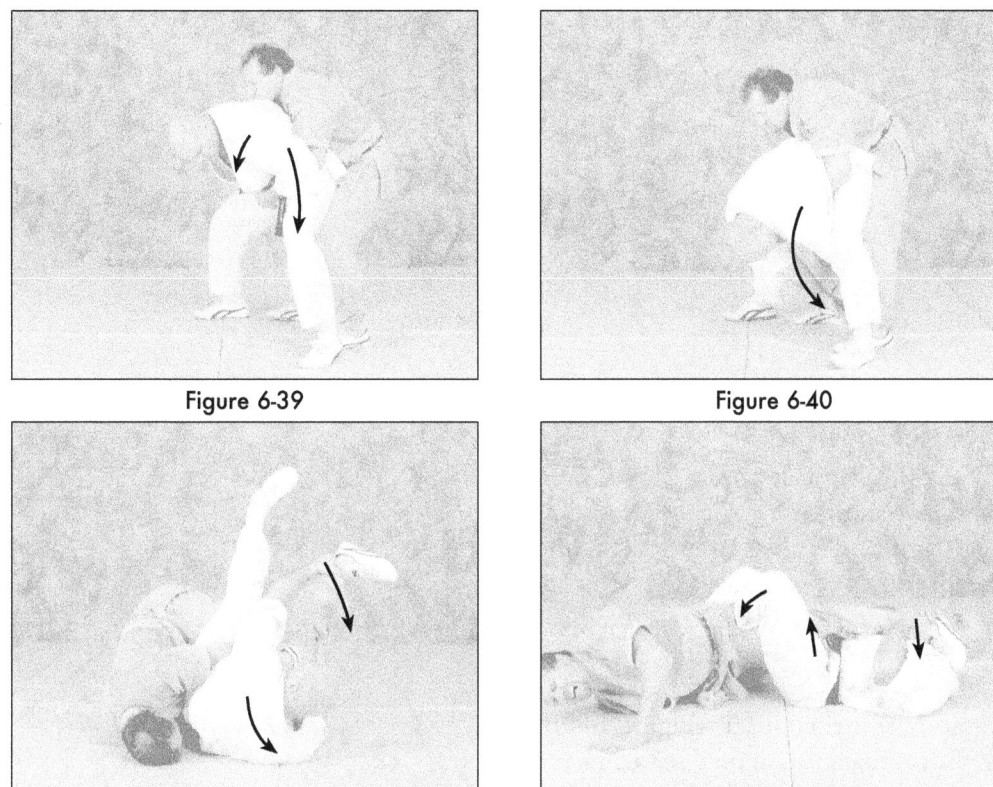

Figure 6-39

Figure 6-40

Figure 6-41

Figure 6-42

Forward Roll to Knee Lock

Grey has White in a rear bear hug. White lowers his center of gravity by bending his knees and he leans forwards in order to make it difficult for Grey to pick up White and slam him to the mat (Figure 6-39). White grabs Grey's left leg with both hands (Figure 6-40), and then executes a forward roll while hanging onto Grey's leg (Figure 6-41). Grey will land on his face/shoulder while White lands on his back. White slides away on his back from his dazed opponent and then figure fours Grey's left leg while pulling Grey's heel backwards towards his chest with both hands, thereby locking Grey's knee out (Figure 6-42).

Key Points

1. This technique works best if your opponent is taller than you are as he would be free to bend over the top of you, otherwise you may be unable to reach his leg freely.
2. You must commit yourself to this technique fully. Be careful in practice, as it can be dangerous for your partner to land on either his shoulder or his face.

Chin Na In Ground Fighting

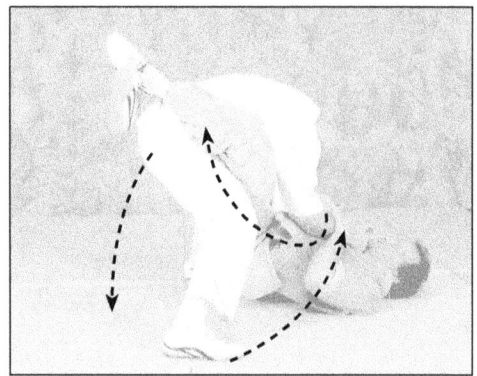

Figure 6-43

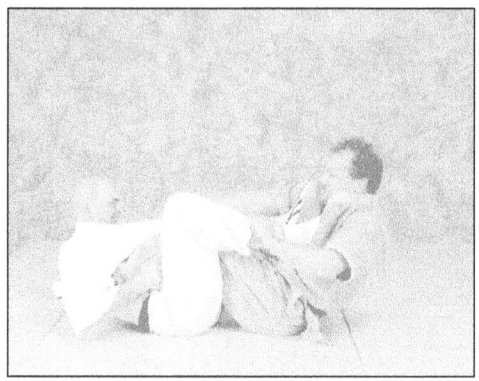

Figure 6-44

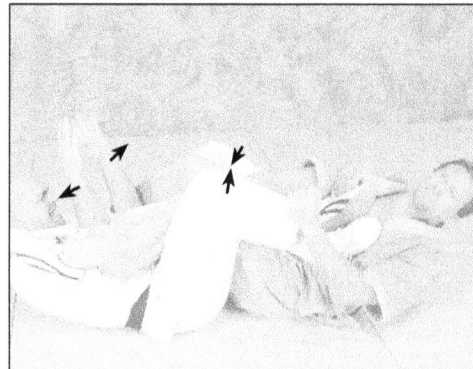

Figure 6-45

Double Knee Lock

White has taken Grey down onto his back and Grey quickly wraps his legs around White's waist as White bends down to choke Grey (Figure 6-43). White sits down unlocking his guard with the weight of his body. White also tucks Grey's feet under his armpits as he sits back (Figure 6-44). Both combatants are now seated facing each other with White's leg on the outside of Grey's legs. White places both of his feet on Grey's chest and pushes strongly against him in order to break out of the guard and to push Grey's torso backwards. White now slides his elbows over the top of Grey's insteps and to the insides of Grey's ankles. Once inside his legs, White can force Grey's lower legs outwards with his forearms as White continues with the inward pressure of his knees (Figure 6-45). This will lock both of Grey's knees sideways.

Key Points

1. Take care not to allow Grey to withdraw his legs in the process of you transferring your elbows from the outside to the insides of the ankles.
2. You can maintain contact by sliding your arms over his legs to help achieve this.
3. You may also squeeze your knees together to further keep the legs trapped in position.

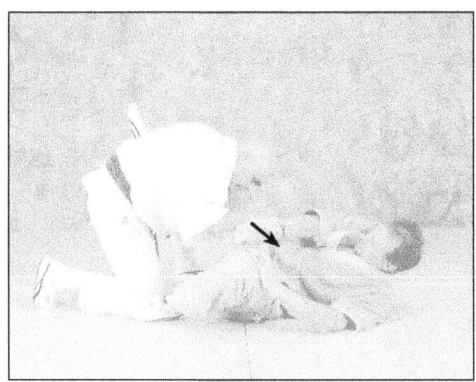

Figure 6-46

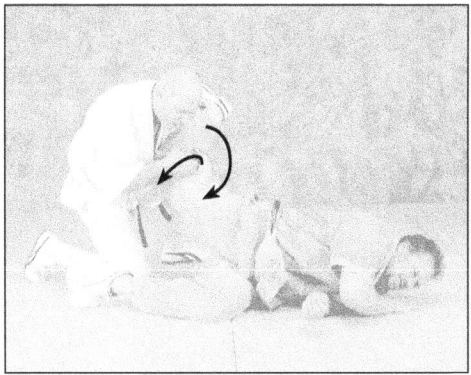

Figure 6-47

6.4. KNEE BLOCKS

Applying Knee Blocks

Most people can bend or flex their legs backward so that their heels touch their buttocks. This allows them to sit in the kneeling position. If a physical block such as a broom handle was placed tight against the inside of the knee joint, and the person were to kneel down on it, he would experience a lot of pain. If enough of his body weight

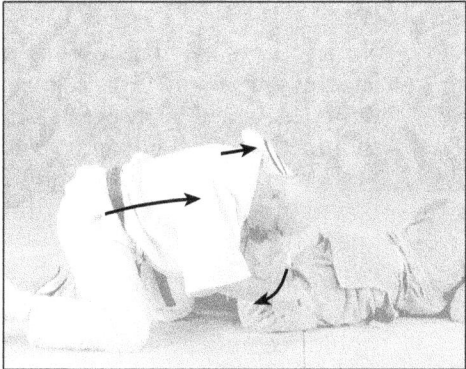

Figure 6-48

were allowed to settle on the blocked knee, his knees would dislocate. Another analogy would be to put a block in a door jam and slam it. The hinges would probably bust apart as the full normal range of motion of the door to the closed position would be impeded or blocked. The knee can be blocked by inserting a body part such as the foot, leg, hand or arm into the crook of the knee and applying external pressure, such as your body weight, to it. The calf muscle will experience much pain and the knee may dislocate. Here are a few ways to block the knee.

Blocking the Knee with the Arm

White has broken Grey's guard and he immediately underhooks the crook of Grey's right leg with his left arm as he steps up with his left leg into a semi-kneeling position (Figure 6-46). White controls Grey's right arm with his right arm to keep from being struck. White then grabs his own left wrist, lifts Grey's right leg onto his left shoulder and torques Grey's leg clockwise as to roll him over onto his chest (Figure 6-47). White keeps his left arm in the crook of Grey's right knee joint and he adopts a power grip, pulling the arm into the knee joint as he presses his body weight forward with his left shoulder (Figure 6-48).

Chin Na In Ground Fighting

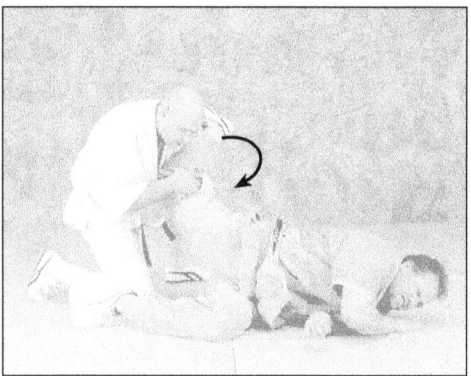

Figure 6-49

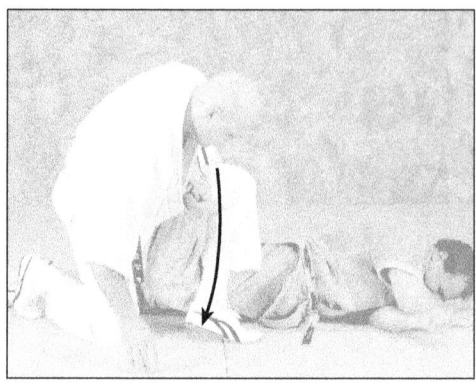

Figure 6-50

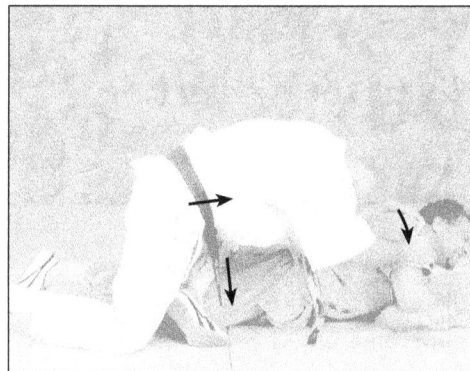

Figure 6-51

Key Points

1. Notice how White uses the levering action of Grey's lower right leg when he uses his left shoulder to push upwards and over to his left while pulling downwards and inwards on the knee.
2. This action will roll him over, for if Grey were to resist, he would feel much sideways stress on his knee. The structure of the knee is ill equipped to handle lateral stress.

Blocking the Knee with the Leg

The leg is used as a block instead of the arm. White turns Grey prone as before (Figure 6-49). Now White steps over Grey's right leg with his left leg, making sure that his leg is as tight as possible to Grey's knee joint (Figure 6-50). White turns into Grey and lets his body weight apply pressure to the blocked knee, pulling on Grey's shoulders for extra forward drive and balance (Figure 6-51). Be careful when practicing this technique that you do not accidentally hyperflex your partner's knee joint.

Key Points

1. This technique is very similar to the previous one, except that the leg is used as the block rather than the arm.
2. Be careful with your partner in training. You can easily dislocate his knee if your leg is deep into his knee joint due to the major blocking effect your leg has on this joint.

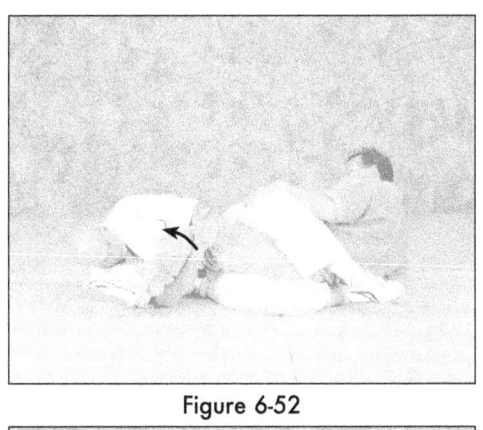

Figure 6-52

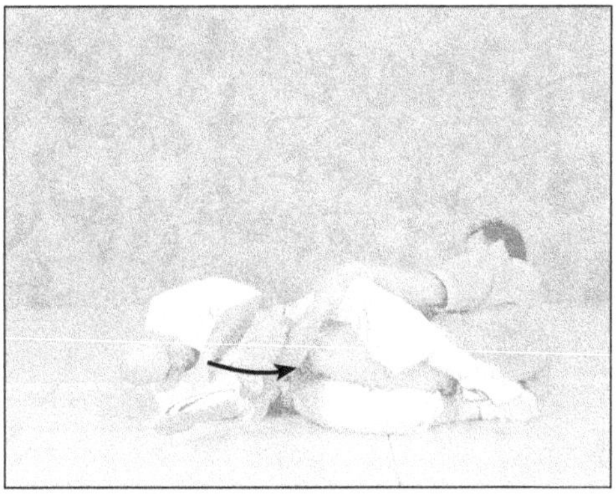

Figure 6-53

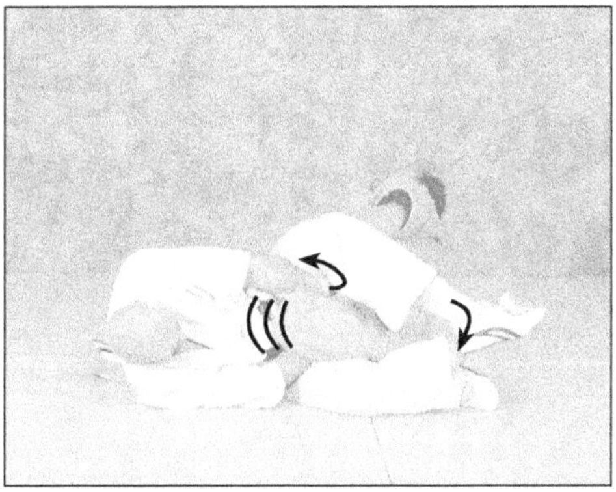

Figure 6-54

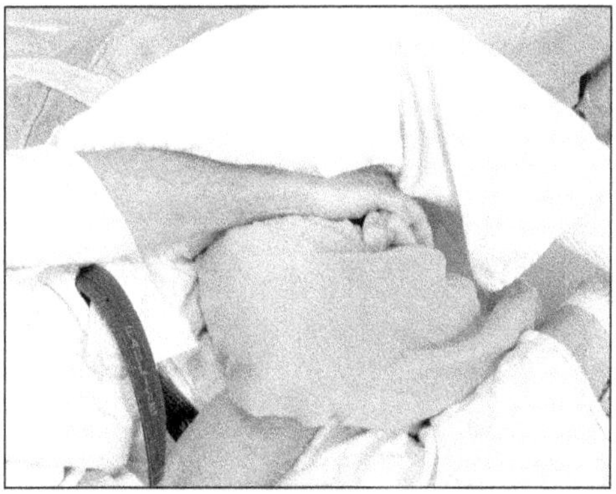

Figure 6-55

Failed Leg Lock to Knee Block

White fails to put on a leg lock (Figure 6-52). In this case, let the knee bend and even help it bend by hooking your right arm around the crook of Grey's knee and taking on a power grip to secure it. Grey may free up his left arm by grabbing his own left leg. Grey can now bend Grey's left leg backward without losing control over this leg at the knee (Figure 6-53). White then hooks Grey's bent left leg and secures it by crossing his own ankles and he adopts a power grip to hold onto the knee (Figure 6-54).

Key Points

1. Sometimes, you try for a leg lock but cannot achieve it because you are too deep into your opponent, or the leg cannot be straightened. Move to another technique rather than to struggle with a failing one.
2. Notice how White frees up his left arm by grabbing his own body/clothing. The grabbing of other body parts (yours or his) or clothing can also solidify and anchor a hold by the grabbing arm.
3. The close-up shows the arm and leg configurations in detail (Figure 6-55). Remember to keep the block tightly into the knee joint so that the block will work sooner by restricting the mobility of the joint to a greater degree.

Chin Na In Ground Fighting

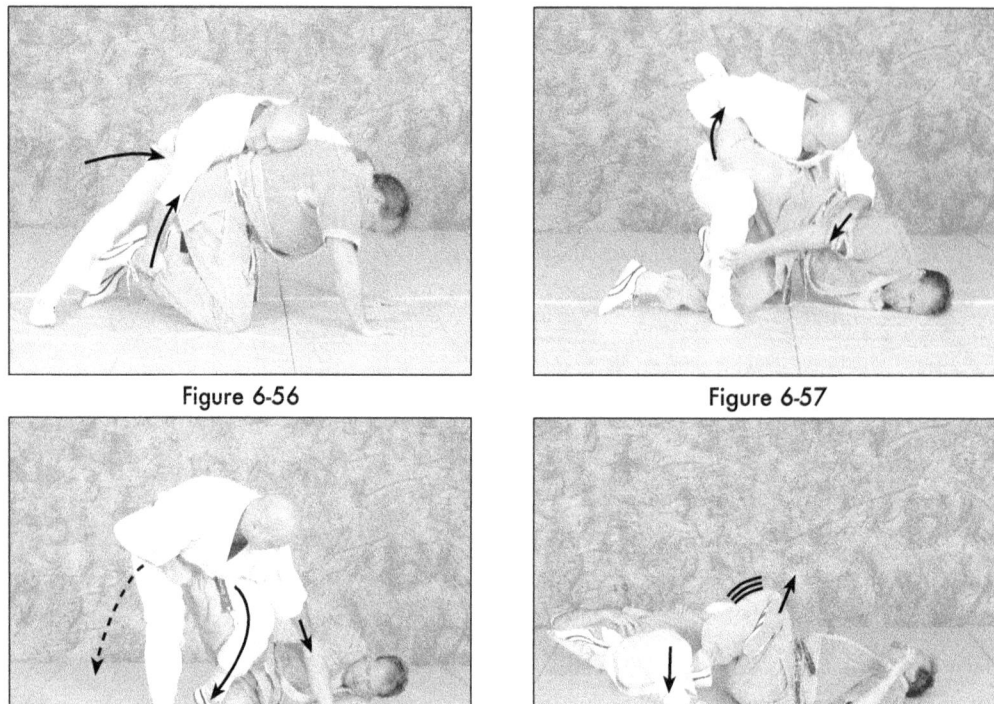

Figure 6-56

Figure 6-57

Figure 6-58

Figure 6-59

Double Leg Knee Block

White has taken down Grey from behind with both landing in kneeling positions (Figure 6-56). White immediately scoops Grey's right ankle with his right hand and takes Grey's left arm with his left arm in a semi-kneeling position. White then picks up Grey's right ankle and he slides his right bent leg under Grey's right thigh while driving Grey forward with his hips, riding him onto his face (Figure 6-57). White also uses his left arm to prevent Grey from backhanding him with his free right arm. White then stands up and steps over Grey's left right leg with his left leg, placing his left foot on the mat behind Grey's left knee (Figure 6-58). White still controls Grey's nearest arm to prevent being struck. Now White simply sits backward and kicks Grey's left knee up with his left leg while pushing down against Grey's left instep with the crook of his right knee (Figure 6-59). This block with the ankle can be supplemented by an ankle lock should White decide to drop his right arm on top of Grey's right instep.

Key Points

1. Notice how White takes away two opposite points of balance from Grey in order to tip him along this axis.
2. Scoop your opponent's furthest leg under the knee to ensure a tightly placed block is in place.

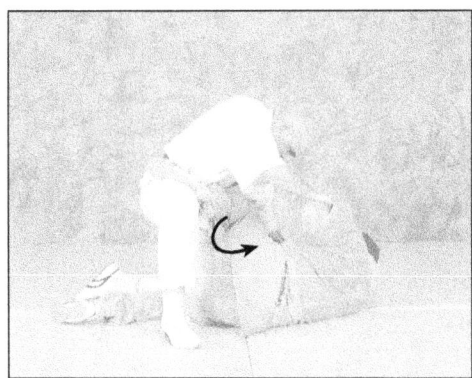

Figure 6-60

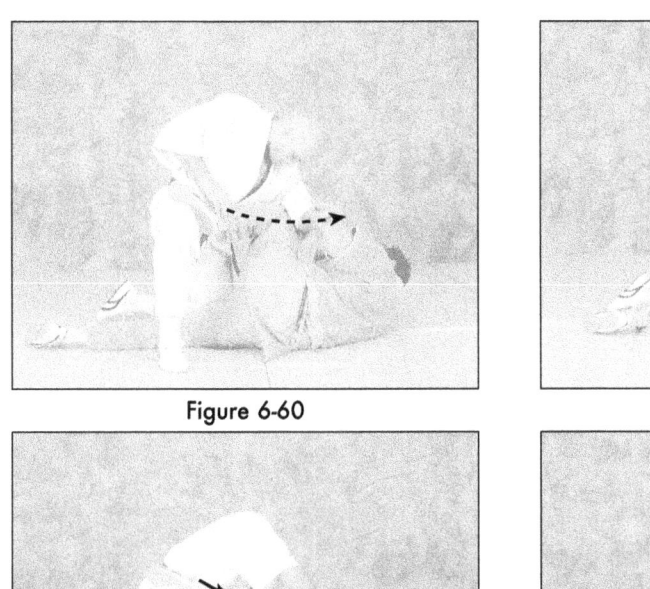

Figure 6-61

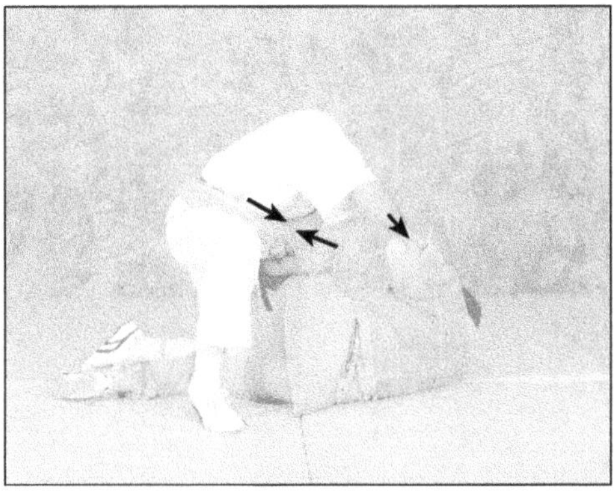

Figure 6-62

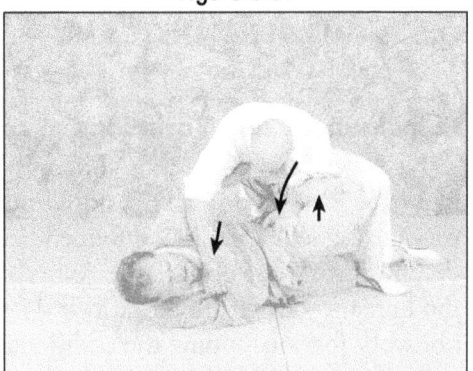

Figure 6-63

3. This ankle block can be supplemented by an ankle lock should White decide to drop his right arm on top of Grey's right instep.

Knee Block from the Half Guard

White has taken down Grey onto his side and is in a semi-kneeling position over Grey in his side guard (Figure 6-60). White holds Grey's left arm with his right hand to avoid being struck. White grabs Grey's left arm with his right hand freeing his left arm so that it may begin to snake around and behind Grey's left knee (Figure 6-61). White places his left hand, palm down on Grey's left hip/thigh area. White now simply presses forward with his legs and hips against Grey's left leg, blocking Grey's left knee (Figure 6-62). Look at the final position from the reverse angle (see Figure 6-63).

Key Points

1. White must control Grey's nearest arm at all times to avoid being struck.
2. White is able to exert lateral pressure on the knee as he levers upward using Grey's own left thigh as a fulcrum.
3. White must ensure that his arm is deep behind Grey's knee joint to effect the block.

Chin Na In Ground Fighting

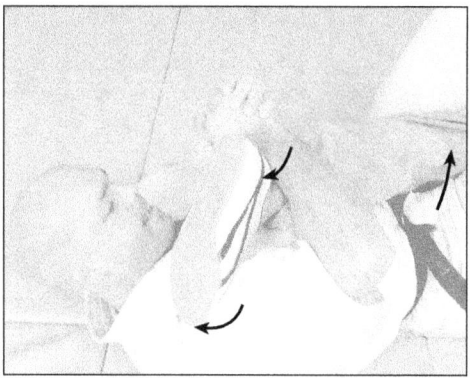

Figure 6-64

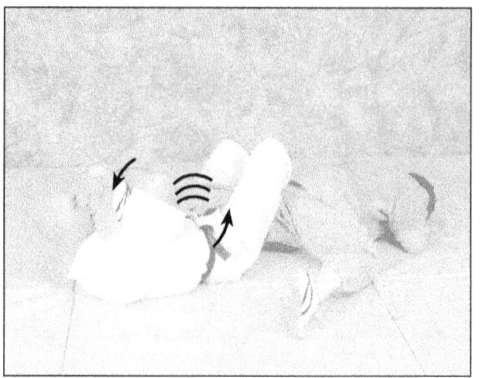

Figure 6-65

6.5. COMBINING ANKLE AND KNEE LOCKS

Combinations and Variations

It is very easy to add an ankle lock to a knee lock as shown in many of the previous leg lock techniques. Remember that the knee is one of the larger joints of the human body. If the knee lock does not work for you, adding the additional pain of the ankle lock may make your opponent submit faster. It makes sense to attack two joints at the same time if

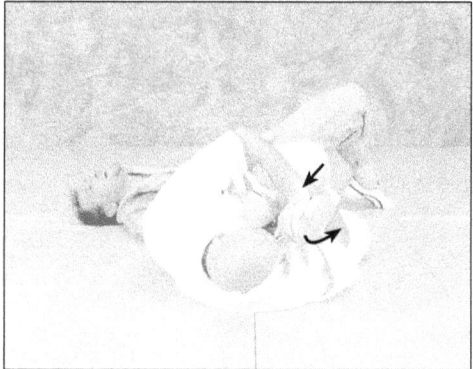

Figure 6-66

possible. Anytime you have your opponent in a straight leg knee lock, you should easily be able to use these following variations of the ankle lock.

White has Grey in a knee lock. Instead of just grabbing a hold of Grey's foot, White uses a power grip and places the bony radial edge of his right wrist against Grey's left Achilles tendon (Figure 6-64). White uses an inward and upward circular motion to grind Grey's tendon as his instep is pressed against White's right shoulder. White may arch backwards and raise his hips to simultaneously attack the knee joint (Figure 6-65).

Another variation is to figure four Grey's right ankle with White's arms (Figure 6-66) while the knee lock is applied. The instep of the foot is hyperextended in addition to the attack on the Achilles tendon. Now White can attack Grey's ankle from two sides as well as the knee.

A final variation is for White to simply twist Grey's right foot with both of his hands in a counterclockwise direction. This move isn't fancy but it is extremely effective (Figure 6-67).

Chapter 6: Controlling the Leg

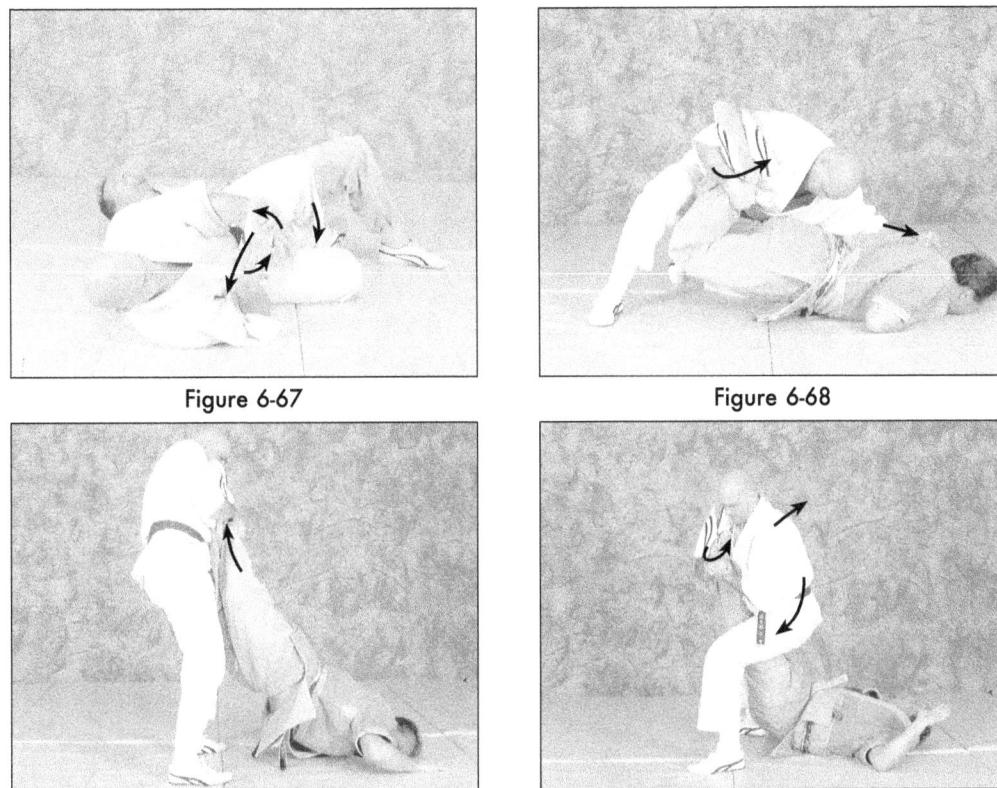

Figure 6-67

Figure 6-68

Figure 6-69

Figure 6-70

Double Ankle and Double Knee Lock

From a semi-kneeling position, White has proned out Grey and has scooped up Grey's crossed ankles with his right arm and pressed them against his left shoulder area (Figure 6-68). White uses both of his hands to keep Grey's ankles in place as he stands up, lifting Grey's lower body off the mat (Figure 6-69). White then steps over Grey with his right leg and places his pelvis against Grey's knees (Figure 6-70). White also arches his back, pushes his hips forward and sinks his weight against Grey's knees to effect a double knee lock.

Key Points

1. Notice how White adopts the power grip allowing his bony portion of his wrist to work Grey's right Achilles tendon.
2. The top of Grey's right ankle presses against the Achilles tendon of his inner ankle to lock it as well.
3. This double knee lock may be difficult to do against a well-muscled opponent.

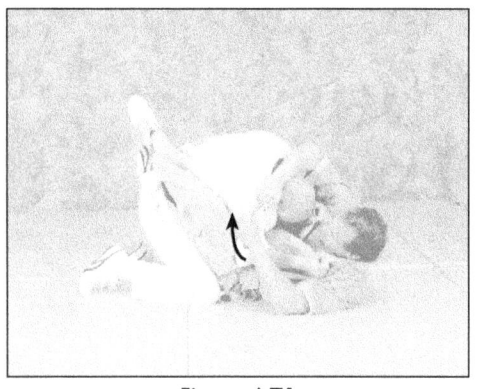

Figure 6-71   Figure 6-72

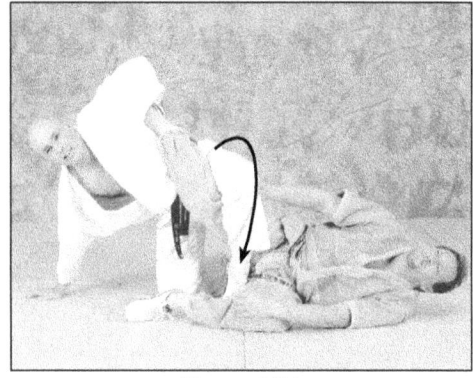 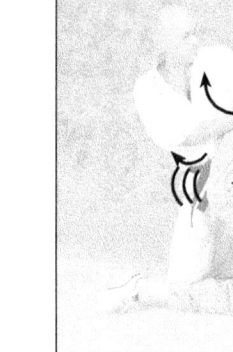

Figure 6-73   Figure 6-74

Kneeling Heel Hook

White is struggling in Grey's guard (Figure 6-71). White breaks Grey's guard and overhooks Grey's right leg with his left arm. White then brings up his left foot up tight to Grey's buttock while pinning his other leg to the mat with his right hand (Figure 6-72). Pivoting on his right knee and balancing himself with his right hand to the mat, White then steps over Grey's right leg with his left leg, placing his right foot beside Grey's groin. White simultaneously hooks Grey's right heel with the radial edge of his left hand (Figure 6-73). White can now complete the ankle lock by using a power grip (Figure 6-74) and applying pressure to the ankle with an inward and upward circular motion.

Key Points

1. This is a dangerous move for Grey because the knee joint can easily be dislocated if White were to twist his hips in a slightly counterclockwise direction.
2. This technique is a little difficult to get into by itself. Once it is in place though, it can be devastating to your opponent because it works both the knee and the ankle.

CHAPTER 7

Controlling the Head/Neck and Body

7-1. INTRODUCTION

Prime Target

According to Dim Mak theory, correctly attacking 36 specific large cavities in the head/neck and torso can result in death and attacking any of an additional 24 specific cavities can cause severe numbing.* The head and neck in particular are target-rich areas of the body and they control vital bodily functions that can be disrupted by attacking them. The neck is very vulnerable as the air passages, arteries, and vital nerves that oxygenate and innervate the brain are susceptible to serious injury. Indeed, some forms of neck restraints are controversial, and all are deemed to be potentially lethal by the forensic community. For this reason, holds like bar arm chokes are banned by all police agencies, in favor of lateral vascular neck restraints, which have a reduced potential for causing death when properly applied. The spinal column is least protected at the neck and can be subjected to strikes, locks, falls, etc., all of which can have lethal consequences. Striking and twisting the neck can easily injure the vertebral arteries or the first cervical vertebrae itself, resulting in serious, if not fatal injuries. As such, there are many cautions given in this section because of the potential lethal consequences that can arise from attacking the neck.

Nervous Systems

The nervous system allows the body to react to and control internal changes and activities of the body as well as to sense external stimuli. Severance of the spinal nerves means paralysis and even death due to the cessation of vital bodily functions. Structurally, the nervous system is composed of the central nervous system (CNS) and the peripheral nervous system (PNS). The CNS consists of the brain and the spinal nerves (31 pairs of nerves making up the spinal cord). The PNS consists of nerve fibers that connect to and are anatomically and operationally contiguous with the CNS, although they are considered to be separate from this nerve group. Functionally, the nervous system may be classified as being either part of the somatic

Practical Chin Na by Zhao Da Yuan, (1993) p. 82

nervous system (SNS) and the autonomic nervous system (ANS). The SNS innervates the skeletal muscles and sense organs of the CNS or PNS to allow voluntary and reflexive actions (movement) to external stimuli. The ANS innervate the involuntary muscles of the visceral organs (like the heart) and glands.

Anatomy of the Head/Neck

There are 36 bones of the head/neck:
28 cranial bones (including those of the ear)
1 hyoid bone (base of attachment for the tongue)
7 cervical vertebrae (neck bones).
The cranium consists of eight bones whereas the face has fourteen bones in it.

The cervical spine consists of seven vertebrae which allows the head 90 degree turning movement from side to side with about 45 degree side bending movement.

We can regard the human body as a mechanical device in order to understand how we can render it inoperable. Using this analogy, the neck can be viewed as a vital conduit between the head (the computer) and the body (the machine). The nerves (electrical lines), windpipe (gas intake line) and the circulatory veins and arteries (gas lines) pass through this narrow structure of the neck. A heavy blow struck to this conduit from any angle will disrupt these lines and the machine will be temporarily or permanently rendered useless.

By starving the device of gas, through either the gas intake line or the gas lines fueling it, the machine must stop. The flow of oxygen to the brain can be shut off, causing unconsciousness (and if withheld long enough-death). Ultimately this is achieved via sealing the breath itself, or more quickly, via the sealing of the veins and arteries in the neck. Death may occur directly through choking or it may arise from the after effects of swelling caused by damage to the relatively delicate structures within the throat, such as the hyoid bone, trachea and larynx. A person can be rendered brain dead if the brain is deprived of oxygen for as little as four minutes.

Terminology Relating to Neck Holds

There is some confusion in the terminology relating to the classes of techniques based upon sealing the vein (vascular restraint) and sealing the breath (respiratory restraint). Choking and strangulation are terms often used to describe both of these classes of techniques. Although they look similar and ultimately yield the same results (unconsciousness from applying pressure to the neck), respiratory and vascular restraints are totally different techniques.

Choke is defined in one martial arts dictionary as follows:

> *Any form of obstructing one's opponent's ability to breathe by using various types of arm and leg leverage to pinch off the air passage or a blood vessel close to the head, causing loss of consciousness. It is most often employed in jujutsu and judo.*

This definition is misleading because it implies that obstructing a person's ability to breathe can be done by sealing the vein. Clearly, the mechanics of the techniques are not well-defined. The word 'strangle' is not defined in this dictionary, and a standard dictionary offers little clarity on this matter either:

"Strangle: squeeze the windpipe or neck of esp. as to kill."

"Strangulate: prevent circulation through a vein by compression."

The main purpose of any neck hold is to mechanically deprive the brain of its oxygen supply (cerebral hypoxia), leading to transient unconsciousness. This may include combinations of airway obstructions (from the tongue covering the epiglottis, or from compression of the trachea and from vascular obstruction (of carotid arteries bringing oxygenated blood to the brain, and of the jugular veins returning de-oxygenated blood from the brain to the heart). Both the airway and vascular obstruction (and heart dysfunction) may overlap but one should be clear as to which type of obstruction your technique will render. While these principles of airway and blood vessel obstruction appear simplistic in nature, the most important additional factors are the unpredictable disorders of the function of the heart, including slowing, stoppage, or rapid ineffectual beating (ventricular fibrillation). A secondary use of a neck hold is just to do that, hold the neck without the intention of rendering a person unconscious. The neck is a great handle to use when controlling a person.

The term 'choke' in this text refers to the act closing off the airway ('obstructing one's ability to breathe'), whereas 'neck restraint' refers to the act of reducing the blood flow to and from the brain (the person's ability to breathe remains unobstructed). The phrase 'choking a person out' loosely (and imprecisely) refers to the rendering a person unconscious by either class of techniques. Similarly, the term strangulation often includes both classes of techniques as well. We suggest that the term 'choke' only be used when referring to sealing the breath techniques (respiratory restraints). Also, we recommend that the term 'neck restraint' be used solely to describe sealing the vein techniques (vascular restraints).

Classes of Neck Hold Techniques

In order to understand the two classes of neck holds, both of which deprive the brain of oxygen but in different ways, one must understand how oxygen is delivered to the brain. Oxygen is brought to the lungs via the windpipe and it is then transferred to the blood stream for circulation to all parts of the body, including the brain, via the blood vessels. Unconsciousness will result if the brain is cut off from its oxygen supply (hypoxia) after as little as three seconds. The most commonly used neck holds attempt to achieve unconsciousness by obstructing the blood supply to the brain (vascular restraints) or by obstructing the airway to the lungs (airway chokes). In order to understand the fundamental differences between sealing the vein techniques (lateral vascular neck restraints or the 'sleeper holds') as shown in Figure 7-1 and sealing the breath techniques (chokes) as shown in Figure 7-2, we must examine the structures within the neck (Figure 7-3). Note the relative position-

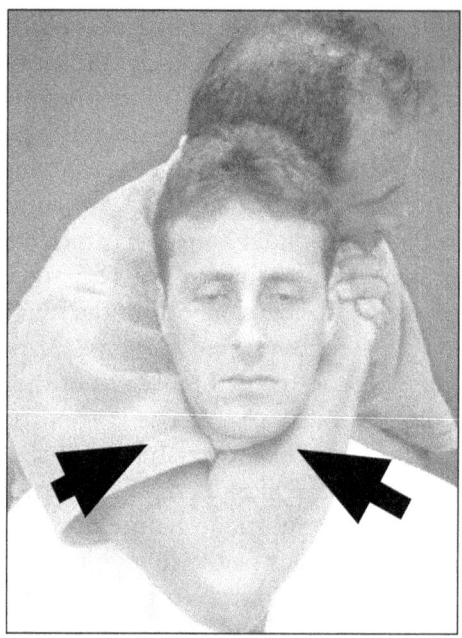

Sealing the Vein
Figure 7-1: This technique uses the pinching pressures
of the lower and upper arm to seal the vein/arteries
in the neck (sleeper hold).

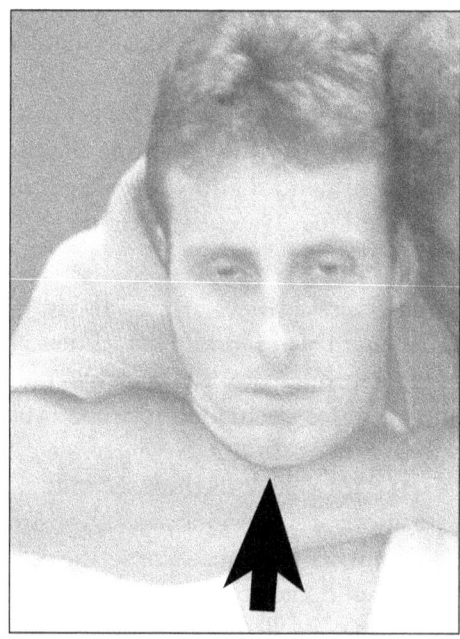

Sealing the Breath
Figure 7-2: This technique is used to seal the breath
by closing the airway. It is a dangerous technique
and should only be used in life and death situations (choke hold).

Chapter 7: Controlling the Head/Neck and Body

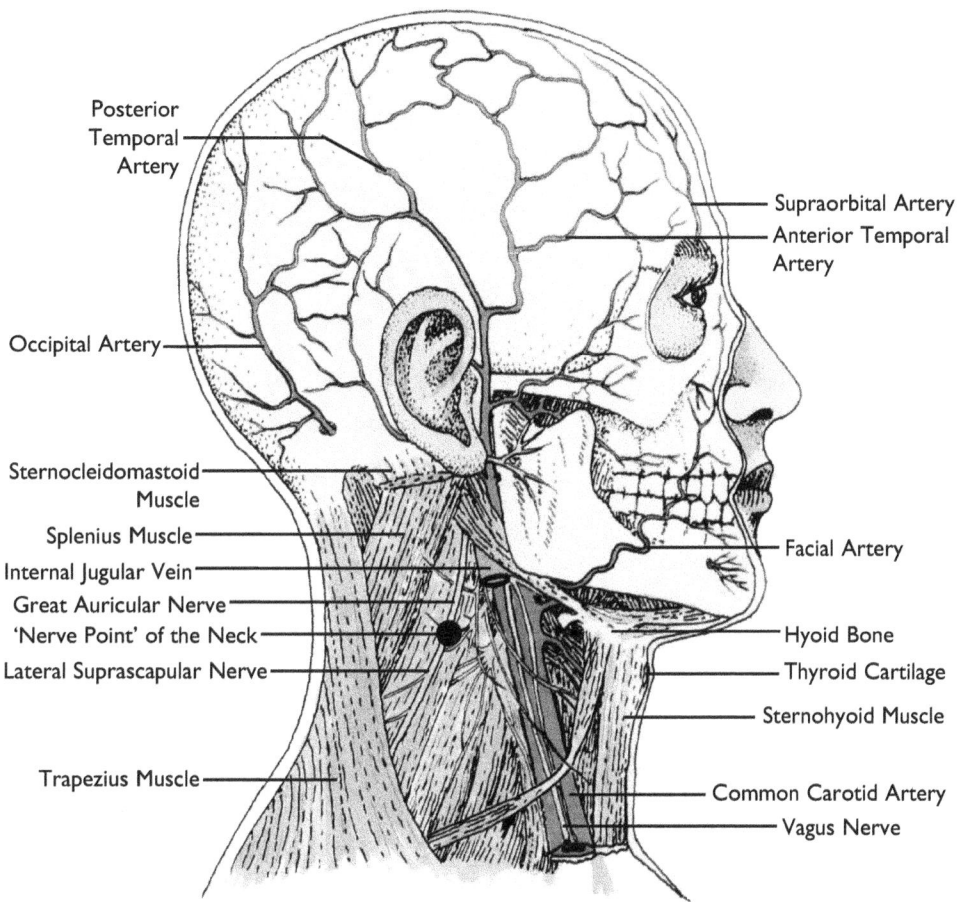

Figure 7-3 Note the relative positioning of the carotid artery, the jugular vein, and the vagus nerve. The nerve point of the neck has many nerves emanating from this spot (S.I. 16).

ing of the carotid artery, and the overlying jugular vein, and the vagus nerve, as well as the position of the windpipe.

Sealing the vein techniques involve attacking the sides of the neck where the jugular vein and the carotid artery lie (Figure 7-5). The brain basically shuts down from the hypoxic effects and the person goes unconscious or 'goes to sleep' (hence the term 'sleeper hold'). A number of physiological mechanisms are at work here, some of which can lead to serious medical problems.

Sealing the breath techniques induces unconsciousness by cutting off the oxygen supply to the brain by stopping air from refilling the lungs. The supply of air can be sealed by a wide variety of choking techniques and unconsciousness ensues after the air trapped in the lungs has been consumed. Notice that the trachea (windpipe) is a narrow, flexible tube made up of 16-20 cricoid cartilages (Figure 7-4). It is readily accessible, as it runs vertically down the front center of the neck and into the lungs.

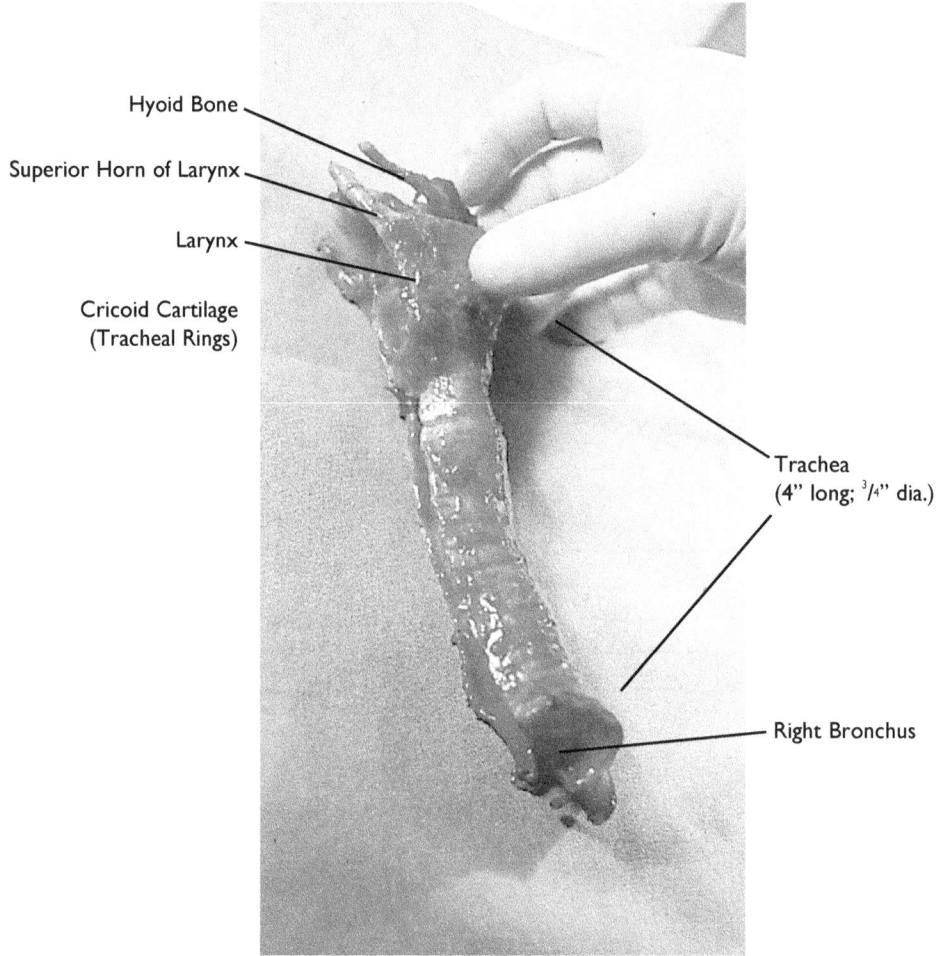

Figure 7-4 The author holds the larynx of the thyroid cartilage. Note that the tracheal cartilage (rings) are actually open-ended posteriorly. His index finger touches the apex of the hyoid bone.

The upper part of the windpipe is most noticeable in men as the Adam's apple (thyroid cartilage or larynx) because it protrudes forwards from the neck below the jaw (REN 23). These structures are highly susceptible to damage when occluding of the windpipe, and the potential for serious medical implications are considerable.

Knockout Punches

Unconsciousness can also be rendered from a percussive shock wave that can be administered in a wide variety of ways to the brain (the 'knockout'). Most people have heard of the 'sweet spot' at the tip of the jaw and have seen boxers 'kiss the canvas' during a knockout (the knockout is due to the percussive shock to the back of the brain and not the spot itself). A lesser-known knockout blow can result when the carotid sinus is struck. This carotid body lies at the bifurcation point of

Chapter 7: Controlling the Head/Neck and Body

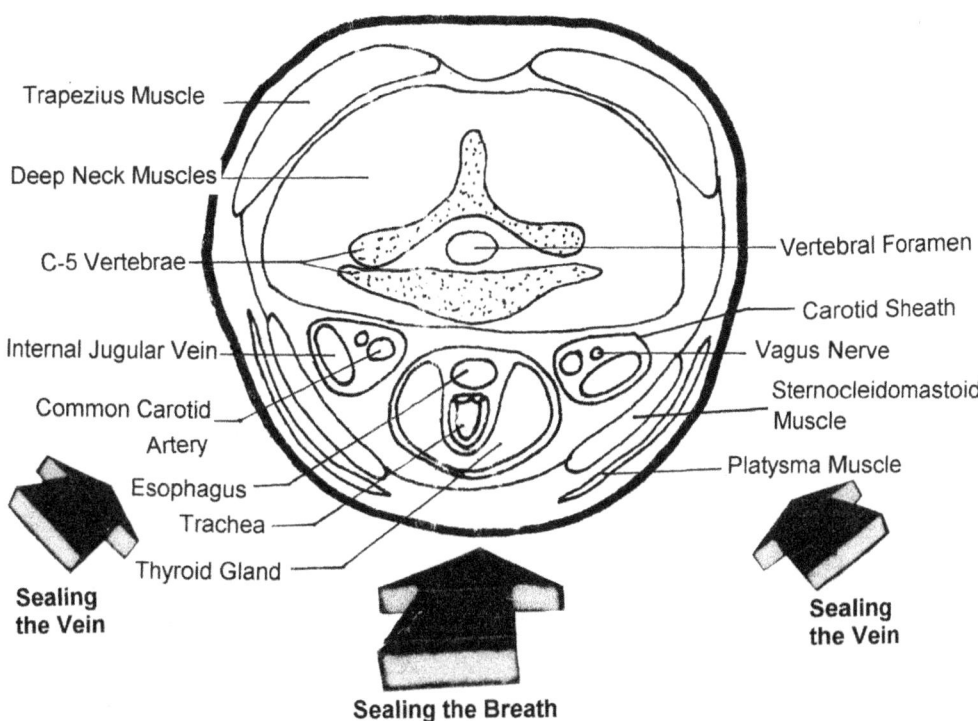

Figure 7-5 Note the correct angles for sealing the breath (choke hold) and sealing the vein (sleeper hold).

the internal carotid artery (feeding the brain) and external carotid artery (feeding to superficial cranium). This point can be located by palpating the carotid artery at the level of the top of the Adam's apple. This sinus is composed of pressure sensitive nerves (baroreceptors) whose purpose is to detect changes in blood pressure that may harm the pressure-sensitive brain. If struck with a blow (or neck restraint is applied) these receptors, not being able to distinguish externally applied pressure from high internal blood pressure, cause the oxygen flow to the brain to diminish, thereby inducing unconsciousness.

The Head as a Target

The head is composed of eight cranial bones and fourteen facial bones (plus other smaller bones of the ear and throat). The calvaria (skull) houses the primary organ, the brain, as well as those organs used for sight and sound: the eyes and ears. Their sensitivity is owed in part with being accessible to the environment, which at times can be a violent and hostile one. The structures are also delicate in design, certainly no match for well aimed and focused blows. Add the annoyances of broken noses, jaws, teeth and bleeding and there is little wonder why our arms are so readily available to protect these vital areas of the body. Predatory animals instinctively go for the throat, because this is the fastest and most efficient way to subdue and kill their prey. In a street fight, the throat is a vital area in need of protection.

With the foregoing in mind, consider the efficacy for the wrestler to thwart a 'pinning' by his opponent by rolling over onto his stomach in order to keep his shoulders well clear of the mat lest he 'lose the match'. The arms have a very limited range of motion beyond the frontal plane of the body, hence we can offer but limited protection to our entire neck and head when our back is turned to our opponent (and there is no direct defensive assistance from our legs). Clearly, the rules pertaining to the sport of wrestling have seriously deviated from the practical applications (and in this case, the deadly consequences) of combat. From a defensive viewpoint, it is sound strategy never to turn your back to your opponent. From an offensive one, it is advantageous to get on your opponent's back to greatly neutralize his weapons and allow you to access the neck and head. This crystallizes the difference between certain aspects of sport versus combat.

7.2. Neck Locks

Susceptibility to Attack

The neck can be attacked from a wide range of positions, using the arms and the legs. Techniques that lever the head forward, backward, or sideward can cause tremendous pain and can cause serious injury to any of the seven cervical vertebrae (Figure 7-6 shows both fighters working each other's necks). The neck may also be locked by rotating it to its maximum (Figure 7-7), roughly 45 degrees in either direction of the medial plane.

Forward Neck Crank

White is fending off Grey's attempt to encircle his neck while in Grey's guard (Figure 7-8). White places both his hands behind the base of Grey's skull and levers Grey's neck forwards after stabilizing his elbows against the top of Grey's chest (Figure 7-9). Grey will experience much pain from both the forward neck crank as well as the double elbow press to the upper chest.

Key Points

1. The cervical spine is the most flexible aspect of the entire spinal column, particularly in the forward direction, but powerful neck muscles can thwart this neck manipulation. White leans forward, transferring his center of gravity towards his elbows to enhance the penetrating effect of the elbows on the torso and increase the power to his arms that is needed to lock the neck.
2. This technique must be done as quickly as possible as White's face can be accessed by Grey's free hands.

Backward Neck Crank

White has mounted Grey from behind, putting both in the prone position

Chapter 7: Controlling the Head/Neck and Body

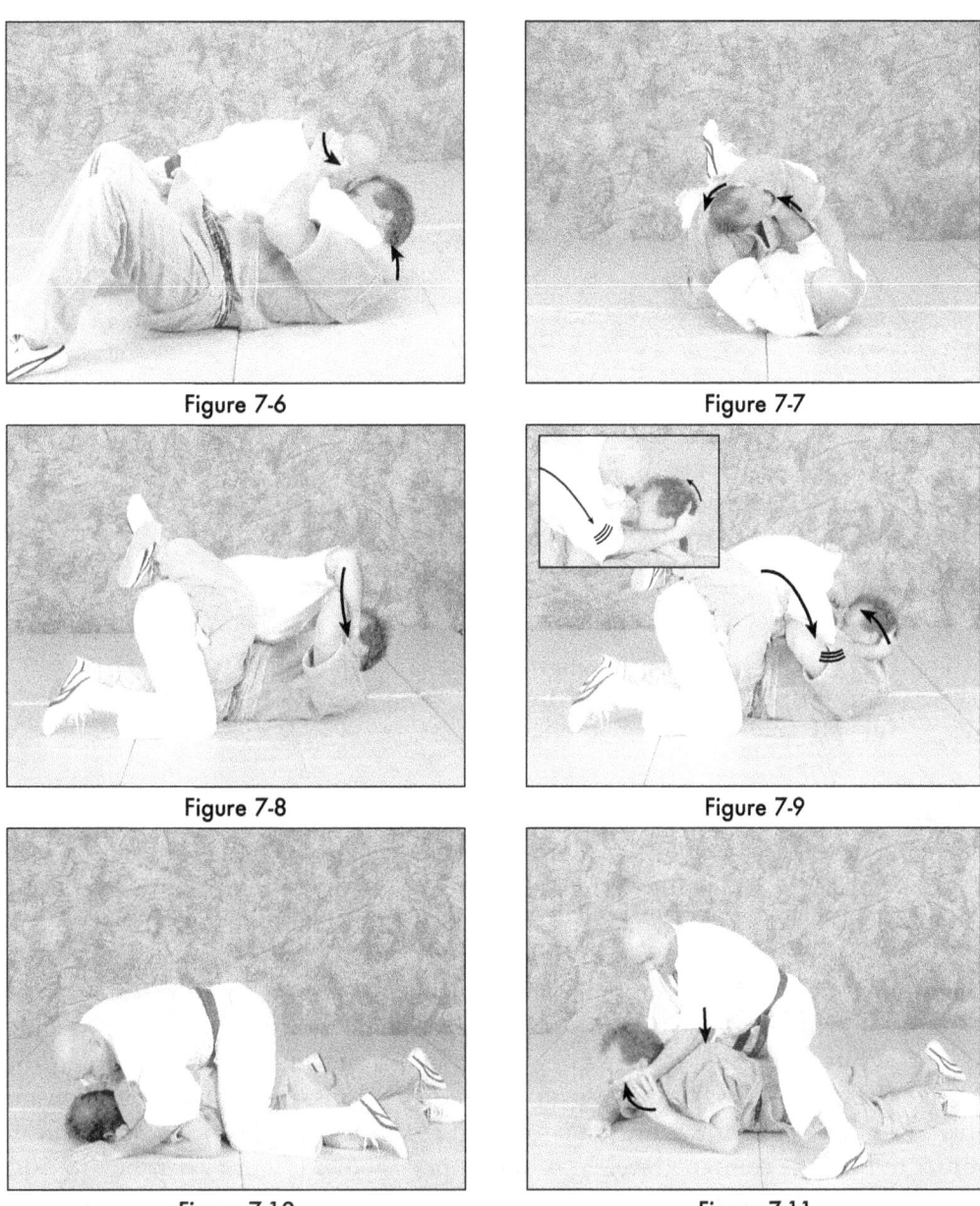

Figure 7-6

Figure 7-7

Figure 7-8

Figure 7-9

Figure 7-10

Figure 7-11

(Figure 7-10). White snakes his hands along the mat and slips them under Grey's jaw, and places his elbows on top of Grey's shoulders (Figure 7-11). White now levers upwards to effect a backward neck crank.

Key Points
1. Grey has placed himself in a relatively defenseless position leaving White to attack with minor interference from Grey's hands.

Chin Na In Ground Fighting

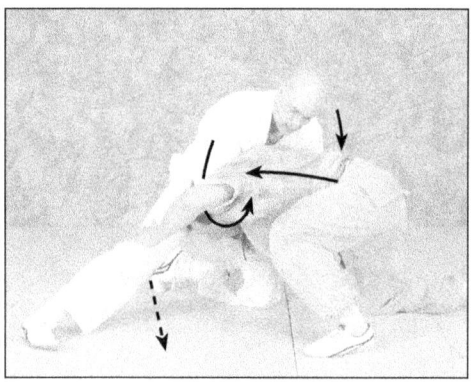

Figure 7-12

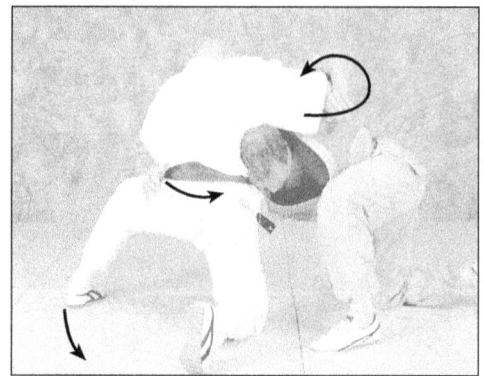

Figure 7-13

2. The fingers may be inserted under the jaw like a hook to access the hypoglossal nerves and to use the jaw line as a handle, both of which will facilitate the backward movement of the head.
3. Grey will lower his body weight onto his elbows to put painful pressure on the shoulder muscles.

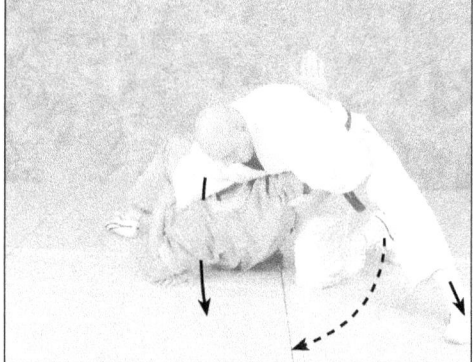

Figure 7-14

Death Lock

From the kneeling position, Grey throws himself headlong into White in an attempt to tackle him. White defends by simultaneously under-hooking Grey's left arm with his right arm and over-hooking Grey's right arm with his left arm (Figure 7-12). White then begins to turn Grey's body counterclockwise by dropping his right knee to the mat, raising his left knee and turning his hips while twisting Grey's upper body in this same direction (Figure 7-13). White takes care to place Grey's head by his ribs under his right armpit. As White completes his 180-degree turn, the hooking action turns Grey over toward his backside. White must ensure that his right arm is firmly planted on the mat in order to bear the combined weight of their upper bodies (Figure 7-14; Figure 7-15 shows the reverse view). Excruciating pressure may be applied to Grey's neck when White sits through with his right leg (Figure 7-16).

Chapter 7: Controlling the Head/Neck and Body

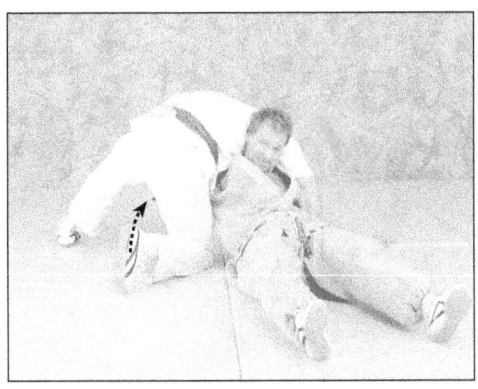

Figure 7-15

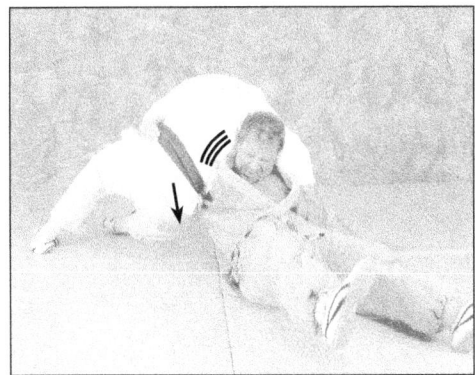

Figure 7-16

Key Points

1. This is not called the death lock in jest. This technique requires only the pressure supplied by your body weight to be effective. **Be extremely careful when practicing this technique** because serious injury to the neck and spine could occur if you were to lose your balance or inadvertently apply excessive pressure when you shoot your leg through.

2. Notice how White uses the over- and under-hooking motions of his arms in conjunction with his hips to turn Grey over.

3. By placing White's right arm on the mat, White can bridge his weight from this arm to his left leg, making his right leg non-load bearing and therefore mobile for the sit through.

4. All White need do is to lean backwards and settle his weight towards the mat by bending his right arm to apply further pressure. This technique tends towards completion as the sit through is being done so it is unlikely that additional pressure would be required.

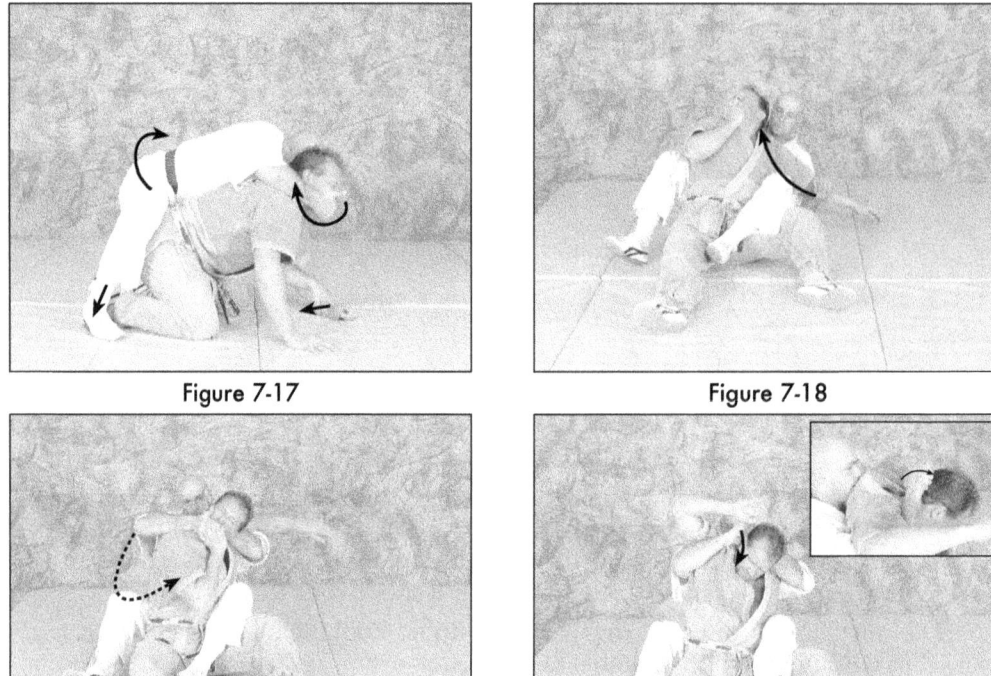

Figure 7-17

Figure 7-18

Figure 7-19

Figure 7-20

Full Nelson

White has taken Grey onto all fours from behind and he kneels on his left knee while grabbing Grey's chin with his right hand and Grey's left wrist with his own left hand (Figure 7-17). White falls onto his right side taking care to remove Grey's supportive left arm and while torquing Grey's head in this same clockwise direction. Both combatants end up in the seated position. Grey tries to remove White's right hand with his own right arm as White slips his left arm under Grey's left upper arm (Figure 7-18). White moves his left hand up to Grey's jaw (Figure 7-19). White releases his right grip and quickly snakes it under Grey's right arm. White then passes both hands behind Grey's neck and joins them in a power grip to effect the hold (Figure 7-20).

Key Points

1. Wherever the head goes, the body must follow. Torquing the head, using the jaw as a lever will move your opponent in the direction of the torque.
2. White kneels in the direction he wishes to turn over his opponent and uses his non-kneeling leg to drive him into the turn.
3. White further ensures that Grey will turn his opponent over by removing one of his points of support in this direction: Grey's left arm.
4. White uses Grey's armpits as fulcrums by leaning back. He also extends both his arms in order to lever Grey's neck forward.

7.3. SEALING THE VEIN

Definition

Sealing the vein techniques refer to the class of techniques that prevent oxygen from getting to the brain by vascular compression and other related mechanisms (carotid sinus stimulation, Valsalva maneuver), resulting in a transient loss of consciousness. Vascular obstruction can be commonly achieved using the upper arm and forearm as a pincher to the sides of the neck, but other methods can also be employed. Clinical studies have shown that proper application of the hold decreases most of the blood flow to the brain within six seconds. Regardless of the technique utilized, the hold should be released once the person has become incapacitated. Complete recovery is generally expected within 30 seconds of the application. It was generally thought that neck restraint worked solely because of the compression of the carotid arteries (hence the term 'carotid sleeper' hold). If this was true, then the techniques would have been more technically correct if they were labeled 'sealing the artery' techniques. After all, it is the higher pressure arteries that bring oxygenated blood to the brain (and all other parts of the body) whereas the lower pressure veins return the de-oxygenated blood back to the heart and lungs. But blood is held mostly in the veins (60%) with smaller amounts in the arteries (25%) and the capillaries (15%). The common carotid artery and the vagus nerve lie underneath the internal jugular vein in the carotid sheath that runs up the front sides of the neck. The jugular vein is, therefore, more susceptible to compression than that of the smaller and more resilient carotid artery. This means that if pressure is applied to the carotid sheath, then the vein would be most readily sealed first. It would be impossible to seal the artery without sealing the vein first, so the term 'sealing the vein' is appropriate after all.

Blood Flow

It makes sense then that sealing both the carotid arteries and the jugular veins aids in a diminishment of circulation to the brain (the brain does have other, albeit relatively minor circulatory routes such as with the vertebral arteries and veins, so total blockage is not possible). The majority of the brain's blood supply (70–80%) comes from the carotid arteries (with 20-30%, or more when the carotid sheath is compressed, coming from the vertebral arteries of the neck). This circulation is bilateral, hence both arteries must be sealed for maximal effect, although results can be obtained from unilateral techniques such as with *kata gatame* (arm-included head lock, a variation of which is shown in Figure 1-41 or *kataha jime* (one-wing strangle as shown in Figure 7-60). This can be accomplished by using various parts of the body such as the arms, hands or legs. Digital pressure can reduce the blood flow in the carotid arteries by 80% at most, but for lateral neck restraints, there is even less reduction in blood flow because of the inefficiency of the neck restraint technique due to the softness of the applied compression tools (muscle mass).* Siddle advocates a shoulder pin method (initially a standing *kata gatame*) that utilizes the bony radial

**Pressure Point and Control Tactics Defensive Tactics Instructor's Manual,* by Bruce Siddle, 1998, pp. 8-2.

edge of the wrist below the mandible to effect compression to the carotid sheath. The airway should remain unimpeded if done correctly, meaning that the person should still be able to breathe as he lapses into unconsciousness. Circulatory restriction may also be achieved using clothing, but your opponent may not always be wearing a shirt or jacket suitable for a decent lapel grab (Figure 7-21).

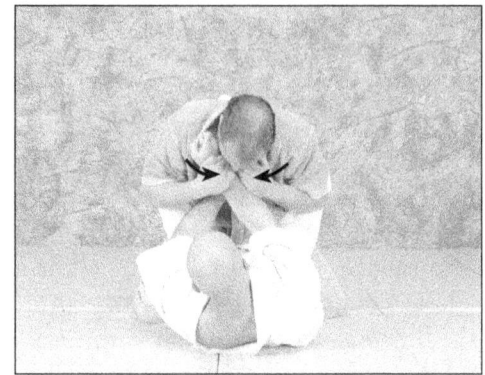

Figure 7-21

Carotid Sinus

The carotid vein and artery can be accessed by pressing into the depression on either side of the larynx and trachea, just under the anterior border of the sternocleidomastoid muscle, which tends to protect this blood flow. This is a commonplace pulse palpation point where people can check their own pulses (also the standard C.P.R. pulse check site). At a point level with the tip of the Adam's apple (St. 9 Man Pulse), the common carotid artery bifurcates into the internal and external carotid arteries.

Just slightly above this splitting of the artery, attached to the somewhat larger (of the split pair) internal carotid artery, is found the carotid body. This chemoreceptor site monitors the level of oxygen in the blood. Low oxygen levels stimulate an increase in heart rate, blood pressure as well as the rate and depth of respiration via the carotid sinus nerve. This nerve further innervates the carotid sinus, a slight dilation within the beginning of the internal carotid artery that is a baroreceptor site (pressure sensitive receptors line the walls of the carotid sinus). It, along with the vagus nerve, allows the brain to make adjustments in the rates of breathing and heart rate as to keep this pressure sensitive organ with a steady pressure of blood, regardless of the head position. This includes the dilation of the blood vessels (vasodilation) to reduce blood pressure. This, and the forced venous pooling of the blood in the face, is what causes the 'purple face' when neck restraint is applied.

It is this latter reaction to an increased pressure that slows down the circulatory system. Neck restraint techniques exploit this reaction to blood pressure reduction in helping to render a person unconscious. The carotid sinus simply cannot distinguish between high blood pressure resulting from internal circulatory problems and that caused by externally applied pressure to the neck. Some people experience 'carotid sinus hypersensitivity', the mere palpation of this spot causing a fall in blood pressure, a slowing of the heart rate, temporary cerebral ischemia (fainting), and in rare cases, death.

A significant reduction of the oxygen tension (and concomitant carbon dioxide tension) in the blood would not occur until after a person has been rendered uncon-

Pressure Point and Control Tactics Defensive Tactics Instructor's Manual, by Bruce Siddle, 1998, pp. 8-2, 8-3.

scious at which point, the carotid body reaction to increase heart, respiration and blood pressure rates would help to revive the person.

Valsalva Maneuver

When a neck restraint is applied properly, the person should be still be able to breathe so there is no great panic for the uninitiated person to escape. Some novices, however, may panic and have an increased susceptibility to the Valsalva maneuver, which involves the pressurization of the thoracic cavity resulting from a person holding his breath while contracting the diaphragm (as with a cough, sneeze, bowel movement strain, or other forced exhalation against a closed airway). This significantly reduces the return of blood from the Vena Cava vessels that pass through the diaphragm, particularly that of the right atrium, which returns de-oxygenated blood from the body back to the heart. It is proper technique to drop the elbow toward the opponent's sternum (if in the recommended seated position), which enhances this pressurization. A person in the fight or flight syndrome will have shorter, quicker breaths making the physiological effect of greatly restricting the amount of blood returning to the heart more pronounced.* Additionally, there is increased stress-induced vascularization to large muscle groups like the legs, in preparation for the perceived need to undertake increased levels of emergency physical activity, which can further reduce blood flow to the head. This stress-induced reaction causes a paleness in the face.

Unconsciousness

As a result of all of these physiological responses, which may be exacerbated by pre-existing medical (heart) problems, the person at the mercy of your flexed arm will quickly feel light-headed and slip peacefully into temporary blackness. Unconsciousness should be reached within three to seven seconds. If not, find out what is incorrect with your technique and make the necessary adjustments. Take care to recognize when your opponent is out cold. The struggle will cease and he will go limp. If this technique is done in a standing situation, it will be readily evident when he is unconscious, as his knees will buckle from under him. A standing application is not recommended because of the stretching effects it can have on the neck and because of the potential for an uncontrolled takedown, both of which can put undue pressure on the neck. It may not be as obvious to you when in a ground fighting situation when your opponent/partner is proned out. In practice, be wary that your partner may fail to tap out if unconsciousness is rapid or unexpected. On the street, relax the pressure immediately when your opponent appears to black out and release the hold entirely when it is safe to do so.

Regaining Consciousness After a Sleeper Hold

In many cases, the judicious application of a properly applied sleeper hold can end a physical altercation quickly and reduce the need to administer the more punishing techniques to a violent offender in need of immediate control. Often the opponent regains consciousness with little desire to resume in his violent behavior.

This is due in part because of the temporary disorientation that comes with his reawakening to consciousness. More rationally, he realizes that he has met his match and does not desire a repeat 'sleep' (particularly if there was an embarrassing loss of bowel/bladder control that sometimes occurs). After all, you have shown complete domination over your opponent by rendering him unconscious, and thereby he was totally at your mercy. It is common for a person to actually snore prior to regaining regaining consciousness, at which point he may start to shake uncontrollably as his brain signs back on ('doing the chicken'). Loud, repetitive, and simple verbal commands may be necessary to gain his voluntary compliance, as the cognitive functions of the brain are initially a little fuzzy. If the person does not regain consciousness within 30 seconds, emergency first aid must be administered

Resuscitation

It is not uncommon that the heart may stop beating after a successful application has been made. In a very few cases, the heart does not restart (carotid sinus syndrome) after the normal 30 second recovery window has passed. Emergency first aid must be administered immediately unless it is your intention to kill your opponent. If a person's heart does stop, cardiopulmonary resuscitation would be required to revive him. A more common effect is the temporary cessation of breathing. This is not an unusual consequence of a fully and successfully applied technique, but respiration will return on its own in the vast majority of cases and consciousness will be quickly regained. The ancient revival techniques (*kappo* or *katsu*) used in judo include seating the unconscious person and sharply slapping the spine in the mid-thoracic area as to stimulate the diaphragm back into action. There are many revival methods, but this one is very commonly used.

Cautions About the Lateral Vascular Neck Restraint

Proper training in lateral vascular neck restraint is essential because of the possibility of lethal consequences. As such, these techniques must only be used if life and death situations. Deaths have occurred at the hands of the police who were improperly trained or who were not trained at all in its usage. As a result, this technique has been banned by many police agencies across the United States in particular over the past two decades. Improper application (a sleeper hold inadvertently turned into a choke hold) can damage the internal structures of the neck like the hyoid bone, larynx, trachea, etc. As such, it is important to line up your elbow with his chin and most importantly, the sternum, keeping his head locked into place looking directly ahead, with your elbow pressing down on the sternum to avoid any dangerous stretching and rotation of the neck. This alignment will help prevent an inadvertent slippage into a choking technique, thereby minimizing an accidental crushing of the relatively delicate throat structures (REN 23).

Other cautions come with using these techniques. Holding the technique too long can cause brain damage. The pressure should be released immediately after a successful application and first aid should be administered if needed (put him in the recovery position and check his vital signs). Pre-existing natural disease significantly increases the likelihood of complications occurring even when the hold was applied correctly. Needless to say, applying these holds on elderly people should be avoided. Men over 40 years of age have marked susceptibility to coronary artery disease that could result in a heart attack.* Underlying heart disease such as narrowing of the coronary arteries or irregular beating patterns can make these individuals very vulnerable to the effects of lack of oxygen and to the effect of the stimulation of the carotid sinus. There may also be a pre-existing disease in the form of atherosclerosis involving the carotid arteries themselves. This involves the deposition of plaque, cholesterol and fatty tissue in the wall of the artery. Pressure applied to such an artery may cause dislodgement of some of this plaque that could go on to produce a stroke by lodging itself in the brain. Also, a stroke may result if the lining of an artery is damaged and a blood clot ensues. Those who become unsafely hyperactive or who are feeling little or no pain from street drug use while in the hold (like cocaine or methamphetamine users, mentally challenged people, or epileptics) may make a technically correct application difficult as well. Stimulant street drugs appear to sensitize the heart for the development of fatal irregularities of the heart. Even prescription medicated people may experience cardiac arrhythmia, also associated with the previously listed pre-existing medical problems. Finally, uncontrollable struggling can tear the vertebral arteries resulting in massive hemorrhaging at the base of the brain leading to immediate collapse and death.

For those acting in a law enforcement capacity, it is advised that others taking control over your restrained and arrested party be aware that a neck restraint hold had been used to subdue him. This will allow the proper medical monitoring of this party lest complications develop while he is in custody. The swelling of the trachea, causing asphyxiation, is the common cause of in-custody deaths relating to the use of neck restraints.

Using Your Tools

Central to applying any kind of neck restraint or choke is your ability to use both of your hands from a stable and safe position while your opponent is in a poor position to defend against it (Figure 7-22). Use the narrower radial and ulnar edges of your wrist to do the work. The thinner the tool, the more penetration will be achieved. Whenever you commit both of your hands to any hold, it is imperative that your opponent cannot easily and powerfully attack you (Figure 7-23).

Visualize using your sealing tool(s) as a thin cord(s). This is not difficult to do when the collar of a jean jacket or gi top is used as a garrote around your opponent's neck (Figure 7-24). One cannot rely on opponents wearing clothing suitable for assistance in your neck restraint techniques (other than in training situations), but

*Reay and Eisele, 1982, p. 257

Chin Na In Ground Fighting

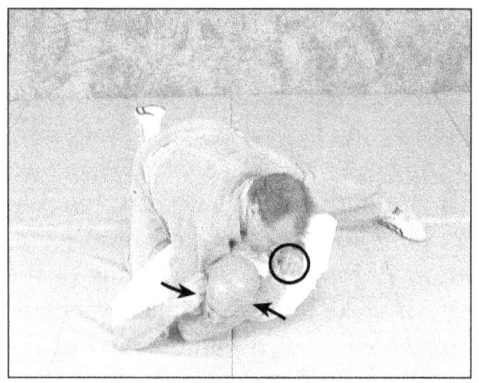

Figure 7-22

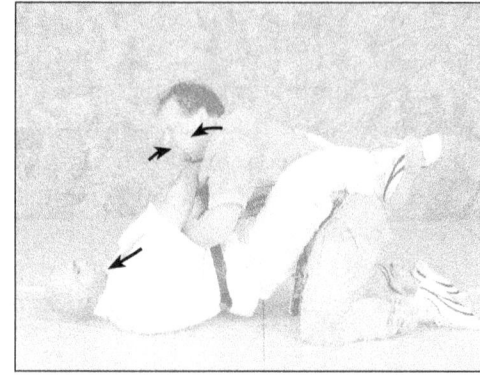

Figure 7-23

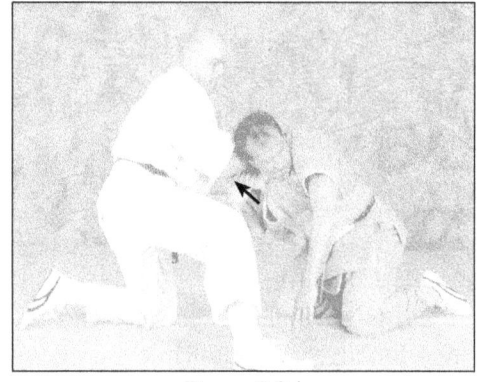

Figure 7-24

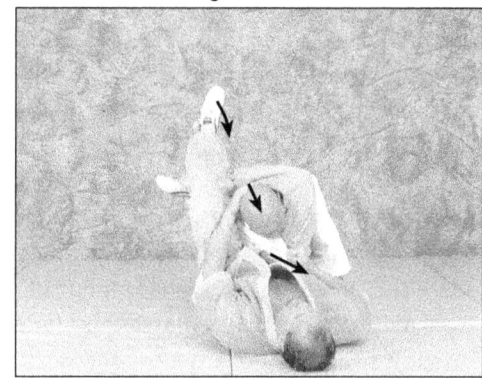

Figure 7-25

take it when you can get it (Figure 7-25). If you are trying for a sleeper but cannot make the grip with your other hand, try gripping your opponent's clothing and turn your body away to cinch up the hold. Also grabbing clothing can help secure or anchor any one-handed hold, especially if your opponent is pulling on your arm and you feel that he is too strong to hold off normally.

Prevention Against Neck Restraint Holds

The best defense against neck restraint holds is to protect your neck at all costs, otherwise the fight may be over in seconds for you. Having well-developed neck muscles, especially the protective sternocleidomastoid muscles, is an asset when protecting yourself from neck attacks. While some attacks to the neck can be diminished by shrugging the shoulders or tightening the platysma and sternocleidomastoid muscles (Figure 7-26), there are ways to overcome these defenses. The snaking of a choking arm around the neck can be achieved by hair pulling (Figure 7-27), eye gouging (Figure 7-28), or the painful rubbing the knuckles of the snaking hand(s) under the jaw line to create some space for the following wrist and arm (Figure 7-29).

Chapter 7: Controlling the Head/Neck and Body

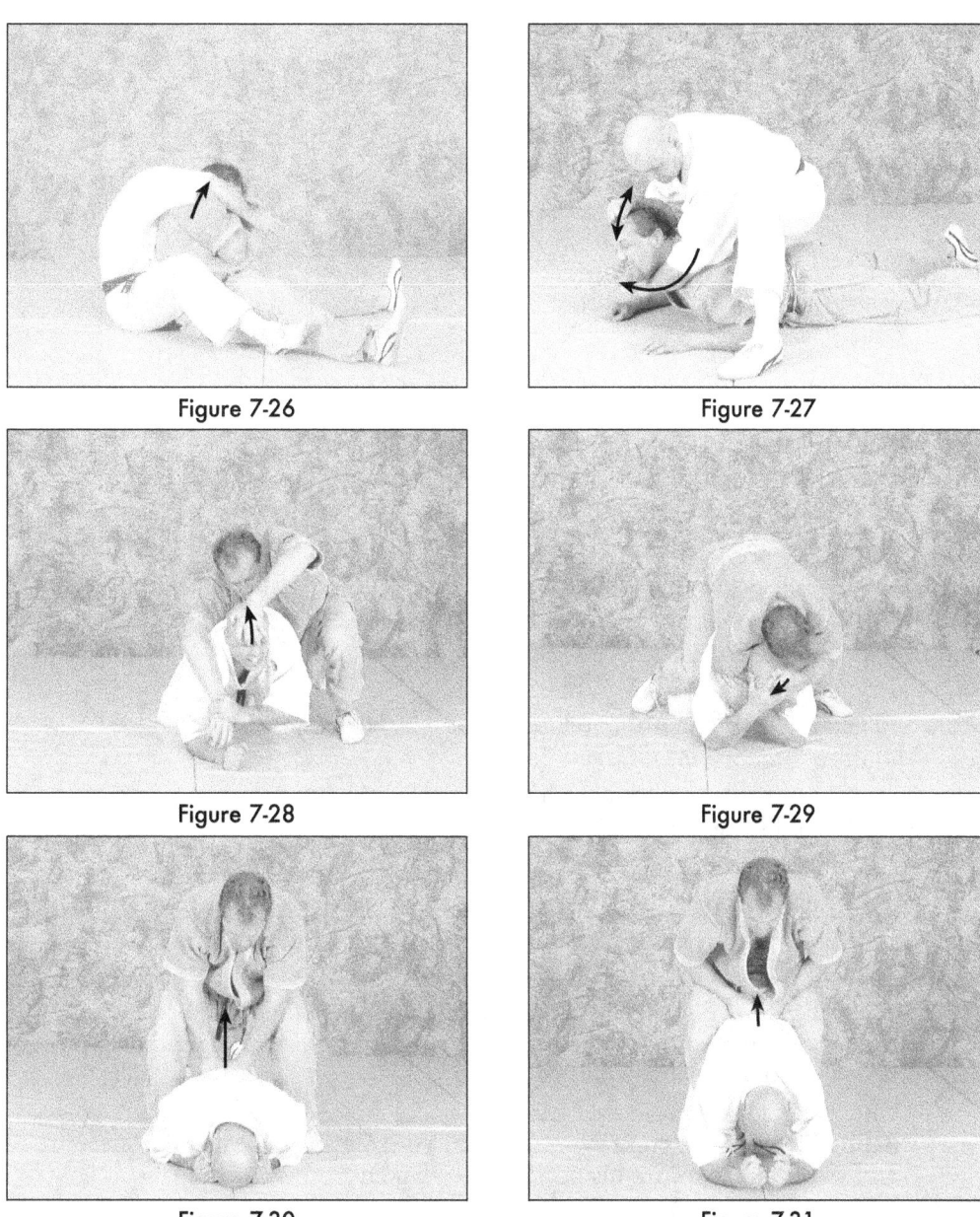

Figure 7-26

Figure 7-27

Figure 7-28

Figure 7-29

Figure 7-30

Figure 7-31

Lateral Vascular Neck Restraint

White is played out and has proned himself out. He has folded his arms at the sides of his neck as a defensive measure against an impending neck attack. Grey straddles him at the waist in the standing position and grabs his belt (waist band) in preparation for lifting him up (Figure 7-30). Grey lifts him up and places his feet as close together (heel to heel) as he can (Figure 7-31). Grey can fall forward if he chooses. Grey reaches down with his left hand and hooks his fingers into White's

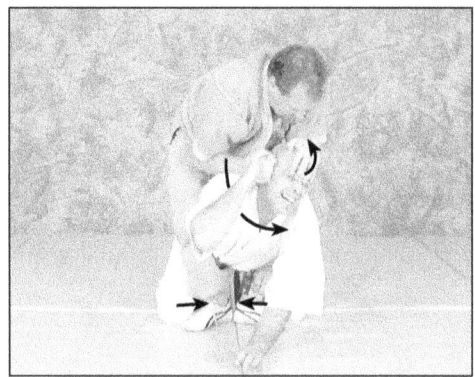

Figure 7-32

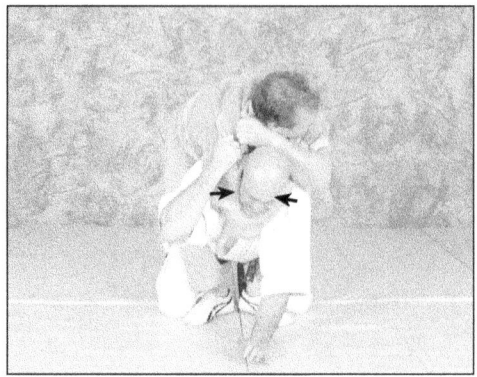

Figure 7-33

eye sockets and pulls upward to expose White's neck (Figure 7-32). Grey then encircles White's neck with his right arm grabbing his own left upper arm/clothing while ensuring that the crook of the elbow is centered to the front of the throat. Grey releases the eye sockets, slides his left arm behind White's head and grasps his own clothing on his right shoulder (Figure 7-33). Grey rolls over onto his right side maintaining his neck restraint hold (Figure 7-34).

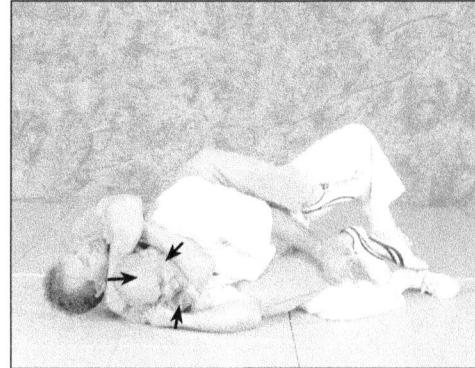

Figure 7-34

Key Points

1. By placing Grey's heels closely together ('rodeo ride' position) White's own body weight will exert pressure from Grey's lower legs into White's floating ribs.
2. Grabbing the eye sockets is an excellent technique when you need to do a rear head crank, and is more reliable than a hair pull crank if your opponent is bald or has little hair to grasp.
3. Your encircled arms act as a triangular neck brace and if you secure your hands by grabbing your own clothing, your opponent can thrash about and you will not injure his neck nor be shaken from your hold, especially if you keep your legs around his waist.

Chapter 7: Controlling the Head/Neck and Body

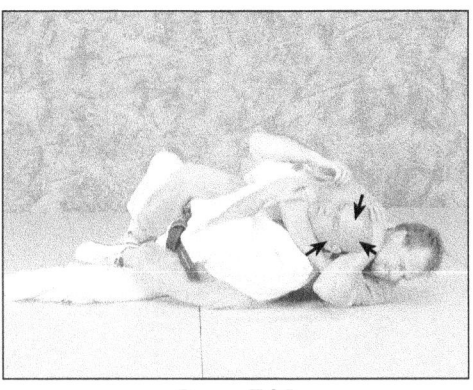

Figure 7-35

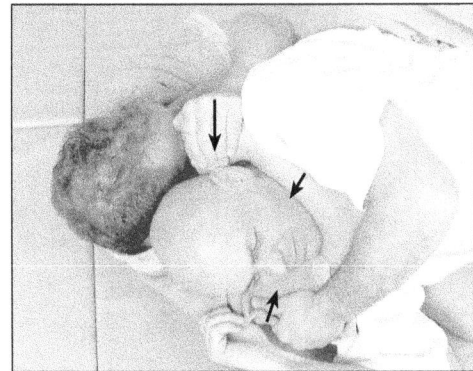

Figure 7-36

4. Centralizing the elbow further minimizes the possibility of inadvertently slipping into a choke hold and thereby causing unwanted structural damage to the neck. It also ensures that circulation on both sides of the neck is being affected.
5. Should you deem that increased pressure to the neck is required, you may shrug your shoulders upward and lever your right and left wrists upwards and downwards respectively. These actions all tighten your hold on the neck.
6. Should further offensive action be required, you may place your left hand on the rear or side of the head and push your opponent's neck against your encircling right arm (neck restraint with chancery) and/or allow your forearm to slide across his throat to strangle him (Figure 7-35).
7. If a person has a large neck, you may elect to use a standard neck restraining hold (Figure 7-36). The free left arm merely grasps the fist of the encircling right arm to pull it in against the side of the neck and anchors it there. Be sure to brace your head against his to prevent a rear head butt.

Chin Na In Ground Fighting

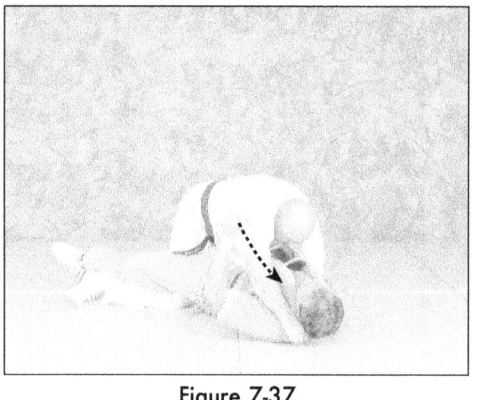

Figure 7-37

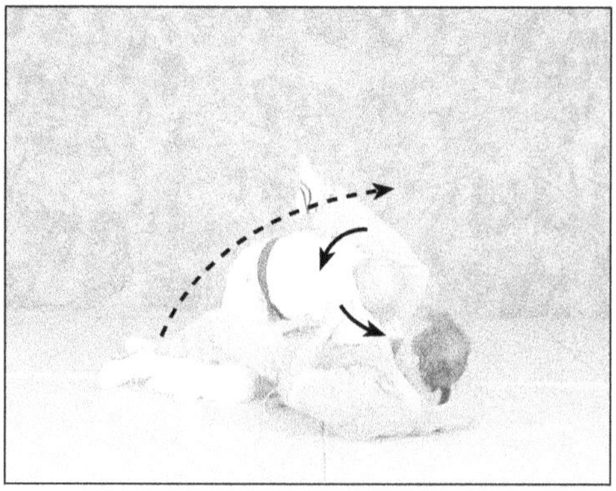

Figure 7-38

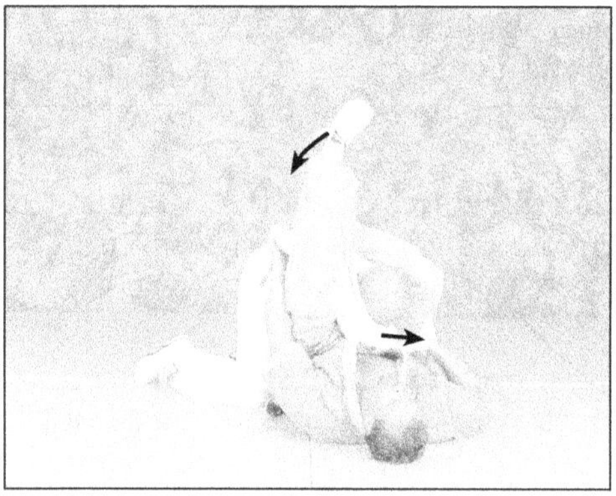

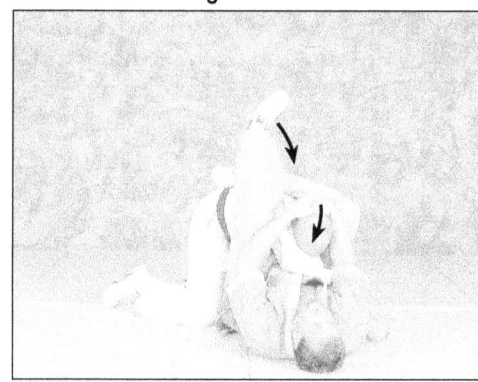

Figure 7-39

Figure 7-40

Triangle Strangle

White is on top of Grey and he reaches down with his right arm to grab Grey's left shoulder (Figure 7-37). Grey passes White's arm over his head and pulls it across White's body as he passes his right leg behind White's neck (Figure 7-38). Grey controls White's right arm by pulling on his jacket as to constrict the right side of White's neck. Grey also raises his left leg and hooks his own right ankle as to further constrict the right side of White's neck as well as the left side of White's neck using his right thigh (Figure 7-39).

Key Points

1. Use both of your legs and one of his arms to strangle him.
2. Notice how Grey uses his left arm to help position his right leg tightly behind White's neck.
3. Grey can also add an element of a choke by pulling down on White's head (Figure 7-40).

Triangle Strangle from Side Position

Grey tries to take White down with a single leg takedown to his advanced left leg (Figure 7-41). White reacts by dropping his weight onto Grey's back by leaning

Chapter 7: Controlling the Head/Neck and Body

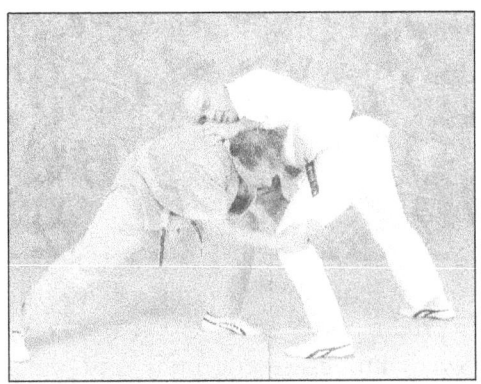

Figure 7-41

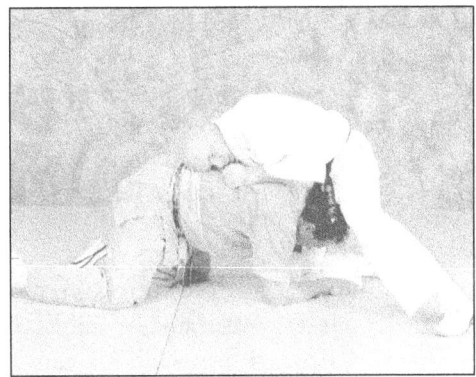

Figure 7-42

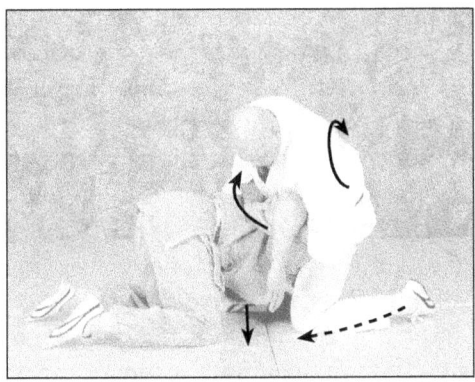

Figure 7-43

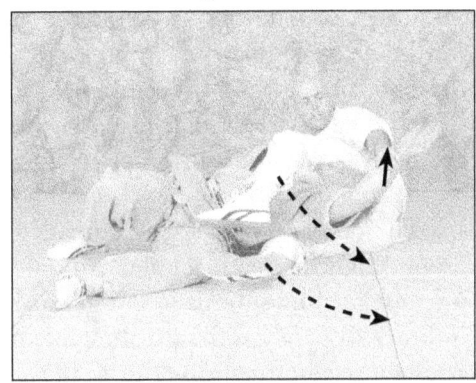

Figure 7-44

over Grey and dropping onto his right knee while he steps backwards with his left leg in order to free it (Figure 7-42). White reaches down and under hooks Grey's right arm pulling it upward (Figure 7-43). White rolls over onto his right side while turning Grey's body over by pulling upward on Grey's right arm (Figure 7-44). White maintains control over Grey's right arm as he secures Grey's left arm and neck by figure-fouring his legs (Figure 7-45).

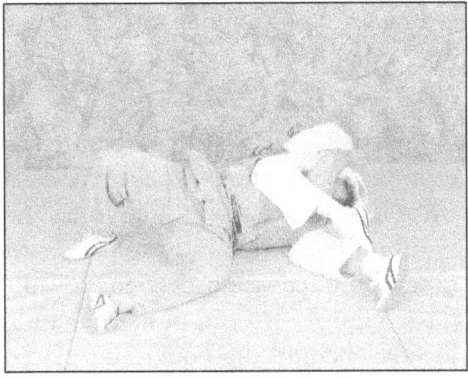

Figure 7-45

Key Points
1. White's right foot must be placed below the line of Grey's shoulders and as far under his body as he can as to allow Grey's upper body (head and shoulders) to roll over onto this leg.
2. White uses Grey's right arm as a lever (like a logger's cant hook) in order to roll him over using his own body weight to do so. He pulls Grey in

towards his groin as he rolls so that Grey is held in tightly between his legs.
3. White can apply pressure to Grey's neck by both using his scissoring thighs and by bending his hooking leg to further tighten the strangle.

7-4. Sealing the Breath

Definition

Sealing the breath techniques refer to the act of inhibiting air from re-filling the lungs (respiratory restraint or chokes) and depriving the brain of oxygen, thereby inducing unconsciousness. This can be achieved through several means. Choking techniques often employ a forearm to apply pressure directly across the front of the throat to painfully close off the airway, using an appreciable amount of force. Additionally, a relatively minor compressive force can displace the tongue into the back of the throat, occluding the free passage of air. Any neck hold recipient should have first aid administered to him immediately, starting by placing him in the recovery position in order to minimize the possibility of this airway occlusion by the tongue.

The other way to seal the breath is to use 'choking' techniques, widely used in ground fighting because they can quickly end a fight (prior to the opponent going unconscious) by submission. The solar plexus (REN 21) can be struck for instance, in order to paralyze the diaphragm, thereby impairing breathing. If the diaphragm does not regain function prior to the air being used up in the lungs, unconsciousness will result. Although the act of sealing the vein is often referred to as 'choking out' as well, it is a misnomer and should not be used. This term 'choking out' should be reserved only to describe 'sealing the breath' techniques.

Choking Bans

All police agencies have banned choke holds in favor of vascular neck restraint techniques, although some agencies (such as the L.A.P.D.) have even banned these latter techniques as well due to a number of deaths in the 1970s and early 1980s. Death often ensued in post-arrest situations when the arrested party lapsed unnoticed into unconsciousness due to suffocation experienced from the swelling shut of the windpipe, or from positional asphyxia as a result of being hog-tied (feet bound together behind the body) and placed in a prone position, thereby restricting (an often overweight/drugged) prisoner's ability to breathe.

Since the bar arm choke places pressure across the front of the throat with the forearm, the larynx (thyroid cartilage or Adam's apple), trachea (cricoid cartilages), and the hyoid bone (floating base of attachment for the tongue) can all be damaged using this hold. The consequences of rendering a struggling opponent unconscious using this relatively painful and slow-acting technique may be lethal (see Figure 7-46 showing the guillotine choke hold). This is the primary reason for this ban (except in

Chapter 7: Controlling the Head/Neck and Body

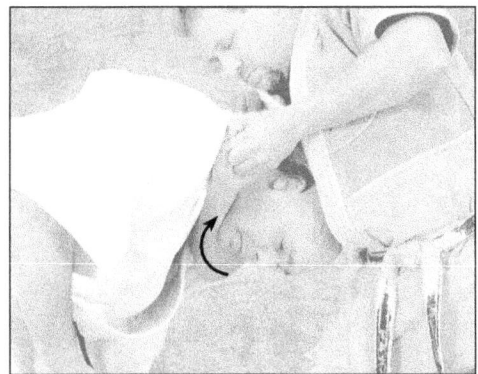

Figure 7-46

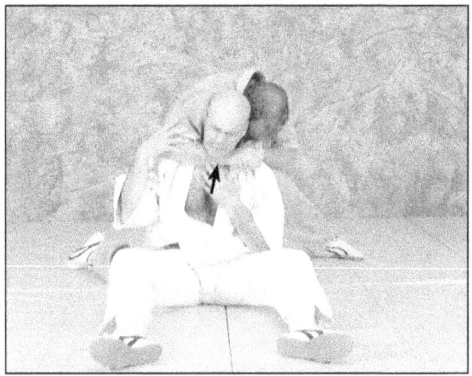

Figure 7-47

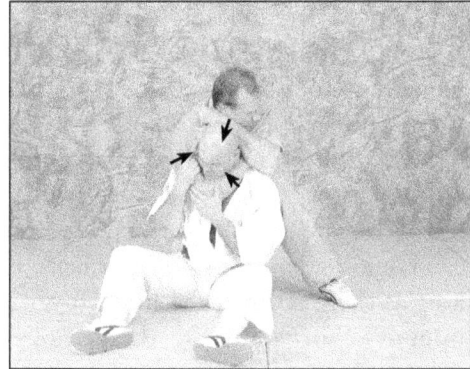

Figure 7-48

deadly threat situations). The police are highly accountable for the amount of force that they use. Indeed, the police should only apply these techniques in special arrest situations and only after considerable training and periodic refresher certification instruction has been undertaken. Civilians may use these techniques at their own risk of criminal and civil liability, hopefully only when the situation merits it.

It should be noted that since the inception of judo in 1882, there have been no recorded deaths associated with the application of any strangle or neck restraint hold. Light applications of the chokes can be made in practice as long as your partner taps out quickly. No doubt, the supervision of healthy and trained athletes by referees and qualified teachers in sporting arenas and training halls account for this unblemished safety record.

Neck Restraints vs. Chokes

Lateral vascular neck restraint (as discussed in the previous section) refers to the act of 'sealing the vein' and should be referred to as 'sleeper holds' or vascular neck restraints. Grey is applying his right arm in a sealing the breath technique (bar arm choke in Figure 7-47) and in a sealing the vein technique (neck restraint with chancery in Figure 7-48). These photos clearly show the difference between the two techniques. The addition of the chancery to the latter technique (Grey's left arm pushing White's neck forward, thereby choking him) actually combines both techniques. Choking techniques can be applied from many angles and body positions, but applying them from the rear offers protection against your opponent's limbs.

*Reay and Eisele, 1982, p. 255-256

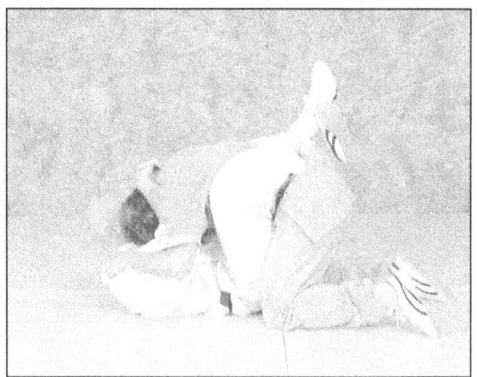

Figure 7-49

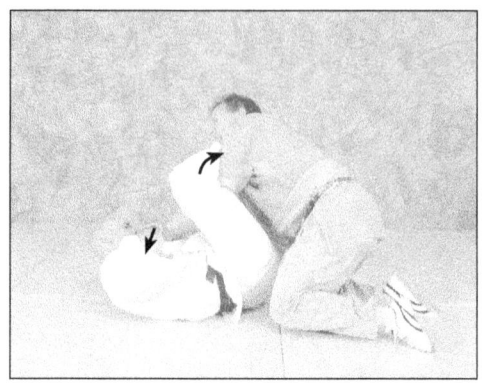

Figure 7-50

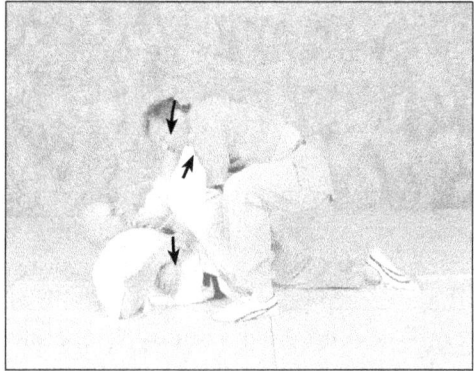

Figure 7-51

Chokes are more painful than sleepers are but they are less efficient in rendering a person unconscious. It has been estimated that it takes six times the amount of force to collapse the cricoid cartilage reinforced airway that it does for the carotid artery.* A person can remain conscious and fight back as long as there is air in the lungs (over a minute?). So painful are these chokes that a person will immediately submit or they will fight wildly, fuelled by an adrenaline dump that accompanies the 'flight or fight syndrome', in order to stop the intense pain and to save their own life (after all, he is being suffocated). This violent struggling can lead to the opponent inadvertently contributing to any damage being done to his own neck. This hyperactivity uses up oxygen held in the lungs at a faster rate than normal, contributing to a more rapid arrival to a hypoxic state. As the entire body is deprived of oxygen, the body may respond by altering the heart rate. The heart muscle, also deprived of oxygen, may go into rapidly fatal ventricular fibrillation or seizure activity may occur. Due to the damage that choking can do to the relatively delicate structure of the neck, and other medical implications, the application of chokeholds should be withheld for life and death situations.

Choke using the Shin

Grey is held in White's guard (Figure 7-49). White gouges at Grey's face prompting him to sit back and to try choking White in return. White grabs Grey's left wrist and swings his right leg over Grey's head, lodging it across Grey's throat (Figure 7-50). With Grey's arm trapped in an arm bar, White reaches up behind Grey's head with his free left hand and pulls Grey's head downwards causing his throat to be pressed against White's shin, thereby choking him (Figure 7-51).

Chapter 7: Controlling the Head/Neck and Body

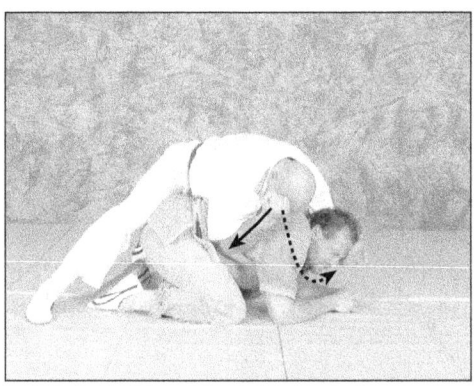

Figure 7-52

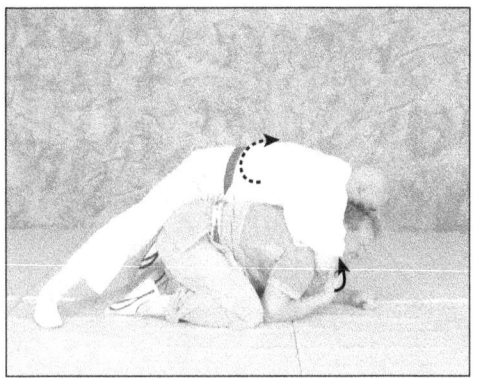

Figure 7-53

Key Points
1. Notice how White trapped Grey's arm to thwart his choke while setting him up for an arm bar.
2. By pulling Grey's head down while White extends his right leg, maximal pressure can be exerted on the neck.

Roll Over Choke

Grey is turtled up with White on top, kneeling on his left knee close to

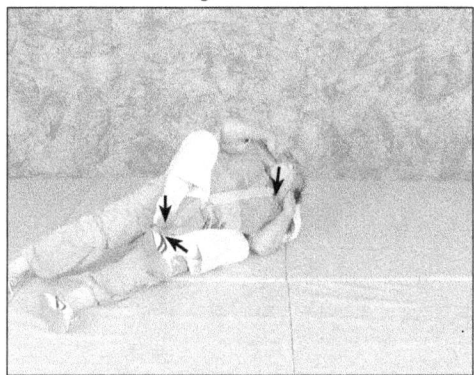

Figure 7-54

Grey's left side. White applies an elbow to Grey's mid-section in order to try and expose Grey's throat (Figure 7-52). White reaches under Grey's throat with his right arm and begins to choke Grey (Figure 7-53). White then elects to roll over onto his left side taking Grey with him between his legs while securing a two-handed grip to seal Grey's breath (Figure 7-54).

Key Points
1. Your opponent's head can be taken off of his chest by using distraction techniques such as eye gouging or hair pulling.
2. Notice how White moves into a more stable and controlling position by rolling onto his side and taking Grey between his legs.
3. By securing the choke with a two-handed grip, White may exert maximal power into the choke, augmenting it by pressing downwards against Grey's body.

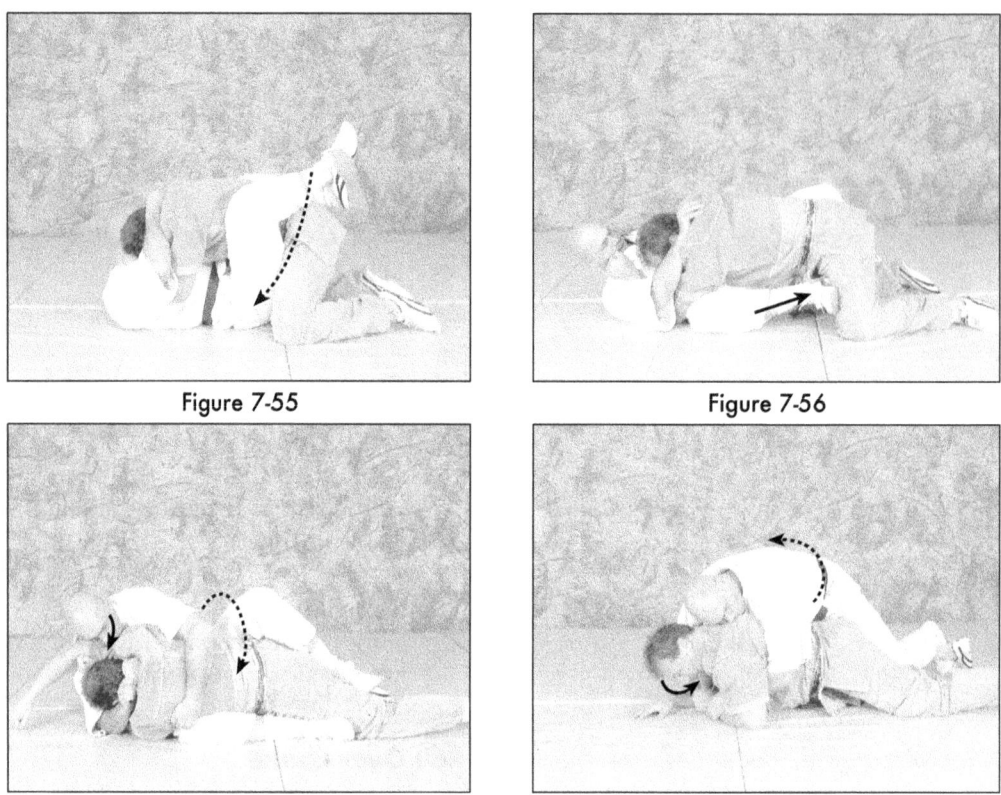

Figure 7-55

Figure 7-56

Figure 7-57

Figure 7-58

One-Wing Neck Choke

White is supine with Grey in his guard (Figure 7-55) and they are at an impasse. White decides to change positions by unlocking his legs, scooting onto his right hip, and using his right foot to push Grey's left thigh backward (Figure 7-56). Notice that White is setting up his choking hand early in this sequence by placing his right hand on White's collar behind the neck (thumb toward the neck) as deep as he can get it. White uses his left leg to hook Grey's right leg and he reaches across Grey's back with his left arm to give him the ability to work his way onto Grey's back (Figure 7-57). White continues to slide fully on top of Grey as he snakes his left hand under Grey's left armpit to take hold of his left wrist (Figure 7-58). White now rolls himself and Grey onto their sides. White locks his legs at the ankles around Grey's waist and continues snaking his left hand behind Grey's head to effectively capture Grey's left arm and to press Grey's neck forward (Figure 7-59). Grey's collar is now pulled taut across the left side of his neck with his right radial edge of his wrist/forearm simultaneously pressing into and across Grey's throat.

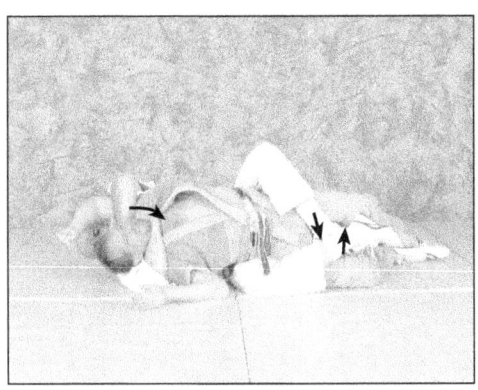

Figure 7-59

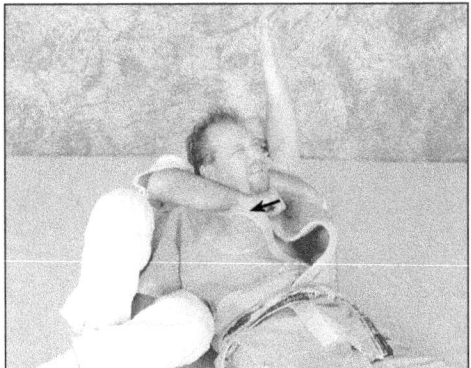

Figure 7-60

Key Points
1. Notice how White uses his legs to control Grey's body by either pushing on a leg or locking his legs around him (controlling the distance and mobility of the hips).
2. By claiming his grip early, it allows White to do so without a struggle and possibly without any attention by the opponent. It also allows all the slack to be removed from the collar as he changes his relative body position.
3. White may easily apply choking pressure to the front of Grey's neck by changing the angle of the wrist. This extra pressure would be advisable should Grey grab White's right arm with his right hand and try to slide out of the hold.
4. The placement of the restraining hand with the thumb side towards the neck ensures that there is proper hand placement for this technique (bony radial edge pressing against the throat).
5. White's left hand can lever against the back/side of Grey's head for additional choking power. It may also grab collar material to lock his arm into place should Grey try to remove it.
6. This technique is known as *kataha jime* in judo (one-wing strangle). It may also be applied crossways from behind (Figure 7-60). Notice how White controls Grey's arm by figure-fouring his legs.

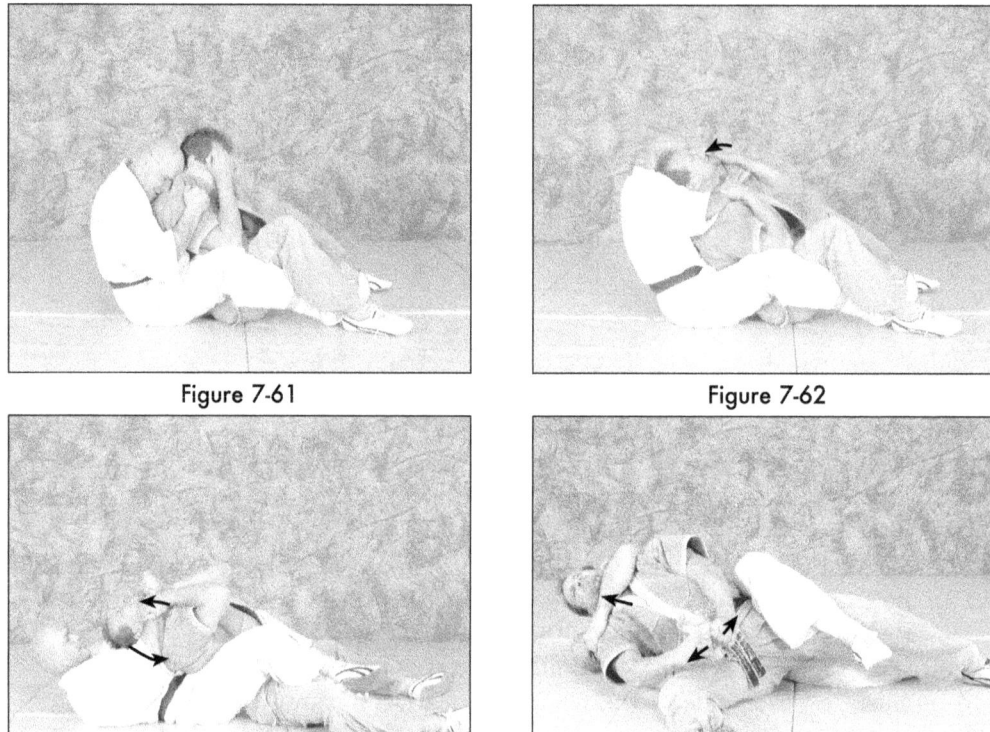

Figure 7-61

Figure 7-62

Figure 7-63

Figure 7-64

Seated Rear Choke

White is seated behind Grey, taking care to avoid a rear head butt by Grey (Figure 7-61). White applies a c-clamp to the left side of Grey's face with his left hand in order for him to access Grey's neck (Figure 7-62). White lets go of the c-clamp to secure his hand in a choke hold, flipping his legs over Grey's legs and leaning back to exert maximum pressure on Grey's neck (Figure 7-63).

Key Points

1. Always be wary of a reverse head butt when you are behind someone. This attack can be dangerous to your dental health.
2. The c-clamp or any facial distracting technique can be used to force your opponent's head backwards and take his mind off of your ambition to choke him.
3. Notice how White traps Grey's legs so that he can better control him and add to his choking power in the opposite direction, using his legs as a base.
4. Securing your own grip with your other hand keeps it away from your opponent's free hands (Figure 7-64), as well as adding power to your technique.

7-5. CONTROLLING THE BODY

Body Locks

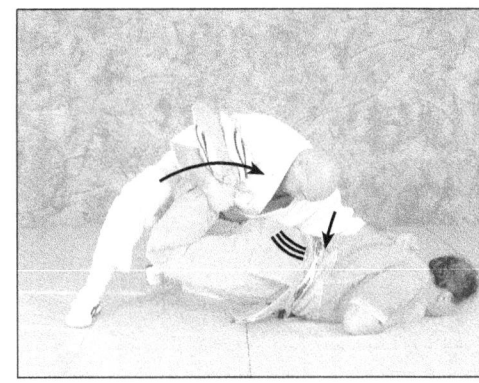

Figure 7-65

Although the movement of the thoracic vertebrae is small, their combined movement is significant. The range of movement is greatest in the lumbar area and least in the thoracic area. The torso is heavily muscled and therefore very difficult to manipulate, particularly since the appendages that stem from it are capable of defense. As such, any attacks to the torso are usually made from the rear as to minimize your opponent's defensive capabilities. The spinal column may be either hyper-flexed or hyper-extended but this requires use of your whole body.

Anatomy of the Torso

There are 44 bones of the torso (from the top of the thoracic spine to the tailbone):

12 thoracic vertebrae (upper spine)   5 lumbar vertebrae (lower spine)
1 breastbone (sternum)   1 sacrum
24 ribs   1 coccyx (tailbone)

The organ-protecting rib cage consists of twelve pair of ribs emanating from the twelve thoracic vertebrae that are connected by ligaments and cartilage. Twelve pairs of nerves follow the length of the ribs. They innervate the muscles of the stomach and chest. Other nerves feed the important internal organs such as the heart, lungs and those of the abdomen and pelvis.

Double Leg Scoop

White scoops Grey's legs with his right arm and hyperextends Grey's spine by leaning forward towards his head while pressing downwards on his spine (Figure 7-65). There is little likelihood of catching a person in this position nor is this a good hold down technique. The Boston Crab is a more likely means of hyper-extending the back.

Chin Na In Ground Fighting

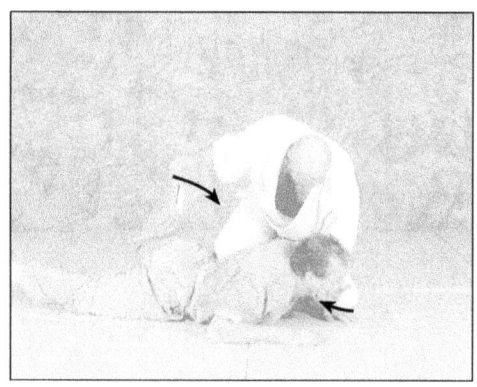

Figure 7-66

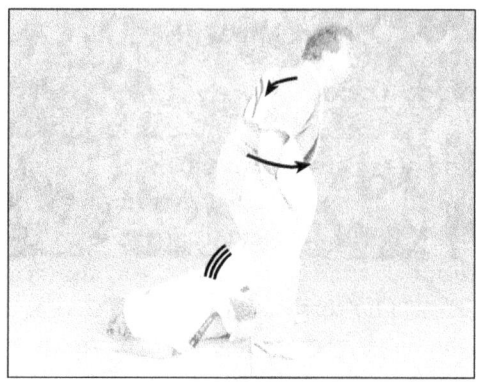

Figure 7-67

Leg Chin Crank

White forces Grey's head upwards with his left hand while lifting upwards on Grey's left leg. White also kneels on Grey's lower spine with his right knee in order to hyperextend Grey's lumbar spine (Figure 7-66). As with the previous technique, the advantage of executing this technique is moot.

Boston Crab

Grey has White in the Boston Crab (Figure 7-67). This technique

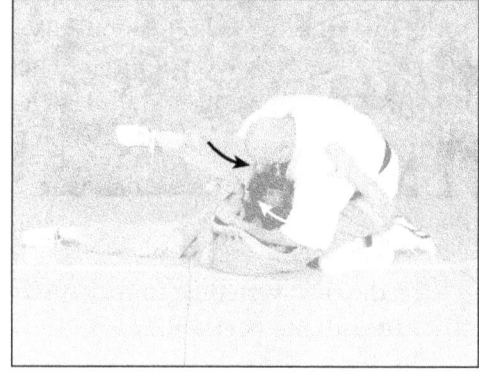

Figure 7-68

places tremendous pressure on the lower back and causes significant pain to the calf muscles as well. Grey arches backwards with Grey's legs in a double calf squeeze in order to hype-extend the lumbar area of the spinal column.

Single Leg Flex

White is hyper-flexing Grey's spine by grabbing Grey's right leg behind the knee with his right arm while he bends Grey's upper body with his left arm behind Grey's neck and squeezing (Figure 7-68). Depending upon the flexibility of your opponent, this technique may work. Be sure to lock your hands tight. This will prevent Grey from merely extending his leg in order to free himself of the hold (the more Grey extends his leg, the more pressure he puts on the back of his own neck).

CHAPTER 8

Fighting Sequences

8-1. Introduction

Combining Techniques

In this section, we will discuss how to utilize the ground fighting and Qin Na (Chin Na) skills we have learned in combination with other skills we may already possess. From a standing position we will see some examples of how blocking, kicking, striking, throwing and finishing holds can be put together in a seamless web of control within the fighting spectrum. We believe that having a good general knowledge of this entire spectrum is important in your ability to adapt to whatever situation you may find yourself in. The Qin Na practitioner just may find himself flat out on the ground because he is tackled from behind or trips and falls in a fracas; the ground fighter may have to deal with someone he cannot or should not take to the ground because of space restrictions or the presence of multiple assailants.

Obviously there are countless combinations of techniques that could possibly be strung together. This task, apart from the restrictions of your own knowledge base, is limited only by your own creative mind. You may have great combinations and applications that you can draw out of your own martial arts experiences that we do not know. We encourage you all to do that and not confine yourself to our narrow interpretation of what will or will not work (for you). As such, view the combinations presented in this chapter with an open and creative mind. We hope they will trigger some of your own combinations that you could share with a training partner. Put whatever techniques you like into your combinations. The only requirement is that they flow smoothly from one to the other. Failing to do so in a real fight could mean defeat. Instead of doing a series of single movements in isolation, think ahead of where each movement will take you or better still where you would like to go with your chosen techniques. This is fight control at its finest.

For example, rather than just throwing a person to the ground and standing over him thinking about what to do next after you realize that your throw did not have the desired results, retain your grip on your fallen foe and immediately apply a follow up move or moves to ensure your victory. You can kick him, lock the arm, slide down, and choke him, whatever. What you do will depend upon how your opponent reacts and what your skill base is. Conversely, if you are taken down by your opponent, you should be initiating your counterattack in thought and possibly in form, even while going down. With practice, your techniques will flow effortlessly.

8-2. Fighting Sequences

Fighting Sequence #1

White attacks Grey with a right roundhouse kick and he defends by stepping off to his right side and executing a butterfly (arm scissors) block in order to capture White's leg (Figure 8-1). Grey turns his hips into White and scoops White's ankle with his left hand while driving his elbow into White's inner thigh (Sp. 11) (or closer to the knee for better leverage) to effect a straight leg take down, dropping onto his right knee as he does so (Figure 8-2). White falls onto his back while Grey follows up with an immediate right backfist strike to White's groin (Figure 8-3). White grabs Grey's right wrist and he swings his left leg across his midline and does a reverse roundhouse kick to the left side of Grey's head, pulling Grey's arm upwards towards his head as he does so (Figure 8-4). Grey falls onto his back and White executes a straight transverse arm bar on Grey's right arm (Figure 8-5).

Key Points

1. Sidestepping is very important in minimizing your opponent's impact power as well as in making target acquisition difficult.
2. Upon executing the butterfly block and capturing the kicking leg, the elbow can be used to press into Sp.11 or it can be struck with a pressing follow-through. White's leg can be rolled to his outside using both the elbow and the capturing hand in order to break the integrity of the stance at the hip, making it easier to take him down.
3. Dropping down onto the right knee adds power to the take down by utilizing body weight into the elbow press.
4. Following up with a technique during or immediately after a take down is wise in case your opponent is not incapacitated by the fall.
5. The reverse roundhouse kick can be done dynamically or in a pressing manner to unbalance Grey backwards.

Chapter 8: Fighting Sequences

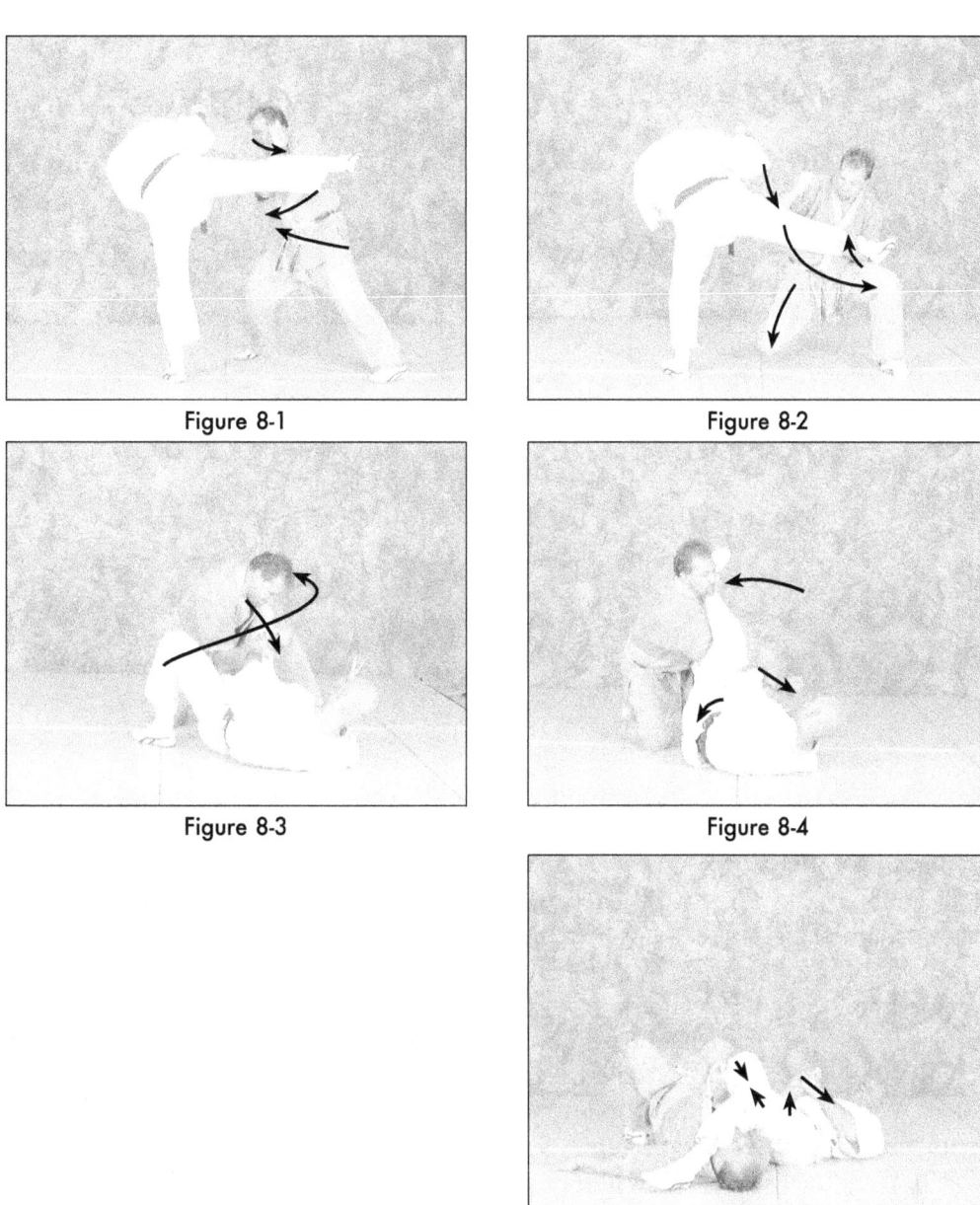

Figure 8-1

Figure 8-2

Figure 8-3

Figure 8-4

Figure 8-5

275

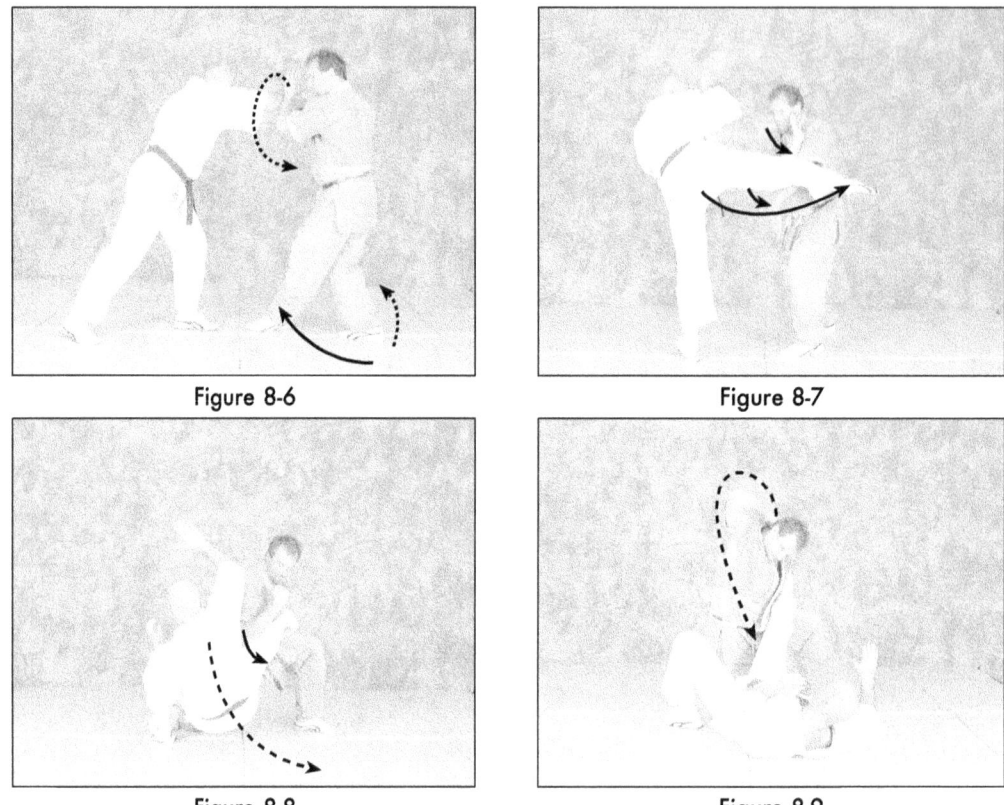

Figure 8-6

Figure 8-7

Figure 8-8

Figure 8-9

Fighting Sequence #2

White attacks Grey with a reverse punch to the head. Grey cross-steps to his right side blocking with a left-pressing cross body block (Figure 8-6). Grey turns his body counterclockwise by sliding his right foot to his right while continuing the clockwise motion of his left arm from the block by dropping it to receive the second attack from White, a right roundhouse kick, in a butterfly block (Figure 8-7). Grey takes White down with a straight leg bar as he drops onto his right knee (Figure 8-8). While maintaining his grip on White's right leg, Grey sets to hit White's groin with a right backfist strike (Figure 8-9). Grey applies this strike to the target (Figure 8-10). Grey then steps over White's right upper thigh with his right leg, placing his lower shin in White's right hip crease as he controls White's right leg with both arms (Figure 8-11). Grey drops onto his own right side and applies a straight leg lock to this leg (Figure 8-12). Grey applies pressure on White's Achilles tendon using the radial edge of his right wrist as he forces White's right leg into hyperextension (Figure 8-13).

Key Points

1. Cross-stepping is useful in this example, to close up your opponent, meaning that Grey blocks to turn White's punching arm to his inside. This will make a follow up punch with White's other arm difficult.

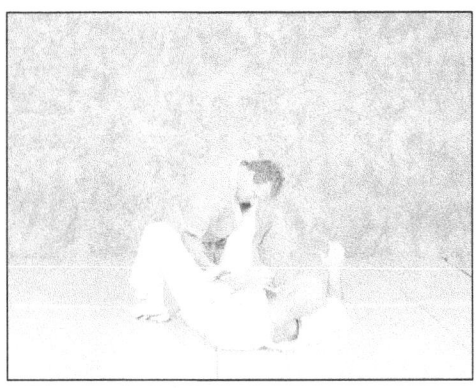

| Figure 8-10 | Figure 8-11 |

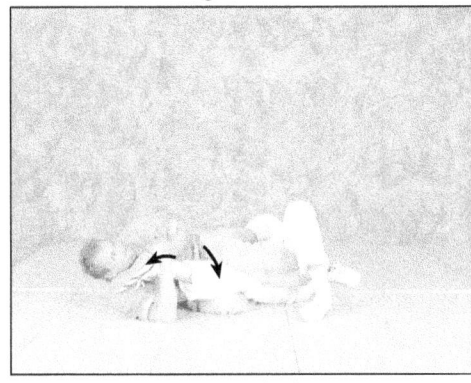

| Figure 8-12 | Figure 8-13 |

2. This does not negate White's roundhouse kick, which is taken at a closer than anticipated range, thereby minimizing the power of this kick, which is absorbed and captured by the butterfly block.

3. Grey uses a smooth circular movement to make his blocks while utilizing simple but evasive footwork to do so.

4. The immediate counterpunch to White's groin distracts White sufficiently to allow him to set up for the straight leg bar.

5. Grey can use his left leg to keep White close for the leg bar should he try to scoot away from the technique.

Chin Na In Ground Fighting

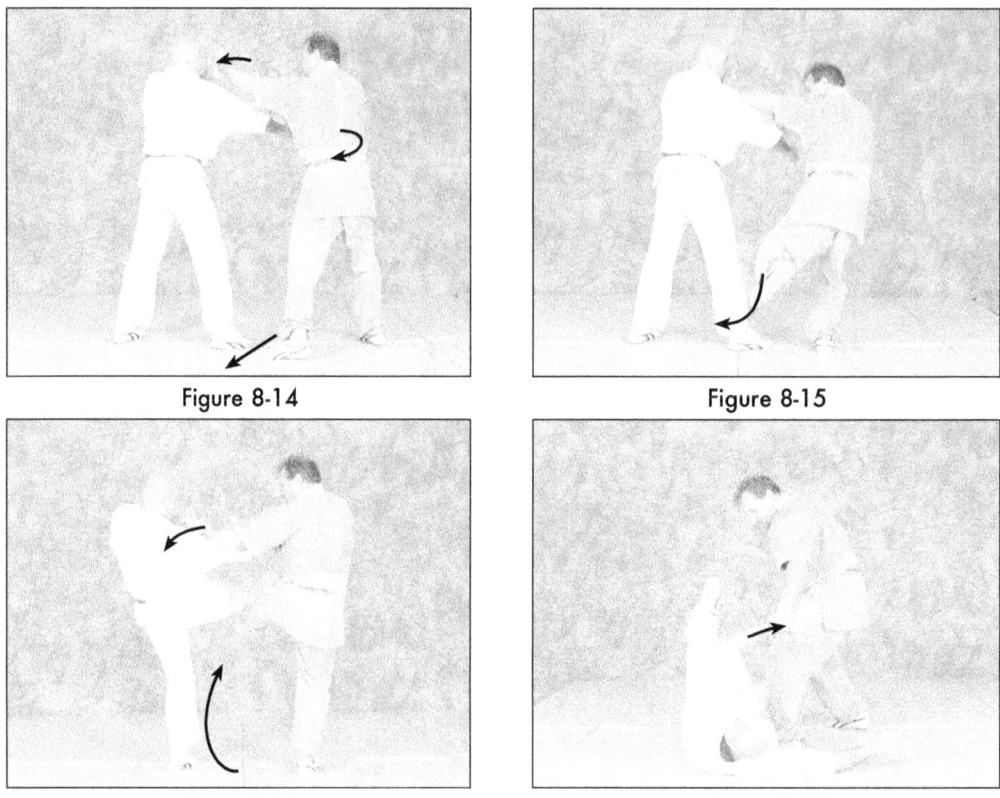

Figure 8-14

Figure 8-15

Figure 8-16

Figure 8-17

Fighting Sequence #3

White throws a straight right hand at Grey's upper body. Grey has responded by sidestepping to his own left, turning his body and blocking the punch with his right hand as he simultaneously attacks with a left back fist strike (Figure 8-14). Grey maintains his control over White's captured right hand as he executes a left low kick to the back of White's right lower leg (Figure 8-15). White has captured Grey's left wrist but Grey uses this contact to push White backward as he sweeps White's right leg from under him and pulls on his right arm to further unbalance him (Figure 8-16). Grey snakes his right hand around White's left wrist as he hits the floor (Figure 8-17). He then pulls White towards himself and rolls him onto his stomach, taking care to put him into a wristlock (Figure 8-18). Grey lowers himself onto his right knee as he transitions for his hold down technique (Figure 8-19). Grey sits through into an armpit hold, maintaining his wristlock on White's left wrist and executes a right elbow strike to the back of White's head (Figure 8-20).

Key Points

1. You can use the contact your opponent has on you to your benefit. White's grab on Grey's left arm is used to help take White down.

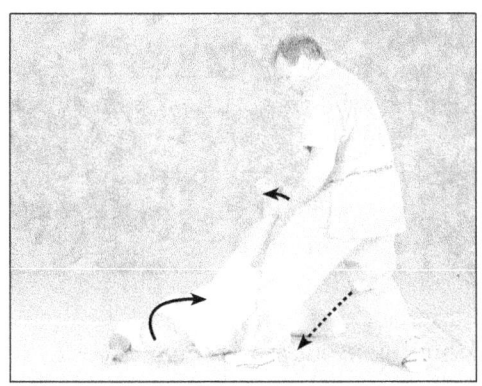

Figure 8-18

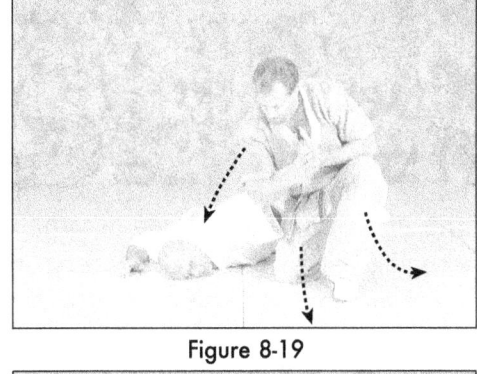

Figure 8-19

2. Grey sweeps away one leg and pushes/pulls him in this direction to unbalance him.

3. Try to maintain control over an appendage while taking your opponent down (or have an immediate follow up technique ready). In this case, Grey grabs White's left wrist in order to roll him over onto his stomach in order to minimize his attacking potential on the ground.

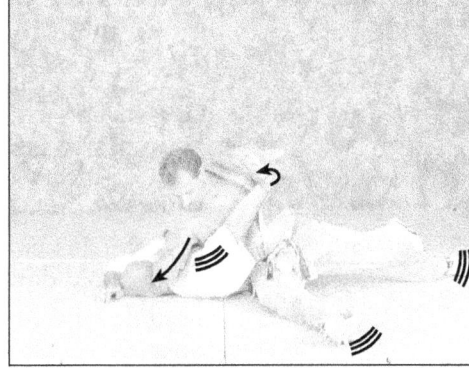

Figure 8-20

4. Grey exerts continuous wristlock control over White's left wrist as he moves into the armpit hold, and even during its application.

Fighting Sequence #4

White attacks Grey with a middle area front kick and Grey responds by cross-stepping to his own right with his left advanced leg as he does a left sweeping block to close him up (Figure 8-21). White follows up with a right straight advanced punch to Grey's head but Grey does a left upper block as he continues to swing counterclockwise around White (Figure 8-22). Grey wraps White's right arm under his left armpit as he continues his counterclockwise body turn as he shoots his right arm down onto the outside of White's right knee in order to keep this leg from stepping (Figure 8-23). Grey utilizes this counterclockwise body rotation to shoulder White over onto his back as he sweeps White's knee upwards and backwards to further unbalance him (Figure 8-24). Grey follows up with a kneeling right knife-hand strike to White's throat while still maintaining control over White's right arm (Figure 8-25). Grey then sits through into a scarf hold (Figure 8-26).

Key Points

1. Grey uses the unbalancing action of reaching for White's knee (pulling White's upper body down) and the counterclockwise movement of his own body to effect his blocks and to add momentum to the takedown (shouldering White counterclockwise onto his back).
2. Notice that Grey maintains control over White's right arm throughout the takedown and the hold down.
3. Grey buries his head downward to prevent his face from being gouged by White's free left hand.
4. Grey maintains a wide and stable leg positioning during the hold down.

Chapter 8: Fighting Sequences

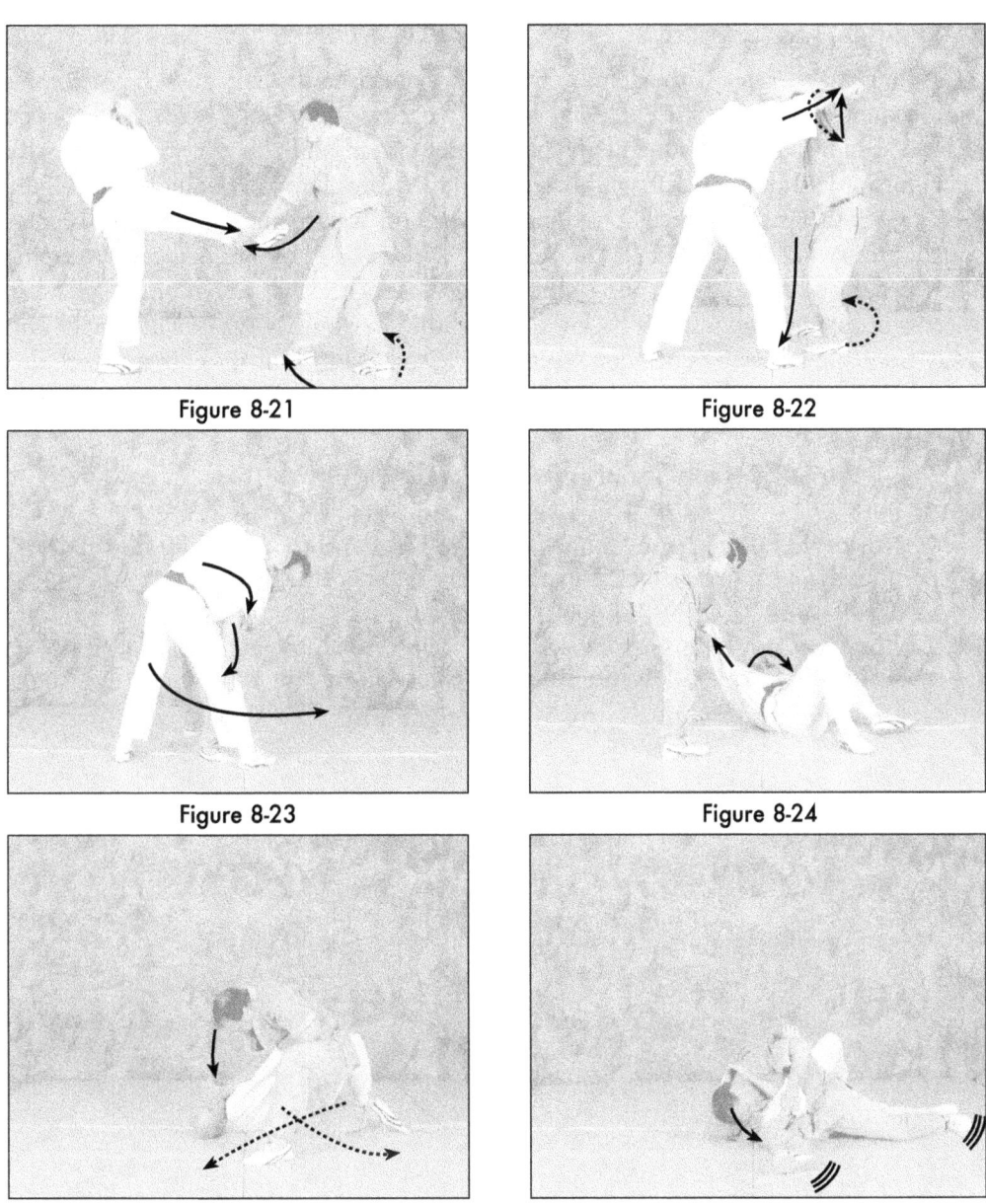

Figure 8-21

Figure 8-22

Figure 8-23

Figure 8-24

Figure 8-25

Figure 8-26

Fighting Sequence #5

White attacks Grey with a left reverse straight punch to the chin and Grey responds with a right inward pressing block as he leans backwards (Figure 8-27). White then delivers a right advanced straight punch to Grey's head and this time Grey shifts his body forwards and to his left while executing a left pressing cross-body block (Figure 8-28). Grey then swings his right leg up and in behind White's right leg while setting for a right-arm swing (Figure 8-29). Grey scissors White's body by simultaneously reaping backward on White's right leg and clotheslining White's neck with a right forearm strike, thereby dropping him onto his back (Figure 8-30). Grey pushes White's held right arm away from himself as he encircles White's neck and places him into an arm-included head lock (*kata gatame*) (Figure 8-31).

Key Points

1. Grey uses the mobility of his upper body to assist in blocking White's punching combinations.
2. Notice that Grey removes one of White's legs and forces White into that quarter. The scissoring effect that Grey's upper and lower body has on White easily takes him down.
3. Grey does not relinquish his left-hand grip on White's right arm until he secures this arm and White's neck in *kata gatame*.
4. Grey uses his head to control White's right arm.

Chapter 8: Fighting Sequences

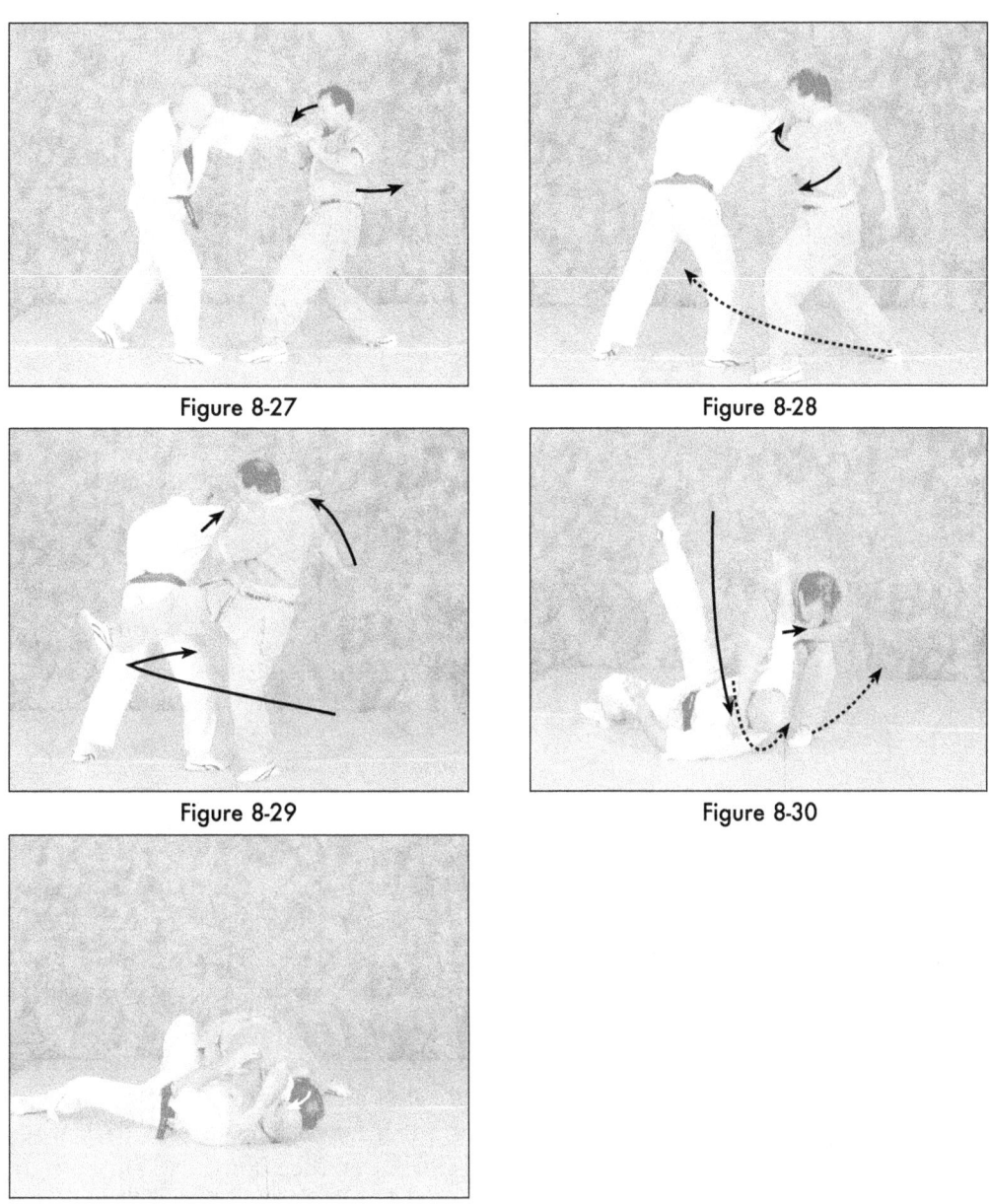

Figure 8-27

Figure 8-28

Figure 8-29

Figure 8-30

Figure 8-31

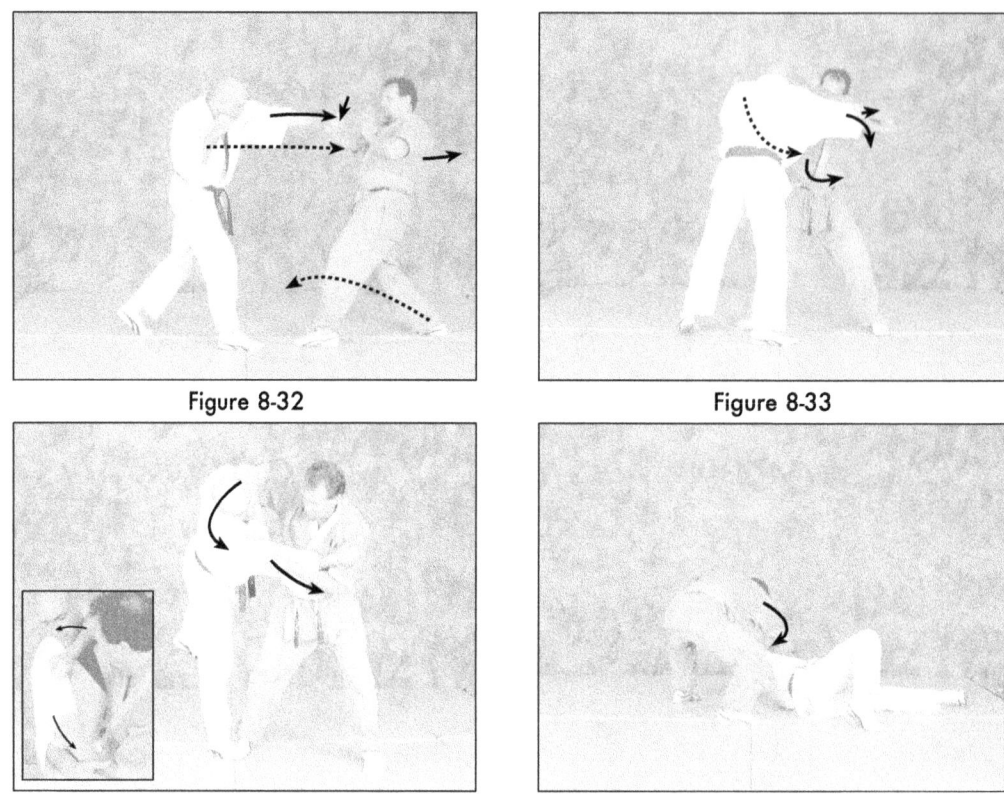

Figure 8-32

Figure 8-33

Figure 8-34

Figure 8-35

Fighting Sequence #6

White attacks Grey with a left reverse straight punch to his chin and Grey defends by shifting backwards and doing a right pressing block (Figure 8-32). White follows up with a right advanced straight punch and Grey defends with a left hooking block which allows him to grab onto White's right sleeve as he applies a right forearm strike to White's throat (Figure 8-33). Grey pulls White's right arm counterclockwise and downwards as he presses his right forearm into White's throat (anchoring his own right hand on White's right shoulder) also in a counterclockwise direction (Figure 8-34), thereby twisting him off balance and onto his back while maintaining hold of his right arm (Figure 8-35). Grey then controls White's right arm in a wristlock (Figure 8-36). Grey steps around White's head and pulls him over into a prone position while maintaining the wristlock (Figure 8-37).

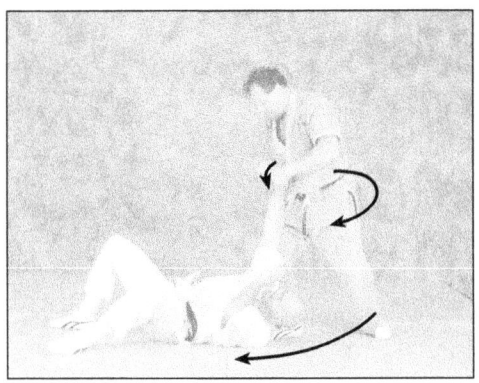

Figure 8-36

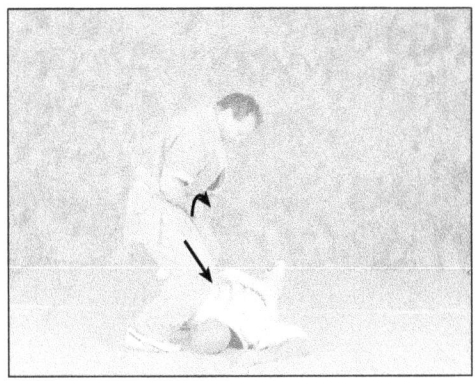

Figure 8-37

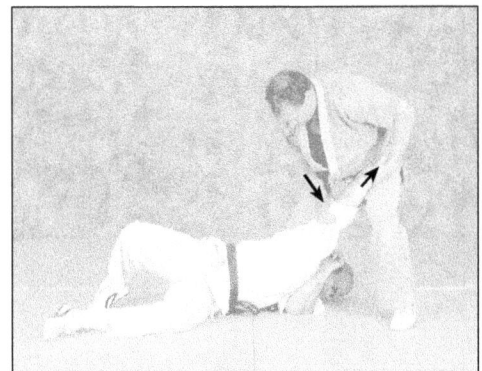

Figure 8-38

Key Points

1. Upper body movement and simple footwork are essential for evading punching attacks.
2. The forearm throat press is an excellent means to take a person to the ground from a grappling situation. Where the head goes, the body must follow.
3. Grey torques his whole body against White's throat (with assistance from the arm pull) to effect the takedown.
4. As Grey steps around White's head, do not change hand positions. Keep White's fingers pointed at his own head as you step to roll him over.
5. It is not as effective to grab White's arm and push him over into the prone position (Figure 8-38). Maintaining a wristlock while pulling him over onto his stomach makes it a useful pain compliance technique should White decide not to cooperate with the rolling over process. Any pushing can be done with the knees without sacrificing the wristlock control.

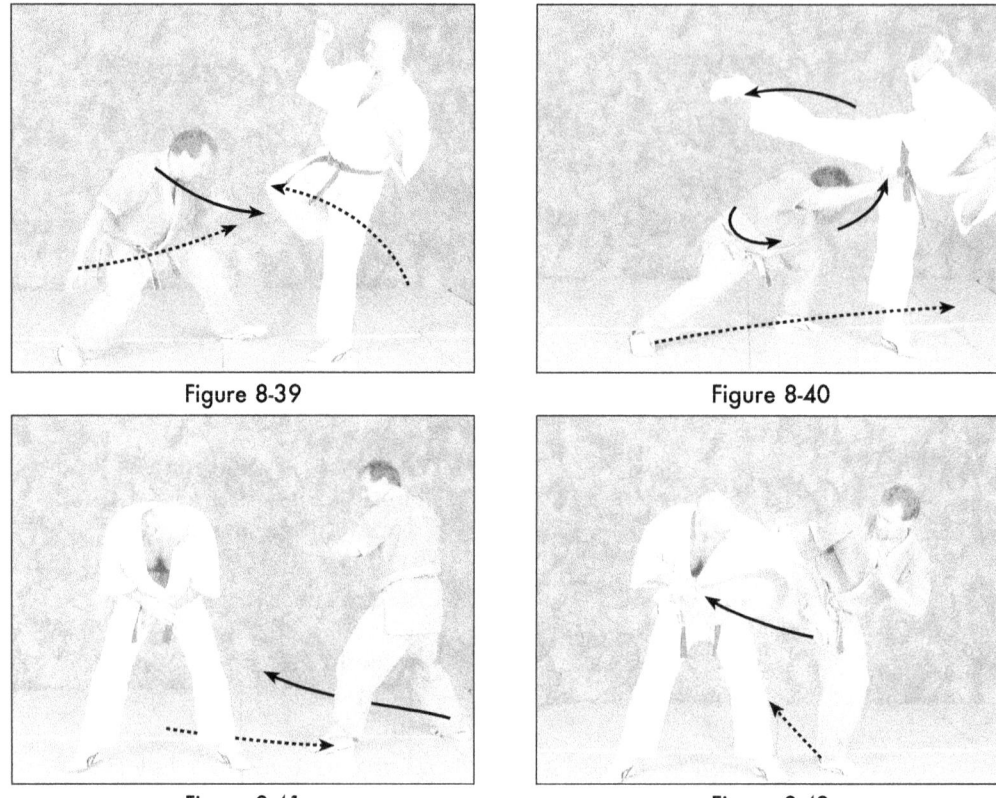

Figure 8-39
Figure 8-40
Figure 8-41
Figure 8-42

Fighting Sequence #7

White attacks Grey with a high right roundhouse kick that Grey decides to duck under (Figure 8-39). As he does so, Grey strikes White in the groin with a right palm heel strike (Figure 8-40). Grey takes two small steps as he ducks under the kick and turns to face White who is distracted by the groin strike (Figure 8-41). Grey then swings the back of his right leg into White's midsection as he grabs onto his left arm (Figure 8-42). White grabs Grey's leg but to no avail as Grey swings up his left leg behind White's knees as he begins to pull White down and backward in preparation for the flying scissors takedown (Figure 8-43). Grey scissors his legs together as he turns his hips backward to topple White onto his back (Figure 8-44). Grey then swings his right leg around White's left leg and scissors it while he applies a sideward ankle lock (Figure 8-45).

Key Points

1. Grey keeps his hands up to protect his face as he ducks under.
2. It is important for Grey to totally commit himself into the scissors takedown in order to get his legs fully around White's body.

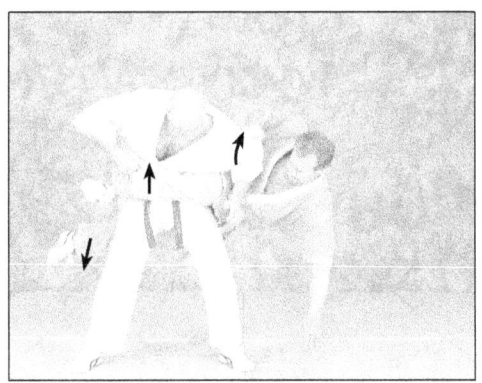

Figure 8-43

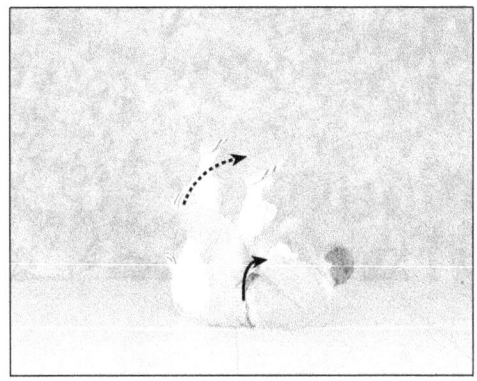

Figure 8-44

3. Care should be taken in training by not fully torquing the hips backward and scissoring powerfully in order to prevent injury to your training partner. (This technique is banned in judo.) Grey can also pull up on White's jacket in order to help keep White's head from contacting the ground.

Figure 8-45

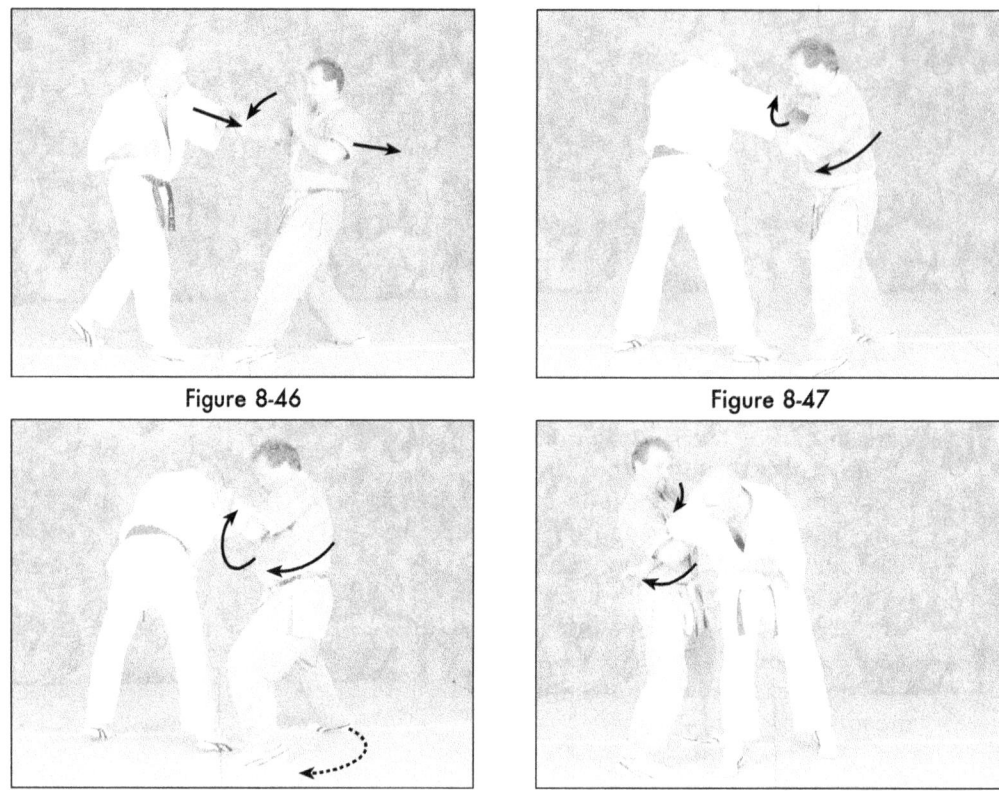

Figure 8-46

Figure 8-47

Figure 8-48

Figure 8-49

Fighting Sequence #8

White attacks Grey's chest with a left reverse straight punch that Grey parries with a right pressing block as he shifts backwards (Figure 8-46). White throws a second straight chest punch that Grey slips while doing a left pressing block as he re-shifts his weight forward and to his left (Figure 8-47). Grey hooks his right arm under White's right arm as he turns and steps clockwise, pulling White with him (Figure 8-48). Figure 8-49 shows the reverse perspective of the arm trap. Grey then quickly reverses his direction and clotheslines White with his right inner arm while White's momentum is still moving him forward (Figure 8-50). White topples onto his back and Grey follows him down to the ground (Figure 8-51). Grey grabs White's right arm and quickly moves his left leg over his head, kicking him in the throat if required (Figure 8-52). Grey then places White's right arm in a shoulder crank (Figure 8-53).

Key Points

1. Grey uses his body weight to swing White around then quickly reverses direction to topple him.
2. When clotheslining White, Grey pushes on White's lower back (in the opposite direction) to further unbalance him.

Chapter 8: Fighting Sequences

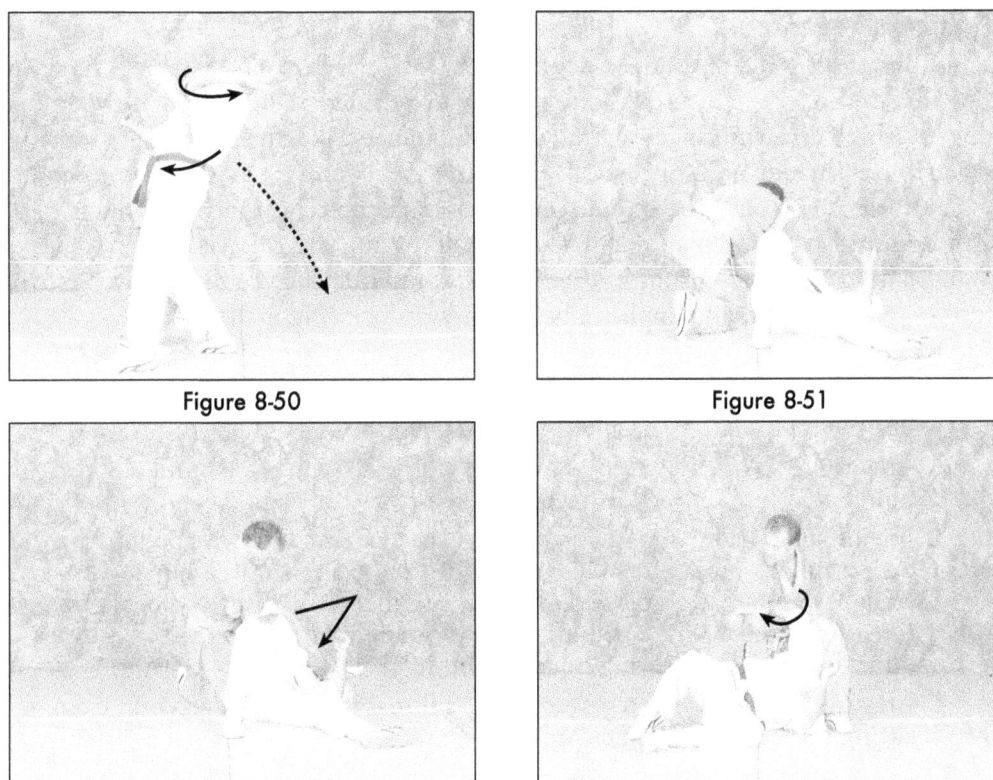

Figure 8-50

Figure 8-51

Figure 8-52

Figure 8-53

3. When on the ground applying the shoulder crank, Grey is free to look around and disengage quickly if other trouble erupts.
4. This shoulder crank is relatively effortless to apply. It is applicable against an opponent who is stronger than you, works well for a shoulder break, or if you just need to hold the position for a long time.

Fighting Sequence #9

White throws a left advanced hook punch at Grey's head and he ducks under it (Figure 8-54). Grey steps into White's follow up left reverse hook punch, wrapping this punching arm with his left arm as he simultaneously applies an inside forearm strike to the left side of White's neck (Figure 8-55). White is spun or thrown counterclockwise down onto the ground and Grey maintains control over White's right arm (Figure 8-56). Grey applies a wristlock to White's right wrist and heel kicks White's head as he sets up for his hold down technique (Figure 8-57). Grey moves to the seated position and applies a bent arm wristlock (Figure 8-58).

Key Points

1. Grey uses his body mobility first to duck under then to close up White's punches. This latter jamming action sets up the subsequent throw.
2. Grey tosses White down in a modified hip toss using the painful clotheslining of White's neck to effect the takedown.
3. The use of a distraction kick to White's head assists Grey in applying his bent arm lock on White. This technique can be applied if White resists a straight arm bar attempt by curling his captured arm. Grey can break the integrity of the wrist by striking the bottom of White's wrist with his fore knuckles, thereby allowing him to bend it.
4. Grey must place his left leg over White's throat in order to keep him from sitting up and out of the technique.

Chapter 8: Fighting Sequences

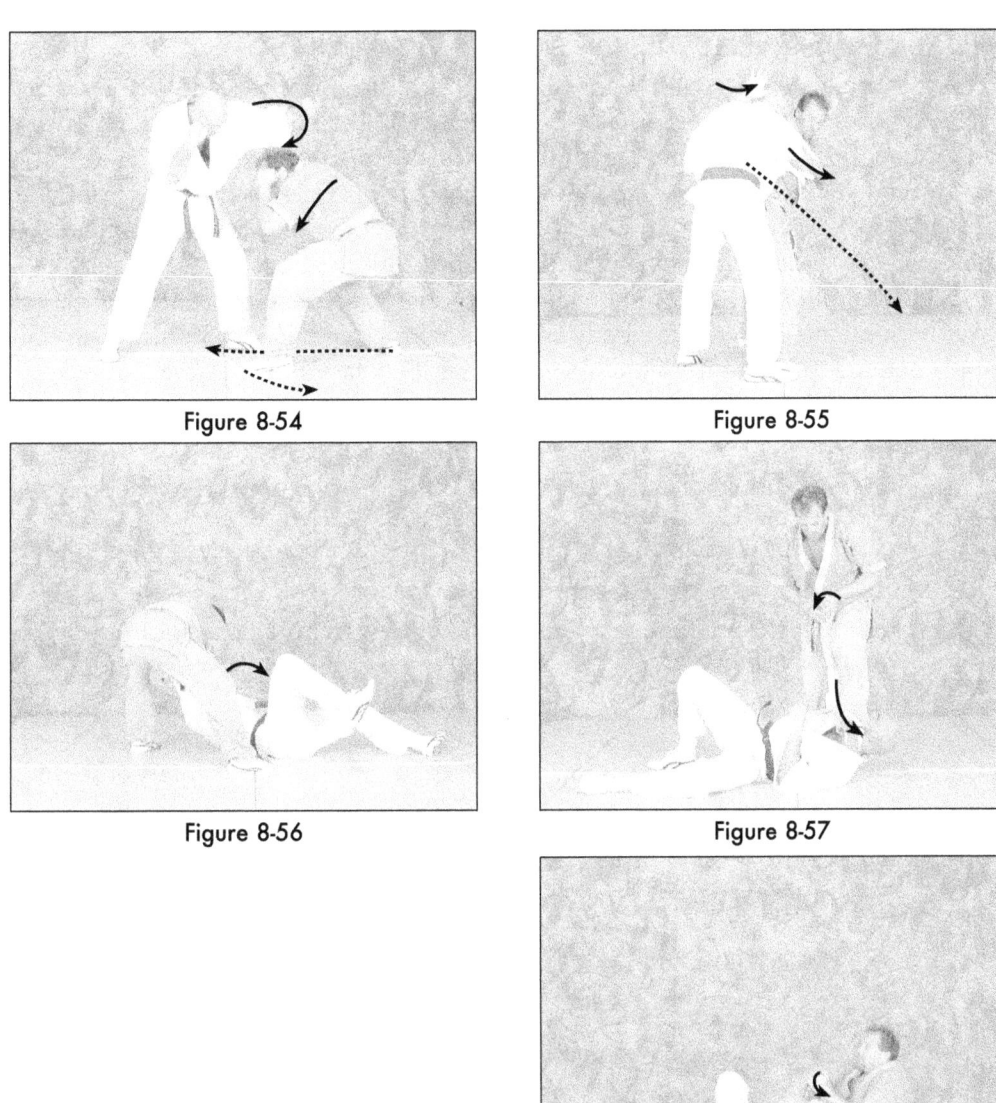

Figure 8-54

Figure 8-55

Figure 8-56

Figure 8-57

Figure 8-58

Fighting Sequence #10

Grey attacks White with a left advanced backfist strike feint to his head that White parries with a left rising block (Figure 8-59). Grey then quickly ducks down and shoots for White's upper legs with both arms (Figure 8-60). Grey takes White down onto his back by pushing White backwards with his head and left shoulder and simultaneously lifting upwards on his legs (Figure 8-61). Grey maintains his hold on White's legs and he applies his forearms into the backs of White's calves as he begins to roll White over onto his stomach (Figure 8-62). Grey continues the roll over by stepping over White's body with his right leg (Figure 8-63). Grey can now apply extreme pressure to White's spinal column as he completes the Boston crab hold on him (Figure 8-64).

Key Points

1. Grey's initial feint gets at least one of White's arms up prior to shooting for White's legs.
2. Grey applies the radial edges of his forearms into White's calves (U.B. 56, U.B. 57) in order to help control White for the turn over.
3. Extreme care should be taken in practicing this technique, as it can easily damage the spine.

Chapter 8: Fighting Sequences

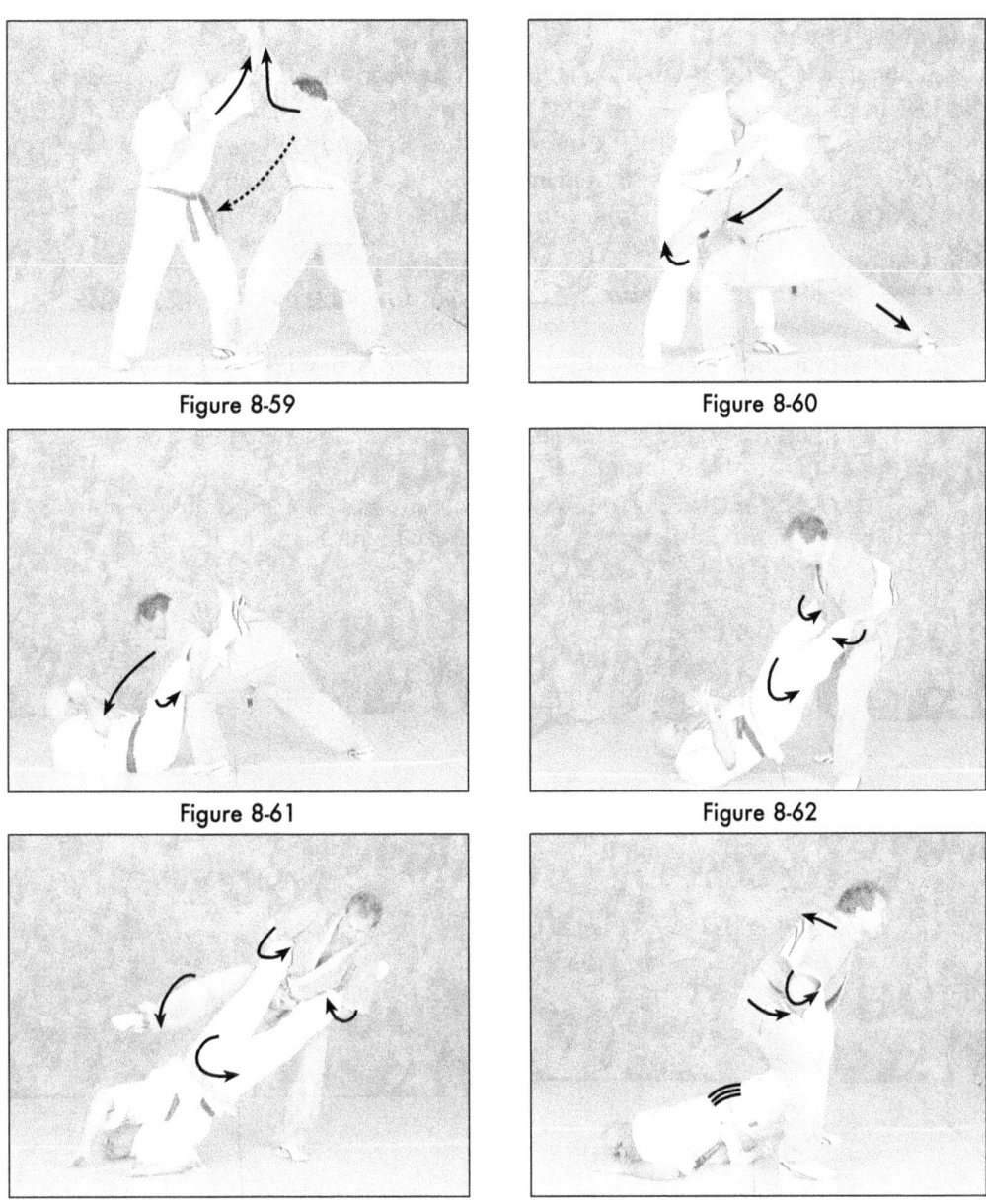

Figure 8-59

Figure 8-60

Figure 8-61

Figure 8-62

Figure 8-63

Figure 8-64

Fighting Sequence #11

Grey attacks White with a right reverse punch to his head that White ducks as he goes to grab Grey's left lower leg (Figure 8-65). White grabs Grey's right punching arm as he scoops Grey's left heel with his right hand (Figure 8-66). White then pulls Grey's left leg upwards in preparation for placing it into an ankle lock (Figure 8-67). White sits down and applies an ankle lock to Grey's left ankle (Figure 8-68).

Key Points

1. White is able to bring down Grey by both picking one of Grey's legs up and pushing him backwards with his other arm.
2. Care must be taken to ensure that Grey does not kick White after the takedown.
3. White controls Grey's other leg after the takedown by pressing on his right thigh with his left foot.
4. Grey arches his back off the floor in an attempt to escape the pressure a little but White can counter this somewhat with his right leg.

Chapter 8: Fighting Sequences

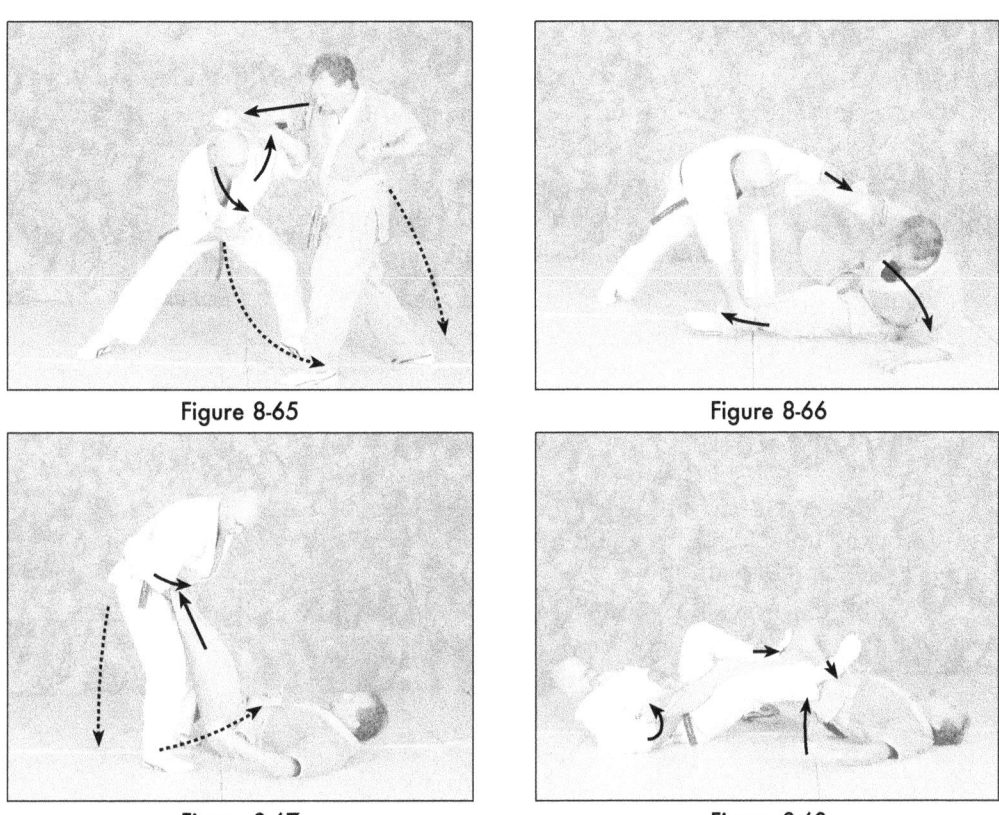

Figure 8-65

Figure 8-66

Figure 8-67

Figure 8-68

Fighting Sequence #12

Grey attacks White with a front kick to his stomach but White sidesteps it to the outside, scooping the ankle as he does so (Figure 8-69). White then pushes on the right side of Grey's body as he turns Grey's captured leg inward to take him down (Figure 8-70). White then leans forward onto Grey's back, trapping Grey's bent right leg as he does so with his own right upper thigh (Figure 8-71). White then pries Grey's chin up with a painful neck crank (Figure 8-72).

Key Points

1. Sidestepping linear techniques in particular replaces the need to block. Here White uses his right arm to scoop Grey's kick at the end of its technique when it is least powerful.
2. By turning the leg, White facilitates Grey's turn over onto his stomach using a left arm push.
3. White traps Grey's left leg with his own, thereby keeping his hands free for the neck attack. White can hyper-flex Grey's knee effortlessly merely by leaning forward more.
4. White digs his elbows into Grey's shoulders while establishing his fulcrums as he levers Grey's neck backward.

Chapter 8: Fighting Sequences

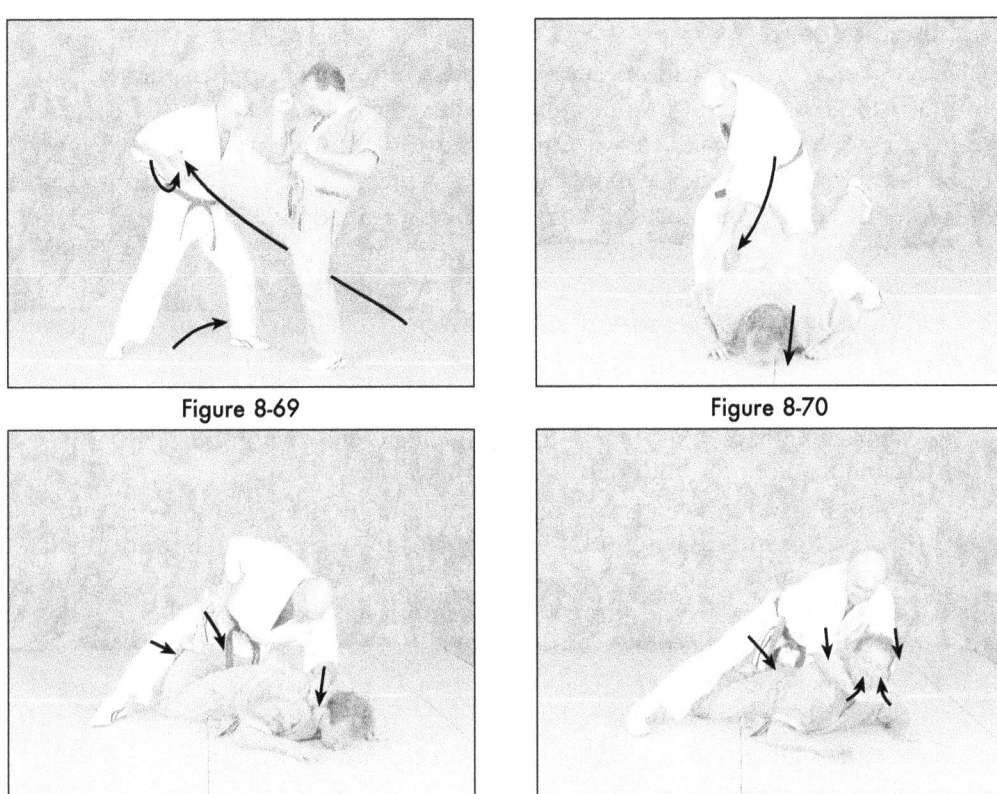

Figure 8-69

Figure 8-70

Figure 8-71

Figure 8-72

Chin Na In Ground Fighting

Fighting Sequence #13

Grey attacks White with an upper area advanced straight punch that he parries with a rising block while simultaneously hitting the solar plexus with a palm heel strike (Figure 8-73). White steps counterclockwise backward with his left leg while he hooks his right arm under Grey's right arm in preparation for a hip throw (Figure 8-74). White pulls Grey forward and down across his right hip/upper leg (Figure 8-75). Grey falls onto his back while White maintains his grip on Grey's right arm (Figure 8-76). White steps over Grey's head and controls Grey's right wrist (Figure 8-77). White then sits down to apply the transverse straight arm bar on Grey (Figure 8-78).

Key Points

1. White simultaneously blocks and punches Grey to minimize the time frame required for both defense and attack.
2. White places himself in a vulnerable position by turning into Grey with his back to him, relying on the paralyzing solar plexus strike to distract Grey.
3. White must step in and throw in one smooth motion in order for it to be effective and to add power to the throw.
4. Continual control over Grey's right arm is essential for a quick post-takedown technique to be applied.
5. Use the squeezing effect of the knees to help control the arm.

Chapter 8: Fighting Sequences

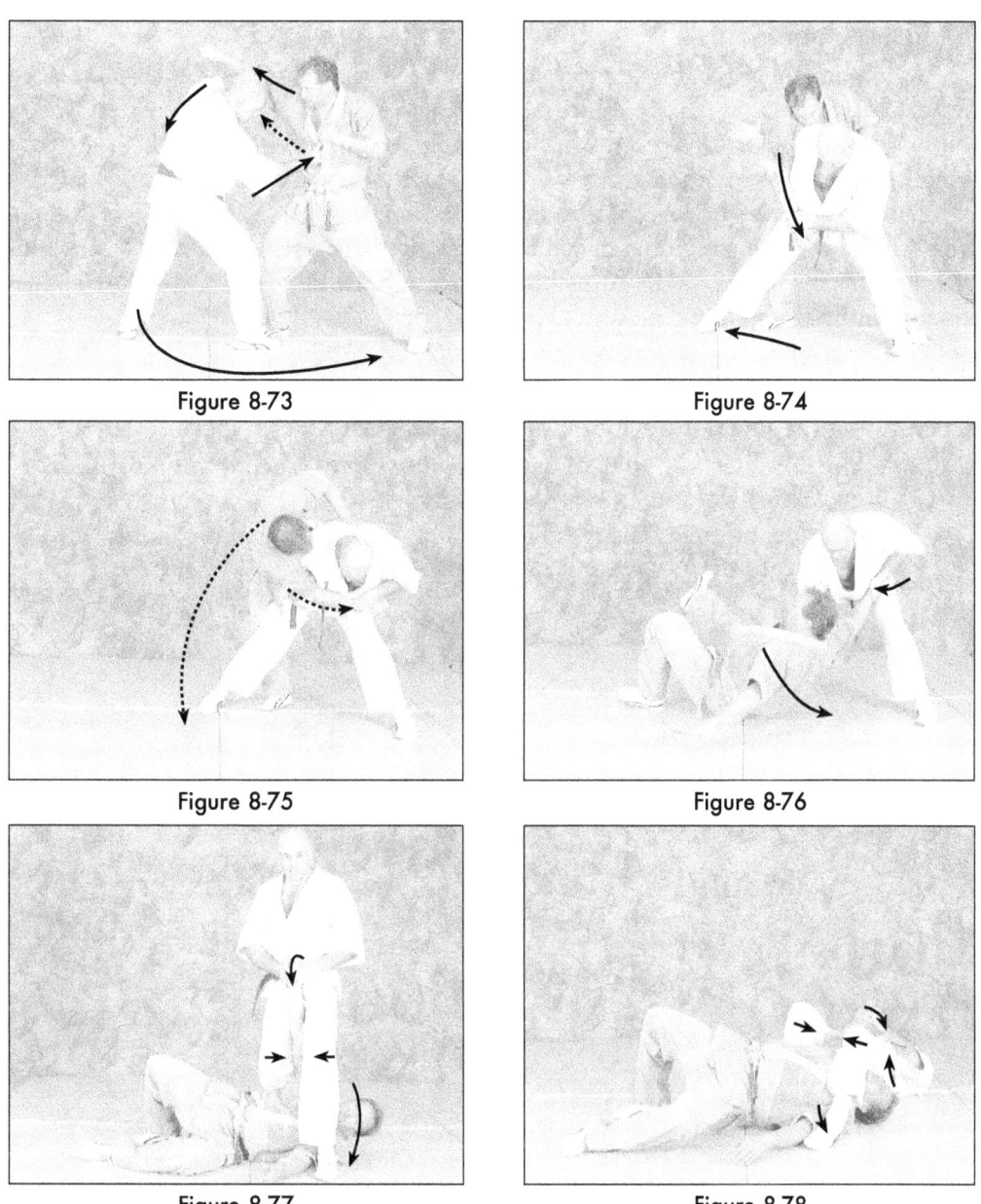

Figure 8-73

Figure 8-74

Figure 8-75

Figure 8-76

Figure 8-77

Figure 8-78

Fighting Sequence #14

White executes a right side kick to Grey's left ribs as Grey tries to land a left advanced straight punch to White's head (Figure 8-79). White then steps down close to Grey, grabs Grey's left arm, and encircles Grey's neck with his right arm (Figure 8-80). White then reaps backwards with his right leg on Grey's left leg while torquing their bodies counterclockwise (Figure 8-81). White follows Grey to the ground while maintaining a grip on Grey' left hand (Figure 8-82). White pulls Grey's left arm straight as he turns his body into him (Figure 8-83). White applies an armpit hold on Grey's left arm (Figure 8-84).

Key Points

1. White evades Grey's punch by leaning backwards and simultaneously using the superior reach of his leg to attack Grey with a kick.
2. White tosses Grey to the ground by reaping Grey's leg and torquing Grey using Grey's left arm and neck as handles.
3. White does not relinquish his hold on Grey's arm to allow for an immediate follow-up technique to be applied.

Chapter 8: Fighting Sequences

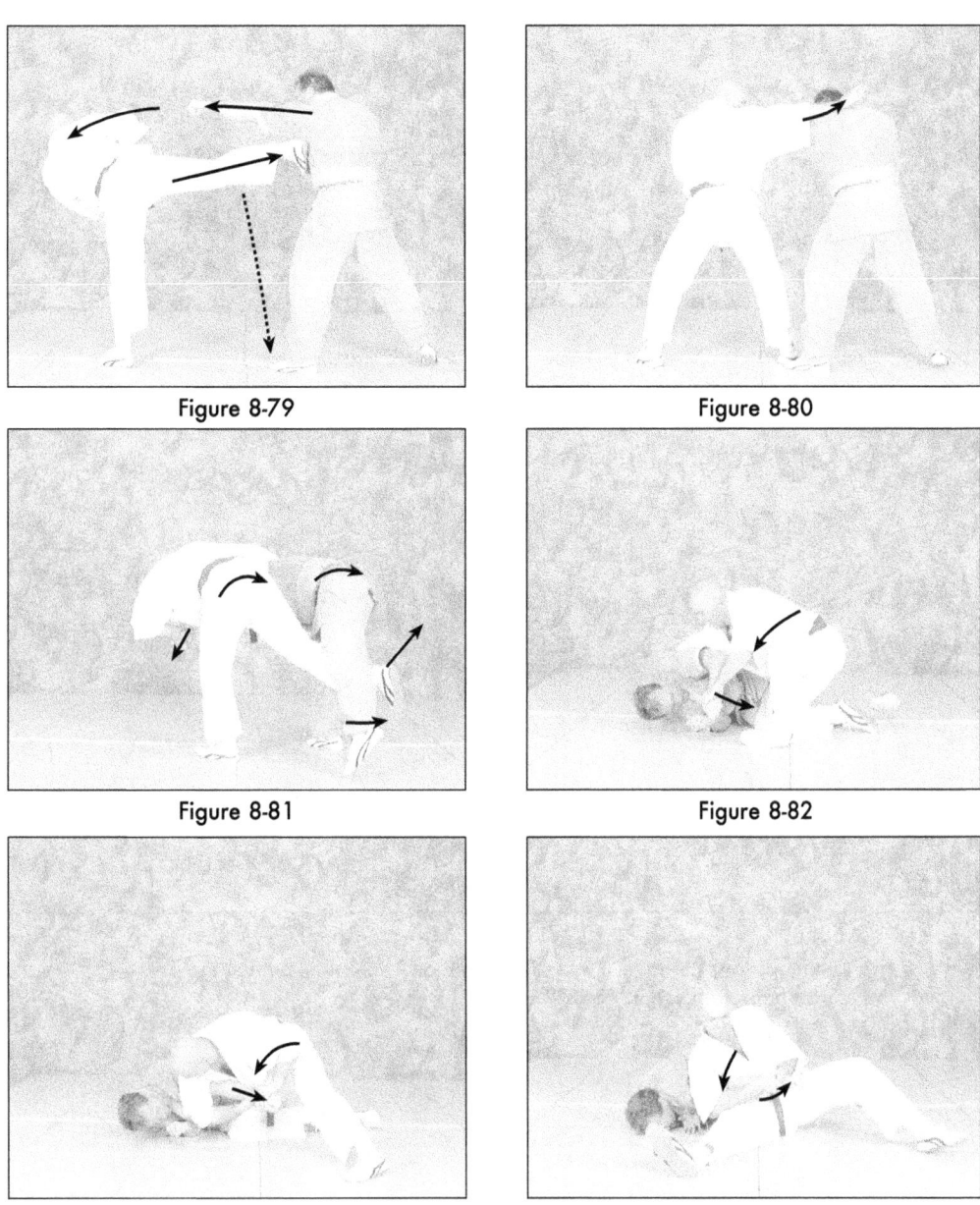

Figure 8-79

Figure 8-80

Figure 8-81

Figure 8-82

Figure 8-83

Figure 8-84

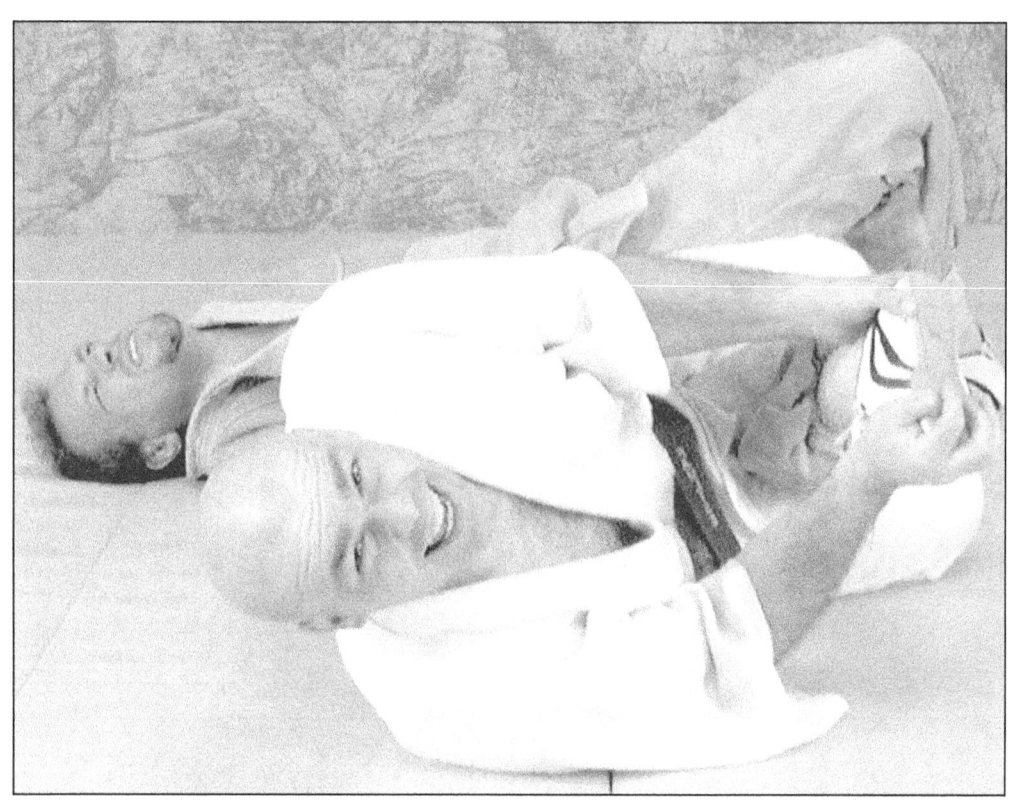

Joe-
Doing this book with you was no mean feat. Thanks for putting the pressure on me to finish it. I say "Uncle!"

-Al

Epilogue

> *All branches of Japanese martial arts have not for their prime object the killing of men; their ultimate purpose is to chastise wicked men. Military virtue is really identical with humanity, and martial arts aim at the attainment of this object.*
>
> E.J. Harrison. The Fighting Spirit of Japan, 1955, p. 113.

It should be evident from reading this book that cross-training in the martial arts is a bonus to fighters. The well-rounded fighter has a better chance of survival in the no-holds barred arena of the street, particularly when he learns techniques beyond the rules of sport. The street is no place to learn of limitations that classical disciplines may offer. There are many ways for the martial artist to augment his street survival skills. By understanding the underlying biomechanical principles of the various martial arts techniques, one can adapt and move forward to creatively fight unfettered by restrictions of sport. Improvisation will be the rule to handle the notorious unpredictability of street confrontations. Having an intimate knowledge of Qin Na (Chin Na) technique can greatly augment one's ability to fight on the ground, whether one wants to be there or not. Acquiring consummate control over one's body's tools and having the knowledge to apply them in an effective and judicious manner on the vulnerable parts of one's opponent, be they located on the arm, legs, neck/head or torso, is an ideal that all pugilists should aspire to.

Knowing the relationship between Qin Na and ground fighting and dynamically applying it, is but a single means to strengthen your fighting skills. Understanding the sometimes subtle and overlapping nature of these disciplines can open one's mind to greater self-defense treasures, as one explores the multi-facetted jewel of martial arts.

APPENDIX A

Glossary of Martial Arts Terms

The meanings for the terms listed here refer to their usage in this book, notwithstanding that many other meanings may exist for them. Italics indicate that the term is also defined in this glossary or the medical glossary.

Ackrocheirismos: is an ancient Greek finger-breaking *technique* that was used to gain *submission* over an *opponent*. It was ultimately banned from *Olympic wrestling contests*.

Acupuncture points: are *points* used in *Traditional Chinese Medicine* to treat physical ailments though the application of needles in order to correct *qi* (energy) imbalances and blockages. There are 361 regular *acupuncture points* (670 in total counting the 309 *bilateral points* with the 52 *midline* ones) that lie on the 14 main *meridians*. There are an additional 20-1500 *extra points*, many of which do not lie on the main *meridians*, although only 30 to 60 of these are in common usage.

Acupressure points: are *acupuncture points* that can be stimulated with fingertip pressure, as with *pressure points*. These *points* are useful for *chin na* purposes.

'Adrenaline dump': is the excretion of *adrenaline* from the *endocrine glands* into the bloodstream via the *flight or fight response*. This survival mechanism supercharges the human *physiology*, making the person under threat very strong, impervious to pain and often narrowly focused to deal with the perceived threat.

Advanced techniques: 1) are *techniques* reserved for more senior and skilled students because of their complexity, difficulty in execution or potential for *injury* to the recipient and possibly to the deliverer of the *technique*; 2) are *techniques* using the leading (most *advanced*) *appendage*. For example, an *advanced straight punch* is a *punch* delivered on the same side as the most forward leg (the leg closest to the *opponent*).

Agility: is the ability to move in a quick and nimble fashion while maintaining good *balance* and *posture*.

Ai: means 'love' or 'harmony' in the sense that all living things in the universe are interconnected by a harmonizing vital *force*.

Aikido: is a more esoteric *martial art* founded by Morihei Ueshiba (1881-1969) in 1942 which uses circular *controlling* and *throwing techniques* to *neutralize* an *opponent*. As the name implies (*ai*:means harmony; *ki* means vital breath; and *do* means the way of), *aikido* stresses the harmony that must be achieved between the breath and the body, mind and moral outlook, in order to attain perfection of *technique* and hence, character.

Aiki jutsu: is the forerunner to *aikido*, which incorporated *bone-breaking techniques* useful in *combat* by *samurai* in 11th- and 12th-century Japan. See *aikido*.

Anchoring: 1) is the act of gripping clothing or a holding a body part to fix a limb firmly in place. This makes overpowering of a limb and subsequent manipulation of it by an *opponent* more difficult; 2) is the placement of fingertips into bodily recesses in order to facilitate a *gripping* or *hooking* action (i.e., the simultaneous placement of the thumb under the jaw and second finger into the eye socket as in *C-clamping*).

Ankle lock: is a painful *joint lock manipulation* of the ankle joint in order to gain control over an *opponent* through *submission*.

Arm bar: is a *joint manipulation technique* in which force is applied to the *opponent's* straightened arm at the elbow in order to achieve a painful *over-extension* of the elbow joint. This is an example of a *first class lever* in action. See *juji gatame*.

Arm hug: is an *arm locking technique* which has the *fighter* push, *hold* or *wrap* the *opponent's* straightened arm at or near the *point* of the elbow in order to *over-extend* it. See *ude gatame*.

Arm locks: is the class of *joint manipulation techniques* that deals with *locking* either the straight or bent arm.

Arm scissors block: is a *block* using both arms pressed together (elbow to elbow) in a *scissoring* action in order to create a *wrapping* type of block. The arm closest to the *opponent* is held low and the other arm is held high like wide-open scissors. See *butterfly block*.

Arm tools: are parts of the arms (fingers, hands, lower and upper arms, elbows) which can be used for *offensive* and *defensive* purposes.

Arm wrap: is the use of the forearms to *wrap* or *control* the movement of an *opponent's* arm, often while applying pressure to the elbow joint. See *ude gatame* and *arm hug*.

Arm-included head lock: is a *head lock* that also captures the near arm of the *opponent*. See *kata gatame*.

Armpit hold: is a *hold* using the armpit to *control* and apply pressure to the back of the upper arm and shoulder. See *waki gatame*.

Assault: is the application of real or perceived *force*, by an act or gesture, against a person directly or indirectly without his consent with the intention of threatening or *injuring* him.

Assaultive behavior: refers to physically aggressive body movement that constitutes an *assault*. This usually has the connotation of physical contact but an assault may include an act *or* gesture.

Attacks: 1) are the actual *blows* that are struck by a *fighter;* 2) is the collective aggressive behaviors exhibited towards a person.

Atemi waza: means 'body *striking techniques*' or '*techniques* for *attacking vital points*'. The ancient knowledge of the body and its *acupuncture points* allowed the hitting *techniques* of *martial arts*, using the hard parts of the body, to be strategically applied to the weak (*vital*) points of the *opponent's* body. Pain-induced *paralysis*, bodily *trauma*, *unconsciousness* and even *death* can result depending on the *vital point* targeted and the amount of *force* used against it.

Augmenting: is the act of using the second and otherwise uninvolved hand to support and strengthen a *technique* being used by the involved arm.

Awareness: is the state of alertness for potential dangers of *attack* that is of paramount importance in trouble avoidance and *self-defense*.

Axe kick: is a *heel kick* directed in a downward direction like an axe chopping firewood.

Axis point: is the *pivot point* or *fulcrum* of a *lever*. In the *martial arts*, it is the point over which you bend a limb in order to *strain* or break it, or over which the *center of gravity* passes in a *throw*.

Back fist strike: is the *hitting* application, using the top of the closed fist, in a circular (*striking*) fashion.

Back hand slap: is the hitting application, using the top of the open rigid hand, in a circular (*striking*) fashion.

Backward breakfall: is a *technique* used for breaking a fall onto one's back that includes *slapping* the *mat* just prior to impact with it, rolling out of the fall and distributing the body weight over the largest area possible. It is known as *ushiro ukemi* in *judo* and *aikido*.

Balance: is the ability to maintain the *center of gravity* over a *base of support*. A larger *base of support* and lower the *center of gravity* of a body will increase its *stability* (*balance*).

Balance displacement: is the movement of the *center of gravity* off of the *base of support*, thereby *unbalancing* the body.

Bagua: an *internal* method of Chinese 'eight hexagram' *boxing* practiced on an imaginary circle (roughly 2.5 meters in diameter).

Base of support: is the area delineated between the *points* of contact of the body with the ground. A wider base of support translates to greater *stability* but decreased *mobility*.

Bear hug: is the encirclement and clasping of arms around an *opponent's* torso from any angle, including his arms or not, so as to forcibly *hold* the *opponent*.

Bent arm lock: is a commonly used class of *restraining holds* that involves the bending of an *opponent's* arm in order to *lock* it at the elbow. See *hammerlock*.

Bent arm wrist lock: is a *wrist lock* that is applied while the arm is bent, like that of a *swan lock*.

Bent wrist lock: is a *wrist lock* that is applied while the arm is straight.

Bi qi: refers to *sealing the breath* or *choking* a person. The resultant deprivation of oxygen to the brain causes *unconsciousness*, *brain* damage and ultimately *death*, depending upon the length of application time. This is one of five *physiological* classes of *chin na technique*. See *fen jin, cuo gu, dian mai* and *dian xue*.

Biomechanical principles: are those physical laws of mechanics relating to movement of the human body.

Biting: is the act of using the use of teeth, normally as a *weapon* of distraction. The human bite can result is serious physical injuries and infections and is considered to be a form of *dirty fighting*. Fingers, noses, ears and other parts of the human body have been subjected to *biting attacks* during *in-close fighting*, usually on the street (Mike Tyson's *ring* antics are the exception, certainly not the rule).

Black belt: is the highly coveted top belt rank in many of the Japanese and Korean *martial arts*, indicating a high level of achievement. Although many believe that a *black belt* is a designation of expert status, in reality, it is the true beginning *rank* of a serious student's *martial arts* training. There are up to ten levels of *black belt* in many *styles*.

Appendix A: Glossary of Martial Arts Terms

Blocking: 1) is the thwarting of an *attack* by deflecting, checking or otherwise *neutralizing* a *punch*, *strike*, *kick* or a *throw* from being applied; 2) is the placing of an appendage into an *opponent's* arm or leg joint prior to *hyper-flexion* in order to *injure* or disable that joint.

Blood sports: refer to ancient Greek *sports* that promoted the *injury* or *death* of its *contestants* for the entertainment of bloodthirsty crowds, such as *wrestling, boxing* and especially *pankration*. Modern equivalents are normally banned as being too brutal and uncivilized, unless *rules of sport* governed by a *referee* are adhered to and medical precautions are undertaken. This is the case in *boxing* where *matches*, though often bloody events, have *ring* deaths only as infrequent and unintentional outcomes (0.13 per 1,000 participants).

Blows: are any powerful applications of *force* made against an *opponent* (normally refer to *punches* and *strikes* or *weapons* held in the hands but could also include *kicks*).

Body bridging: is the act of arching the *supine* body upward and sideward using the shoulders/neck and the explosive power of the legs. This *technique* is often used in *wrestling* to remove the shoulders from the *mat* in order to thwart a *pinning* and as a more practical *defensive* move, to displace the *opponent* from his *superior position* on top of him. See *bucking*.

Body guards: are people trained to protect V.I.P.'s, dignitaries and other vulnerable people from personal armed or *unarmed attacks*.

Body mass: is the weight of a person's body. The location of the *center of gravity* for the upright body approximates that of the *tanden*, the energetic and spiritual center of the body.

Body mechanics: is the study of how the body moves using the principles of physics. See *biomechanical principles*.

Body movement: refers to the use of the body (or control over an *opponent's* body) in a deliberate *offensive* or *defensive* manner.

Body positioning: is the placement or *positioning* of the body relative to that of the *opponent*.

Body tools: refers to the use of parts of the arms, legs, torso and head/neck as tools in which to apply *force* offensively or *defensively* to an *opponent*.

Bone breaking techniques: are those *offensive* and *defensive martial arts* moves which snap *bones* (or less accurately, *dislocate joints*), often ending a *street fight*.

Bone misplacement techniques: are those *offensive* and *defensive* moves which *dislocate bones* from their *joints*. See *cuo gu*.

Boston crab: is a painful *wrestling finishing hold* in which a *fighter* picks up his opponent's legs while standing astride his *supine torso* (facing his feet) and *hyper-extends* the *spine*.

Bottom position: is the person who is lying directly on the *mat* (usually face up). See *inferior position*.

Bout: is a *pugilistic match* that could have any number of rounds (3-15 is common), duration of *rounds* (3 minutes is common) and a set length of breaks (2-3 minutes is common). At least one *referee* (and up to five judges) presides over a *match*.

Boxer's hug: is a protective stalling *technique* of *wrapping* the arms over an *opponent's* arms. This ploy is often used by tired or *injured boxers* to smother an aggressive *puncher's attacks*. It is also known as 'the clench', *clinching* or *tying up* in *boxing*.

Boxing: a form of *pugilism* that involves solely the use of the *fists* to *out-point* an *opponent* over a number of predetermined *rounds* or to deliver a *knockout* blow that ends the *fight*. Modern *matches* have *fighters* wearing *boxing* gloves and they generally obey strict *rules of sport* as enforced by a *referee*. Ring deaths occur only at a rate of 0.13 per 1,000 participants (compared to scuba diving, for example at 1.1 per 1,000).

Brachial plexus clavicle notch pressure point: is a *Pressure Point and Control Tactics* (PPCT) *target point* (St. 12) that is located in the hollow spot behind the mid-*clavicle*, the gouging of which will access the *brachial plexus*, a *nerve* bundle innervating the arm.

Brachial plexus origin pressure point: is a *Pressure Point and Control Tactics* (PPCT) *target point* (EX-HN 19) that is located near the source of the *brachial plexus*, a *nerve* bundle that runs from the lower neck and under the *clavicle* in order to innervate the arm.

Brachial plexus tie-in motor point: is a *Pressure Point and Control Tactics* (PPCT) *target point* (Lu. 2) that is located on the *brachial plexus* where the chest, arm and shoulder *muscles* meet.

Brachial stun: normally refers to the effects of a *strike* to the *brachial plexus* at its *origin* (the side of the neck). This could include intense pain, concomitant *mental stunning* and dysfunction of *median*, *radial* and *ulnar nerves* feeding the arm and hand.

Brazilian Jiu Jitsu: refers to the *jiu-jitsu* introduced to the *Gracie* family in 1914 by Japanese *judo* / *jiu-jitsu* expert Mitsuyo *Maedakama* (Count Komo). Refinements of this *style* by *Gracie* family members led to the creation of *Gracie Jiu-jitsu*.

Bridging: refers to the arching of the *supine* body, making a bridge from the feet to the shoulders/head. See *body bridging* and *bucking*.

Bubishi: is an old Chinese text, called the 'bible of karate', because it was highly regarded by past *karate masters*. There are actually two texts (one is a treatise on the art of war while the other 'Okinawan Bubishi', relates to the *fighting* traditions of White Crane *boxing* and *Shaolin* monk fist). The latter document was first translated into English by Patrick *McCarthy* in 1987, but the name, date or place of publication of the *bubishi* still remain unknown.

Bucking: is the act of quickly and forcefully pushing the hips upward (using the legs), while lying in a *supine* position, against a straddling *opponent* in order to unseat him. See *body bridging*.

Budo: means 'way of *combat*', a term given to modern *martial arts* in general. *Bu* infers 'confrontation' and *do* refers to a 'way or path' hence both the physical and spiritual sporting aspects of the *martial arts* are reflected in this term. See *bugei*.

Budokan: is a *martial arts* training center. The *Kodokan* (1882) in Tokyo was replaced by the *Budokan* in 1962. It is a multi-disciplinary *dojo* and a mecca for *martial arts* students. The *Budokan* in London was established in 1918.

Bugei: means the 'art of *combat*' as practiced by the ancient *weapon*-bearing, *Bushido*-governed *samurai*.

Bujutsu: is a generic term for the Japanese 'military arts' used almost exclusively by the *samurai warriors* prior to their disbanding in 1867. These *jutsu* (skills) became the forerunners for all modern Japanese *martial art* ('*do*') systems.

Bulldozing: is the act of pushing against an *opponent* using the head/shoulders while in the *all fours position* in order to turn him over onto his back.

Bushi: are warriors who evolved as a distinct class of families (clans) in northern *feudal* Japan in response to having to protect their lands from invaders.

Bushido: means 'way of the warrior', a code of honor and conduct that was initiated in the 1600s and adhered to by the *samurai* until their disbanding in 1867.

Butterfly block: refers to a *block* that uses the crossed wrists or even elbows to *trap* or *wrap* an *attacking* limb. See *arm scissors block*.

Caestus: is an ancient Greek set of *knuckle dusters* designed to protect the user's hands, and to give the hand integrity and weight while inflicting damage to the recipient's body by virtue of the hard *striking* face. Around the time of 480 B.C. a Greek gladiator named Theogenes, from the island of Thasos, killed 1,425 opponents in *death matches* using the *caestus*. The *combatants* were strapped in close proximity, in a seated position, to blocks of stone with their hands wrapped in special leather thongs.

Catch-as-catch-can wrestling: is a loose *wrestling style* that developed (along with *free style wrestling*) from Lancashire *wrestling*. Contestants grasp each other's neck with the right hands while standing head to head and one *wrestler* grabs the left wrist of his *opponent* with his free left hand. A *win* is awarded when the *opponent's* shoulders have been *pinned* to the *mat* for two seconds. *Rules* were added to make the *sport* safe and exciting to watch by relaxing the necessity of *pinning*, awarding penalties for inactivity and awarding *wins* in pointless *matches* for aggressiveness and *style*.

Cavities: refers to the *acupuncture* or *pressure points* that are linked to internal organs of the body via their corresponding *meridians*, the pathways for *qi* circulation.

C-clamping: is the act of applying *finger scissors* to the throat or parts of the head by inserting the tip of the thumb and opposing finger tips (usually the first two fingers) into an *anchoring point* (i.e., in the hollow under the ear and opposite side of the nose). The availability of opposing *anchor points*, especially when used with *pressure points*, enhances the effects of pain-inducing *gripping* pressure.

Center of gravity: is an imaginary *point* (located in the abdomen below the level of the navel for a standing person, near the *tanden*) that best approximates a body's center of mass. It is the intersection of the *x,y*, and *z axes* making it the point where the body mass is perfectly *balanced* in all directions. An understanding of the concept of *center of gravity* assists in the mastering of *balance, stability* and *mobility* since changes in *body positioning* affects its location. Stance and body positions in particular, affect the *center of gravity*, because the *base of support* and positional attitude of the torso vary for each type of position adopted.

Ch'an Buddhism: is a form of Buddhism developed by Buddhist teacher Bodai Daruma *Daishi* (460-534 A.D.). It is believed that he traveled overland from India to China in 525 A.D. He is credited with establishing the *Ch'an Buddhist* sect in the *Shaolin Temple* of China (later to become the *Zen Buddhist* religion in Japan).

Chancery: is the act of *holding* the *opponent's* head (as opposed to *holding* the neck).

Chi: is the vital energy of life (*qi* in Chinese, *ki* in Japanese) that is thought to originate in the *tanden* (approximately *the center of gravity*).

Chicken head wrist strike: is a *striking technique* using the top of the wrist while the hand is bent down with the finger tips bunched together (hand position resembles a chicken's head).

Chin: means to seize or catch (an appendage in order to control it).

Chin twist: is the act of twisting the head in a plane roughly perpendicular to the *cervical spinal column* using the palm of the hand to cup the chin, assisted by the other hand at the antipodal position (top back of head). This is an effective *release technique*, since there is a sense of urgency when it is applied, given the serious consequences of resisting it. Wherever the head goes, the body must follow.

Appendix A: Glossary of Martial Arts Terms

Chito Ryu karate: is a style of traditional Japanese/Okinawan *karate* that is a blend of Goju Ryu and Shorin Ryu. It was founded by Tsuyoshi (Gochoku) Chitose (1898-1984) in 1952.

Chivalry: is the medieval knight's code of conduct, similar to that of *Bushido*; it is a combination of high moral and religious standards, as well as exemplary social qualities such as courage, honor, courtesy, justice, loyalty, and protection of the weak.

'Choking out': is a slang term for the act of applying a form of *neck restraint* or *strangulation* to render a person *unconscious*. See *doing the chicken, sealing the vein and sealing the breath*.

Choking techniques: are one of three main categories of *judo grappling techniques* (along with *pinning* and *joint locking techniques*) that refers to the *sealing the breath* (and less accurately- *sealing the vein*).

Cinema of violence: is an expression for the proliferation of Chinese *martial arts* action films in the early 1970's that became known as 'Kung Fu (Gong fu) movies', 'chop sockies', and 'chop suey westerns'. Starting with 'King Boxer' ('Five Fingers of Death' [1971]) and films starring *Bruce Lee* ('Fist of Fury' [1972]; 'Enter the Dragon' [1973]), these films featured well-choreographed and extended *fight* scenes that were exotic and thrilling to sell-out western audiences.

Circular techniques: are non-linear *techniques* including *spinning attacks* and *throws*, many *kicking techniques* and by definition, all *striking techniques*.

Classes of levers: are defined by the relative arrangement of the *force point* (point of force application), *resistance point* (load) *and axis point* (*fulcrum* or pivot *point*) which creates *first, second* and *third class levers* with varying degrees of *mechanical advantage*. See *speed levers* and *force levers*.

Clinching: is a means of *tying up* an *opponent* by staying very close to him, using the arms to do so. See *boxer's hug*.

Close quarters: refers to the *in-close fighting* range where *elbowing, head butting*, etc. are employed.

Clotheslining: is the act of applying the forearm in a forceful manner backward across the throat of an *opponent*, thereby knocking him on his back as if he ran unknowingly into a clothesline.

Combat: refers to the act of *fighting*, particularly with armed soldiers while in a *warfare* situation.

Combatants: are those persons engaged in a *pugilistic* altercation or *fight*. This term usually refers to persons in actual *street fight*s or soldiers in *combat*.

Combative: refers to those persons who show a readiness or eagerness to fight or who are actually engaged in *fighting*.

Competitors: are persons who are engaging in a sporting *contest*.

Compliance: is the act of being obedient and therefore submissive and willing to be *controlled*. For initially *combative* but relatively sober persons, some kind of *pain compliance technique* can represent an offer that the *combatant's* brain cannot refuse (less struggling reduces the pain and vice versa).

Contests: are sporting *bouts* where *competitors* (*fighters*) are pitted against each other under the control of at least one *referee* who officiates according to the *rules of the sport*.

Control: refers to the use of a *joint manipulation technique* to subdue an *opponent*. *Pain compliance techniques* are invaluable to police in preventing a person from mounting an *attack* or escaping lawful custody, while minimizing the chances for *injury* to the arrested party.

Control tactics: are those techniques used by police to *control resistive* and *combative* behavior. See *Pressure Point and Control Tactics* and *taiho jutsu*.

Controllability: is a *fight control* factor that applies to the movement of the *opponent's* body. See *mobility* and *vulnerability*.

Controlled escape: refers to the guiding of a *controlled* person in the direction of the *controlling force*, so that he is motivated by pain relief to move in the direction of the applied *joint lock technique*. See 'directionality of technique'.

Controlling force: is the direction in which the *load* is being applied to the body part being used in a *joint manipulation technique*. See *directionality of technique*.

Cornish style wrestling: is an old English style of *wrestling* (Devon style *wrestling*), one of three to develop from *English wrestling*, along with *Westmoreland* (or Cumberland) *wrestling* and Lancashire *wrestling* (which incorporated *ground work* with the aim of *pinning*). This style was named after the *wrestlers* who lived in Cornwall and Devonshire who wore linen or leather jackets to allow for grips that facilitated *throwing techniques*. Basically a *match* was won by tossing an *opponent* flatly on his back.

Counterattacking: is the act of applying a *technique* to thwart an *offensive* move. It can involve direct interference to an *attack* (i.e., blocking the hip during a *judo throw*) or be an outright *counterattack* itself in order to beat the initial *attack* (i.e., slapping the ears while a choke is being applied).

Counterpressure: is the force that is required to be applied (in the opposite direction of the initiating pressure) for any *chin na hold* or *joint manipulation technique* to be effective. If pressure is applied to a joint and there is no *counterpressure* exerted, then the *opponent* will simply respond by moving the affected *appendage* in the direction that the force is being applied. This will *neutralize* the pressure and allow an *escape* to occur.

Counterpressure may be generated by another body part, by an immovable object (such as the ground or a wall), or by using the force of gravity.

Crane head strike: is an *attack* using the top of the bent wrist joint as the *striking* surface.

Cranial pressure points: are *pressure points* that are applied exclusively to the *cranium*.

Crank: is a *wrestling* term that refers to the *rotational torque* applied to *joints* in the body such as those of the shoulder and neck.

Creating distance: in the active sense, is the act of moving the *opponent* away from you, usually by applying a low level *use of force* (i.e., by applying *pressure* into the *jugular notch pressure point*). In the passive sense, it is retreating from the *opponent* in order to *escape* his *in-close attacks*.

Crescent kicks: are circular straight-legged *kicks* using the inside or outside edges of the foot.

Critical incident: in police jargon, is usually an event that is traumatic in nature such as an incident involving *death* (a homicide), threat to life, or *grievous bodily harm*. Life and *death* situations requiring intervention are critical events.

Cross mounted position: is a *wrestling position*, usually a *transitional* one, which has an *attacker* lying on top of his *inferior opponent* at right angles.

Cross-mark hold: is a *straight arm lock* in which the *opponent* is at right angles to the *attacker*. See *juji gatame*.

Cross training: usually refers to the simultaneous or complementary study of several *martial art* disciplines so that the *fighter* is versatile in *fighting* at a broader range of the *fighting spectrum*.

Cuo gu: refers to the *misplacing of the bone*, one of five *physiological* categories of *chin na techniques*. See *fen jin, bi qi, dian mai* and *dian xue*.

Cupping: is a *holding technique* used in *wrestling* to loosely *hold* the back of an *opponent's* head for the purpose of pushing the head forward.

Da: is one of four essential components of the Chinese *martial arts* that refers to the *striking* and *punching* aspects. See *ti, shuai* and *na*.

Daishi, Bodai Daruma (460-534 A.D.**):** was a Buddhist teacher, also known as Bodhidharma or Da Mo, who was believed to have traveled overland from India to China in 525 A.D. He is credited with establishing the *Ch'an Buddhist* sect in the *Shaolin* Temple of China (later to become the Zen Buddhist religion in Japan). It is hypothesized that he originated a breathing and *fighting style* to strengthen the mind and bodies of his monks, as well as to afford the monks a means of *self-defense*.

Damo: is the Chinese name for Bodai Daruma *Daishi*.

Dan grades: are the levels of *black belt* that are awarded to those *martial arts* practitioners who are seriously studying to improve their skills. There are five to twelve levels of *black belt*, depending upon the *style*. The highest level is reserved for the founding *master* and his successors.

Dantien: refers to a *point* ('elixir field') in the abdomen a few inches below the navel, where *qi* is thought to be stored. Known as *hara, tanden*, and *qihai* ('energy sea': REN 6).

Da peng qigong: is *Iron Shirt training* that consists of the development of protective muscle and '*qi*' armoring. This is achieved through the incremental toughening of the body by high intensity body pounding and breath control for *qi* development.

Dead weight: is the effect of being *rooted* to the ground using *qi*, so that the person cannot be lifted easily. The term gets its name from the comparison in lifting a dead body that lacks rigidity.

Deadly force: is any physical force that is applied to another person (not necessarily using a *weapon*) that causes *death* (or even *grievous bodily harm*). In police circles, this usually refers to the use of a firearm. It is the highest *use of force level* within the police *use of force spectrum*.

Deadly threat: is a situation that a person faces that could cause his death. It is not a death threat.

Death lock: is a very dangerous *wrestling technique* that *cranks* the *opponent's* head forward using the weight of the torso.

Death matches: were *blood sport matches* held in ancient Greek, which saw man pitted against fellow man (these gladiators were often slaves) or against dangerous and often exotic beasts (e.g., lions and panthers). Sometimes the *winners* gained their freedom; the *losers* lost their lives *fighting*.

Death touch: is an almost mystical set of Chinese *martial art techniques* that *attacks vital points*, allegedly causing the *death* of an *opponent* within hours, days or weeks after the *attack*. This allegedly requires specific knowledge about the best times of the day to *attack* the selected *cavity points* to bring on *death* in such a delayed manner. See *dim mak* and *kyusho jitsu*.

Defensive: describes anything that is done to repel an *attack* (real or perceived). These may be *blocks* or *counterattacks* that are meant to *neutralize* the *attacks* before they are landed. See *offensive*.

Dialogue: is the use of words in an attempt to generate voluntary *compliance* from people. *Dialogue* is the second *use of force level* in the police *use of force spectrum*.

Dian mai: refers to the pressing of a *blood vessel* (jugular vein and underlying *carotid artery*). It is also known as *dim mak*. This category, known also as *vascular neck restraint*, is one of five *physiological* categories of *chin na techniques*. See *fen jin, bi qi, cuo gu* and *dian xue*.

Appendix A: Glossary of Martial Arts Terms

Dian xue: refers to the 'pressing of the *chi cavity*' (*pressure point attacks*), one of five *physiological* categories of *chin na* techniques. See *fen jin, bi qi, cuo gu* and *dian mai*.

Digital penetration: refers to the application of the finger tip(s) into a *pressure point* of a person who is offering low levels of resistance for the purpose of generating *pain compliance*.

Dim mak: is the Cantonese term for *dian mai* and refers to the art of *attack*ing the *vital points*. See *delayed death touch*.

Directionality of technique: refers to the direction in which the *load* is being applied to the body part being used in a *joint manipulation technique*. Knowledge of this principle will allow the *chin na* practitioner to steer his *opponent* in any direction he chooses by allowing a *controlled escape*. The person being controlled is allowed to move in a direction that slightly alleviates the pressure on the *controlled joint*, thereby reducing the pain he is experiencing. See *controlling force*.

Dirty fighting: refers to *techniques* used on the street that are considered to be nasty and unfair in an unwritten *fighting* code of moral conduct. Prior to the popularization of *striking arts* such as *karate* and *tae kwon do*, *kicking* someone was done so in bad form. *Hair pulling, eye gouging, spitting, biting*, all have a negative stigma attached to them. Some *rough play* tolerated in the *grappling arts* can be considered to be *dirty fighting* in the sports venue.

Disengaging: is the act of retreating from an *opponent* while at *close-quarters* for *tactical* reasons.

Distraction technique: is any *attack* that causes the recipient to lose concentration on his own method of *attack*. Ideally, it contains elements of both surprise and pain. Distraction techniques by definition, are not strong enough on their own to *incapacitate* the *opponent*, rather they facilitate a *release* or they create a lapse in the *opponent's defensive* capabilities so that an opportunity for a stronger *attack* may be launched. See *slapping*.

Do: means the 'way' or 'path' in Japanese ('dao' in Chinese). It is a suffix that is attached to *martial art* disciplines with a philosophical base in order to differentiate them from methods of *combat* that are lacking in moral and spiritual dimensions (as indicated by the suffix *jutsu*).

'Doing the chicken': is a slang phrase for a person who is moving involuntarily in a spastic manner, while regaining *consciousness* after having a *neck restraint* applied or after being otherwise *knocked out*. It is the neurological effect of having the *brain* 'sign back on'.

Dojo: is the place to 'train in one's way'. It refers to a Japanese *martial arts training hall*.

Dragon fist: is the *punching* fist made by extending the middle knuckle of the middle finger beyond the plane of the other knuckles of the closed *fist*.

Elbowing: is the act of forcefully applying the *elbow joint* to an *opponent's* body. It is a very powerful and versatile *in-close fighting technique*.

Empty hand control: is the middle *use of force* level in the *use of force spectrum* employed by police. It involves actual physical contact with a person, using *joint lock manipulations, punching, kicking*, etc., but without using *weapons* and normally without causing *grievous bodily harm* or *death*.

English wrestling: was also known as 'loose wrestling' popular since the thirteenth century in England (the earliest recorded *matches* were held in London in 1222 A.D.). The nature of this *style* is somewhat obscure, but it is thought to have been similar to the ancient *Olympic* upright style of *wrestling*. See *Cornish style wrestling* and *Westmoreland style wrestling*.

Escape: refers to the act of extricating oneself from the *grip* or *hold* of an *opponent*, using more passive methods like *reversals* or *positional changes* to do so. The use of *releases* infers *hitting* or the use of *chin na* to actively weaken the *opponent's grip* or *hold*.

Etruscan-based wrestling: is an ancient form of Roman *wrestling* that originated from the ancient Etruria area of west-central Italy (north of Rome). The Etruscans came to Italy in the 9th century B.C. from Asia Minor. Their *wrestling* (and *boxing*) style was an unsophisticated *blood sport*.

Excessive force: refers to a *level of force* used that is in excess of what is required to subdue an *attacker* under the given *combative* circumstances.

Exhibition bouts: refer to *demonstrations* of *martial art* skills, during the *golden age of wrestling*, that included *wrestlers* 'taking on all comers'. These popular *bouts* were undertaken in traveling shows with 'wrestling booths' at fair grounds and on music hall stages.

Expert: is a label given to those professing superior knowledge and skill but often wrongly attributed to anyone who simply achieves the *black belt* level.

External martial arts: are those *martial arts* that heavily emphasize *strength* and *power* in their *techniques*, such as with the *southern styles* of *Kung Fu (Gong fu)*. See *internal martial arts*.

Extreme fighting matches: are 'no holds barred' contests where *pugilists* from all styles can test their skills in venues like the *Ultimate Fight Championship's* octagon (fenced *ring*).

Eye gouging: is the act of inserting fingers into the eye socket(s) of an *opponent*. This is a high level *use of force* because of the probability of blinding someone, hence it should be reserved for *deadly threat* situations.

Fair fight: is a term given to a physical altercation in which certain *attack*s, considered to go against an unwritten *fighting code*, are not utilized (*dirty fighting techniques* like *spitting, biting, hair pulling, groin kicking, eye gouging*, etc.). Serious *fighters* feel that there is no such thing as a fair fight, just survival.

Fall: 1) is the judgement (*win*) received for *pinning* of a person's shoulder blades to the *mat*; 2) is the term loosely given to a *throw down technique*.

Feint: is a deceptive move of faking a *punch* (or other *technique*) meant to cause the *opponent* either to erroneously await for the *technique* to unfold or to react prematurely to it. This can create an opening for a real *attack* to be launched even prior to the completion of the feint itself.

Femoral nerve motor point: is a *Pressure Point and Control Tactics* (PPCT) target *point* (Sp. 11) that is located on the *midline* of the middle inner thigh.

Fen jin: refers to the splitting or dividing of the *muscles* or *tendons*, one of five *physiological* categories of *chin na techniques*. See *dian mai, bi qi, cuo gu* and *dian xue*.

Feudal combat: refers to the *style* of *fighting* done in medieval periods. Feudalism was not contemporaneous in all cultures but significant *martial* knowledge was acquired and practiced in these times. Parallel codes of conduct were experienced in England with knights (*chivalry*) and in Japan with their *samurai* (*bushido*). Strategies of *warfare* and *fighting techniques* changed with the invention of gunpowder and the firearm.

Fight: 1) is a *pugilistic match* or *contest* under *rules of sport*; 2) is a *combat* situation on the street, usually lacking any rules (i.e., a *street fight*).

Fight control: is a *fighting* concept that utilizes aggressive, decisive and strategic moves in order to shape the *fight* to the user's advantage.

Fight fixing: is the illegal practice of 'throwing a fight', or predetermining the winner, usually through cash payoffs to the *losing fighter*. Such action can obviously render the betting odds worthless but to all the crooked gambler (to him this inside knowledge as to the outcome of the *fight* is invaluable). This practice has tarnished many sports where betting is commonplace. This practice even occurred in the ancient *Olympic games* in Greece.

Fight or flight response: is a high stress defense mechanism that causes *adrenaline* to be released into the bloodstream, involuntarily preparing the body for survival by either *fighting* or fleeing in *a critical situation*. Physiological changes include increased heart rate and blood pressure, increased rate and shallowness of breathing, tunnel vision, and auditory exclusion. The net result is, amongst other things, a reduction in reaction and response times.

Fighting: 1) is the physical act of applying bodily force to another person by any means, including the use of non-firearm weaponry for the purpose of assaulting that person. 2) a generic term for military combat.

Fighting spectrum: is the range of *fighting* that exists between two *combatants*. Distance dictates what kind of *techniques* can be effectively used, and this often dictates the style of *martial art* that dominates at a given range. This is why *cross training* is so important in bouts like *Ultimate Fight Championships* where few *rules* exist and *martial artists* from different *pugilistic* backgrounds 'do battle'.

Fighting spirit: is the display of courage and mental toughness exhibited by *fighters* who refuse to give up the *fight* or back down from an *opponent* regardless of the odds against them. In *boxing* it is called 'having heart'.

Figure-four hold: is a *holding technique* that uses one arm to grip the opponent's lower arm (usually) while the other arm snakes under the arm being controlled and *anchors* itself onto the holding arm itself, thereby *augmenting the hold*. The resultant intermeshing of arms resembles the number '4' figure.

Finger grabbing: is a popular *chin na technique* that utilizes the availability and weakness of the fingers to being grabbed and painfully manipulated in order to control a person. See '*ackrocheirismos*'.

Finger jab: is the application of a *finger poke* into a weak part of the *opponent's* body (i.e., a finger into the eyeball).

Finger lock: is a popular set of *chin na techniques* that involve the grabbing, bending and twisting of the fingers. See *fen jin*.

Finger poke: See *finger jab*.

Finger scissors: is another name for the *c-clamp* which uses the thumb and first few opposing fingers to squeeze together like the blades of a pair of scissors.

Finishing holds: is a class of *wrestling holding techniques* that are meant to end a *match* by way of *submission*.

First class lever: is the simplest of the three classes of *levers* as exemplified by the pry bar. See *second class levers* and *third class levers*.

Fish hooking: is a *dirty fighting technique* that involves the act of inserting the fingers into the side of the mouth (outside the teeth) and ripping into the side of the cheek, like a fish with a hook in its mouth.

Fist: is a tightly closed or clenched hand that can be used for *punching*.

Fist press: is the use of the *fist* as a tool to push onto a part of the *opponent's* body, usually at a *pressure point*.

Flying scissors: is a *technique* which is delivered by jumping at a sideways *opponent*, and catching his waist and the backs of his knees between *scissoring* legs in order to effect a backward *takedown*.

Appendix A: Glossary of Martial Arts Terms

Follow-up technique: usually refers to a *technique* that is applied shortly after a *takedown* or immediately after a primary *attack*.

Force: 1) refers to muscular *power*, *strength*, or an application of the same in a pugilistic manner to a person; 2) refers to an external entity, act or, gesture, that causes a body or person to move or be influenced into compliance. See *use of force spectrum*.

Force arm: is the part of a *lever* from the *axis point* to the *force point*. See *resistance arm*.

Force lever: is a *lever* that has a *force arm* longer than the *resistance arm*. See *speed lever*.

Force point: is the *point* where *force* is applied to the *force arm* of the *lever*.

Forearm chop: is the *striking* application of the forearm to a *vital area* such as the throat. See *brachial stun*.

Fore knuckle press: is the *pressing* application of the middle knuckles of the fist to a tender spot such as the *triceps tendon*.

Fore knuckle strike: is the *punching* application using the middle knuckles of the *fist* as the impact area.

Forward breakfall: is a *breakfall* that uses a forward rolling motion in order to dissipate the energy of a forward fall.

Foul play: are those *techniques*, beyond *rough play*, that are considered to be against the *rules of sport*. A *foul* may be worthy of a penalty *point* or disqualification if the *referee* considers it to be a serious enough infraction.

Fouls: are *techniques* done in contravention of *rules of sport*, such as *eye gouging* in *judo*, hitting below the belt in *boxing*, and excessive contact in *karate point* sparring.

Framing: is the act of placing one forearm against an *opponent's* hugging body (neck) and *gripping* one's own wrist so as to fix this forearm against his neck. The more the *opponent* squeezes the defender into him while applying a *head lock*, the more pressure he puts on his own neck because of the frame created by the defender's arms.

Free Fighting: is the practice of sparring continuously, without interference, and without stoppage to award points, etc.

Free style wrestling: is a style of *Olympic wrestling* that allows for *holds* below the waist, *tripping*, and tackling. Like *Graeco-Roman wrestling*, the object is to simultaneously *pin* both of the *opponent's* shoulders onto the mat. See *catch as catch can wrestling*.

Front kick: is the forceful application of the ball or heel of the foot straight into the *opponent*. See *kicking*.

Fulcrum: is the *pivot* or *axis point* on a *lever* arm. Many *body tools* can be used as *fulcrums* when applying *joint locks*.

Gi: is the traditional training apparel of Japanese *martial artists*, consisting of loose-fitting pants, a long-sleeved top and a belt indicating *ranking*.

Going to the ground: is the act of taking the *stand-up fighter* off of his feet and onto the *mat*, for the purpose of continuing the *fight* using *ground fighting techniques*.

Goju Ryu Karate: is one of the four main Japanese styles of *karate* created by Chojun Miyagi (1888-1953) and so named in 1933. It is known for its 'hard-soft' approach to *attack* and *defense*.

Golden age of wrestling: is the short time period from 1900-1914 when *wrestling* was at its zenith in the English-speaking world. Music-hall stages and traveling *wrestling* booths saw the likes of George *Hackenschmidt* and American Frank *Gotch* (who unexpectedly defeated this 'Russian Lion' in 1908).

Goshin Jitsu: is an obscure offshoot of Shotokan *karate* (Kensho Kan).

Gouging: is the act of forcefully inserting fingers into tender and often *vital areas* of the body, such as the eyes, throat and testicles in a *penetrating* or squeezing manner.

Grabbing techniques: is one of three classifications of *chin na* application involving the *holding* of limbs in order to attain *joint lock manipulations* and the effects of *muscle/tendon stretching (fen jin)*. See *pressing techniques* and *striking techniques*.

Gracie Jujitsu: is a powerful style of *Brazilian Jiujitsu* created by Carlos *Gracie* and popularized by his sons in the *Ultimate Fight Championships*.

Grading: is the process of testing *martial arts* students to determine their suitability for promotion to a higher belt *rank*.

Grappling techniques: are hand- or arm-based *techniques* done in *ground fighting* situations by *wrestlers* and *judoka* as part of their *fighting* method, including the setups for *throwing* and *tripping*. These *techniques* can be categorized into *pinning*, *choking* and *joint locking techniques*.

Graeco-Roman wrestling: is a style of *Olympic wrestling* that prohibits all *tripping* and leg *holds*. Once both shoulders simultaneously touch the *mat*, a *fall* is obtained. See *free style wrestling*.

Greek wrestling: is an ancient upright style of *wrestling* that was blended with *Etruscan-based* style of *wrestling* to form *Graeco-Roman wrestling*.

Grievous bodily harm: is considered to be a *deadly use of force level*, even though *death* does not ensue. This includes the breakage of major *bones* in the body, or injuries that could have caused *death* or that result in permanent disfiguration.

Grinding: is the act of applying a hard body part, such as the knuckles, chin, head or elbow to a hard area of an *opponent* lacking protective fat and muscle like the temple, chin, sternum, etc.

Grip augmentation: refers to the use of a hand *grip* on another body part or piece of clothing in order to secure or *anchor* this hand in place. Doing so will assist in overcoming attempts by an *opponent* to remove it.
Gripping: 1) are those *techniques* that utilize a gripping action of a *body tool* to affect a *pressure point*, as opposed to a *striking* or *pressing* action; 2) is the act of grabbing onto a person's body or clothing for the purpose of obtaining a secure *hold*.
Groin kicking: is the act of using the top of the foot to hit the *testicles*. It is considered to be a *dirty fighting technique* in some sectors of society. It is a well-known *self-defense target area*, but as a *vital point*, it has mixed results.
Ground: is a term given loosely to any flat surface upon which people *fight*, be it a *mat*, roadway, floor, or grass.
Ground fighting: is the act of fighting while on the *ground*, during which *grappling techniques* are commonly employed.
Groundwork: is the term used by *ground fighters* to denote the practice of *ground fighting techniques*. See *grappling*.
Guard position: is the *defensive position* adopted such that the *opponent* is in the *superior position* but between the *supine defender's* legs.
Guillotine choke hold: is the hip-to-hip *choking hold* that positions the back of the *opponent's* head in the 'executioner's' armpit while the forearm is placed across the *opponent's* throat. A lifting action on the holder's forearm causes the *sealing the breath* of the *opponent*.
Hair pulling: is the use of hair as a distraction *technique* or more importantly, for use as a handle to direct an *opponent's* movement. Wherever the head goes the body must follow.
Hakudo: is one of dozens of ancient forms of Japanese *jujutsu* from the Tokugawa period (1615-1867).
Half guard: is a *position* adopted by the *defender* lying semi-*supine* on one hip such that the *defender's* upper leg is drawn across the *attacker's* body so as to prevent the *attacker's* full entry into the *guard position* (between the *defender's* legs).
Half Nelson: is an arm *holding technique* that belongs to a group of *wrestling holds* (quarter Nelson, three-quarter Nelson, full Nelson, etc.) that were popularized by a *wrestler* named Nelson in the *golden age of wrestling* at the turn of the twentieth century.
Hammer fist strike: is a closed *fist strike* in which the baby-finger side of the hand is utilized as the *striking tool*, in much the same way as a hammer is used to pound a nail.
Hammer lock: is a *wrestling hold* that is attained by twisting the *opponent's* arm upward behind his own back. The bent arm can be *levered* upward and outward in order to generate *pain compliance*. See *bent arm lock*.
Hand techniques: are *martial arts techniques* using the hands as the primary tools for *attack* or defense.
Hand tools: refers to parts of the hand used as implements for *offensive* and *defensive* purposes.
Handcuffing: is the act of placing a restraining device around the wrists of an arrested party.
Hand-to-hand combat: is an armed forces term referring to the art of *close quarter combat* that could include the use of hand-held *weapons*, excluding the actual use of firearms.
Hara: refers loosely to the area of the abdomen approximating the *center of gravity* but on a deeper level, thought to be the seat of the soul, or the center of *qi*. See *tanden, dantien* and *qihai*.
Head butting: is the act of bashing one's skull onto weaker parts of the *opponent's* head for the purpose of *injuring* or *incapacitating* him. This devastating *in-close fighting technique* is often overlooked by inexperienced *fighters* on the street, or is disregarded as being a *dirty fighting technique*.
Head tools: refers to the use of various parts of the head for *offensive* and *defensive* purposes.
Headlock: is a *holding technique* that consists of the *attacker* encircling the *opponent's* neck with one arm with the *holding grip* being *augmented* with the other hand.
Heavy bag: is an elongated canvas or leather bag filled with pieces of cloth, water, sand, sawdust, etc. that is suspended vertically at body level for the purposes of honing *punching* and *kicking* skills.
Heavy-handed: is a term given to the practice of using *excessive force* against a person, especially when done in a mean-spirited manner.
Heel hook: is a *pain compliance technique* that presses the *radial* edge of the forearm across the *opponent's* Achilles tendon.
Heel kick: is a *kicking technique* that utilizes the heel of the foot as the contact point.
'Hell dojo': is the nickname given to *Morihei Ueshiba's* early pre-*aikido dojo* that saw many *fighting injuries* from the *combat* effective *jujutsu* being taught prior to the Second World War.
Hip toss: is a *judo technique* that tosses an *opponent* over the hip (from behind) and onto his back.
Hit: is a term loosely given to a *punch, strike* or a hand held *impact weapon* that makes contact with an *opponent*.
Hold: 1) is a *technique* that maintains control over a part or parts of an *opponent's* body, most effectively achieved through *joint lock manipulation*. See *finishing holds*. 2) refers to a grip on an *opponent's* clothing or body part such as the wrist, hair or testicles.
Hold down technique: is a *technique* that is meant to *immobilize* or pin an *opponent* on the ground.
Hook punch: is a *punch* delivered at close range to an *opponent*, usually to the side of the head or ribs.

Appendix A: Glossary of Martial Arts Terms

Hoplology: is the study of the nature and use of weaponry.

Hyper-extension: is the forced movement of a joint past the usual range of motion, which results in limb dysfunction and pain.

Hyper-torsion: is the forced of a joint past the usual range of motion, which results in limb dysfunction and pain.

Hypoglossal nerve pressure point: is a *Pressure Point and Control Tactics* (PPCT) *target point* (St. 5) that is located inside the midline of the mandible.

Incapacitate: means to render an *opponent's defensive* abilities useless by *knocking him out* or by *injuring* the *opponent* badly.

Immobilize: 1) is the affectation by a *motor dysfunction* such that effective *offensive* and *defensive* movement is not possible; 2) to apply a *hold down technique, pin* or otherwise use a *chin na technique* to effectively limit the *opponent's* ability to *attack* you and *escape* your control.

Impact weapons: are hand-held *weapons*, such as a baton or club, which are used to *strike* an *opponent*, generally for the purpose of *controlling* or *injuring* him. It is the fourth *use of force level* in the police *use of force spectrum*.

Indian wrestling: 1) is an ancient form of *fighting* akin to *free style wrestling*. The golden age of *Indian wrestling* began in the 16th century with the support of the reigning Moghul rulers; 2) is a *contest* that pits two *opponents* supine on their backs, hip to hip, but facing in opposite directions. The *contestants* simultaneously raise their near legs on a signal and forcefully interlock them to see who can pull the other out of their resting position through the downward action of the leg.

Inertia: is the property of matter that resists a change in motion (a change in course or a change from a resting position into motion) brought on by an externally applied *force*.

Inferior position: is the *bottom position,* yet it can be capably *defended*, unless the *defender* is in the *prone* rather than *supine position*.

In-close fighting: is close range *combat* using *kneeing, elbowing, hook punching, head butting* and *throwing techniques*. See *close quarters combat*.

Infraorbital nerve pressure point: is a Pressure Point and Control Tactics (PPCT) *target point* (DU 26) that is located under the nose at the *philtrum*.

Injure: is to do physical harm or damage to oneself or to another person, intentionally or by accident.

Injury: is physical harm or damage resulting from applying *force* to another person, be it purposeful or by accident. In practice, the safety of a training partner usually depends upon the person applying the *technique*.

Instructors: are teachers within a *martial arts* school, usually *black belt* holders.

Internal martial arts: are those *martial arts* that heavily emphasize the cultivation of *qi* through breath control and concentration on the *dantien*, such as with *northern styles* of *Kung Fu (Gong fu)*. See *external martial arts*.

Inverted arm bar: is an upside down *hold* done when the *opponent* tries to *escape* a hold like the triangle choke. It leaves the *attacker* almost in an upside down position when he converts the choke into an arm bar.

Iron shirt training: is *da peng qigong* training consisting of the development of protective muscle and *qi* armoring through progressive body pounding and conditioning, coupled with breath control *techniques*.

Jamming: refers to the act of stepping into an *opponent's technique* prior to it unfolding. This crowding renders the *technique* useless due to a lack of distance required for it to unfold.

Japanese wrestling: are *styles* of *wrestling* in Japan such as *sumo, judo* and *jujitsu*. The *samurai* used various forms of *wrestling* as part of their *self-defense* training. The ritual of *sumo* is believed to predate 200 B.C. as documented in the Japanese chronicle Nihongi (Nihon Shoki). This chronicle was completed in 720 A.D. but it covered early Japanese history. According to this document, the first recorded *wrestling match* took place in 23 B.C.

Jeet Kune Do: means 'way of the intercepting fist'. It is an eclectic *martial arts style* developed by *Bruce Lee* (1940 -1973), or rather a gathering of 'what is useful' in the *martial arts*.

Jin: refers to *martial arts power* generated by the combination of *external* (muscular) and *internal* (qi) power.

Joint dislocation: is the forceful displacement of a *bone* from the *joint capsule*, rendering the corresponding limb or appendage *dysfunctional*.

Joint lock manipulation techniques: are one of three main categories of *grappling techniques* that involve the *hyper-flexion*, extension, and/or *torsion* of appendages. See *pinning* and *choking techniques*.

Jujitsu: is an ancient form of Japanese *martial arts*. 'Ju' means 'soft', 'yielding' or 'harmonizing' and 'jitsu' means 'science' or 'art'. Hence, this *martial art* can be called the 'art of softness'. The terms *ju jitsu* and *ju jutsu* are often used interchangeably but the former term is more commonly used to depict a more refined and sports-oriented style of *martial art*.

Judge: is usually a *black belt* holder who presides over a *fight* or other competition and awards *points* or scores *contestant* performances, based on the relative skills exhibited.

Judicious application of force: is a term given to a reasonable amount *force* in a given *self-defense* situation. In other words, the *force* is legally defensible because it would be deemed appropriate and justifiable in a court of law.

Judo: is a form of *self-defense* and a *sport* developed by Jigoro *Kano* in 1882 from *jujutsu*. It means the 'gentle way', and includes *standing techniques* (*throwing*), *ground fighting techniques* (*grappling, joint locking* and *choking techniques*) as well as *vital point striking techniques* (*atemi waza*).

Judoka: is a person who practices *judo*.

Jugular notch pressure point: is a *Pressure Point and Control Tactics* (PPCT) *target point* (REN 22) that is located in the hollow behind the upper border of the mid-*sternum*.

Juji gatame: is a well-utilized *judo hold-down technique* that is basically a *straight arm bar* which utilizes the pelvic area as a *fulcrum*. See *cross-mark hold*.

Jujutsu: is an ancient method of Japanese *combat* that was used extensively by the *samurai* to *throw, choke* and *joint lock* their *opponents*. This art also uses *striking techniques,* skills that were passed on to *judo* as *atemi waza*. *Ju* means 'gentle', 'soft' or 'yielding', and *jutsu* means 'methods' or 'techniques', hence it can mean 'to conquer by yielding'. Over 700 schools of *jujutsu* were developed in Japan. The terms *jujutsu* and *jujitsu* are often used interchangeably.

Jumping kicks: are *kicks* launched from an aerial position in order to increase the distance, height and *power* of a *kick*. They are favored by *Tae Kwon Do* practitioners.

Junsa: were Japanese policeman in the days of yore. Modern Japanese police officers are required to study *judo* and *kendo* (for male officers) or *judo* and *naginata* (for female officers).

Karate-do: means the 'way of empty hand' *fighting* that includes *kicking techniques*. It is a Japanese *martial art* that evolved from Okinawan indigenous *fighting* arts that were heavily influenced by Chinese *martial art* forms. The ideograms were changed from 'Tang (China) hand' to 'empty hand' in 1936 by Gichin Funakoshi, the father of modern karate, in order to minimize the Chinese influence.

Kata: are set patterns of *blocking, punching, kicking* and *throwing* used by Japanese *martial artist*s in order to practice important *techniques* of the given style. Collectively, *kata* can be considered to be a textbook of *technique* for a *style*. The strict adherence to perfection of execution of all movements in *fighting* imaginary *opponents* can develop *power, speed, agility* and *balance*. Many *martial art*s have such dance-like, ritualized forms for solo practice by their practitioners.

Kata bunkai: are the practical aspects of the *kata technique.* These applications are revealed through the practice of *kata* using real *opponents* choreographed into the demonstration.

Kata gatame: is a side to side *head lock* that also captures the *opponent's* near arm while the *opponent* is on his back. The *controller* kneels on his near leg beside the *opponent* and extends his far leg outward for *balance* control. See *arm-included head lock*.

Kataha jime: is a 'single wing lock', a type of *judo stranglehold* that utilizes the collar of a jacket to *choke* an *opponent* with one arm while using the other arm to control one of the *opponent's* arms (the 'single wing').

Katsu: is a resuscitation system for reviving an unconscious person (due to *strangulation* or *knockouts*), including slapping the mid-*thoracic vertebrae* to stimulate the *diaphragm* or stimulating the *pressure points* of the pertinent *meridians* to stimulate the heart and lungs. The *revival method* that uses *kiai* is known as *kappo*.

Kempo: means 'way of the fist'. This ancient Chinese *martial art* (ch'uan fa) was strongly influenced by indigenous Okinawan *karate* styles after its introduction to these islands in the late 1500s. The evolution continued in Japan through the mid-1900's with the birth of modern *karate-do*.

Kendo: means 'the way of the sword'. Its predecessor, *kenjutsu* ('warrior art of the sword'), was developed by warriors of feudal Japan, the *samurai*, as early as the 1200s. After the *samurai* were disbanded in 1867 and sword carrying was prohibited in 1876, Kendo became the sporting replacement for this 'too warlike' *martial art*. The first Kendo academy was founded in Tokyo in 1906. The 'live' blade was replaced by the *shinai* (sword consisting of four long bamboo strips bound by leather strips) so that non-lethal *contests* could be held with *combatants* wearing lightweight armor.

Keroma: is a specially prepared *ground fighting* area in the ancient Greek *palaestra* that had a soft sticky surface over a leveled-off sand pit, which was the forerunner to the *mat*.

Kesa gatame: is a *judo scarf hold* that is basically a reclining *head lock* on a *supine opponent* (with the near arm of the *opponent* included in the scarf-like neck *hold*).

Ki: is a Japanese term meaning 'spirit', referring to *internal* energy or *qi* (*chi*). Most forms of *martial arts* embrace this concept of cultivating mental and physical energies.

Kiai: is the 'harmony of energy' in the form of a 'spirit shout'. Such a loud and forceful auditory *technique* serves to do several things. It assists in the total concentration of physical and mental energy upon the physical *attack* or task at hand; it unnerves the *opponent* while psychologically empowering the user; it ensures proper breath control; and it tightens the abdominal region *defensively* when in the process of *attacking*.

Kicking: is the act of using different parts of the legs to *attack* an *opponent*.

Killing: is the act of rendering a person lifeless by a deliberate and overt physical act. See *death*.

Kinesthetic sense: is the awareness of the spatial relationship of one's various body parts.

Appendix A: Glossary of Martial Arts Terms

'Kissing the canvas': is a colloquial term given to the involuntary act of falling unconsciously to the *prone position* in a *boxing ring* as a result of being *knocked out*.

Knee block: a group of *techniques* that employs the insertion of an appendage into the crook of the knee prior to the forced leg *flexion*. This *block* destroys the integrity of the knee *joint*.

Kneeing: is the act of forcefully applying the kneecap to an *opponent's* body in an *offensive* manner.

Knee locks: is a set of *leg locking techniques* that focus on destroying the integrity of the knee *joint*.

Kneeling arm bar: is an *arm bar* (*ude garumi*) that is applied from a *kneeling position* (with one knee resting on the *opponent's* head or neck).

Knife hand strike: is the forceful application of the blade of the hand (baby finger side of the open rigid hand) to an *opponent*.

Knockout: is the rendering of an *opponent unconscious* (or *semi-conscious* in a technical *knockout*), usually via a *blow* to the head.

Knuckledusters: are prohibited *weapons* that consist of a hard material, usually of metal (classically brass), that cover the *root knuckles* of the hand. See *caestus*.

Kodokan: is the 'hall for teaching the way' in the *martial art* of judo. The original *Kodokan* in Tokyo (Eisho-ji temple) consisted of only twelve mats for use by nine students in 1882. In 1962, the multi-disciplined *Budokan* replaced the *Kodokan*.

Kugusuku: is one of scores of ancient forms of *jujutsu* from the Tokugawa period (1615-1867).

Kumiuchi: is one of scores of ancient forms of *jujutsu* from the Tokugawa period (1615-1867).

Kung fu (Gong fu): means many things such as *skill*, *strength* or work. It is often generically refers to Chinese *martial arts*. They may be broadly classified into soft, *internal*, *northern styles* and hard, *external*, *southern styles*.

Kyusho jitsu: is the art of *attacking* the *vital points*. See *delayed death touch*.

Lateral femoral nerve motor point: is a *Pressure Point and Control Tactics* (PPCT) *target point* (G.B. 31) that is located along the outside mid-*point* of the thigh.

Lateral vascular neck restraint: is a *technique* that employs the *radial* edge of the forearm and the same-side biceps (or nub of the shoulder) to apply pressure ideally to both sides of the neck as a method of *sealing the vein*. See *sealing the breath*.

Leg lever: is the use of the leg to apply *leverage* to the back of the *joint* of a straightened appendage such as the arm or leg.

Leg locks: are the generic *joint locks* derived from the application of *force* to the *joints* of the legs, specifically the knee and ankle.

Leg pick: is the *scooping* of a leg and maneuvering of it so as to cause the *opponent* to fall down.

Leg scissors: is the squeezing application the legs (crossed at the ankles) around the *opponent's* neck or torso.

Leg tools: are those parts of the leg that can be used for *offensive* and *defensive* purposes.

Lever lock: is a *lock* using the elbow to *pin* a body part while also using it to serve as a *base of support* for the *levering* action of the forearm (via contraction of the biceps muscles).

Leverage: is the *mechanical advantage* gained by the use of a *lever*.

Linear techniques: are those *punching* and *kicking techniques* that deliver the *force* of the *blow* in a roughly straight (non-spinning) line.

Load: refers to the weight of the object being being acted on by a *lever*. Often, where leverage is applied in *ground fighting* and *chin na* situations, this *load* is the impossibly heavy weight of the *opponent's* body. If sufficient *force* is applied to the appendage serving as the *lever arm*, the *lever* breaks at the weakest point, the *joint* (*fulcrum*).

Lock: 1) is a generic term given to any *joint lock manipulation* that achieves full range of motion; 2) refers to the act of completing a full *joint lock manipulation*.

Losers: are the *contestants* relegated to placements below top spot in competition.

Losing a match: is the failure to win a *pugilistic bout* under *rules of sport*, by being *pinned*, *knocked out*, *out-pointed*, etc.

Low level stunning: is a mild and temporary disruption of the thought process with concomitant *neuromuscular dysfunction*, occurring when a *pressure point* is *attacked*. Such *stunning blows* allow creates a window of opportunity for *attack* using follow-up *techniques*.

Mandibular angle pressure point: is a *Pressure Point and Control Tactics* (PPCT) *target point* (S.J. 17) that is located in the hollow behind the ear lobe.

Manipulate: means to bend or twist a portion of a limb or appendage, as with a *joint lock*, as to place stress on the *muscles*, *tendons* and *joints*. Since these *bones* are physically connected in a *structural chain*, their *manipulation* up to and past their full ranges of movement will allow for the *control* of an *opponent* through *pain compliance*.

Martial arts: refers to all *fighting* disciplines, whether *weapons* are used or not, that have a philosophical base. 'Martial' comes from the Latin word 'martialis' pertaining to 'Mars', the god of war. There are an estimated one thousand *martial arts* being practiced in the world.

Mass: is the quantity of matter in a body that can be represented as its weight.

Master: refers to a long-term *martial arts* practitioner who attains the highest *rank* within a given *style*.

Mat: is an area of protective layering that softens the floors of *dojo* where practice the *grappling arts* occur. These *mats* reduce the potential for injuries. Three-foot by six-foot covered straw mats (*tatami*) are widely used in *judo dojo*, whereas large roll-out, dense, foam *mats* are commonly used in *wrestling* gyms. See *keroma*.

Match: is a *pugilistic bout* consisting of a number of *rounds* dictated by the *rules of sport* for that particular type of *fighting* event.

Mat work: is the general term given to the practice of *ground fighting*.

Mechanical advantage: is the ratio of the exerted *force* to the applied *force* in a machine such as a *lever* (*force arm/resistance arm*).

Median nerve motor point: is a *Pressure Point and Control Tactics* (PPCT) *target point* (EX-UE 11) that is located at the mid-*point* of the bottom of the forearm.

Mental stunning technique: is a powerful *blow* that causes a temporary *neuromuscular dysfunction*, affecting movement. The *mental stunning* arises from the overwhelming sensation of pain and concomitant shock. This is also known as *softening up* the *opponent* or *distracting* him.

Meridian theory: is the science dealing with the location and medical application of hundreds of *acupuncture points* along fourteen main *qi meridians* in the body. It is the basis for *Traditional Chinese Medicine*.

Meridians: are the pathways of *qi* throughout the body. There are twelve regular (*bi-lateral*) *qi* paths (corresponding to *internal* and *external organs*), two main *extra meridians* (plus six others), and a host of collateral *meridians* that control the flow of *qi* throughout the body.

Militarism: refers to the spirit or tendencies of a professional soldier, or to the undue prevalence of military spirit or ideals.

Military training: is the regimented and rigorous training of troops to get them into *fighting* shape and spirit. 'Obedience to orders' and 'never giving up' are several military credos that are instilled into the training regimen.

Minimum force: refers to the lowest *use of force* level possible under the circumstance of controlling a person's *resistive* or *combative* behavior. The softer approach sometimes requires a maximum of effort in order to avoid hurting an *opponent*.

Misplacing the bone: is the forcible and painful removal of a *bone* from its *joint capsule*. See *cuo gu*.

Mobility: is the ability to use the legs (and arms if on the *mat*) to move about with a degree of *speed* and *agility*. With an increase in *mobility*, brought about by decreasing both the center of gravity and the *base of support*, comes a decrease in *stability*.

Momentum: is the impetus of an object gained by movement (mass multiplied by the velocity).

Motor dysfunction: refers to the temporary disruption of a portion of the *neuromuscular system* that renders the affected limb or body part partially or totally inoperable. This *incapacitation* is achieved through an *attack* on a *motor nerve point* or *pressure point*.

Motor nerve points: are *nerve plexuses* and other sensitive *points* on the body and limbs that are susceptible to an *attack* that renders the associated muscles temporarily dysfunctional.

Motor nerve pressure point: is a key *nerve point* that is targeted to create a *motor dysfunction* with the corresponding muscles when struck or forcefully *penetrated*.

Mounted position: is the *superior position* in *ground fighting* that has the aggressor straddling his *supine opponent's* abdomen.

Mounting: is the act of straddling a *prone* or *supine opponent*.

Multiple assailants: refers to a situation involving more than one *opponent*. The ultimate strategy in a *swarming* situation is to *fight* only one person at a time, by staying very *mobile*, by not letting your *opponents* surround you, and by not engaging them with *holding techniques* (hit hard and as quickly as possible and keep moving!). When dealt with properly, *opponents* become 'stacked', making a series of 'one-on-ones' possible.

Muscle/tendon splitting techniques: are those *chin na techniques* that *strain*, *sprain*, and rip the *muscles* and *tendons* from their corresponding attachments, usually by *manipulation* of the attached *bones*. See *fen jin*.

Muscle/tendon stretching: is a principle of *chin na technique* application that uses the physical *manipulation* (dysfunction through *hyper-flexion-extension*, and/or *torsion*) of (often) minor body parts like the fingers and wrists in order to effect *pain compliance* control over an *opponent*.

Na: refers to the 'seizing' and 'controlling' aspects of *chin na*. It is one of four essential components of the Chinese *martial arts*. See *ti, shuai* and *da*.

Naginata: is a type of halberd (long spear tipped with a single-bladed cutting edge) used by foot soldiers and by wives of the *samurai* to kill enemy horses. This *weapon* is popular amongst young Japanese women and female police officers and is practiced using a six- to nine-foot bamboo pole. See *junsa*.

Neck holds: are any techniques that encircle the neck, be they *neck restraints, neck locks, head locks*, etc.

Neck locks: are those *joint manipulation techniques* that are applied to the *cervical spine*. See *death lock*.

Neck restraint: is a category of *techniques* that focus on *sealing the breath* or *sealing the vein* with the use of the bare arms.

Appendix A: Glossary of Martial Arts Terms

Neck restraint with chancery: is a *vascular neck restraint* that uses the non-*restraining* shoulder or *bicep* as a base for *anchoring* or locking in the *technique*. The non-*restraining* arm presses the back of the *opponent's* head forward in *chancery*, adding a *choking* component to the *hold*.

Neuromuscular dysfunction: is the temporary disruption of the *neural pathways* that innervate the *muscles*, the contraction of which is necessary for movement to occur. The resultant inability to move properly is called *stunning*.

Neutralize: refers to the nullifying of an *opponent's offense* by landing an *incapacitating blow*, by *blocking* or *sidestepping* the *attack* itself, or by the *holding* of an *opponent* in such a way that his ability to *attack* is eliminated.

Nisei Karate-do: 'second generation' *karate*, meaning that the art did not come directly from Japan.

No holds barred contests: are those *matches*, such as found in the *Ultimate Fight Championships*, whereby there are few *rules of sport* guiding the type of *fighting* to be done. A true no holds barred contest would basically be a *death match*.

Northern styles: are those *martial arts* that evolved in northern China. These *internal* forms of *Kung Fu (Gong fu)* typically use softer, more flowing *techniques* with an emphasis on legwork. See *southern styles*.

Nutting: is a Scottish term for *head butting*. This much overlooked and devastating *dirty fighting technique* is also known as the *Scottish handshake*.

Octagon: is the infamous eight-sided *ring* surrounded by a mesh fence, in which the *Ultimate Fight Championships* are held.

Offensive: is the term given to aggressive *techniques* that are launched either without initial provocation or not directly in response to an *opponent's attack*. See *defensive*.

Okinawan karate: are the indigenous *martial arts* of the Ryukyu Islands, including Okinawa (*tode* or Okinawa-te), that are the forerunner to modern Japanese *karate*.

Olympic games: are those sporting events that originated in ancient Greece, perhaps as early as the thirteenth century B.C. The Greeks based their chronology on four-year periods called Olympiads and started these periods with a festival. The first real Olympiad was held in 776 B.C. (a single 200 yard race called a 'stadium'). Events were later added, including *pugilistic sports* such as *wrestling* (708 B.C.), *boxing* (688 B.C.) and *pankration* (648 B.C.). These were known as the 'heavy events' as there were no weight classes, no time limits, and not an over-abundance of rules.

Olympic wrestling: consists of two forms: *Graeco-Roman wrestling* (no leg *holds* and *tripping* allowed) and *free style wrestling* (leg *holds* or *tripping* allowed). These *contests* are held separately because of variances in the *rules of the sport*.

On all fours position: is the *position* of being on one's hands and knees (but not *turtled up*).

One finger punch: refers to the use of a single lead knuckle while *punching*.

One wing strangle: is a *judo strangle* (*kataha jime*) that also *neutralizes* one of the *opponent's* arms ('wing').

One knuckle press: is the use of a single knuckle as a *pressing tool* for *attacking* a *pressure point*.

Opponent: is a person with whom one is *fighting* either in practice, for *sport*, or on the street. The founder of *judo*, Jigoro Kano, replaced the word 'enemy' in his teaching and writing with the softer terms '*opponent*' and 'adversary' indicating a shift from *militarism* to *sport*.

Out-pointing: is the act of having more *points* scored against the *opponent* ('*out-pointing* him') or having had more *points* scored against you (being *out-pointed*) in a *pugilistic contest*. See *point systems*.

Outrigging appendage: refers to that arm or leg of a person in the *superior position* that is extended to the side in the direction that the *opponent* is trying to roll you, in order to prevent a forced *positional change*.

Overhooking: is the act of scooping an *opponent's* appendage being seized from over top of it.

Owning your opponent: is the phrase referring to the *neutralization* of an *opponent* via a *restraint and control technique*. This is the first and most essential step of the *handcuffing* procedure. The *owning* of an *opponent* stems from the ability of the *restraining* party to cause the *opponent* sufficient pain (and threat of a higher degree of pain) to gain his *compliance*. This generation of *pain compliance* prevents the arrested party from successfully mounting an *attack* or *escaping* because of the superior *control* being executed.

Ox jaw hand strike: is an outside snapping wrist *strike* using the *ulnar* side edge of the blade of the hand/wrist.

Pain compliance: is the cooperation gained through the use of pain, or more accurately, via the reduction of the degree of pain as a reward for such cooperation.

Pain compliance technique: is a *restraint and control technique* that owes its success in *controlling* a person's violent behavior to the discerning and judicious use of pain. Pain is increased with continued resistance and decreased in accordance with the cooperation shown to the *controller*. The brain is basically given an offer that the body cannot refuse, unless the person is under the influence of drugs or who is suffering from mental problems ('the lights are on but no one is home').

Pain tolerance level: is the level of pain that a person can reasonably withstand. This level varies from person to person and is influenced by such factors as prior experiences with pain, use of drugs, emotional focus, and mental health.

Palaestra: was the place housing the *skammae* upon which the ancient Greeks practiced their combatives. It is derived from the Greek verb *palaio* meaning 'to *wrestle*'. Privately owned *palaestrae* preceded public ones, which did not become available until the fifth century B.C.

Palm heel strike: is the use of the heel of the palm to *attack* an *opponent*. This type of *punch* or *strike* is recommended over a normal closed fist *punch* when *hitting* the mouth, as there is less chance of sustaining a cut hand than with an open hand *blow*. *Pathogens* can be transmitted from the mouth if the knuckle skin is broken on teeth (particularly if the mouth is bleeding).

Palm press: is use of the palm as a tool to press against a part of the *opponent's* body.

Palm slap: is use of the palm in a *striking* fashion as a *technique* of *distraction* or against the eardrum to puncture the eardrum.

Pankration: means the 'game of all powers' (*pancratium*) and refers to the early combined Greek sports of *boxing* and *wrestling*. Introduced into the *Olympic* games in 648 B.C., this brutal *sport* even allowed *kicking* but it excluded *biting* and *eye gouging*.

Pankrationist: is a person who practices *pankration*.

Penetration: is the forcible insertion of a relatively small body part into a larger, softer body part for the purpose of inflicting pain.

Perceived threat: is the determination or anticipation of an impending *attack* or merely the perception that an *attack* may take place.

Pinching: is the act of grabbing a nerve-rich (tender) spot of the body (such as the inside of the thigh as with a 'horse bite') or a minor body part (ear lobe) that can be used to *control* a person's movement.

Pinning: is the act of forcing a *competitor's* shoulders onto the *mat* for a given period of time (a few seconds) as in *judo* and *wrestling*.

Play-fighting: is the act of pretending to *fight*, often seen in children's behavior (particularly with males).

Plyometrics: is the training of *power* and explosiveness through rapid *eccentric muscle* contractions.

Points: 1) is the award given to a *contestant* in a *pugilistic* contest for *scoring* with a *technique*, be it a *throw, pin, kick, punch, reversal,* etc. *Judo* allows for quarter- and half-*points* to be given out; 2) are specific areas or spots of the body, as with *pressure points, acupuncture points* and *vital points*.

Point systems: are the award systems, according to the different *rules of sport*, that allow *referees* and judges to score the contestant's *techniques* thereby allowing them to determine who the *winners* are in a fair manner. A *contestant* can win a *match* by obtaining a given number of *points* prior to his *opponent* doing so (as in *wrestling* and *judo*). A win can also occur by acquiring the highest number of *points* after a given time period (*wrestling, judo,* and *boxing*- the latter allows for an unlimited number of points to be scored).

Position: is the *posture* adopted relative to an *opponent*.

Positional change: is the change from one *position* to another for *tactical* and strategic reasons.

Posting: is the use of a body part like the lower leg and foot to prevent an *opponent* from moving past or out of the *position* of the 'posted' (and immovable) leg for strategic reasons. This action could also include *pinning* a body part or clothing to the ground with the foot or even by *spiking* the shoulder into the ground using the *opponent's* own straightened arm (like driving a post into the ground). Posting prevents the person being *controlled* from squirming out of *position* while he is being *manipulated* from one *position* to another, thereby *escaping*.

Posture: refers to the relative *positioning* of body parts for functional and/or *stylistic* purposes.

Power: is the combination of *speed* and *strength*.

Power grip: is the mutual grasping of both hands (palm to palm) at right angles to each other. A grip with interlocking fingers is never recommended because of the potential of finger breakage, difficulty in disengaging, and ease for opponent in *locking* your hands together.

Pre-assault cues: are body gestures, often unintentionally exhibited by an *opponent*, that telegraph the possible intent to *attack*. These include adopting a *combative* stance, the clenching of *fists*, blading of the body, *target* glancing, etc. Enraged people can disguise many *pre-assault cues* but some leak out. When a discordant piece of body language is detected (clenching the teeth under a friendly smile), believe the minor element to be important in assessing the person's true intentions.

Presence: refers to the appearance and reputation of a police officer which affects the behavior of people that they are dealing with. It is the lowest *use of force level* in the police *use of force spectrum*.

Pressing cross body block: is the use of the bottom of the forearm to deflect and push an *attack* across to the opposite side of the body.

Pressing techniques: are those *techniques* that utilize a *pressing* action (as opposed to a *striking* or *gripping* action) of a *body tool* to effect a *pressure point* or apply pressure to a *lock*.

Pressure locks: are any *holds* that utilize a squeezing action of the arms or legs about an *opponent's* body (*head lock*, body *scissors*, *bear hug*, etc.).

Appendix A: Glossary of Martial Arts Terms

Pressure Point and Control Tactics: is a scientifically researched and tactically sound training system used by criminal justice workers, that focuses on inherent weaknesses of the human body in order to control *resistive* or *combative* behavior. This legally defensible and morally responsible *control tactics* system was developed by Bruce Siddle from non-lethal force research started in 1980. He serves as the PPCT Executive Director.

Pressure points: are often *acupuncture points* that are used for hurting as opposed to healing. See *vital points* and *vulnerable points*.

Pressure point attacks: are those *attacks* (*hitting*, *gouging*, etc.) that *target pressure points* on the body.

Primary targets: are those readily accessible and easy to locate *target areas* of the body that are reliable in terms of *incapacitating* a person if properly *attacked*. Some *self-defense* trainers set the *attacking* priorities as being 'vision, wind and limbs' (eyes, throat, *joints*) in decreasing severity and ease of execution for life-threatening situations. Other trainers regard *target areas* like the *testicles*, *solar plexus*, and *eardrums* as being both reliable and easy to locate *primary targets*.

Professional wrestling: refers to the highly colorful and well-choreographed *bouts* of *wrestling* that is a form of the theatre-in-the-*ring*. The period 1900-1914 was the short-lasting *Golden Age of professional wrestling*, eclipsing *boxing* and all other *sports* for popularity. Interest in *wrestling* soon spread to America. Gimmick *matches* and showmanship abounded, with *wrestling* reaching its zenith in the early 1960s. These dramatized *matches* are still very popular today.

Progressive overloading: refers to the incremental challenging of the body in order to achieve desired *physiological* improvements. Most competitive training sessions see an increase of weights lifted, distances run, *rounds* fought, etc. in order to attain a positive training effect.

Prone position: the *position* adopted when lying face down on the ground.

Proning: is the act of having an *opponent* lie face down. For a police officer, this is a *tactically* sound *position* to place a suspect prior to *handcuffing* him, as it greatly diminishes his ability to *fight* (as opposed to having him lie in the *supine position* which allows him to *punch* and *kick* at will).

Pugilism: refers to the act of *hand-to-hand* type *fighting* (fisticuffs), but can refer to *fighting* in general.

Punching: is the act of using the hand to deliver a *blow* whose *force* is transmitted linearly along the forearm. It normally refers to the use of the *fist* as the actual impact tool, but the usage of any part of the hand, whose *force* delivered in this manner, is considered to be a *punch*. See *strike*.

Push hands: is a series of standing arm-to-arm *tai chi* (*taiji*) exercises designed to develop the ability to sense, deflect, *neutralize* and *attack* the training partner without breaking contact with him (unless required to do so for the direct *hit* that has been lined up).

Qi: refers to the universal energy that exists in all living organic matter. Such energy may be *bio-electrical* in nature and is thought to stream through our *internal organs* via *meridians* in the body.

Qin (Chin): means to 'seize' or 'catch', in the sense of a police officer apprehending a criminal.

Qin na (Chin na): refers to the art of 'seizing and holding' a person in the way a police officer apprehends and holds a criminal. This ancient Chinese *fighting* method utilizes *muscle/tendon splitting (fen jin)*, *bone misplacement (cuo gu)*, *sealing the vein/artery (dian mai)*, *sealing the breath (bi qi)* and *pressure point attacking techniques (dian xue)*.

Qigong: is the study of *qi* for the purposes of healing or use in the *martial arts*. See *da peng qiqong*.

Radial nerve motor point: a *Pressure Point and Control Tactics* (PPCT) *target point* (L.I. 10) that is located on top of the forearm a few inches below the elbow.

Rank: 1) is the level of personal skill achievement within a *martial arts* style, as indicated by the colour of the belt (i.e., increasing skill levels are awarded white, yellow, orange, green, blue, brown and *black belts*) or degrees of *black belt* (first degree, second degree, etc. in increasing skill levels); **2)** is the relative rating of *contest* skills displayed by a *fighter* within an organization (i.e., top ranked, second ranked, etc. in descending order of skill positioning).

Reap: is the act of using a *sweeping* leg *technique* to remove an *opponent's* leg from the ground, often done in conjunction with a *throwing technique*.

Rear bear hug: is the act of encircling an *opponent* (including his arms or not) from behind with the arms for the purpose of forcefully *holding* him.

Rear guard: is the *seated* or *supine position* taken from behind an *opponent*.

Reclining arm bar: is an *arm bar* applied while lying *supine* at right angles to the *opponent*. The *opponent's* arm is held down (at the wrist) between the attacker's open legs with the pelvis/upper thigh acting as the *fulcrum*. See *juji gatame* and *cross-mark hold*.

Reclining guillotine: is a *choking technique* that is executed from the *inferior position* while leaning backward to create extreme pressure on the *opponent's* throat with the forearm.

Referee: is the official who ensures that the *rules of the sport* are being adhered to by being present in the *ring* during a *match*. He does not score the *match*, but he can award *points* to the recipient of *fouls*. He declares a winner from scorecards of the judges, who are at ringside.

Release technique: is any *attacking technique* (not an *escape*), that is applied for the specific purpose of weakening the *opponent's grip* or *hold* to facilitate extrication from it.

Resistance arm: is the arm of a *lever* that bears the *load*.

Resistance point: is the *point* on the *lever* where the *load* is focused.

Resistive: refers to a person's behavior who offers a small amount of passive or active (as opposed to *combative*) resistance to being *controlled*.

Respiratory restraint: is a *technique* that *seals the breath* (*chokes*) the *opponent*.

Restraint and control techniques: is a general police term given to *techniques* that are designed to *hold* or *incapacitate* an arrested party. The object of using such *techniques* is to apply the minimum amount of *force* possible in order to minimize the possibility of *injuring* him, unless higher levels of *force* are required to subdue him. In Japan, *taiho jutsu* was developed just for such purposes.

Reversal: is the *wrestling* term given to a *positional change* stemming from an *escape*, whereby the defender becomes the attacker.

Reverse guard: is the *ground fighting position* that places the *opponent* in front of and facing in the same direction (between his legs) as the attacker. See: the *guard position*.

Reverse roundhouse kick: is a circular *kick* that utilizes the heel or sole of the foot as the *striking* area. See *roundhouse kick*.

Reverse techniques: 1) are *techniques* using the trailing (least *advanced*) appendage. For example, a *reverse straight punch* is a *punch* delivered on the same side as the rear leg (the leg furthest from the *opponent*); 2) are *techniques* that are delivered from the opposite (weaker) side than they are normally delivered from.

Reverse waki gatame: is the *technique* of *waki gatame* that has the person applying the *hold* doing so from the head side (*reverse* side) of the *controlled* arm rather than from the standard torso side.

Revival techniques: are resuscitation methods for *reviving* an *unconscious* person (due to *strangulation* or *knockouts*). See *katsu*.

Ridge hand: is the *striking* area of the rigid, flat hand that is exposed when the thumb is tucked under the palm.

Ring: is the area (usually circular or square) in which a *pugilistic contest* is held. The *contest* area varies with each type of *bout*. It may be bounded by ropes or delineated by marks on a bare floor or *mat*.

Rodeo ride position: is the *position* that can be adopted on a *prone opponent* by straddling him (in the same direction he is facing) and pulling up on his *belt*. By putting one's heels close together, before lying on top of him, his lower torso will be squeezed and his inner upper thigh will be pushed upward and outward.

Roll over: is the act of turning over an *opponent*, usually from the *prone position* to the *supine position*.

Root: is the concept of being grounded or having good *balance* through superior control over one's *center of gravity*.

Root knuckle punch: refers to *punching* with the knuckles of the first two fingers where they join the hand. (phalanges/metacarpal bone joint).

Rough play: refers to *foul play* such as *gouging*, *kneeing*, *elbowing* and *punching* with a clenched *fist* (while holding the *opponent's gi*). These *techniques* can be considered to be *foul play* but they are difficult to see and be distinguished from truly accidental contact in physically rough *sports* like *judo*.

Roundhouse kick: is a circular *kick* that utilizes the ball or top of the foot as the *striking* surface. See *reverse roundhouse kick*.

Round: is an amount of time allotted for *fighting* in a *contest*, usually varying from one to three minutes in length. The number of *rounds* is also predetermined in accordance to the *rules of sport*. One to fifteen *rounds* are fought, unless a *knockout* occurs or one *fighter* is unable to continue due to fatigue or *injury*.

Rules of sport: are the regulations that ensure that *fights* are as fair and safe as possible. There are rules governing conduct in the *ring* such as *fouls*, *scoring* of *points*, selecting a *winner*, use and type of equipment, etc.

Samurai: were feudal warriors of Japan, renowned for their *combat* ability (particularly with the sword) and adherence to the *bushido* code. Disbanded in 1867, this warrior class played an important part in the protection of and *fighting* for the warlords of the 12th to 19th centuries, a service which helped shape modern Japan.

San Shou Kuai Jiao: is the Chinese *martial art* that means 'fast *wrestling* for *free fighting*'. This type of *fighting* uses rapid and clean *throws* and *takedowns* to handle an *opponent* without becoming ensnared with him.

San shou: means 'random hands' referring to the act of *free sparring*. See *Wushu San Shou Dao*.

Scarf hold: is a *judo hold* that involves an arm encircling the *supine opponent's* neck (like a scarf) as the *holder* lies at right angles across the near side of the *opponent's* body. See *kesa gatame*.

Scissoring: is the act of crossing the legs (at the ankles) or arms (at the wrists) and applying pressure to an *opponent's* body part that is between the two *scissoring* appendages. The hands must be *anchored* to clothing (like the lapel) in order for the technique to work, whereas the legs utilize the crossing of the ankles.

Scooping: is the act of *sweeping* with an arm in order to locate and *trap* an appendage.

Scoring: is the attaining of a successful *technique* in a *pugilistic match*, rewarded by a *point* or portion thereof.

Appendix A: Glossary of Martial Arts Terms

Scottish handshake: is a Scottish term for *head butting*. It is also known as *nutting*.

Scrap: is a colloquial term for a *street fight*, usually minor in nature.

Sealing of the breath techniques: refers to *choking* a person. The resultant deprivation of oxygen to the brain causes *unconsciousness*, brain damage and ultimately *death* depending upon the length of application time. This is one of five *physiological* classes of *chin na technique* known as *bi qi*. See *fen jin, cuo gu, dian mai* and *dian xue*.

Sealing the vein: refers to the pressing of a *vein* and underlying *artery*. This category, known also as *vascular neck restraint*, is one of five *physiological* categories of *chin na techniques* (also known as *diam mai*). See *fen jin, bi qi, cuo gu* and *dian xue*.

Seated position: is the *position* adopted whereby a person rests his weight on his buttocks, usually with the legs extended in front of him.

Second class lever: is a *force lever*, meaning that the *force arm* is greater than the *resistance arm*, as with a wheelbarrow or nutcracker. See *first class levers* and *third class levers*.

Secondary targets: are those *target areas* of the body that are less reliable in terms of *incapacitating* a person if *attack*ed. They are generally less readily accessible and more difficult to locate than *primary targets*.

Seize: means to physically capture a person, usually by grabbing onto a piece of clothing or a body part. See *Chin*.

Self-defense: is the term given to an aggressive act of defending oneself. By law, the amount of *force* used in such an act must be proportional to the amount of *force* used against the defender. (Bearing in mind disparities in size, skill, age, etc.).

Semi-kneeling position: is the position adopted whereby a person kneels on one knee while the foot of the other leg rests on the ground.

Shaolin priest: were 'young woods' Chinese Buddhist monks who lived in the *Shaolin* Temple of the Henan province of China. These priests, initially taught by *Bodhidharma* (460-534 A.D.), were renowned for their *fighting* abilities based upon the animal forms such as the leopard, snake, tiger, crane, and dragon. Their training was meant to *combat* bandits as well as to strengthen them for the rigors of meditation.

Shime waza: is a class of *judo holds* that use *strangulation techniques* to deprive the brain of oxygen, (thereby inducing *unconsciousness*).

Shin kick: 1) is a *kick* targeting this part of the *anterior* portion of the lower leg; 2) is a *kick* that uses this *tibial bone* as the *striking* surface.

Shin press: is the *technique* that uses the *anterior* portion of the *tibia* to press against a part of the *opponent's* body.

Shogunate: were hereditary generals for the Emperor of Japan. They were part of the elite and true ruling class of Japan prior to 1868 (the 'Restoration of the Meiji era'). After this time, the real power was returned to the Emperor.

Shoot fighting: is a term coined by Bart Vale of Miami. It is a recent eclectic hybridization of *stand up fighting* (muay thai), *throwing*, and *ground fighting (jiu jitsu)*. This rough and tumble *sport* is a fairly popular spectator *sport* in Japan, where *professional* heavy weight *matches* can last up to 30 minutes.

Shooting: is the act of diving to capture one or both of the *opponent's* legs as an initiation to *ground fighting*.

Shotokan Karate: is one of the four main styles of Japanese *Karate* ('Shoto's house') founded by Funakoshi Gichen (1869-1957). (This master used 'Shoto' as his calligraphy pen name).

Shoulder crank: is a class of *finishing holds* that involve the turning of the upper arm so as to compromise the integrity of the shoulder *joint*.

Shoulderlock: is a *technique* that compromises the integrity of the shoulder *joint* by *torquing* the upper arm to its limit of movement.

Shuai: is one of four essential components of the Chinese *martial arts* that refers to their *wrestling* (*throwing* and *tripping*) aspects. See *ti, da* and *na*.

Shuai Jiao: is Chinese *wrestling* more akin to the *throwing* aspects of *judo*, in that there is no *ground fighting* component to it. In fact no part of the body, other than the feet, are allowed to touch the ground under the *rules of sport* that govern this *martial art*.

Shubaku: is an ancient form of *jujutsu*.

Shudo Kan Karate: is a minor karate style founded by Akira Shiomi, who has been graded to 8th degree black belts in both *Goju* and *Shotokan Karate*.

Side kick: is a sideward, *linear kicking technique* that uses the outside edge of the foot (with emphasis on the heel) as the contact area.

Sidestepping: is the act of using lateral movement to defeat a *linear attack*, jam a *technique* by moving into it, or gain an advantageous position to launch or enhance an *attack*. It is an ideal way to avoid *blocking* while simultaneously providing the positioning needed for *counterattacking*.

Signal of defeat: refers to *tapping out*, a physical indication that the *opponent* is conceding to the loss of the *point* due to his inability to *escape* the *hold*, or more urgently, his *submission* due to its painful application.

Single leg takedown: is the bringing down of a standing *opponent* to the *mat* by *leg picking* one of his legs.

Sitting out: is the act of rotating the torso from an *all fours position* towards a *seated position*. 'Sitting through' a *technique* adds the *torque* of the body into a *technique*. See *death lock*.

Skamma: is a leveled off area of sand on which ancient Greeks held their *wrestling matches*.

Skill: refers to the physical proficiency of *technique*. It is said that it takes 3,000 repetitions to perfect a *technique* and ten years or 10,000 hours (at 20 hours per week) to perfect a *sport*.

Slack: refers to looseness in the *muscle* attached to an appendage to which *torque* is being applied or to looseness in the *technique* that is being applied. By removing the slack prior to the actual application of the *technique*, it will start to take the intended effect sooner and with a greater effectiveness.

Slapping: 1) is the act of applying an open hand briefly and broadly across a *target*. Such relatively soft *striking blows* are generally used when damage to the *striking* hand cannot be chanced or when the creation of a mere *blow* of *distraction* is required. A *slap* can be used to control damage done to *vital areas* like the neck but it can cause serious damage to *targets* like the eardrums or testicles; 2) is the action done to a *mat* in the early stage of a *breakfall* in order to dissipate the force of the fall.

Sleeper hold: is the layman's term for the class *of restraint and control techniques* known as *vascular neck restraints* that *seals the vein* and starves the brain of oxygen to cause *unconsciousness* (as if inducing 'sleep').

Softening up: is the use of a painful *distraction technique* to weaken an *opponent's* resolve in *defending* himself.

Southern styles: are *martial arts* originating in southern China. These kinds of *external Kung Fu (Gong fu)* emphasize hard *techniques* that are steeped in *strength* and *power*. See *northern styles*.

Specificity of training: refers to the adoption of training *techniques* that mirror the conditions under which a *martial artist* is required to perform. This provides maximal training benefit.

Speed: is the rapidity of movement of a *technique*. Training can improve a person's *speed* to the extent of the degree of *fast twitch* muscles present in his body.

Speed lever: is a *third class lever* whose *resistance arm* is greater than that of the *force arm*, such as with a shovel.

Spiking the weight: refers to the use of the body weight to its fullest advantage by resting it maximally on the *opponent* in a focused manner, as opposed to resting it unnecessarily on the ground or even broadly across the *opponent's* torso. The resultant 'spiked' feeling is one of crushing *immobilization*, making breathing difficult.

Spitting: is the act of expectorating upon an *opponent*. It can be used as a *distraction technique*, particularly if the eye is targeted successfully. Such an act is considered to be a huge and dirty insult to the recipient, especially if the face is hit.

Splitting the fingers: is the act of taking two fingers and ripping them apart in opposite directions. See *cuo gu*.

Sport: in reference to *martial arts* refers to *fighting contests* that are bound by *rules of sport* so as to safely allow a mimicking of *combat* under the supervision of a *referee*.

Stability: is the quality of being firmly fixed or not easily moved off base. *Stability* can be increased by lowering the *center of gravity* and by increasing the *base of support*. An increase in *stability* brings a decrease in *mobility*.

Stamina: refers to endurance, which is dependent upon the energy system being used and the *specificity of the training* used to enhance the relevant system. *Ground fighting* places substantial demands on the *anaerobic system*. It is a key component of fitness along with *strength* and *suppleness*.

Standing position: is the *position* adopted by most *fighters* at the beginning of a *fight*, usually with some distance separating the *combatants*, unless the *sport* promotes the use of *throwing* and *ground fighting*.

Standing techniques: are those *techniques* done in the *standing position*, usually referring to *throwing techniques* in *judo*.

Stand up fighting: is the act of *pugilism* from the *standing position*, such as in *boxing*.

Stomp: is a short range, powerful downward *kick* to the *opponent's* lower extremities or a stamping *kick* to any part of the body while he is on the ground.

Straight arm bar: is a basic *arm lock* that applies pressure to the elbow when the arm is in the extended position. There are a great many ways to achieve this *lock* using many *body tools* to apply pressure on the elbow. See *juji gatame*.

Straight punch: refers to the use of the 'square *fist*' in delivering a *linear punch*. See *hook punch*.

Strangle: 1) is the act of rendering a person *unconscious* or *dead* by squeezing the neck with the hands or arms (either by *sealing the breath* or by *sealing the vein techniques*); 2) is a colloquialism used by *ground fighters* for a type of *neck hold* that induces *strangulation*. This class of *techniques* is known as *shime waza* in *judo*.

Strangleholds: are *neck holds* leading to *unconsciousness* or *death* (if oxygen flow to the brain has been cut off for about four minutes).

Strangulation: is a confusing term that has been used to describe both the acts of *sealing the vein* and *sealing the breath techniques*. Commonly it refers to the act of placing the hands around the neck and squeezing forcefully until *unconsciousness* or *death* occurs.

Appendix A: Glossary of Martial Arts Terms

Street fight: refers to an unsanctioned physical brawl between two or more persons, where no rules of conduct exist, regardless of the venue. Alcohol and egos frequently fuel these senseless and often destructive altercations.

Strength: refers to the ability of a person to use his *muscles* in a concentrated and focused manner. Weight training can significantly improve a person's *strength* by progressively overloading the body, but such training does little to improve one's ability to *fight*. It is a key component of fitness along with *stamina* and *suppleness*.

Striking: is the act of *hitting* an *opponent* in a *circular* manner, such that the *force* of the *blow* is not transmitted linearly down the forearm as with a *punch*. This term can loosely include *punching* and *impact weapon* use.

Striking arts: are those pugilistic arts such as *boxing*, muay thai, *karate*, etc. that employ *punching*, *striking* and *kicking techniques*.

Striking techniques: are those *techniques* that utilize a striking action of a *body tool* to effect a *pressure point*, as opposed to a *pressing* or *gripping* action.

Structural breakdown: refers to the destruction of the *structural integrity* of the body: the *bones*, *joints*, *musculature* and other *physiological* systems that allow the human machine to function and therefore defend itself. The breaking of the knee, for example, can reduce a person's ability and will to *fight* by severely hampering his *mobility*.

Structural chain: is the physical linkage of various connected *bones* through *joints*, *muscles* and *tendons*. By *manipulating* one *bone* in the link to its full *range of motion*, the limiting *joint* becomes *locked* causing rotation to the adjacent joining *bone* to be transferred to it, and so on until no further movement can be tolerated. Any further rotation will cause structural damage to the weakest link in the *structural chain*.

Structural integrity: is a normal state of functioning of the human body in terms of its *mobility*, due to its ability to exhibit proper *joint articulation* and *muscular* expenditure. In short, the human machine is ready to *fight* or flee.

Stunning technique: is a *technique* that *attacks* a *motor nerve point* thereby temporarily overloading the *neuromuscular system*. The resultant mental and physical confusion impedes normal *physiological* responses.

Styles: are classifications of *martial arts* that differentiate one *martial art* from the other. For example, 'northern legs and southern hands' is a saying that relates the relative emphasis of *technique* placed on the *northern* and *southern styles of Wushu*. *Styles* are often hybridizations of several *martial arts*.

Submission: is the act of admitting defeat by *tapping out*, usually as a *pain compliance* signal.

Submission holds: are superior *holds* that result in the *opponent* stopping the *fight* for fear of being *injured*. Sometimes a person may also *tap out* and concede defeat when he cannot break out of a *hold*.

Sucker punch: is an aptly named method of assault given to the unsuspecting victim of a 'cheap shot' (i.e., a short range, unanticipated, or unseen *punch* in the head by an aggressor). Many *sucker punches* are just that, because the 'sucker' failed to read his *opponent's* body language or allowed an aggressor inside his personal *defensive* space.

Sumo: is an ancient Japanese method of stand-up *wrestling* that pits two large men covered only in loin cloths against each other in an elevated circular ring. A winner is declared if a person is pushed or *thrown* out of the *ring* using any of the forty-eight approved *techniques* or if he causes any part of his *opponent's* body to touch the floor.

Superior position: is the 'on top' position, usually straddling his *supine opponent*. A person is very capable of defending from the *inferior position*, so such terminology is misleading, notwithstanding that the person in the *inferior position* has to deal with his *opponent's* body weight on top of him.

Supine position: is the face up position adopted when a person lays on his back.

Suppleness: refers to flexibility, a key component of fitness along with *strength* and *stamina*.

Suprascapular motor nerve pressure point: a *Pressure Point and Control Tactics* (PPCT) *target point* (S.I. 16) that is located at the base of the side of the neck at the lower juncture of the *trapezius muscle*.

Swarming: is the cowardly act of overpowering a victim through the use of *multiple assailants*.

Swan lock: is a *bent arm wrist lock* that resembles a swan's neck when being *manipulated*.

Sweep: 1) in *Judo*, it means to use a foot to destabilize one or both of the opponent's feet in order to *throw* him. 2) in *Karate*, it means to use a hand to press an attack laterally.

Sweet spot: is a *boxing* term referring to the *point* of the chin that results in a *knockout* when one is struck there, due to the *concussive shock* received by the brain.

Sword hand: is the name given to the *striking* application of the baby finger side of the rigid open hand.

T'ai Chi Ch'uan (Taijiquan): means 'Supreme Ultimate Fist', which is an ancient *internal* form of *Kung Fu (Gong fu)* now regulated more as a system of very slow motion exercises designed to promote the growth and circulation of *qi*.

Tactically sound: is a police term referring to the safety consciousness of an approach to a potentially dangerous situation.

Tae Kwon Do: is the Korean 'art of hand and foot *fighting*' that places special emphasis on the use of *kicking techniques*. It was developed in 1955 (and coined by General Choi Hong Hi) from the ancient indigenous *martial art* of 'tae kyon', hence it can be called Korean *karate*.

Tag team: is a pair of *professional wrestlers fighting* together to defeat another pair of *wrestlers*. One *wrestler* from each *tag team* stays inside the *ring* and one outside the *ring*. The *fighters* on each team can spell their partners off if they can get to the edge of the *ring* close enough to touch (tag) their partner. The constant change of *opponents* makes for exciting and more unpredictable *wrestling matches*.

Taiho jutsu: is a system of *restraint and control techniques* developed in 1947 by Japanese police. It is a synthesis of *techniques* taken from *martial art* disciplines such as *karate, aikido, ju jutsu, judo, kendo*, etc.

Taijutsu: is an ancient form of *jujutsu* that was modified in 16th-century Japan.

Takedown: refers to the felling of an *opponent* without using a *throw* or without knocking him down by a *punch* or a *kick*. It usually involves the *grabbing* of a leg or other body part such as the hair or neck and forcing him to the ground by *unbalancing* him or using a *pain compliance technique*.

Takenouchi Ryu: an original *jujutsu* style founded by Toichiro (Hasamori) *Takenouchi (Takeuchi)* in 1532.

Tanden: is the area within the lower abdomen about one and a half inches below the belly button (at the level of the L3 vertebrae). It is known as *qihai* or 'energy sea' (REN 6), one of three *qi* reservoirs within the body that is thought to be the spiritual center of man. See *dantien*.

Tang Soo Do: the 'way of the knife hand' is a form of Tae Kwon Do that was developed in 1949 by Hwang Kee from the ancient Korean *fighting* arts of 't'sang su' and 'subak'.

Tapping out: refers to the act of *submitting* to an *opponent's joint lock manipulation* using the universal signal of two or more rapid light but firm *taps* (usually with the hand) on the *controlling opponent's* body. If the body cannot be accessed, then the *submitting* body or *mat* may be *tapped*, although these are less reliable signals given that there is often considerable noise in *training halls* (if all else fails, a 'verbal tap out' by screaming to halt the *locking pressure* is appropriate).

Target areas: refers to any *vital* or *secondary areas* of the body to which an *attack* is directed. These areas are given consideration based upon the type and nature of the threat being perceived.

Third class levers: are *speed levers*, meaning that the *force arm* is less than the *resistance arm*, as with a shovel. See *first class levers* and *second class levers*.

Threshold of training: refers to the minimum amount of individualized physical training required to have a positive training effect on the body. By incrementally exceeding this *threshold in training*, the body is *progressively overloaded* forcing the body to adapt by getting stronger.

Throw down technique: is any *technique* that uses a *throw* to force the *opponent* to the ground. See *takedown*.

Throwing technique: is any *technique* that uses a combination of *gripping, unbalancing*, and the forceful displacement of the *opponent's center of gravity* in order to hurl him to the ground.

Thrusting kick: is any *linear kick* in which the hips are *extended* into the *kick*, giving it a heavy (non-snapping) feel.

Ti: one of four essential components of the Chinese *martial arts* that refers to the *kicking* aspects. See *na, da* and *shuai*.

Tibial nerve motor point: a *Pressure Point and Control Tactics* (PPCT) *target point* (U.B. 56) that is located mid-calf between the two heads of the calf *muscles*.

Torite: is a *ju jutsu*-like Japanese system of ancient *unarmed combat* that was a predecessor to *judo*.

Torque: that type of *force* causing rotational movement about an *axis*.

Torsional movement: rotational or twisting movement caused by a *force* not aligned with the *axis* of rotation.

Torso tools: the use of portions of the torso to apply force to your *opponent* in an *offensive* or *defensive* manner.

Traditional Chinese Medicine: is a type of oriental medicine that is based upon *meridian theory* and the existence of *qi*.

Training drills: repetitive exercises meant to strengthen movements central to the execution of *martial art techniques*.

Training hall: a place where the *martial arts* are practiced. See *dojo*.

Transitional phase: a *position* that is between the initiation and completion phases of a *technique* or the between *postural changes*.

Transverse arm bar: is a *straight arm lock* that uses the pelvis as the *fulcrum*. Normally the *combatants* are in the *supinated position* at a ninety-degree angle to each other. See *juji gatame*.

Trapping: is the act of ensnaring an *opponent's attacking appendage*, normally using the forearms or wrists rather than the hands to do so. See *wrapping*.

Triangle choke: is a *judo* strangle hold, known as 'sankaku jime', that uses both legs to encircle one of the *opponent's* arms and his neck in order to *seal the vein*.

Tricks: was the term given to *jujutsu techniques* in the English literature at the turn of the nineteenth century. There may have been a degree of ethnophobic mistrust of these *techniques* and an egotistic perception of unfairness revolving around the fact that a small oriental man could take a larger Englishman to his knees merely by *manipulating* a few fingers. In Hancock and Higashi's (1905) book on Kano Jiu-jitsu, the 'Rules Governing Jiu-Jitsu Contests in Japan' section (pp. x-xi) states that 'serious trick …such as kicking and the breaking of arms, legs or neck are barred'.

Tripping: is the act of using the foot to unexpectedly *sweep* an *opponent's* leg in mid-stride, causing him to cross-step or otherwise impede his normal leg movement such that he stumbles or falls to the ground.

Tude Vale: is a form of *shoot fighting* where 'anything goes'.

Turkish wrestling: the Turks of the Ottoman Empire were revered for their *wrestling*, archery and horseracing abilities. Traditional *wrestling* games have been held at Kirkpinar, with stand-up *wrestlers* (naked from the waist up and wearing only leather pants) oiling themselves up from head to foot while *grappling*.

Turning: 1) is the act of causing a rotation along the long *axis* of an *appendage* through a *gripping* action; 2) the act of rotating the body around the *spinal axis*, so as to impart angular momentum into a *spinning kick*.

Turning kicks: are (non-linear) *spinning kicks*.

Turtling up: the *defensive* act of collapsing from an *on all fours position* to that position which sees the defender sitting on his haunches while covering the sides of his neck with his forearms. This is done so as not to allow the easy insertion of an *appendage* into the *frontal* portion of the torso. It also makes acquiring a limb or accessing the neck difficult.

Tying up: is the act of *clinching* or otherwise smothering an *opponent's* available *attacking* limbs in order to buy recuperation time needed when either extreme fatigue sets in or a when a heavy *blow* was received. It can also be used to keep a physical altercation from escalating should *fighting* not be a desirable outcome.

Ude garumi: is an 'entangled arm lock' used in *judo*. This type of *arm lock* applies pressure to the elbow and shoulder joints when the arm is bent either upward or downward by the *opponent's* side or behind his back, as with a *hammer lock*. See *bent arm lock*.

Ude gatame: is a *judo hold* that applies pressure to the elbow of the *opponent's* straight arm by pressing on the back of the elbow with the hands or forearms while using a part of the torso as a *fulcrum*. See *arm hug* and *arm wrap*.

Ultimate Fight Championships (UFC): are *no-hold barred* types of *contests* fought in a special fenced octagonal *ring* called the *octagon*. These professional *matches* underscore the value of *cross-training* in *martial arts* for *street fighting*, and have popularized the *grappling arts*. UFC 1 was held in Denver, Colorado (1993) and was won by Royce *Gracie*.

Unarmed combat: is an armed forces term given to *hand-to-hand combat* that may include *close quarter combat* using non-firearm weaponry such as the knife or bayonet.

Unbalancing: is called *kuzushi* in *judo* and is the act of displacing the *center of gravity* close to, or beyond, the edge the *opponent's base of support*. The *opponent* is vulnerable to a *throw* when in this precarious and unstable position.

Uncontrolled takedown: is a *takedown* whereby the person being thrown, tripped or otherwise taken off his feet, cannot be taken down under his *opponent's* total *control*. A hard landing with some unanticipated movement is typical.

Underhooking: is the act of scooping an *opponent's appendage* being seized from underneath it.

Uprooting: is the act of displacing the *opponent's center of gravity* or minimizing his *base of support* in order to destroy his solid connection with the ground.

Use of force level: refers to the amount of physical and non-physical *force* used within the *use of force spectrum*.

Use of force spectrum: is a police term given to the range of interactions that can be applied to a suspect. It ranges from soft to hard non-physical and physical *techniques* and these can be classified into five levels of force, ranging from *presence, dialogue, empty hand control, impact weapons* to *deadly force*. The *techniques* chosen by an officer preclude the appropriateness or effectiveness of lesser force options based upon numerous situational factors. A judicious application of *force* predicated by the level of resistance offered by the suspect is not only desirable, it is required by law.

Vascular neck restraint: is a class of *sealing the vein techniques* that restricts the flow of oxygenated blood to the brain, causing *unconsciousness*.

Verbal commands: are the words authoritatively spoken to suspects being arrested or having their behavior *controlled* through non-physical means. It is a form of *dialogue*, the second use of force level in the *use of force spectrum*.

Vital organ: is any organ that that is essential to life, such as the *brain* or *liver*. These would be classified as *primary targets* based upon their relative importance in sustaining life but not necessarily for ease of access, in the case of the *liver*.

Vital points: are *pressure points, vital organs* and other *vulnerable points* within the body, that are both accessible and devastating when *attacked*. Strictly speaking, these are *points* causing *death* when properly struck.

Vulnerability: is the state in which a person's *defenses* are not tight, meaning that opportunities for *attack* are available. A person can be made to be *vulnerable* if *injured*, distracted, frozen with fear or anger, or is out positioned, etc.

Vulnerable points: are areas of the body susceptible to *attack* by virtue of the difficulty in *defending* such areas, such as the *kneecap* and groin. They need not be *vital points*.

Waki gatame: a *judo hold down technique* involving the *combatants* lying back to back at right angles to each other, with the *controlling* party lying partially on his *opponent's* back with the near arm under the *controller's* armpit (normally the arm closest to the opponent's head). The *controlling* party has an effective *arm bar* on his *opponent* when using this *hold down* and he is free from *counterattack* by his *proned-out opponent*. See *armpit hold*.

War: refers to armed hostilities between nations.

Warfare: refers to the state of *war* or engaging in *war*.

Warrior: refers to the soldier who is trained to engage in *war*. See *samurai warrior*.

Waza: refers to *martial art 'technique'* in Japanese.

Weapons: are anything that is used (or threatened to be used) against a person to cause *injury* or *death*, regardless if it was designed for such a purpose. An innocuous or utilitarian object can be converted to a *weapon* by the use of, or intention to use, it as a *weapon*.

Weapons disarming: is the ability to forcefully remove from an *opponent* an object that is meant to *injure* or kill a person. Many *martial arts styles* teach *weapons disarming techniques* as part of their *self-defense* curriculum.

Weight classes: are the ranges of weight categories that *fighters* are grouped into, in accordance with the *rules of sport*, to ensure a fair *contest*. In *full contact fighting*, size does matter.

Westmoreland style wrestling: or 'Cumberland *wrestling*' is an old *English style* of stand-up *wrestling* that originated in the north of England, and has the *contestants* clasp their hands behind each others backs until a fall is attained. It is one of three styles to develop from *English wrestling* (although it has changed little since its codification in the 1820's), along with Cornish (or Devon style, that involved 'barbaric hugging and kicking') *wrestling* (which utilized linen or leather jackets for *gripping*) and Lancashire *wrestling* (which incorporated *ground work* with the aim of *pinning*).

Winning a match: in *tournaments* refers to the accumulation of a predetermined number of *points* or the most *points*, in a number of given *rounds*, in accordance to the *rules of sport*. A *winner* may be found by knocking out an *opponent* or *fighting* him until his *opponent's* corner 'throws in the towel' or the *opponent* himself concedes defeat by *tapping out*.

Winning mindset: refers to the state of mind, the mental toughness required to win a *fight* at all costs, particularly a *street fight* where there is no *referee* to ensure that a clean and *fair fight* is fought.

World champion: is supposedly the top *fighter* of a given *weight class* in a given *style* of *fighting*. There are many factions claiming to be the governing body of many *sports* including *professional wrestling* and *boxing* that confer such titles to *fighters* within their organization. As such the titles are often meaningless, other than for show.

World Wrestling Federation: is a governing body for one faction of the *sport* of *professional wrestling*. It is a popular television extravaganza in North America.

Wrapping: is the act of *holding* onto an *opponent's appendage* without using the hands. The forearms are used to hold the *appendage* against the body or against themselves, usually for an *offensive* purpose, whereas *trapping* infers a *defensiveness* arising from intercepting and *holding* an *attacking* limb.

Wrestling: is the art of *grappling* with and throwing an *opponent* to the ground. The rules vary in accordance to the *rules of sport* for each particular form of *wrestling*, be it *Graeco-Roman* or *free style wrestling* (both forms of *Olympic wrestling*). *Wrestling* was introduced to the *Olympics* in 704 B.C. (18th Olympiad).

Wrestling choreography: refers to the fake *wrestling* done purely for entertainment purposes in *professional wrestling*.

Wrestling festivals: were *demonstrations* of *wrestling* held by the ruling classes and the masses throughout medieval Europe for entertainment purposes. Local fairs and traveling fairs were breeding grounds for *contestants* in international *matches*, a practice that continued into the nineteenth century.

Wrist lever: is the *technique* that uses the non-supporting wrist (in a *power grip*) to tighten up a hold by *flexing* the wrist inward towards the body part being held, after the *slack* has been removed. This has the subtle but forceful effect of maximally cinching up the *hold*.

Wrist lock: is a class of *joint lock manipulations* that bend and/or twist the wrists.

Wushu: means 'war arts' and is the generic term for all Chinese *martial arts* or *Kung Fu (Gong fu)*, whether *northern style* or *southern style*.

Wushu San Shou Dao: is an 'applied *free fighting*' art that includes short and long range *techniques*, *punching*, *kicking*, *grappling*, *throwing* and *pressure point attacking* using both *internal* and *external power*.

Yang: is the active, sufficient, male, positive counterpart and complement to the metaphysical element of *yin* that permeates the universe according to *yin-yang theory*.

Yawara: 1) is an ancient form of *ju jutsu;* 2) is a short rod used in *blocking*, and *striking*, and used for *penetrating pressure points*.

Appendix A: Glossary of Martial Arts Terms

Yin: is the passive, deficient, female, negative counterpart and complement to the metaphysical element of *yang* that permeates the universe according to *yin-yang theory*.

Yin/Yang theory: Daoist philosophy regards the two metaphysical elements of *yin* and *yang* as being complementary and inseparable *forces* that permeate the universe. One cannot exist without the other, in fact a little of each always exists in the other. *Yin* gradually becomes *yang* just as night becomes day.

Zen Buddhism: is the Japanese religious doctrine that emphasizes meditation, discipline and discipleship. These teachings, introduced to Japan in the late twelfth century, descended from Chinese *Ch'an Buddhism* and the Indian Buddhist Dhyana sect.

APPENDIX B

Glossary of Medical Terms

The meanings for the terms listed here refer to their usage in this book, notwithstanding that many other meanings may exist for them. Italics indicate that the term is also defined in this glossary or the martial arts glossary.

Abdomen: is the part of the body between the hips and the chest, informally known as the 'belly'.
Abdominal cavity: is the space in the body that contains the *internal organs* referred to colloquially as the 'guts'. This is below the *thoracic cavity* of the chest.
Abduction: refers to the movement of a body part such as an arm or leg away from the body's *median plane*.
Achilles tendon: is a band of fibrous *tissue* connecting the *calf muscles* to the back of the heel. It is the thickest, strongest *tendon* in the body. It is also known as the *calcaneal tendon*.
Adam's apple: is a large structure of *cartilage*, located on the mid-front line of the neck. Known also as the *laryngeal prominence*, this *thyroid cartilage* functions to keep the airway open, along with other *cartilage* in the upper *respiratory* tract.
Adduction: refers to the movement of a body part such as an arm or a leg towards the body's *medial plane*.
Adrenaline: is a hormone released by the body in response to stress and fear. It helps the body to perform by increasing *heart rate*, *blood pressure*, *blood* sugar, and *blood* flow to the *muscles*.
Aerobic: describes a process that requires *oxygen*. For example, aerobic exercise requires increased *oxygen* in the *blood*, versus *anaerobic* exercise such as weight lifting, which does not require an increase in *oxygen* levels.
Anabolism: is a process that produces energy though the conversion of simple substances into complex matter as in *muscle* building. Compare with '*catabolism*'.
Anaerobic: describes a process that occurs in the absence of *oxygen*. Only relatively short-term *muscular* activity can be performed under anaerobic conditions.
Anastomose: refers to cross-connection of *blood vessels*, particularly with reference to *arteries* and *veins* around the *skull*. This accounts for the profuseness of *bleeding* when even a minor head *wound* is sustained.
Anatomy: is the science of the body's structure, and of how body parts relate to each other. See '*physiology*'.
Angina pectoris: is a *heart disease* in which pain felt across the chest, and sometimes in the neck, shoulder blades, and arms, caused by a lack of *oxygen* to the *heart*. It is often caused by a narrowing of the *arteries* (arteriosclerosis).
Angular vein: is a short *vein* running between the eye and the side of the back of the nose on both sides of the face.
Ankle: is the juncture of the two lower leg *bones* (tibia and fibula) with the talus *bone* of the *foot*.
Ankle joint: is the juncture of the *tibia*, *fibula bones* of the leg and the talus *bone* of the *foot*, where it forms a *hinge joint*.
Antebrachial cutaneous nerves: are those *nerves* feeding the arm, consisting of the *medial* and *lateral* branches, that can be accessed by pressing deeply near the *elbow joint*.
Anterior: refers to location towards the front, or belly, surface of the body (opposite to *posterior*). For example, the chest is *anterior* to the back.
Anterior cervical triangle: is the area bounded by the *anterior* border of the *sternocleidomastoid*, the *anterior midline* of the neck and the *mandible*. Compare with '*posterior cervical triangle*'.
Anterior ethmoidal nerves: are two *nerves* running the length of the nose, whose distribution includes the mucous area of the nasal *cavity* and the tip of the nose. See *external nasal nerves*.
Anus: is the terminal opening of the *digestive system*, from which solid waste is eliminated.

Appendage: is something added on to something else (e.g., a limb is an appendage of the body *torso*).
Artery: is a *blood vessel* carrying *oxygen*-enriched *blood* away from the *heart* to the rest of the body.
Articulate: means to unite so as to form a *joint*, making *skeletal* mobility possible.
Asphyxiation: refers to *suffocation*, *injury* or *death* due to lack of *oxygen* in one's air intake.
Atherosclerosis: is a common disorder of the arteries that sees fat and cholesterol (plaque) deposited in the walls of the large - and medium - sized arteries. The walls become thick and hardened. The vessel narrows.
Autonomic nervous system: is that part of the *nervous system* concerned with automatic bodily functions, such as the activities of *heart muscles*, glands, and *smooth muscles* of the *internal organs*.
Axillary artery: is the shoulder *artery* that supplies each arm. Above it at the *clavicle*, it is known as the *subclavian artery* and below it where it crosses the *biceps*, it becomes the *brachial artery*.
Axillary vein: is one of a pair of veins that run from the top of the arm near the bicep to the *collarbone* where it becomes the *subclavian vein*.
Ball and socket joint: is a type of *joint* in which one of the *bone* surfaces is smooth and round (the "ball"), and the other surface is a *cavity* (the "socket") which receives the ball. An example is the *hip joint*.
Baroreceptor: is a type of *nerve ending*, such as those found in the *carotid sinus*, which sends information to the brain, via the *carotid sinus nerve*, about changes in *blood pressure*.
Biceps brachii tendon: is a *tendon* attaching the *biceps muscle* of the upper arm to the head of the *humerus*.
Biceps femoris: is a long *muscle* at the back of the thigh, which *flexes* the leg and *extends* the thigh.
Bifurcation: means to split into two branches, such as with the *windpipe* dividing into the two bronchi of the lungs.
Bilateral: means having two sides, referring to symmetrical patterns of *nerves*, *circulatory system* and *meridians*.
Bioelectricity: is the small electrical current that is generated by living tissues like the *nerves*, brain, heart, and muscles.
Bleeding: is the escape of *blood* from the *circulatory system* due to damage to one or more *blood vessels*. *Internal bleeding* is usually the result of a traumatic blow to the body where the *skin* itself is not perforated or cut. *External bleeding* has visible *blood* loss outside of the body.
Blood: is the fluid that carries *oxygen* and nutrients to the body, through the *heart*, *arteries*, *veins* and *capillaries*. There are about ten pints of *blood* in the average human body.
Blood pressure: is the force of *blood* being pumped through the *circulatory system* by the *heart* (the pressure of *blood* against the walls of the arteries). A healthy *blood pressure* is 120 over 80 (mmHg), where the first number is the "systolic" or maximum pressure, and the second is the "diastolic" or minimum pressure, during a beat of the *heart*.
Blood vessels: are the 100,000 miles of tubes that carry *blood* throughout the body such as *arteries*, *veins*, and *capillaries*.
Bodily fluids: are any liquids produced by the body, most commonly *blood*, *urine*, saliva and mucous.
Bone: is a piece of hard (and somewhat flexible) *tissue* making up the *skeleton* in invertebrates. The human body has 206 *bones* that account for 35% of the body weight (1/3 organic protein and 2/3 inorganic calcium and phosphorous). *Bones* are very strong and are the hardest of all living *tissue*s. See '*skeleton*'.
Brachial: refers to the arm.
Brachial plexus: is a large network of *nerves* extending from the lower side of the neck and upper *spine* to the armpit. The *nerves* supply areas of the chest, the shoulder, the upper arm and *forearm*, and the *hand*.
Brachialis muscles: are two *muscles* that attach to the front of the *humerus* and the upper tip of the *ulna*, and *flex* the *forearm*.
Brachioradialis muscle: is a *muscle* attaching to the side of the *humerus* and the lower end of the *radius* that is involved in *flexing the forearm*.
Brain: is that delicate *organ* made up of the *cerebellum*, *cerebrum*, pons, *medulla oblongata*, midbrain and *spinal cord* contained within the *skull* that controls the function of the *central nervous system*.
Breathing: is the process of *respiration*, whereby air is cyclically taken in and expelled from the *lungs* using the *diaphragm* and *intercostal muscles*. The normal *respiratory* rate is between 12-16 breaths per minute, a function that is controlled by the relative amount of *blood* gases (*oxygen* and *carbon dioxide*) in the *blood*. See '*carotid body*'.
Breastbone: is a long, flat bone at the middle and front of the chest, running from the *collarbone* to the seventh *rib*. In adults, it has three pieces, and is on average 7 inches long; it tends to be longer in males than in females. It is also called the *sternum*.
Buccal nerve: is a *nerve* supplying the cheek, including the *skin*, mucous lining of cheeks, gums and some of the teeth.
Buttocks: is the *muscular* mass at the base of the back (the rump) which includes the gluteal *muscles* or "glutes".
Calcaneal tendon: See *Achilles tendon*.
Calf muscle: is the *muscle* mass, composed of more than one *muscle*, at the back of the lower leg.

Appendix B: Glossary of Medical Terms

Calvaria: is the dome-like upper portion of the *skull* (skull cap), from just above the eyebrow ridge to above the notch at the bottom rear of the *skull*.

Canthus: is the angle formed at either end of each eye, where the upper and lower eyelids meet.

Carbon dioxide: is a clear, colorless, odorless gas that is a byproduct of *respiration*.

Cardiopulmonary resuscitation: is a method of reviving someone whose *heart* has stopped beating, by using a combination of compressions to the *heart* region ("cardio-") and blowing of air into the *lungs* through the *mouth* ("pulmonary"). For adults, the ratio of compressions to breaths is 5:2.

Cardiorespiratory endurance: is the ability of the *cardiovascular* and *respiratory systems* to work together for an extended period by providing *oxygen* and nutrients to the cells of the body while eliminating *carbon dioxide* and other waste products.

Cardiovascular system: is the body's *circulatory system*, consisting of the *heart*, *blood vessels*. Arteries take *blood* away from the *heart* whereas *veins* return the de-oxygenated *blood*, and *capillaries* allow gas and nutrient exchanges to occur. Circulation is regarded as either being pulmonary (through the *lungs*) or systemic (through the body) in nature.

Carotid sinus nerve: is a branch of the *cranial nerve* (CN IX) associated with the portion of the *carotid artery* at or just beyond the point where the *artery* divides into inner and outer branches (side of the neck at the level of the top of the *Adam's apple*). See '*carotid sinus reflex*' and '*carotid body reflex*'.

Carotid artery: is the *artery* running from near the *heart* to the base of the neck (*common carotid artery*), then dividing into two parts - *internal* and *external carotid arteries*. The *internal carotid artery* is the direct continuation of the *common carotid artery* (with no cervical branches) that enters the *skull* through the *temporal bone* near the middle ear. The *external carotid artery* supplies *blood* to the face, neck and *skull*, the inner to middle ear, *brain* and eye via eight major branches.

Carotid body: is a small ovoid mass of *tissue* located at the *medial* (*deep*) side of the *bifurcation* of the *internal* and *external carotid arteries*. It is a *chemoreceptor*, a combination of the *carotid sinus nerve* (CN IX), *vagus nerve* (CN X), and *blood vessels*, that respond to changes such as decreased *blood-oxygen* levels by stimulating *respiration*, along with cardio and vascular adjustments. See '*carotid body reflex*'.

Carotid body reflex: is the chemical reaction through a *chemoreceptor* at the *carotid body* to the sensing of *blood* gas (*carbon dioxide* and *oxygen*) changes in the *common carotid artery*. When *oxygen* levels drop, the *carotid body* initiates a reflexive action *by sending nerve impulses to the brain's breathing center via the carotid sinus (CN IX) nerve*. This accordingly increases the rate and depth of *respiration*, *heart rate*, and *blood pressure* (through *vasodilation* and *vasoconstriction*), all via the *vagus nerve*.

Carotid sinus: is the slight enlargement of the wall of the *proximal* part of the *internal carotid artery* (where the *common carotid artery bifurcates* into the *internal* and *external carotid arteries*). This pressure sensitive *baroreceptor* varies *heart rate*, via the *carotid sinus*, to protect the *brain* from destructive over-pressurization. See '*carotid sinus reflex*'.

Carotid sinus reflex: is the decrease in *heart* rate in response to an increase in *blood pressure* sensed by *baroreceptors* in the *carotid sinus*.

Carotid sinus syndrome: refers to a temporary swoon or fainting due to over-activity of the *carotid sinus reflex*. Pressure on the *carotid sinus* causes a reflexive slowing of the *heart rate*, leading to loss of consciousness and sometimes to *convulsions*.

Carpals: are the 16 *bones* that form the base of the *wrist* in each *hand* (8 per *hand*). Compare with '*tarsals*'.

Cartilage: is a specialized form of relatively tough and non-elastic connective *tissue* that connects and supports. It contains no *blood* supply or *nerves* making *injury* not as readily noticeable and recovery time lengthy. Most of the nose, for example, is made up of *cartilage*.

Cartilaginous: refers to *tissue* consisting of *cartilage*.

Catabolism: refers to the chemical breakdown of complex substances into simple compounds that release energy for work, storage and heat production. See '*anabolism*'.

Cavities: are hollow spaces in the body or in an *organ*. This term also refers to the *acupuncture* or *pressure points* that are linked to *internal organs* of the body via their corresponding *meridians*, the pathways for *qi* circulation.

Celiac plexus: is also called *solar plexus* or "pit of the *stomach*". It is a large but compact network of nerves at the front and sides of the abdominal aorta behind the *stomach*. When forcefully struck just below the *breastbone*, the *phrenic nerves* can be stunned, causing the *diaphragm* to be temporarily paralyzed.

Central nervous system: is the *brain* and *spinal cord* portion of the *nervous system*.

Cerebellum: is a part of the *brain* at the lower back portion of the *skull*, which co-ordinates movement. It is typically three to four inches wide, two inches high and two inches thick.

Cerebral cortex: is a thin layer of gray matter covering the surface of the *brain*. This *cerebrum* is only three millimeters thick, yet is the control center for general movement, perception, *internal organ* functions, behavioral reactions, higher mental functions, and the co-ordination and integration of all these functions.

Cerebrum: See *cerebral cortex*.
Cervical plexus: is the network of *nerves* formed by divisions of the first four *cervical nerves* (C1-C4) in the neck.
Cervical vertebrae: are the top seven *vertebrae*, which form the neck (C1-C7). It is capable of *rotating* ninety degrees as well as bending forty-five degrees. The chin to chest movement is called *flexion*; the back of the head towards the *spine* is called *extension*.
Chemoreceptor: is a sensory *nerve* cell that is activated by chemicals. For example, an increase in *carbon dioxide* or a decrease in *oxygen* levels in the *carotid artery* is sensed at the *carotid body* (at its *bifurcation* point). A *nerve* signal is sent (via the *carotid sinus nerve*) to the *brain* to alter the *breathing rate* accordingly (via the *vagus nerve*).
Circulatory system: is the network that includes the *heart* and *blood vessels*, which enable the *circulation* of *blood* throughout the body.
Clavicle: is the *collarbone*. There are two clavicle *bones*, left and right, each of which *articulates* with the breastbone (*sternum*) and the shoulder blade (*scapula*) on either side of the *medial plane*. It is one of the most frequently broken *bones* in the body.
Clavicular notch: is the hollow area at the midpoint of the *clavicle*.
Coccyx: is the *tailbone*, consisting of four fused *vertebrae* at the very bottom of the *vertebral column*.
Collarbone: See *clavicle*.
Collateral: is a side branch of, for example, a *nerve*, *vein*, or *meridian*.
Common carotid artery: See *carotid artery*.
Common fibular nerve: is a *nerve* in the lower part of the thigh, supplying the *biceps femoris muscle*, the knee and the shin.
Concussion: is a medical condition where a loss of consciousness caused by a blow to the head or violent shaking of the head is experienced.
Concussive shock: is a blow or movement of the head leading to a *concussion*.
Convulsion: is a sudden, violent and uncontrollable contraction of *muscle* groups experienced during an epileptic attack, a post-*concussion* episode, or a post-*neck restraint* regaining of consciousness.
Coracoid process: is a strong prominence on the shoulder blade, or *scapula*, overhanging the shoulder *joint*.
Costal cartilages: are the pieces of *cartilage* attaching the *ribs* to the *sternum*.
Cranium: is the part of the *skull* that houses and protects the *brain*. It is comprised of eight *bones* (single *frontal*, *occipital*, *sphenoid*, *ethmoid bones*, and paired *temporal* and *parietal bones*). An additional fourteen *bones* make up the facial *skeleton*.
Cranial cavity: is the space occupied by the *brain* within the *skull*.
Cranial nerves: are the twelve pairs of *sensory* and *motor nerves* (numbered with Roman numerals CN I- CN XII) that emerge from the *cranial cavity* through openings in the *skull*.
Cricoid rings: are the 16-20 pliable *cartilaginous* rings that, in part, form the *trachea*. These ossify with age.
Crook of knee: refers to the back of the knee.
Cutaneous nerve: is any nerve that is close to the *skin* surface.
Death: is the absence of life. Apparent death is the end of life as indicated by the absence of a *heart beat* and *breathing*. Legal death refers to the irreversible cessation of all *brain* function, and of the spontaneous functioning of the *respiratory* and *circulatory systems* as declared by a physician. Typically, death will occur once the *brain* has been deprived of *oxygen* for more than four minutes.
Deep. means away from the surface of the body. Compare with '*superficial*'.
Deep peroneal nerve: is an alternative name for the *deep* portion of the *common fibular nerve*.
Deep temporal arteries: are *arteries* in the region of the temple, feeding the *temporal muscles*.
Deltoid muscles: are three thick, powerful shoulder *muscles* that cover the *shoulder joint*. They originate at the *scapula* and *clavicle* and insert at the *humerus*, giving it a triangular shape and a rounded shape to the shoulder.
Diaphragm: is the dome-shaped musculo-tendinous membrane separating the *abdominal cavity* from the *thoracic cavity* (where the *lungs* and *heart* are). Innervated primarily by the *phrenic nerve* (C3-C5), it is the primary *muscle* used for breathing, accounting for æ of the *respiratory* flow. See '*intercostal muscles*'.
Digestive system: consists of the *organs* associated with eating, chewing, food absorption, and solid waste elimination.
Digital nerves: are the *nerves* in the fingers.
Disease: is a condition of abnormal functioning of any structure, body part or system of an organism, or a specific illness relating to the same.
Dislocation: is the displacement of any body part, particularly of a *bone* from a *joint* (for example, *dislocation* of the *hip*, of the shoulder, of the knee).
Distal: refers to a location (arms and legs) that is further from the *median plane* or limb root. For example, the fingers are distal to the *wrist*. Compare with *proximal*.

Appendix B: Glossary of Medical Terms

Dorsiflexion: is the movement of foot that points the toes towards the shins. Compare with '*plantarflexion*'.
Dorsal cutaneous branch of the ulnar nerve: is the part of the *ulnar nerve* which supplies the little, ring, and middle fingers.
Dorsal nerves: are twelve *nerves* on each side of the back, supplying most of the *muscles* of the back.
Dorsum: is the back side of any anatomical structure.
Eardrum: is a thin membrane dividing the outer from the middle and inner ear *cavities*. It can be punctured if the outer ear is struck in such a way as to send a percussive shock wave into the ear canal.
Elbow: is the point of the *flexed* arm formed by the *proximal* end of the *ulna* (*olecranon*).
Elbow joint: is the juncture of the *humerus* with the *radius* and *ulna bones* forming both *hinge* and *pivot joints*.
Endocrine glands: are *organs* which secrete hormones into the *circulatory system* (for example, the testes, the ovaries, the pituitary gland, the thyroid gland).
Endocrine system: is the network of *endocrine glands* that secrete hormones into the *circulatory system*.
Endocrineous: refers to the *endocrine* system.
Epicondyle: is a knuckle-like projection at the end of a *bone*, such as found on the *humerus* and *femur*.
Epiglottis: is the cartilage-like structure that overhangs the windpipe like a lid. It closes while swallowing in order to prevent food from entering the windpipe.
Esophagus: is the nine and a half inch long *muscular* canal (gullet) or digestive tube that extends from below the *tongue* to the *stomach*.
Ethmoid bone: is the cubical-shaped *bone* between the eyes, at the root of the nose.
Exhalation: refers to the expulsion of air out of the *lungs*. This is done through the relaxation of the *diaphragm* and contraction of *internal intercostal muscles*.
Extension: is the action of bending, or being bent such that the angle between two connecting *bones* is increased. See '*flexion*'.
Extensor: is a *muscle* that *extends* or straightens out part of the body.
Extensor carpi radialis muscles: are the long (longus) and short (brevis) radial *extensor muscles* of the *forearm* which *extend* and *abduct* the *hand* at the *wrist joint*.
External: means outer or *muscular*. Compare with '*internal*'.
External malleolus: is the lower end of the *fibula*, forming the *ankle bone*.
External nasal nerves: are those *nerves* that run in the nasal *cavity* under the bridge of the nose to its tip. See *anterior ethmoidal nerves*.
External oblique muscles: *muscles* in the *abdomen*, by the lower eight *ribs*, which compress the *abdominal cavity*, and also *flex* and *rotate* the *vertebral column*.
Facial nerve: is a *motor nerve* (seventh *cranial nerve*) which supplies the *muscles* controlling facial expression.
Femur: is the thigh *bone*, the largest, heaviest, and strongest *bone* in the body.
Femoral artery: is a major *artery* supplying the *abdominal* wall, genitals and lower body that can be palpated at the inner upper thigh.
Femoral nerve: is the *nerve* supplying the front thigh muscles, hip and *knee joints*, and the *skin* of the leg.
Fibula: is the smaller, *laterally*-positioned of the two *bones* of the lower leg (the other being the *tibia*).
Fibular nerve: is a *nerve* running the length of the *fibula*, dividing into *superficial* and *deep* branches.
Flexion: is the action of bending, or being bent such that the angle between two connecting *bones* is decreased. Compare with '*extension*'.
Flexor carpi radialis muscles: are *muscles* that flex and *abduct* the *wrist*.
Floating ribs: are the two lowest *ribs* on either side of the *spine*, which do not attach to the *sternum*.
Foot: is comprised of 26 *bones* and has mobility and weight-bearing functions. These *bones* form three arches that absorb shock, balance the body, and give spring to the step.
Fore knuckles: are the middle knuckles or second *joints* of the fingers and the thumb.
Forearm: is the part of the arm from the *wrist* to the *elbow*, consisting of the *radius* and the *ulna bones*.
Fracture: means to break, specifically a *bone*.
Frontal bone: is one of the *bones* that make up the front of the *skull* (around the forehead).
Frontal plane: is the plane that divides the body into the *anterior* (front) and *posterior* (rear) sections.
Frontal lobes of the brain: is the forward portion of the *brain*, responsible for the processing of vision and language.
Gall bladder: is a sac-like structure attached to the surface of the *liver*, in which bile is stored and released into the bile duct. Bile functions to digest fats.
Gastrocnemius muscle: is the main, two-part *muscle* forming the *calf*. It *flexes* both the knee and the *ankle*.
Glabella: is the flat area of the forehead, between the eyebrow arches. A blow to the glabella can cause *concussion* or *death* due to the damage of the *frontal lobes*.
Great auricular nerve: is a *sensory nerve*, supplying the *skin* over the back of the jaw, and the surface of the ear.
Great occipital nerve: is a *sensory* and *motor nerve*, supplying the neck *muscles* and the *skin* of the *scalp* as far up as the top of the head.

Hamstrings: are *muscles* running from the bottom *posterior* of the hip to either side of the top of the lower leg. They are responsible for *extension* of the lower leg from the *knee joint*.

Hand: is a sophisticated set of 27 *bones*, including an opposing thumb that has an exceptional *range of movement* that allows us, on the most basic level, to grasp and manipulate tools.

Heart: is the fist-sized *muscular organ* located slightly to the left center of the chest whose expansions and contractions cause the *circulation* of the *blood*. The *heart* is actually a double pump that annually beats 40 million times to *circulate* 650,000 gallons *blood*.

Heart rate: is the number of *heartbeats* per minute. The heart rate can be checked by placing finger(s) over the point of a major *artery* so that the pulses can be palpated and counted over a given short time period (and extrapolated over a minute). The maximum theoretical *heart rate* (beats per minute) can be calculated by subtracting a person's age from 220.

Hematoma: is a localized collection of *blood* in *tissue*s or body spaces, known colloquially as a bruise.

Hemorrhage: is *bleeding*; caused the escape of *blood* from *blood vessels*.

Hinge joint: is a fluid-filled *joint* that allows for extensive movement in one plane (i.e., finger *joints*).

Hipbone: is made up of the ilium, ischium and pubis *bones*. Known also as the coxal *bone*, the pair of *hipbones* constitutes the *pelvic girdle*.

Hip joint: is where the head of the *femur* meets the ilium to form a *ball and socket joint*.

Humerus: is the *bone* of the upper arm, from shoulder to *elbow*.

Hyoid bone: is the u-shaped *bone* just above the *thyroid cartilage*, which serves as the floating base of attachment for the *tongue*.

Hyper-flexion: refers to the forceful over-*flexion* of a limb or *joint* resulting in *muscle*, *tendon*, *ligament* and *joint capsule* damage.

Hypoglossal: means under the *tongue*.

Hypoglossal nerve: is a *motor nerve* which supplies the *tongue muscles*. It can be accessed by hooking the fingers under the jaw line.

Hypoxia: is the state of having too little oxygen in the cells (person turns blue). Mild hypoxia increases heart rate and respiratory rates. Severe hypoxia results in respiratory failure leading to death.

Ilioinguinal nerves: are *sensory nerves* supplying the groin region and the upper portion of the inner thighs.

Incontinence: is the inability to control one's *urinary* or bowel functions.

Infection: is the invasion of the body's *tissue*s by microorganisms (e.g., bacteria, viruses, fungi) which multiply, often producing toxins which cause illness.

Inferior: refers to the location below something else (opposite of *'superior'*). For example, the foot is inferior to the knee.

Infraorbital nerves: are *sensory nerves* supplying the lower portion of the eye sockets.

Inguinal crease: is the region where the scrotum or labia major adjoins the thigh.

Inhalation: refers to the intake of air into the *lungs*. This is done through the contraction of the *diaphragm* and the *external intercostal muscles* (while the *internal intercostal muscles* are relaxed).

Injury: is physical harm or damage done to the body.

Innobinate bone: See 'hipbone'.

Insertion point: is the place (further from the *midline* of the body) where a *muscle* attaches to a *bone* that it moves. See *'origin point'*.

Intercostal: means between the *ribs*.

Intercostal muscles: are the three layers of *muscles* joining the *ribs* together that account for º of the *respiratory* flow. See *'diaphragm'*.

Intercostal nerves: are the *nerves* that supply the *intercostal muscles*.

Intermaxillary suture: is the fibrous seam joining together the two *bones* that form the upper jaw.

Intermediate supraclavicular nerves: are the *sensory nerves* that pass over the *collarbone*, supplying the chest and shoulder *muscles*.

Internal: refers to having to do with the inside of the body or of a specific part of the body or what is of a non-muscular nature.

Internal carotid artery: is that portion of the *carotid artery* supplying *oxygen*ated *blood* deeply to the *brain*, the middle ear, and the eye socket.

Internal jugular vein: is that portion of the *jugular vein* carrying *blood* from a large portion of the head and neck returning back to the *heart*.

Internal oblique muscles: are the *muscles* running from the lower edge of the *rib* cage to the pelvis, involved in *rotating* the *vertebral column* and pulling in the *abdomen*.

Involuntary muscles: are the *muscles* whose movements are not subject to one's will or control (i.e., the *muscles* of the *internal organs*).

Ischemia: is the condition of having poor blood supply to an organ or part of the body.

Appendix B: Glossary of Medical Terms

Jaw hinge: is the point at which the upper (*maxilla*) and lower (*mandible*) *bones* of the jaw *articulate*.
Joint: is a point at which the ends of two or more *bones* meet.
Joint capsule: is any structure, usually composed of *cartilage*, which encloses a *joint*.
Jugular notch: is the point of indentation immediately above the centre-point where the *bones* of the *clavicle* (*collarbone*) meet at the base of the neck. This is an effective point at which to exert pressure using one or more digits, to repel an opponent's advance in a conflict requiring lower levels of force.
Jugular vein: is one of the major *veins*, which brings *oxygen*-depleted *blood* from the head and neck back to the *lungs* and *heart* for re-oxygenation and re-circulation.
Kidney: is one of a pair of *organs*, located in the lower *posterior torso* region, which filter the *blood* to remove toxic by-products of metabolism, such as urea (in the form of *urine*). The kidneys are also critical in regulating the level of essential salts such as potassium, sodium, and phosphates, and hydrogen in the body. Forceful impact to one or both kidneys can result in permanent, potentially fatal, *injury* to the victim.
Knee cap: is the piece of *cartilage* in both legs which covers the *anterior joint* between the upper and lower *bones* of the leg.
Knee joint: is the junction of the *femur* and the *tibia*. The *anterior* portion of this *joint* is protected by the *knee cap*. Although it is well-constructed primarily a *hinge joint* (with some gliding, rolling and rotational abilities), it is susceptible to *injury* by *hyper-extension*.
Labiomental groove: is the area between the chin and lower lip.
Large intestine: is also called the lower intestine. This is the second 'half' of the intestinal tract, called 'large' because of its larger diameter rather than its greater length (the *small intestine* is actually much longer). The main function of the large intestine is to reabsorb most of the water from the body's solid waste material before evacuation (defecation). Rupture of the large intestine can lead to *death* due to contamination of the *abdominal cavity* and *internal organs* by the toxins in fecal matter.
Laryngeal nerves: is a complex set of *nerves* supplying the *larynx*, *trachea* and *esophagus*.
Laryngeal prominence: See *Adam's apple*.
Larynx: is commonly known as the 'voicebox'. This *cartilaginous* and *muscular* structure both contributes to one's voice quality and, more critically, controls the passage of air to the *lungs* via the *trachea*.
Lateral: refers to the location to one or the other side of the *median plane* (center) of the body, or of a bodily structure.
Lateral cutaneous nerve: is a *sensory nerve* supplying the *skin* of the side (lateral) and front portions of the thigh.
Lateral femoral cutaneous nerve: is a *sensory nerve* supplying the *muscle* of the side and front portions of the thigh.
Latissimus dorsi muscle: is the *muscle* of the outermost (i.e., most *lateral*) portion of the lower back (known colloquially as 'lats' or 'swimmer's muscle').
Lesser occipital nerve: is a *sensory nerve* supplying some of the *skin* on the head and around the ear.
Ligament: is tough, flexible fibrous *tissue*, which connects and supports *bones* or other *internal* body structures. They are less elastic and more prone to tearing than *tendons*.
Lingual lacerations: are cuts or tear *wounds* to the *tongue*.
Lips: are the fleshy, *external* portions of the *mouth*.
Liver: is a large and critical *internal organ*, situated in the upper right portion of the *abdominal cavity*. The liver has many functions, including filtering the *blood*, secreting bile and other metabolic substances, and conversion of sugars into glycogen (a storage unit of sugars).
Lumbar: refers to the lower region of the back.
Lumbar vertebrae: are the five *vertebrae* (L1-L5) located in the lower-most section of the back. They are larger than the other *vertebrae* because they must support more weight.
Lung: is one of a pair of light spongy *organs* in the chest, which are critical for life. Being the main part of the body's breathing system, the highly elastic *lungs* take in air, absorb the *oxygen* from that air, and pass on that *oxygen* into the *blood* stream for the rest of the body. On each deep breath, the *lungs* exhale on average four quarts of unabsorbed *oxygen* and *carbon dioxide*, a waste product of the body.
Mandible: is the large *bone* forming the lower jaw.
Manubrium: is the widest, thickest and uppermost section of the three parts of the *sternum* that is fixed between the first two *ribs*.
Mastoid process: is the projection of the *temporal bone* behind the ear canal that serves as the attachment for various *muscles*.
Medial: refers to the location that is closer to the *median plane* (midline) of the body. For example, the nose is medial to the ear.
Median nerve: is a major *motor* and *sensory nerve* of the arm that runs along the *forearm* and *hand* from the *brachial plexus*.
Median plane: is a body plane that is also called the midline. It divides the body symmetrically into left and right sides. The terms '*lateral*' and '*medial*' refer to this plane.

Medulla oblongata: is the top of the *spinal cord*, that forms the base of the *brain*. It contains important *nerves* that deal with vital functions such as *breathing* and the *circulation* of the *blood*.

Meninges: are the three membrane layers covering the *brain* and *spinal cord*. Inflammation of the meninges, due to bacterial infection, is called meningitis.

Mental nerve: is a *sensory nerve* of the chin and lower lip.

Mental stunning: refers to the temporary confusion, accompanied by dizziness, due to *nerves* in the head being overloaded, usually due to a strong blow to the head.

Metacarpals: are the 10 *bones* (5 per *hand*) that make up the palms of the *hands* (excluding the fingers). See 'metatarsals'.

Metatarsals: are the 10 *bones* (5 per foot) that make up the main part of the *foot* (excluding the toes). See 'metacarpals'.

Middle meningeal artery: is an *artery* supplying *blood* to the *bones* of the head, and to the outer layer of the *meninges* (called the dura mater).

Middle meningeal vessels: are the *blood vessels* branching from the *middle meningeal artery*.

Midline: See 'median plane'.

Motor nerves: are those *nerves* that are responsible for *muscular* contractions producing body motion. See *sensory nerves*.

Mouth: is the *anterior* opening of the alimentary canal; also one of the two openings to the airway (the other being the nose).

Muscle fiber types: are the two types of *muscle* fibers: striated or voluntary, the contraction of which is usually under one's control (with the exception of the *heart muscle*, which is striated but not voluntary); and non-striated, smooth, or involuntary, the contraction of which is not under one's control.

Muscular system: consists of *muscle* groups that allow for motion to occur, stabilize body movements, produce heat, regulate *organ* storage (*urine* and fecal matter), and are responsible for the movement of substances throughout the body. There are over 650 *muscles* in the body (making up 36% of body weight for women and 42% for men). There are 430 voluntary (*skeletal*) and 220 involuntary *muscles* (controlling bodily functions).

Muscles: are the *organ tissues* in the body that produce body movement through cooperative and coordinated antagonistic *muscular* contractions.

Muscular branch of the femoral nerve: is a *sensory* and *motor nerve* that supplies the *muscles* of the front of the thigh.

Nasal bone: are either of the two *bones* which form the bridge of the nose.

Nasal cavity: the area in the *skull* from the nares (*nostrils*) to the opening of the pharynx (throat).

Nasolabial groove: the indentation in the *bone* (and marked by a trough in the *skin*) between the bottom tip of the nose and the upper lip.

Natural range of motion: is the area of movement of which a limb or other body part is capable without excessive *strain*, pain, *fracture* (of bone) or tearing/rupturing of *muscles, joints, or tendons*.

Nerve endings: are the points of *nerve* cells which receive information (in the case of *sensory nerves*) or send information commands (in the case of *motor nerves*) to the regions they innervate.

Nerve: is one or more bundles of signal-carrying fibers between the *brain* and *spinal cord* with other parts of the body. There are twelve pairs of *cranial nerves* and thirty-one pairs of *spinal nerves* on both sides of the body.

Nerve plexus: Is a group of joined *nerves* such as the *solar plexus, cervical plexus*, etc.

Nervous system: is the network of cells and *tissues* that convey and record information throughout the body, by chemical and electrical means. The main parts of the nervous system, from which the other parts derive and with which the rest of the system interacts, are the *brain* and the *spinal cord*.

Nostrils: are the *external* portions (nares) of the nose that serve as opening for *breathing*.

Obstruction: refers to something that blocks or clogs a passage or opening or the condition of being blocked or clogged.

Obturator nerve: is a *sensory* and *motor nerve* supplying the middle thigh area, and the *knee* and *hip joints*.

Occipital arteries: the arteries supplying the neck and *scalp muscles* and the *mastoid process*.

Occipital bone: is the large, roughly trapezoidal-shaped *bone* at the rear of the *skull*.

Occipital nerves: *sensory* and *motor nerves* supplying the *skin* in the occipital area.

Oculomotor nerve: is the third *cranial nerve*; a *sensory* and *motor nerve* with branches serving the upper eyelid, the *muscle* which moves the eye inward, and the *muscle* which constricts the pupil.

Olecranon: is the *proximal* end of the *ulna*, which forms the *elbow*.

Orbicularis oris muscle: is the *muscle* that moves the lips.

Orbit: one of a pair of *bony* concave openings in the *skull* that house the eyeballs.

Organ: is an organized set of *tissues* that performs specialized functions in the body.

Origin point: is the place on the *bone* (closer to the *midline* of the body) to which a *muscle* attaches. This is usually to a larger and more stable *bone*. See 'insertion point'.

Appendix B: Glossary of Medical Terms

Oxygen: is a tasteless, odorless and colorless gas which comprises approximately 20 percent of the Earth's atmosphere at surface level, and which is essential for the survival of animals and plants.
Palmar cutaneous branch of median nerve: is a *sensory nerve* supplying the palm of the *hand*.
Palmaris longus muscle: is a *muscle* running from the lower end of the *humerus* to the palm, responsible for *flexing* the *wrist* and tensing the palm.
Paralysis: refers to the inability to voluntarily move a part of the body normally under voluntary control.
Parietal bones: are the main side *bones* of the *skull*.
Patella: is the *kneecap*, a flat triangular-shaped *bone* that protects the front of the *knee joint*.
Pathogens: are any agents of *disease*, usually microorganisms such as bacteria, fungi and viruses.
Pectoral: refers to the breast or chest.
Pectoralis major muscles: are the large chest (*pectoral*) *muscles* that cover the upper front of the *torso*, and which *flex* and *rotate* the shoulder/arm.
Pectoralis minor muscles: are the smaller *pectoral muscles*, attaching at the top of the *scapula* (*coracoid process*) and at the 3rd, 4th, and 5th ribs. They function in the movement of the shoulder blades and shoulder.
Pelvic girdle: is made up of the two *hipbones*.
Pelvis: is the lower part of the trunk of the body that is comprised of four *bones*: two *hipbones*, the *sacrum* and the *coccyx*.
Pericardium: is a fibrous double-layered *tissue* sac enclosing the *heart*.
Perineum: is the area between the anus and the scrotum or vulva.
Peripheral nervous system: is the portion of the *nervous system* outside of the *brain* and the *spinal cord* (which form the *central nervous system*).
Phalanges: are the 28 *bones* of the fingers (3 per finger and 2 per thumb) and the 28 *bones* of the toes (3 per toe and 2 per big toe).
Philtrum: is the area between the bottom of the nose and the upper lip.
Phrenic nerves: are *sensory* and *motor nerves* (C3- C5) in the *diaphragm* region, involved in the control of breathing.
Physiology: is the study of the physical and chemical processes in the workings of the human body. See '*anatomy*'.
Pivot joint: is a *joint* that allows for back and forth *rotational* movement, like the *elbow joint*.
Plantarflexion: is the movement of the *foot* that points the toes away from the shins. Compare with '*dorsiflexion*'.
Platysma: is a *muscle* originating from the upper portion of the chest, and inserting at the lower *mandible* and face. It functions to wrinkle the *skin* of the neck and to depress the lower face and chin.
Pleura: is the thin membrane forming the outside of the *lungs*, and lining the *thoracic cavity*. The pleurae protect and cushion the *lungs*.
Popliteal fossa: is the hollow region behind the knee.
Positional asphyxia: is the severe loss of *oxygen* that is induced by placing a (usually overweight and drugged) person on his belly. If a person is *hog-tied*, it further exacerbates the difficulty he can have trying to breath.
Posterior: refers to a position that is the back (rear) of the body or is behind a body structure (opposite to '*anterior*'). For example, the spine is posterior to the chest.
Posterior antebrachial cutaneous nerve: is a *sensory nerve* supplying the *skin* of the rear of the *forearm*.
Posterior brachial cutaneous nerve: is a *sensory nerve* supplying the *skin* on the rear of the upper arm.
Posterior cutaneous femoral nerves: are *sensory nerves* supplying the *skin* of the buttocks, genitalia, and the rear of the thigh and *calf*.
Posterior interosseous nerves: are *sensory* and *motor nerves* between the two *bones* of the *forearm*, supplying *muscles* that *extend* the thumb and second finger, and the *wrist*.
Posterior scrotal nerves: are *sensory nerves* supplying the *skin* of the scrotum.
Posterior cervical triangle: is the triangle formed between the *posterior* border of the *sternocleidomastoid*, the *trapezius* muscles and the *collarbone*. Compare with '*anterior cervical triangle*'.
Process: is a part of a structure that sticks out, or projects, from the structure.
Prone: means to lie face down. Compare with '*supine*'.
Proximal: refers to the location that is nearer to the *median plane* or limb root (opposite of *distal*). For example, the *wrist* is proximal to the fingers.
Pterion: is the point where all the major *bones* of the *skull* (*frontal, parietal, temporal, sphenoid*) meet in the temple area.
Pubic symphysis: is the area at the front of the *pelvis* where the two pubic *bones* meet.
Pudendal nerve: is a *sensory, motor,* and *parasympathetic nerve* supplying the *skin, muscles* and erectile *tissues* in the *perineal* region.
Pulse: is the dilation of an *artery*, directly corresponding to the beating of the *heart*.
Quadreplegic: refers to having the loss of the use of all four limbs.
Radial artery: is an *artery* supplying the *forearm, wrist,* and *hand*.
Radial edge: is the inner portion of the *forearm* formed by the *radius*.

Radial nerve: is a *sensory* and *motor nerve* with many branches, supplying the *skin* on the back of the arm, the *forearm*, and the *hand*, *muscles* on the back of the arm and *forearm*, the *elbow joint*, and other *joints* in the *hand*. It is the direct continuation of the *posterior* cord of the *brachial plexus* and its largest branch.

Radius: is the *bone* that runs along the inner side of the *forearm*.

Range of movement: refers to the maximal degree of movement in all directions possible without experiencing an *injury*.

Reproductive system: is the system of genital *organs* (ovaries, testes, *external* genitalia) that is responsible for *reproduction*.

Respiratory system: are the *organs* and associated structures involved in *breathing*, including the nose, throat, *larynx*, *trachea*, bronchi and *lungs*. This system supplies *oxygen* to the body and eliminates *carbon dioxide* via the *circulatory system*.

Resuscitation: is the action of restarting someone's *respiratory* and/or *cardiovascular systems* after they have ceased to function.

Rib: is one of the 12 pairs of *bone* that make up the protective rib cage. The first seven pairs of ribs are 'true ribs' as they attach to the *sternum* and *vertebrae*. The other five pairs of ribs are 'false ribs' because the first three pairs join the ribs above and the last two pairs are free at the *lateral* ends and are called 'floating ribs'.

Rotation: is the movement of a body part around its longitudinal axis.

Sacral vertebrae: is the lower portion of the *spine* formed from the natural fusion of five *vertebrae*.

Sacrum: is the large, triangular-shaped *bone* at the bottom of the *spinal cord* and above *coccyx*.

Sagittal plane: is any plane running parallel to the *median plane* of the body.

Saphenous nerve: is a *sensory nerve* supplying the *knee joint*, *kneecap* region, and the *skin* on parts of the leg and *foot*.

Scalp: is the *skin* of the head, excluding ears and face.

Scapula: is the shoulder blade.

Sciatic nerve: is a *sensory* and *motor nerve* with several branches supplying numerous regions of the lower body. It is the largest *nerve* of the body running down the back of the entire leg.

Seimitendinosus muscle: is a *muscle* at the back of the thigh, which *extends* the thigh, and *flexes* and *rotates* the leg.

Sense organs: are any of the *organs* involved in sensory reception (i.e., taste, touch, smell, sight, and hearing).

Sensory nerves: are nerves that carry sense signals from parts of body to the *brain* or *spinal cord*. See 'motor nerves'.

Shoulder joint: is the juncture of the *proximal* end of the *humerus* (head of the greater tubercle) with the *scapula* (acromion process), forming a *ball and socket joint*. The *joint* is a shallow one, making *dislocation* relatively easy but it allows for excellent mobility.

Skeletal muscles: are striated *muscles* that typically attach to *bones* and cross one or more *joints*.

Skeletal system: is the supporting frame for the body, consisting of 206 *bones*. These *bones* protect the *internal organs*, provides attachments for *muscles* which enables body movement, serve as *blood* reservoirs and sources of red *blood* cells. There are two classifications of skeletons: 1) axial skeleton (80 *bones* arranged along the vertical body axis as a support structure), and 2) appendicular skeleton (126 *bones* that allows for body movement).

Skin: is the tough, supple membrane consisting of five layers of cells covering the entire body. It is also a sensory *organ* and is the largest *organ* of the body.

Skull: is the bony structure of the *cranium* (8 *bones*) and the 14 *bones* of the face that houses the *brain*.

Small intestine: is the upper portion of the intestinal tract. Although it is much longer than the *large intestine*, it is called "small" because it has a smaller diameter than the *large intestine* (or bowel).

Smooth muscles: are one of two kinds of involuntary *muscle* as found in the *stomach* and intestines.

Solar plexus: is also known as the *celiac plexus*, a dense cluster of *nerve* cells and supporting *tissue*, located behind the *stomach* in the region of the celiac *artery*, just below the *diaphragm*. The solar plexus is the largest autonomic *nerve* center in the *abdominal cavity*. A blow to the solar plexus can cause significant pain and may also temporarily halt intestinal and respiratory activity.

Somatic nervous system: is that portion of the *nervous system* controlling *muscles* that are under voluntary control.

Sphenoid bone: is a wedge-shaped (sphenoid) bone in the *skull* just *posterior* to the *orbital* region, but *anterior* to the *temporal* region.

Spinal column: consists of 33 *vertebrae* separated by spongy disks that make up the *spine* or *backbone*. The spine is divided into five regions: 7 *cervical vertebrae* (C1-C7), 12 *thoracic vertebrae* (T1-T12), 5 *lumbar vertebrae* (L1-L5), 5 *sacral vertebrae* (fused) and the 4 *coccyx vertebrae* (fused). This *vertebral column* is a strong, flexible (capable of bending in all directions and rotation) housing for the *spinal cord*. It also serves as an attachment site for the *ribs*, pelvic girdle *muscles* and the head.

Appendix B: Glossary of Medical Terms

Spinal atlas: is the first *cervical vertebrae* (C1) which connects the head to the spine and sits atop the *spinal axis* (C2), the second *cervical vertebrae*. The head can *rotate*, *extend*, and *flex* at this lower *joint*.

Spinal axis: is the second *cervical vertebrae* (C2) on top of which is the *spinal atlas* (C1), the first *cervical vertebrae*. The head can *rotates*, *extends*, and *flexes* on this *vertebrae*.

Spinal cord: consists of 31 pairs of *spinal nerves* which run from the base of the *skull* to the upper part of the lower back within the *vertebral* canal of the *spinal column*. It averages less than a half of an inch in diameter, and 16.5-18.0 inches in length with a total weight of one ounce.

Spleen: is an *organ* in the upper left *abdominal* region, which filters *blood* and produces lymphocytes (white *blood* cells, essential for the body's immune system).

Sprain: is an *injury* to the *muscles*, *tendons*, or *ligaments* around a *joint*. Compare with 'strain'.

Sternal angle: is the angle formed where the body of the *sternum* meets the *manubrium* above it.

Sternal shield: is the name given to the *sternum* because of the protection it gives to the *internal organs* like the *heart* that underlie it.

Sternocleidomastoid muscle: is a *muscle* extending from the *sternum* and *clavicular* head to the *mastoid process* of the head, which *rotates* the head and *flexes* the upper portion of the *vertebral column*.

Sternum: is the *breastbone* that is composed of three parts: the *manubrium* top section), the sternal body, and the *xyphoid process* (bottom section).

Stomach: is an *organ* of the body involved in the digestion of food. Once food passes from the *mouth* into the *esophagus*, it then proceeds to the *stomach*, where it is further broken down and mixed with gastric juices, forming a liquid, which then passes to the *small intestine* for further digestion.

Strain: is an *injury* to a *tendon* or *muscle*, caused by trauma or overuse. See 'sprain'..

Styloid process: is a spike-shaped projection at the *medial* base of the *skull*, to which three *muscles* and two *ligaments* attach.

Subclavian artery: is an *artery* supplying the neck, *thoracic* wall, *spinal cord*, *brain*, and upper limbs (via the *brachial artery*).

Subclavian vein: is the continuation of the *axillary* (armpit) *vein* in the upper body where it runs under the *clavicle*.

Suffocation: is also called asphyxiation: *death* due to lack of *oxygen* in the air one breathes.

Superficial: means near the surface of the body. An equivalent term is *external* (opposite of *internal*). Compare with 'deep'.

Superficial branch: is the branch of an *artery*, *vein* or other body structure that is closer to the surface than other branches.

Superficial carotid arteries: are the *carotid arteries* that are closer to the body's surface than the *internal carotid arteries*.

Superior: refers to the location above something else (opposite of *inferior*). For example, the knee is superior to the foot.

Superior cervical ganglion: a cluster of *nerve* cells and fibers near the second and third *cervical vertebrae*. It passes *nerve* fibers to the *heart*, *pharynx*, *larynx* and head.

Superior laryngeal nerve: is a nerve with several, complex, functions originating at the *vagus nerve* and supplying *muscles* of the *pharynx* and *larynx*, and the mucous membranes at the back of the *tongue*.

Supinator longus (brachioradialis) muscle: is a *muscle* originating along the *humerus*, inserting at the lower end of the *radius*, and functioning to *flex* the *forearm*.

Supine: means to lie flat on the back. Compare with 'prone'.

Supraclavicular fossa: is an indentation or depression in the neck, just above and behind the *clavicle*.

Supraclavicular nerves: is the collection of *nerves* in the region above the *clavicle* (in the *posterior cervical triangle*), supplying the regions around the *collarbone*, and the *pectoral* and *deltoid muscles*.

Supraorbital nerves: are *sensory nerves* supplying the upper eyelid, forehead, and front portion of the *scalp*.

Suprasternal notch: is the notch on the *sternum*, between the *clavicular notches*.

Sural nerve: is the *nerve* formed by the union of branches of the *tibial* and common *fibular nerves*. This *nerve* supplies the *lateral* side of the leg and *ankle*.

System: is a series of interconnected parts (e.g., *organs*) which function together and produce results which would not be possible through the action of the parts in isolation.

Tail bone: is the *coccyx*; the lower end of the *vertebral column*.

Tarsals: are the 14 *bones* of the *ankle*s (7 per foot). Compare with 'carpals'.

Teeth: are the 32 hard, conical structures set in the upper and lower jaws in the *mouth* that are used for biting and chewing.

Temple: is the flat region on either side of the head, between the forehead and the ear.

Temporal: having to do with, or in the region of, the *temple*.

Temporal bone: is one of a pair of large *bones* of the lower head that underlies the ear.
Temporal muscle: is the *muscle* covering the side of the head that elevates the *mandible*.
Temporomandibular joint: is the *joint* that hinges the lower *mandible* of the jaw to the *temporal bone* of the *skull*. It is one of the most frequently used *joints* in the body.
Tendon: is a tough, flexible (but inelastic) fibrous *tissue* joining a *muscle* to a *bone*.
Testicles: are the pair of male sex glands located in the scrotum.
Thenar eminence: is the mound of *muscle* and *tissue* at the base of the thumb, on the palm of the *hand*.
Thoracic cavity: is the chest *cavity* that contains the *heart* and *lungs*.
Thoracic nerves: are the twelve pairs of *nerves* arising from the *thoracic* segments of the *spinal cord*, supplying the *thoracic* wall and upper *abdominal* region.
Thoracic vertebrae: are the (usually) twelve *vertebrae* (T1- T12) located between the *cervical* and the *lumbar vertebrae* (roughly in the mid-back region).
Thoracoabdominal nerves: are the *inferior intercostal nerves* that run from between the *ribs* and between the *internal* oblique and transverse *abdominal muscles* to innervate the *abdominal skin* and *muscles*.
Thorax: is the chest area of the body.
Thyroid cartilage: is the largest piece of *cartilage* forming the *larynx*; it forms the *laryngeal prominence*, or *Adam's apple*.
Tibia: is the larger, weight-bearing, *bone* of the lower leg (the other bone is the *fibula*).
Tibial nerves: are multi-branched *sensory* and *motor nerves*, originating from the *sciatic nerve*, supplying the *knee joint*, the *muscles* and *skin* of the *calf*, the sole of the *foot*, and the toes.
Tissue: is a collection of similar cells that act together in doing a particular function.
Tongue: is the *muscle* located and anchored in the *mouth* (and throat by the *hyoid bone*). It is the main taste *organ* and is used for eating, and related activities.
Torso: is the *thoracic* (chest) and *abdominal* (belly) regions of the body (i.e., the body, excluding the head and limbs).
Trachea: is the tube forming the airway from the back of the throat through to the point where it branches into the left and right bronchi that open into the *lungs*.
Transverse plane: is the plane that divides the body into *superior* (upper) and *inferior* (lower) sections.
Transverse cervical artery: is a branch of the *cervical artery*, supplying *muscles* of the shoulder blade (*scapula*) and *trapezius* regions.
Transverse cervical nerve: stems from the C2 and C3 *vertebrae* to feed the *skin* in the front of the neck.
Transverse crease: any crease or fold that runs across an area of *skin*.
Transverse cubital crease: is the crease at the inner part of the *elbow*, where the arm bends inward.
Transverse foramina: is the passage in the *cervical vertebrae* through which the *vertebral blood vessels* pass.
Trapezius muscles: are *muscles* running from the neck to the *clavicle* and *scapula*, rotating the *scapula* and elevating the shoulder.
Triceps muscle: is the *muscle* in the arm that *extends* (straightens) the *elbow*.
Triceps tendon: is the *tendon* attaching the *triceps muscle* to the *proximal* end of the *ulna* (*olecranon*).
Ulna: is the larger of the two *bones* forming the *forearm*, on the side of the little finger.
Ulnar edge: is the outer edge of the *forearm* formed by the *ulna*.
Ulnar nerve: is the larger of two terminal branches of the *medial* cord of the *brachial plexus*. It can be accessed by applying pressure to the *medial epicondyle* ("funny bone") and *medial* portion of the *olecranon*.
Umbilicus: is the belly button or navel.
Unconsciousness: is the temporary partial or complete loss of consciousness, due to a temporary reduction in *blood* flow (and hence in *oxygen* supply) to the *brain*.
Urinary system: is the system responsible for filtering *blood* and consequently producing (*kidneys*), transporting (ureters), storing (*urinary bladder*) and intermittently excreting (urethra) *urine*.
Urinary bladder: is the sac in which the body holds *urine* prior to voiding it from the body.
Urine: is the fluid secreted by the *kidneys*.
Vagus nerve: is either of a pair of complex, multi-functional and multi-branched *nerves*, arising from the *brain* (as the tenth *cranial nerve*: CN X), and branching through the neck and thorax into the abdomen. It supplies such varied regions as the ear, *tongue*, *pharynx* and *larynx*, the *esophagus*, and the *thoracic* and *abdominal cavities*.
Valsalva maneuver: is the forcible attempt at *exhalation* whilst keeping the passages to the *mouth* and nose closed (i.e., when one is *straining* to lift a heavy weight). This increases *thoracic cavity* pressure which temporarily reduces *blood* flow (a condition which assists in rendering a person *unconscious* in *lateral vascular neck restraint*) and increases *blood pressure*.
Vasodilation: refers to the widening of the *blood vessels*, a condition that is helpful in lowering *blood pressure*. The *vagus nerve* innervates the *lungs*, *heart* and *blood vessels*. See *carotid body reflex*.

Appendix B: Glossary of Medical Terms

Vasoconstriction: refers to the narrowing of the *blood vessels* in response to cold, fear, stress, and drugs like nicotine.
Vein: is a *blood vessel* that carries *oxygen*-depleted *blood* back to the *lungs* and *heart* for reoxygenation and recirculation to the body, via the *arteries*.
Vena cava vessels: are two large veins (inferior and superior) that returns blood from the lower body and upper body respectively, to the heart.
Ventricular fibrillation: is a condition of fast erratic heart beats, resulting in a complete lack of a regular heart beat and no blood pressure. Unconsciousness will quickly ensue and death may occur within four minutes.
Vertebral column: See *spinal column'*.
Vertebral subluxation: is the displacement of a *vertebra*.
Vertex: is the top of a body or structure (i.e., crown of the head).
Visceral organs: are the *organs* of the body located in the chest and *abdomen*.
Whiplash: is an *injury* to the neck, caused by *hyperextension* of the neck *muscles*.
Windpipe: is the *cartilaginous* and *bony* tube in the throat through which air passes to the *lungs*. It is also called the *trachea*.
Wounds: is any physical *injury* involving a break in the *skin*.
Wrist: is comprised of eight *carpal bones* arranged in two rows.
Wrist joint: is the juncture of the *radius* and *ulna* bones with several of the *carpal bones* in the *wrist*.
Xiphoid process: is the small, pointed *bone* at the lower end of the *sternum*.
Zygomaticotemporalis nerve: is the *sensory nerve* supplying the *skin* of the *temple* and adjacent parts of the face.
Zygoma: is that part of the *temporal bone* of the *skull* forming the "cheekbone".
Zygomatic arch: is another term for the *zygoma*, the cheekbone.

Bibliography

Adams, Brian. *Deadly Karate Blows: The Medical Implications.* Burbank: Unique Publications, 1985.
Allen, R.E., ed. *The Concise Oxford Dictionary of Current English.* Oxford: Clarendon Press, 1991.
Anon. *Dick's Art of Wrestling.* New York: Fitzgerald Publishing Corp., 1887.
Arsenault, Alan D., *Neck Restraint.* Vancouver, BC: Unpublished Internal Police Report, Vancouver Police Department, 1986.
Banister, E.W., I.B Mekjavic, R.C. Amundson, and R. Ward. *Laboratory Experiments in Human Structure and Function.* Burnaby: Simon Fraser School of Kinesiology, 1990.
Butler, Pat. *Judo Complete.* London: Faber and Faber Ltd., 1963.
Corcoran, John, and Emile Farkas. *Martial Arts: Traditions, History, People.* New York: Gallery Books, 1983.
Craig, Darryl Max. *Japan's Ultimate Martial Art. Jujitsu Before 1882: The Classical Japanese Art of Self-Defense.* Boston: Charles E. Tuttle Co. Ltd., 1995.
Dillman, George, and Chris Thomas. *Kyusho-jitsu: The Dillman Method of Pressure Point Fighting.* Reading: Dillman Karate International Books, 1992.
—. *Tuité: Advanced Pressure Point Grappling.* Reading: George Dillman Karate International, 1995.
—. *Pressure Point Karate Made Easy.* Reading: George Dillman Karate International, 1999.
Dorland's Illustrated Medical Dictionary. 29th ed. Philadelphia: W.B. Saunders Co, 2000.
Dratz, John P., Manly Johnson, and Terry McCann. *Winning Wrestling.* Englewood Cliffs: Prentice-Hall Inc., 1966.
Farkas, Emile, and John Corcoran. *The Overlook Martial Arts Dictionary.* New York: The Overlook Press, 1983.
Farrar, Robert Hobart. *American Judo.* New York: Padell Book Co., 1943.
Frederick, Louis. *A Dictionary of the Martial Arts.* Rutland: Charles E. Tuttle Co. Inc., 1991.
Garrud, WH. *The Complete Jujitsuan.* London: Methuen and Co. Ltd., 1953.
Glaessner, Verina. *Kung Fu: Cinema of Vengeance.* Norfolk: Lorrimer Publishing Ltd., 1974.
Goldberg, Stephen. *Clinical Anatomy Made Ridiculously Simple.* Miami: MedMaster Inc., 1984.
Gray, Henry. *Anatomy, Descriptive and Surgical.* T. Pickering Pick and Robert Howden, eds. Philadelphia: Running Press, 1974.
Griffith, H. Winter. *Complete Guide to Sports Injuries: How to Treat Fractures, Bruises, Sprains, Strains, Head Injuries.* Tucson: The Body Press, 1986.
Hackenschmidt, George. *Complete Science of Wrestling.* London: Health and Strength Ltd., 1909.
Hancock., H. Irving, and Higashi, Katsukuma. *The Complete Kano Jiujitsu.* New York: Dover Publications, 1905.
Harrison, E.J. *The Fighting Spirit of Japan.* Woodstock: The Overlook Press, 1955.
Harrison, E.J. and Yuko Tani. *The Art of Ju-jitsu.* London: W. Foulsham and Co. Ltd., circa 1930.
Hewitt-Zaitlin, Margaret. *The Fitness Knowledge Home Study Program.* Nelson: Canadian Fitness Education Services Ltd., 1996.
Hewett-Zaitlin, Margaret, Heather Bourchier, Claudia Bianca-DeBay, and Rick Tobin. *The Canadian Fitness Knowledge Course Student Resource Manual.* 5th Ed. Summerland, B.C.: Canadian Fitness Education Services Ltd, 2002.
Hewitt-Zaitlin, Margaret, and Paula Stockdale. *The Weight Training Instructor: Level 1 Student Resource Manual.* Nelson: Canadian Fitness Education Services Ltd., 1996.
Hollinshead, William, Henry. *Textbook of Anatomy.* Maryland: Harper and Row Publishers, Inc., 1974.
Keen, C.P., C.M. Speidel, and R.H. Swartzt. *Championship Wrestling.* Toronto: Coles Publishing Co. Ltd., 1978.
Kent, Graeme. *A Pictorial History of Wrestling.* Middlesex: Spring Books, 1968.
Kudo, Kazuzo. *Dynamic Judo: Grappling Techniques.* Tokyo: Japan Publications Trading Co., 1967.
Kuhaulua, Jesse. *Takamiyama: The World of Sumo.* Tokyo: Kodansha, 1973.
Kurihara, Tamio, and Howard Wilson. *Championship Judo: Original and Development, Techniques, Training, Self-defence.* London: Kingswood and Crawley Bookprint Ltd., circa 1960.

Lawson-Wood, Denis, and Joyce Lawson-Wood. *Judo Revival Points, Athletes' Points and Posture.* Sussex: Health Science Press, 1960.
LeBell, Gene. *Gene LeBell's Grappling World: The Encyclopedia of Finishing Holds.* Santa Monica: Pro-action Publishing, 1998.
—. *Pro-wrestling Finishing Holds.* Santa Monica: Pro-action Publishing, 1985.
Li, Ding. *Acupuncture, Meridian Theory, and Acupuncture Point.* San Francisco: China Books and Periodicals Inc., 1992.
Liang, Shou-Yu, and Tai D. Ngo. *Chinese Fast Wrestling for Fighting: The Art of San Shou Kuai Jiao.* Jamaica Plain: YMAA Publication Center, 1997.
Liang, Shou-yu, and Wen-Ching Wu. *Qigong Empowerment.* Providence: The Way of the Dragon Publishing, 1997.
Liederman, Earle. *The Science of Wrestling and the Art of Jiu-jitsu.* New York: Earle Liederman, 1924.
Linck, S.R. *Combat Jiu Jitsu for Offense and Defense.* Portland: Stevens-Ness Law Publishing Co., 1943.
Long, Hei. *Advanced Dragon's Touch: 20 Anatomical Targets and Techniques for Taking Them Out.* Boulder: Paladin Press, 1995.
—. *Dragon's Touch: Weaknesses of the Human Anatomy.* Boulder: Paladin Press, 1983.
—. *Gouzao Gongji: Seven Neurological Attacks for Inflicting Serious Damage.* Boulder: Paladin Press, 1992.
Long, Joe. "Jujutsu: The Gentle Art and The Strenuous Life." *Journal of Asian Martial Arts.* Vol.6, No.4: 62-75.
Maliszewski, Michael. *Spiritual Dimensions of the Martial Arts.* Rutland: Charles E. Tuttle Co. Inc., 1996.
Mashiro, N. *Black Medicine: The Dark Art of Death.* Boulder: Paladin Press, 1978.
McCarthy, Patrick. *The Bubishi.* Kanagawa Ken: International Ryukyu Karate Research Society, 1990.
—. *Bubishi: The Bible of Karate.* Tokyo: Charles E. Tuttle Co. Inc., 1995.
Montaigue, Earle. *Dim-mak: Death Point Striking.* Boulder: Paladin Press, 1993.
Moore, K.L. *Clinically Oriented Anatomy.* NY: Lippincott Williams and Wilkins, 1999.
Morehouse, Laurence E., and Leonard Gross. *Maximum Performance.* New York: Pocket Books, 1977.
Mosby Medical Encyclopedia. Editors and writers: Glantze Walter d., Kenneth N. Anderson, and Lois E. Anderson. Revised Edition. St. Louis: Plume (Penguin Group), 1992.
Musashi, Miyamoto. *A Book of Five Rings.* Woodstock: The Overlook Press, 1974.
Noble, Graham. "An Introduction to W. Barton-Wright (1860-1951) and the Eclectic Art of Bartitsu." *Journal of Asian Martial Arts.* Vol.8, No.2: 50-62.
Nothiger, Andreas. *World History Chart.* Toronto: Penguin Books Canada Ltd., 1991.
Obata, Toshishiro. *Samurai Aikijutsu: The Techniques of the Samurai Swordsmen.* Essex: Dragon Books, 1987.
Poliakoff, Michael B. *Combat in the Ancient Sports World: Competition, Violence and Culture.* New Haven: Yale UP, 1987.
Ratti, Oscar, and Adele Westbrook. *Secrets of the Samurai: A Survey of Martial Arts of Japan.* Tokyo: Charles E. Tuttle Co. Inc., 1981.
Reay, Donald T. and J.W. Eisele, "Death From Law Enforcement Neck Holds." *The American Journal of Forensic Medicine and Pathology.* Vol 3, No. 3: 253-258, 1982.
Shapiro, Amy. *Running Press Glossary of Martial Arts Language.* Philadelphia: Running Press, 1978.
Shaw, R. Paul and Yuwa Wong. *Genetic Seeds of Warfare: Evolution, Nationalism, and Patriotism.* Boston: Unwin Hyman, 1989.
Siddle, Bruce K. *Pressure Point and Control Tactics: Defensive Tactics Instructor Manual.* Millstadt: PPCT Management Systems Inc., 1999.
Skinner, Harry H. *Jiu-jitsu: The Wonderful Japanese Method of Attach and Self-defense.* New York: Japan Publishing Co., 1904.
Spry, Leverton, and Peter Kornicki. *Japan.* London: Michael O'Mara Books Ltd., 1987.
Serizawa. *Tsubo: Vital Points for Oriental Therapy.* New York: Japan Publications Inc., 1989.
Stone, Henry A. *Wrestling: Intercollegiate and Olympic.* New York: Prentice-Hall Inc., 1939.
Sugawara, Tetsutaka, and Jujian Xing. *Aikido and Chinese Martial Arts: Its Fundamental Relations.* Tokyo: Japan Publications, 1996.
Swaddling, Judith. *The Ancient Olympic Games.* London: British Museum Publications Ltd., 1980.

Tedeschi, Marc. *Essential Anatomy*. Turnbull: Weatherhill Inc., 2002.
Torrey, Lee. *Stretching the Limits: Breakthroughs in Sports Science That Create Super Athletes*. New York: Dodd, Mead & Company, Inc., 1985.
Trias, Robert A. *The Hand is My Sword*. Tokyo: Charles E. Tuttle Co., Inc., 1974.
Uyehara, M., ed. "Kano, Founder of Kodokan Judo." *Black Belt Magazine*. Vol.1, No.1: 7-13.
Watanabe, Jiichi, and Lindy Avakian. *The Secrets of Judo*. Tokyo: Charles E. Tuttle Co. Ltd., 1981.
Watts, Emily, and G.W. Beldam. *The Fine Art of Jujitsu*. London: William Heinemann, 1906.
Yamanaka, K. *Jiu-jutsu or Jiu-do: Selection from Kodokwan* [sic] *Method*. Atlantic City: Kondo and Co., 1920.
Yang, Jwing-Ming. *Analysis of Shaolin Chin Na*. Jamaica Plain: YMAA Publication Center, 1982.
—. *Chinese Qigong Massage*. Jamaica Plain: YMAA Publication Center, 1992.
—. *Comprehensive Applications of Shaolin Chin Na: The Practical Defense of Chinese Seizing Arts For All Styles*. Jamaica Plain: YMAA Publication Center, 1995.
—. *The Essence of Shaolin White Crane: Martial Power and Qiqong*. Jamaica Plain: YMAA Publication Center, 1996.
—. *The Root of Chinese Chi Kung: The Secrets of Chi Kung Training*. Jamaica Plain: YMAA Publication Center, 1989.
—. *Shaolin Chin Na: The Seizing Art of Chin Na*. Burbank: Unique Publications Inc., 1982.
—. *T'ai Chi Chin Na*. Jamaica Plain: YMAA Publication Center, 1995.
Zarrilli, Phillip B. "The Vital Spots in Two South Indian Martial Traditions." *Journal of Asian Martial Arts*. Vol.1, No.1: 36-67.
Zhao, Da Yuan. *Practical Chin Na*. Pacific Grove: High View Publications, 1993.

About the Author, Alan D. Arsenault, B.Sc., B.Ed.

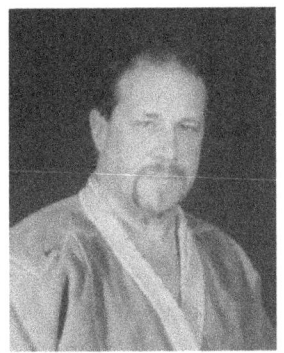

It was 1971 when Mr. Arsenault began his martial arts training in North Bay, Ontario under the watchful eye of Sensei Duane Sawyer in Kenshokan Dharma, Goshin Jutsu. At this time, he had yet to hear of Bruce Lee who became a screen idol in the early 70's and started the 'Kung Fu craze' here in North America. He knew about the existence of judo, as it was an Olympic sport. Karate was just a word that he associated to a newly introduced fighting style and kung fu was relatively unheard of.

Mr. Arsenault threw himself intensely into karate during his university years (1972-78) at McMaster University in Hamilton, Ontario. He attained the rank of first kyu brown belt in Eastern's rough and tumble Goju Ryu Karate. After dabbling in Chito Ryu karate and obtaining his teaching degree at Queen's University in Kingston, he moved to Vancouver, British Columbia.

He joined the Vancouver Police Department in 1979, a career he continues today. In Vancouver, he met Master Wong, Yuwa his karate instructor, or colleague as Yuwa now wishes to be called, and the true essence of karate unfolded under his expert and humble tutelage. Al was awarded his 3rd degree black belt from Dr. Wong in 1986. Al had never known such a technically brilliant yet utterly humble martial artist before. Master Wong encouraged his students in Nisei Karate-do to study all facets and styles of the martial arts and to utilize only what was useful for our temperaments and body types. Indeed, it was because of this freedom that one of Yuwa's long time karate students, Michael Levenston, came to study T'ai Chi Chu'an (Taijiquan) with Master Liang, Shou-Yu. In 1989, Michael introduced Master Liang to Yuwa and Al as being a 'living treasury of martial arts skill and knowledge'. Master Liang proved to be indeed just that. Al stopped teaching karate, preferring to train with Master Liang. Soon the concept of Wushu Sanshou Dao was born in a gym at the University of British Columbia, where the few of them trained together (see early training photo). Sanshou Dao is basically the hybridization of the extensive and collective knowledge of these two masters with Michael and Al assisting in the meshing process whenever they could. This process still continues to grow worldwide today as they seek new skills to absorb into the slowly evolving sanshou style.

As his experience in the martial arts and street policing grew, Mr. Arsenault became interested mainly in the practical applications of the martial arts. He fought continuously with the students in his club despite a chronic back problem. Now at 50 years of age he still enjoys vigorous workouts. He obtained his black belt in judo under Tim Laidler, Brian Shipper, Toby Hinton and Wes Fung who head the Vancouver Police Judo/ Jiu Jitsu Club and he serves as an assistant instructor at this club. Al is actively involved in teaching his fellow officers about police restraint and control tactics (within the judo club), he was a founding member of a Crowd Control Unit and he has been used extensively by the courts as an expert in non-firearm weaponry over the last two decades.

Today, he is also beginning to explore the creative side of his personality through writing and visual arts such as 'Odd Squad' filming of documentaries and educational videos like 'Through a Blue Lens' [1999], 'Flipping the World' [2000] and 'Beyond the Blue Lens' [2004] (see www.oddsquad.com).

Cst. Arsenault has had to arrest many violent offenders throughout the course of his career as a police officer. He has learned to read pre-assault cues and with the utmost speed, take the fight to his would-be assailant and put him quickly down to the ground without causing unnecessary harm. He likes to say that 'there is a time for talk and a time for action'. Not knowing the difference could mean a trip to the hospital to treat his injuries or to police Internal Affairs to explain his actions. He has always fought smarter, not harder and he only fights when he has to. Cst. Arsenault has chosen to stay exclusively on the street as opposed to taking the softer inside 'desk jockey' positions. A 'carpet cop' he is not. He takes pride in being a 'career constable' and being up to his elbows in the seedy and often violent part of society (in Vancouver's notorious skid road- the Downtown Eastside) where drug-induced human misery and surviving by instincts are the norm.

Having said this, Al advocates for a strict code of non-violence to his students other than for reasons of self-defense. If they must fight a righteous and unavoidable battle, he teaches them that there is no 'fair' fight, only personal survival. The amount of force they use must be proportionate to the amount of force used against them, in accordance with our laws. With such a training environment, few bullies or hot heads are attracted. These types soon leave or are shown the way out. And so our students must learn the distinction between self-serving violence and the judicious application of force for the common good of all.

For over a decade, Al has served as the President of the International Wushu Sanshou Dao Association that Master Liang, Shou-Yu, Dr. Wong, Yuwa and Dr. Yang, Jwing-Ming formed in 1988. In 1997, Master Liang awarded Al a 5th degree black belt in Sanshou Dao, a degree that is humbly acknowledged as being largely an honorary one. The SYL Institute in Vancouver is immensely popular and our students successfully compete internationally. Indeed, Master Liang has a large contingent of both local (see group photo) and international students. Sanshou Dao has spread to China and elsewhere, taking on the flavors of other styles of martial arts to give it additional strength and depth.

It is Al's sincere hope that the cross training in martial art styles flourishes in the new millennium and that this book in some small way serves to assist in this endeavor.

About the Author, Joseph Faulise

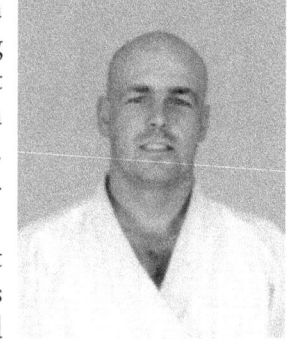

Mr. Faulise has been training and has had an interest in the martial arts since the age of thirteen. He began training in 1973, when he was encouraged by his mother to try out for the wrestling team at school. He learned that the coach also owned a judo school and began training there as well. He did wrestling in the winter months and judo in the summer months until 1977.

In 1978 Mr. Faulise started training at a school that emphasized striking and kicking techniques, as well as throwing and ground fighting. It was here that he learned to apply his judo and wrestling skills in a more realistic and practical way. He began learning as many different facets of fighting as he could, always looking at the practicality and effectiveness of what he was learning.

In 1983 he moved to Alaska and settled in the small community of Tok. He was looking for a change from city life and as he have always enjoyed fishing and hunting. What better place he thought, than Alaska to do so. He began teaching a self-defense class for the University of Alaska through their rural education program. He taught these classes for two years, working mostly with adults. It was also in these classes that he met his wife Tess.

In 1985, with the encouragement of his wife, Joe opened up his own school. It has been her continual support that has helped Joe get where he is today. After his first year or so of teaching he found himself starving for more knowledge. It was at this point that he felt he needed more training in order to progress as a martial artist. He has always believed that if you want to get better at the martial arts, you must train with people better than yourself. As his school grew and the students progressed, they began going to tournaments in Fairbanks, Alaska, a city approximately two hundred miles distant. This was the nearest location for other martial arts schools or tournaments of any kind. It was at one of these tournaments that he met Master Larry Wick, who runs a Tang Soo Do school.

They began sharing their knowledge and developed a lasting friendship. Master Wick introduced him to many in the Fairbanks martial arts community, including Master Charles Scott who was an 8th dan in Shudo Kan Karate. He put on a yearly open tournament. Mr. Faulise was impressed with these two men and the way they ran their schools. He was encouraged to continue his quest in martial arts studies.

Mr. Faulise continued training on his own and teaching at his school, but felt he needed a teacher and some outside influence. Because most of the clubs in Alaska only practiced one style and 90% of them were striking styles of either Japanese or Korean lineage, he considered looking outside Alaska. During one of his many trips to Fairbanks, Master Wick sensed his frustration and encouraged him to find a system and teacher he liked and to stick with it.

In the fall of 1992 he went to Vancouver B.C. to train with Master Liang, Shou-Yu for nine months. It was here that he also met Al Arsenault and Master Wong, Yuwa along with Michael Levenston. He began training in Bagua and T'ai Chi Ch'uan (taijiquan) with Master Liang. After a month or so he recommended that he try the Wushu classes that led him to train in Sanshou Dao. In Sanshou Dao there are no rules other than not to injure your training partner. Needless to say this class was fairly rough. Al and Joe immediately hit it off; they were yin and yang. While their skills and backgrounds were opposites, they complemented each other. Al helped Joe with his kicking and striking combinations whereas Joe assisted Al with his throwing and ground fighting techniques. At the end of his stay in Vancouver he was graded by Master Liang and Master Wong to second degree black belt in Sanshou Dao.

Mr. Faulise returned to Alaska and reopened his school in the spring of 1993. He continues to teach and train in Alaska still exploring all aspects of the martial arts, but now he has a system and teachers to always return to, which is a great feeling.

INDEX

abnormal movement 27-28
ackrocheirismos 11
acupuncture 97-98, 104
acupuncture points 97-98, 103-104
adrenaline 32
airway chokes 243-246
all fours position 92-93
anatomy, leg 217
ankle joint 218
arm bar 77-79, 84-85, 195-196, 200
arm holds 207, 208
arm lock 195-196
arm wrap 211-212
arm, anatomy of 74-77, 194
armpit hold 82-83
atemi waza 6-7, 12-13, 14-15, 19-20
awareness 28-30
axis (pivot) point (AP) 58-61, 69-72
Backward Neck Crank 248-249
Baihui 109-111
bar 46
base of support 66-67
Basic Ankle Lock #1 219
Basic Ankle Lock #2 220
Basic Ankle Lock from a Defensive Position 222
Basic Ankle Lock from the Guard 221
Basic Knee Lock 228
baton strikes 132
bear hug 88-90
bent appendage techniques 57
Bent Arm Locks 209, 213
bi qi 24-25
biomechanical principles 48, 57, 144, 196, 209-210, 217
Bizhong 141
Blocking the Knee with the Arm 233-234
Blocking the Knee with the Leg 234
blows to vital points 24
Bodhidharma 15
body bar 48
body control 28
body locks 271
body positions 85
body tools 35, 68, 102-103, 143, 193
body weight, controlling 38, 44
Boston Crab 272
bugei 17-18
bulldogging 80
C.V. Conception Vessel 112-113

cardiopulmonary resuscitation 256
carotid artery 245, 254
carotid sinus stimulation 253-254
cavities 97-98, 101-102, 241-242
center of gravity 38, 71-72
Changqiang 109
Chengjiang 115
Chengjin 131-132
Chengqi 128
Chengshan 132-133
chi cavities 23-26
Chinese martial arts 15
Chize 117-118
choke holds 80-81, 264-265
Choke using the Shin 266-267
chokes 257-258, 266
choking 242, 264
choking bans 264-265
choking to unconsciousness 24-25
Chongmen 136
Conception Vessel (C.V.) 112-113
conditioning 52
controllability 44
controlling body weight 38
controlling the distance 33
controlling the leg 217
controlling the limbs 39
controlling the mind 43
counterholds 55-57
counterpressure 82
countertorque 80
cross mount 90-92
cross training, value of 4-7
cross-mark hold 78-79, 83-85
cuo gu 24-25
da 4
Dabao 136-137
Daying 128
dead weight 72
Death Lock 250-251
death touch 104
dian mai 24-26
dian xue 25-26, 101-102
dim mak 101-102
Dim Mak theory 241-242
dirty fighting techniques 4
distance 33
distance, controlling 44
distraction 28-29

dividing the muscles or tendons 24
Double Ankle and Double Knee Lock 239
Double Ankle Lock 226
Double Knee Lock 232
Double Leg Knee Block 236
Double Leg Lock 224-225
Double Leg Scoop 271-272
Double Lever Lock 212
DU 1 Changqiang 109
DU 16 Fengfu 109
DU 20 Baihui 109-111
DU 26 Renzhong 111-112
Du Meridian 105
Dumai Meridian 109
elbow joint 194-195
elbow, anatomy of 74-77
elbow, hyper-extension of 77
electrical skin resistance 104
escapes 55-57
escapes, preventing 30-31
EX-HN 19 Jingbi 140
EX-HN 2 Yingtan 140
EX-UE 11 Bizhong 141
excercising, recuperation 52
excessive force 32
explosive power 72
F.I.T.T 53
Failed Leg Lock to Knee Block 235
fall, wrestling 11
fen jin 24
Fengfu 109
Fengshi 135
fight control 273-274
fight control factors 33, 44
fighting machine, body as 144-145
fighting spectrum 5-6, 32-33, 273
figure four leg lock 220
figure four lock 80, 150, 196-197, 238-239
finger pressure 127
flexibility 52
force arm (FA) 69-72
force components in Qin Na 22
force lever 59-63, 63-64
force point (FP) 58-61, 69-72
force, application types 22-23
force, applying 144-145
force, direction of 57
force, use of 54
fore knuckles 80-81
forearms, hugging with 78-79
Forward Neck Crank 248

Forward Roll to Knee Lock 231
fu (Yang) organs 104
fulcrum 46, 57-61, 196
Full Nelson 252
G.B. 24 Riyue 134
G.B. 31 Fengshi 135
G.B. 34 Yanglingquan 136
G.B. 6 Xuanli 133
G.V. Governor Vessel Meridian 109
Gall Bladder Meridian 133
Governor Vessel Meridian (G.V.) 109
grabbing techniques 22-24
Gracie ju jitsu clan 22
Graeco-Roman wrestling 10
grappling arts 26-27
Greek society, wrestling 9-10
grip augmentation 72-74
ground fighting,
    control factors 33
    defined 3
    Gracie clan 22
    principles of 32-33
guard position 85-86
H. 3 Shaohai 119
half guard position 90
half Nelson 93-95
Hammer Lock 215
hand 195
handcuffing 54
head as a target 247-248
head, anatomy 242
Heart Meridian 119, 120
Heart Palace 114
heart rate, training and 53
Hegu 121
hip joint 218
hook, heel 223-224
Huagai 114
hugging with forearms 78-79
hypercontraction 46
hyperflexion 46
hypoxia 243-246
indentations 101-102
inertia 70-72
instructors 54
inverted straight arm bar 201
Japanese martial arts 15
Japanese martial arts, post WWII years 19-20
Jiache 129
Jimen 136
jin 26

Index

Jingbi 140
Jingqu 118-119
joint dislocation 24-25
joint locks,
    arms 193
    knee and ankle 238
    maneuvers 22-24
    physical principles of 57
joint slack 50-51
joints, body tools and 144
ju jitsu, history of 14-15, 16
ju jutsu 12-13
judo 6-7,
    from the ju jutsu styles 12-13
    recent history 21-22
judoka 196
jugular vein 245
juji gatame 78-79, 83-85
Juque 114
K. 3 Taixi 138
karate 21-22
Kempo 12-13
kesa gatame 83
Kidney Meridian 137-138
Knee Block from the Half Guard 237
knee blocks, application 233
knee joint 218
knee locks, application 228
Kneeling Ankle Lock 227
Kneeling Heel Hook 240
kneeling positions 92-95
Kneeling Straight Arm Hold 207
knockout punches 246-247
knuckle digs 80-81
Kongzui 118
Kung Fu (Gong fu) 21-22
kyusho jitsu 101-102
L.I. 10 Shousanli 121-122
L.I. 11 Quchi 122-123
L.I. 4 Hegu 121
Large Intestine Meridian 120-122
lateral femoral nerve motor point 135-136
lateral vascular neck restraint 256-257, 259-260
Lee, Bruce 21-22
leg Blocks 218
Leg Chin Crank 272
leg locks 217
leverage 46, 57-61
Lianquan 115
ligament 46
limbs, controlling 39

Liv. 13 Zhangmen 139-140
Liver Meridian 139
load 69-72
low oxygen levels 254-255
Lu. 10 Yuji 119
Lu. 2 Yunmen 116-117
Lu. 5 Chize 117-118
Lu. 6 Kongzui 118
Lu. 8 Jingqu 118-119
Lung Meridian 116, 117
mandibular pressure point 126-127
massage 104
mat work 95-97
mechanical advantage 59-64, 69-70
mechanics, lever 57-61
median nerve motor point 141-143
meridian theory 97-98, 103-104
meridian triplets 104
meridians, nomenclature 104
misplacing of the bone 24-25
mobility 44
momentum 70-72
mounted position 87-89, 91-92
movement chain 77
movement chains 46
moving your opponent 57
muscle fiber types 53-54
muscle/tendon stretching 22-24
muscles 46
muscles/tendons tearing 24
muscular strength 26
Na, defined 3
neck 248
neck holds 242, 243-246
neck restraint 257-258, 265-266
neck restraint holds, defense 258-260
neck, anatomy 242
neck, structure 243-246
Neiguan 119-120
nerves 23-24
nerves, motor 99-101
nerves, voluntary 99-101
nervous system 241-242
One-Wing Neck Choke 268-269
P. 6 Neiguan 119-120
pain compliance techniques 46, 102-103
pankration 9-11
Pankrationis, defined 10
partner, training with 50, 54
pelvis, levering with 83-84
penetrating ability 68

355

Pericardium Meridian 119, 121
physical traing 53
physical training 51-52
physics, in fighting 46
pinning 11
plyometric power 72
points, superficial 103-104
police officers, controlling suspects 54, 264-265
police officers, spread-eagled position 67-68
police, lateral femoral nerve motor point 135
police, mandibular pressure point 126
police, median nerve motor point 141
police, Qin Na as a tool 26-27
position, controlling 44
position, rear guard 88-90
positional change 89-90
positional changes 35, 85-86
positioning 95
positions, mount 87-89
practice 54-55
pressing of an artery 24-26
pressing techniques 23-24
pressure on body bar 48
pressure points
    attacks 23-24, 25-26, 101, 102-103, 143
    locations 99-101
    fighting strategies 102-103
    for martial arts 105-106
    nomenclature 97-101
pressure, applying to joints 57
pressure/counterpressure 27-28
professional athletes ancient history 10
progressive overload 52
Prone Bent Arm Lock 209-210
prone position 90-91
pugilism 26-27,
    early history 8
    recent history 22
punches, knockout 246-248
qi 103-104
qi, flow of 101-102
qigong 104
Qihai 113-114
Qin Na,
    application of 27-28, 28-29
    components of force 22
    defined 3
    history of 15
    leverage in 46
    physiological effects 24
    speed in 50

    value of 26-27
Qin, defined 3
Qinglengyuan 126
Quanliao 125
Quanliao-zygomatic crevice 87-89
Quchi 122-123
Quepan 130
Rear Bent Arm Lock 214
rear guard position 88-90
Reclining Straight Arm Hold 208
recuperation 52
regaining consciousness 256
relaxing 72
REN 14 Juque 114
REN 17 Tanzhong 114
REN 20 Huagai 114
REN 22 Tiantu 115
REN 23 Lianquan 115
REN 24 Chengjiang 115
REN 6 Qihai 113-114
Ren Meridian 105, 112-113
Renying 130
Renzhong 111-112
resistance point (RP) 58-61
respiratory restraint 242
rest after exercise 52
restraint and control techniques 26-27
resuscitation 256
Riyue 134
Roll Over Choke 267
rotational movement 68-70
Rugen 130-131
S.I. 16 Tianchuang 124
S.I. 17 Tianrong 124-125
S.I. 18 Quanliao 125
S.J. 11 Qinglengyuan 126
S.J. 17 Yifeng 126
S.J. 23 Sizhukong 127-128
S.J. 3 Hand Zhongzhu 126
safety 54
Sanjiao Meridian 126
scarf hold 83
scissoring arms 81-82
sealing of the breath 24-25
sealing the artery 253-254
sealing the breath 242, 243-246, 264
sealing the vein 242-246, 253-254, 265-266
Seated Rear Choke 270
sensitivity 48
Shaohai 119
Shenmai 133

Index

Shoulder Crank 210
shoulder joint 194-195
Shousanli 121-122
shuai 4
shuigo 111-112
Single Leg Flex 272-273
sit out 205
Sizhukong 127-128
slack in joints 50-51
sleeper holds 243-246, 255, 265-266
Small Intestine Meridian 124, 125
Sp. 11 Jimen 136
Sp. 12 Chongmen 136
Sp. 21 Dabao 136-137
speed 28-30
speed levers 61-64
speed of application 50
Spleen Meridian 136, 137
splitting the muscles or tendons 24
spread-eagled position 67-68
St. 1 Chengqi 128
St. 12 Quepan 130
St. 18 Rugen 130-131
St. 43 Xiangu 131
St. 5 Daying 128
St. 6 Jiache 129
St. 7 Xiaguan 130
St. 9 Renying 130
stability 66-67
stand up fighting 34
stand up fights 32-33
Stomach Meridian 128, 129
Straight Arm Bar from a Single Leg Takedown 196-197
Straight Arm Bar From a Sit Out 205
Straight Arm Bar From the Reverse Guard 204
Straight Arm Bar Using a Leg Lever 203
straight arm lock 202-203
straight arms 82
strangulation 242
strength 28-30
stress response 32
stretching muscle/tendon 22-24
striking techniques 24
superior position 29-31
surface contact 68
surprise 28-29
Tae Kwon Do 6-7
taiho jitsu 14-15
Taixi 138
tanden 64-66

Tanzhong 114
tapping out 32, 54
target areas 241-242
techniques, conceptualizing 57
telegraphing tension 72
tendon 46
tense body 72
threshold, physical training 53
ti 4
Tianchuang 124
Tianrong 124-125
Tiantu 115
tibial nerve motor point 132
torsion 46
torsional movement 68-70
torso, anatomy 271
Traditional Chinese Medicine (TCM) 103-104
training schedule 52
training zones, target 53
training,
    F.I.T.T. 53
    physical 51-52
    target zones 53
    threshold of 53
Transverse Arm Bar From a Roll Over 200
Transverse Arm Bar From the Guard 198
Transverse Arm Wrap 211-212
triangle choke 83-85
Triangle Strangle 262
Triangle Strangle from Side Position 262-263
triceps muscle 59-63
Triple Burner Meridian 127
Triple Heater/Warmer/Burner Meridian 126
U.B. 40 Weizhong 131
U.B. 56 Chengjin 131-132
U.B. 57 Chengshan 132-133
U.B. 62 Shenmai 133
ude garumi 47, 207
ude gatame 78-79
unconsciousness 255, 264-265
Urinary Bladder Meridian 131, 132
vagus nerve 245
Valsalva maneuver 253-254, 255
vascular compression 253-254
vascular neck restraints 242, 265-266
vital areas, protecting 34
vital points, blows to 24
waki gatame 82-83
waza 15
Weizhong 131
whole body action 72-74

winning mindset 43
wrestling,
    early history 8
    far east 11-13
    Graeco-Roman 10
    Greek history 9-10
    in Europe and America 13-14
wrist joint 195
Xiaguan 130
Xiangu 131
Xuanli 133

Yang organs 104
Yanglingquan 136
Yifeng 126
Yin organs 104
Yingtan 140
Yuji 119
Yunmen 116-117
zang (Yin) organs 104
Zhangmen 139-140
Zhongzhu 126

BOOKS FROM YMAA

- 101 REFLECTIONS ON TAI CHI CHUAN
- 108 INSIGHTS INTO TAI CHI CHUAN
- A WOMAN'S QIGONG GUIDE
- ADVANCING IN TAE KWON DO
- ANALYSIS OF GENUINE KARATE
- ANALYSIS OF GENUINE KARATE 2
- ANALYSIS OF SHU HA RI IN KARATE-DO
- ANALYSIS OF SHAOLIN CHIN NA 2ND ED
- ANCIENT CHINESE WEAPONS
- ART AND SCIENCE OF STAFF FIGHTING
- THE ART AND SCIENCE OF SELF-DEFENSE
- ART AND SCIENCE OF STICK FIGHTING
- ART OF HOJO UNDO
- ARTHRITIS RELIEF
- BACK PAIN RELIEF
- BAGUAZHANG
- BRAIN FITNESS
- CHIN NA IN GROUND FIGHTING
- CHINESE FAST WRESTLING
- CHINESE FITNESS
- CHINESE TUI NA MASSAGE
- COMPLETE MARTIAL ARTIST
- COMPREHENSIVE APPLICATIONS OF SHAOLIN CHIN NA
- CONFLICT COMMUNICATION
- DAO DE JING: A QIGONG INTERPRETATION
- DAO IN ACTION
- DEFENSIVE TACTICS
- DIRTY GROUND
- DR. WU'S HEAD MASSAGE
- ESSENCE OF SHAOLIN WHITE CRANE
- EXPLORING TAI CHI
- FACING VIOLENCE
- FIGHT LIKE A PHYSICIST
- THE FIGHTER'S BODY
- FIGHTER'S FACT BOOK 1&2
- FIGHTING THE PAIN RESISTANT ATTACKER
- FIRST DEFENSE
- FORCE DECISIONS: A CITIZENS GUIDE
- HOMECOMING
- INSIDE TAI CHI
- JUDO ADVANTAGE
- JUJI GATAME ENCYCLOPEDIA
- KARATE SCIENCE
- KEPPAN
- KRAV MAGA COMBATIVES
- KRAV MAGA FUNDAMENTAL STRATEGIES
- KRAV MAGA PROFESSIONAL TACTICS
- KRAV MAGA WEAPON DEFENSES
- LITTLE BLACK BOOK OF VIOLENCE
- LIUHEBAFA FIVE CHARACTER SECRETS
- MARTIAL ARTS OF VIETNAM
- MARTIAL ARTS INSTRUCTION
- MARTIAL WAY AND ITS VIRTUES
- MEDITATIONS ON VIOLENCE
- MERIDIAN QIGONG EXERCISES
- MINDFUL EXERCISE
- MIND INSIDE TAI CHI
- MIND INSIDE YANG STYLE TAI CHI CHUAN
- NORTHERN SHAOLIN SWORD
- OKINAWA'S COMPLETE KARATE SYSTEM: ISSHIN RYU
- PRINCIPLES OF TRADITIONAL CHINESE MEDICINE
- PROTECTOR ETHIC
- QIGONG FOR HEALTH & MARTIAL ARTS
- QIGONG FOR TREATING COMMON AILMENTS
- QIGONG MASSAGE
- QIGONG MEDITATION: EMBRYONIC BREATHING
- QIGONG GRAND CIRCULATION
- QIGONG MEDITATION: SMALL CIRCULATION
- QIGONG, THE SECRET OF YOUTH: DA MO'S CLASSICS
- ROOT OF CHINESE QIGONG
- SAFEST FAMILY ON THE BLOCK
- SAMBO ENCYCLOPEDIA
- SCALING FORCE
- SELF-DEFENSE FOR WOMEN
- SHIN GI TAI: KARATE TRAINING
- SIMPLE CHINESE MEDICINE
- SIMPLE QIGONG EXERCISES FOR HEALTH, 3RD ED.
- SIMPLIFIED TAI CHI CHUAN, 2ND ED.
- SOLO TRAINING 1&2
- SPOTTING DANGER BEFORE IT SPOTS YOU
- SPOTTING DANGER BEFORE IT SPOTS YOUR KIDS
- SPOTTING DANGER BEFORE IT SPOTS YOUR TEENS
- SPOTTING DANGER FOR TRAVELERS
- SUMO FOR MIXED MARTIAL ARTS
- SUNRISE TAI CHI
- SURVIVING ARMED ASSAULTS
- TAE KWON DO: THE KOREAN MARTIAL ART
- TAEKWONDO BLACK BELT POOMSAE
- TAEKWONDO: A PATH TO EXCELLENCE
- TAEKWONDO: ANCIENT WISDOM
- TAEKWONDO: DEFENSE AGAINST WEAPONS
- TAEKWONDO: SPIRIT AND PRACTICE
- TAI CHI BALL QIGONG: FOR HEALTH AND MARTIAL ARTS
- TAI CHI BALL QIGONG
- THE TAI CHI BOOK
- TAI CHI CHIN NA
- TAI CHI CHUAN CLASSICAL YANG STYLE
- TAI CHI CHUAN MARTIAL APPLICATIONS
- TAI CHI CHUAN MARTIAL POWER
- TAI CHI CONCEPTS AND EXPERIMENTS
- TAI CHI DYNAMICS
- TAI CHI FOR DEPRESSION
- TAI CHI IN 10 WEEKS
- TAI CHI PUSH HANDS
- TAI CHI QIGONG
- TAI CHI SECRETS OF THE ANCIENT MASTERS
- TAI CHI SECRETS OF THE WU & LI STYLES
- TAI CHI SECRETS OF THE WU STYLE
- TAI CHI SECRETS OF THE YANG STYLE
- TAI CHI SWORD: CLASSICAL YANG STYLE
- TAI CHI SWORD FOR BEGINNERS
- TAI CHI WALKING
- TAI CHI CHUAN THEORY OF DR. YANG, JWING-MING
- FIGHTING ARTS
- TRADITIONAL CHINESE HEALTH SECRETS
- TRADITIONAL TAEKWONDO
- TRAINING FOR SUDDEN VIOLENCE
- TRIANGLE HOLD ENCYCLOPEDIA
- TRUE WELLNESS SERIES (MIND, HEART, GUT)
- WARRIOR'S MANIFESTO
- WAY OF KATA
- WAY OF SANCHIN KATA
- WAY TO BLACK BELT
- WESTERN HERBS FOR MARTIAL ARTISTS
- WILD GOOSE QIGONG
- WING CHUN IN-DEPTH
- WINNING FIGHTS
- XINGYIQUAN

AND MANY MORE . . .

VIDEOS FROM YMAA

ANALYSIS OF SHAOLIN CHIN NA
ART AND SCIENCE OF SELF DEFENSE
ART AND SCIENCE OF STAFF FIGHTING
ART AND SCIENCE STICK FIGHTING
ART AND SCIENCE SWORD FIGHTING
BAGUA FOR BEGINNERS 1 & 2
BEGINNER QIGONG FOR WOMEN 1 & 2
BEGINNER TAI CHI FOR HEALTH
BREATH MEDICINE
BIOENERGY TRAINING 1&2
CHEN TAI CHI CANNON FIST
CHEN TAI CHI FIRST FORM
CHEN TAI CHI FOR BEGINNERS
CHIN NA IN-DEPTH SERIES
FACING VIOLENCE: 7 THINGS A MARTIAL ARTIST MUST KNOW
FIVE ANIMAL SPORTS
FIVE ELEMENTS ENERGY BALANCE
HEALER WITHIN: MEDICAL QIGONG
INFIGHTING
INTRODUCTION TO QI GONG FOR BEGINNERS
JOINT LOCKS
KUNG FU BODY CONDITIONING 1 & 2
KUNG FU FOR KIDS AND TEENS SERIES
MERIDIAN QIGONG
NEIGONG FOR MARTIAL ARTS
NORTHERN SHAOLIN SWORD
QI GONG 30-DAY CHALLENGE
QI GONG FOR ANXIETY
QI GONG FOR ARMS, WRISTS, AND HANDS
QIGONG FOR BEGINNERS: FRAGRANCE
QI GONG FOR BETTER BALANCE
QI GONG FOR BETTER BREATHING
QI GONG FOR CANCER
QI GONG FOR DEPRESSION
QI GONG FOR ENERGY AND VITALITY
QI GONG FOR HEADACHES
QIGONG FOR HEALTH: BETTER DIGESTION
QIGONG FOR HEALTH: HEALING QIGONG EXERCISES
QIGONG FOR HEALTH: IMMUNE SYSTEM
QIGONG FOR HEALTH: JOINT REHABILITATION
QIGONG FOR HEALTH: MERIDIAN EXTREMITIES
QIGONG FOR HEALTH: SITTING QIGONG EXERCISES
QIGONG FOR HEALTH: SPINE AND BACK
QI GONG FOR THE HEALTHY HEART
QI GONG FOR HEALTHY JOINTS
QI GONG FOR HIGH BLOOD PRESSURE
QIGONG FOR LONGEVITY
QI GONG FOR STRONG BONES
QI GONG FOR THE UPPER BACK AND NECK
QIGONG FOR WOMEN WITH DAISY LEE
QIGONG FLOW FOR STRESS & ANXIETY RELIEF
QIGONG GRAND CIRCULATION
QIGONG MASSAGE
QIGONG MINDFULNESS IN MOTION
QI GONG—THE SEATED WORKOUT
QIGONG: 15 MINUTES TO HEALTH
SABER FUNDAMENTAL TRAINING
SAI TRAINING AND SEQUENCES
SANCHIN KATA: TRADITIONAL TRAINING FOR KARATE POWER
SCALING FORCE
SEARCHING FOR SUPERHUMANS
SHAOLIN KUNG FU FUNDAMENTAL TRAINING: COURSES 1 & 2
SHAOLIN LONG FIST KUNG FU BEGINNER-INTERMEDIATE-ADVANCED SERIES
SHAOLIN SABER: BASIC SEQUENCES
SHAOLIN STAFF: BASIC SEQUENCES
SHAOLIN WHITE CRANE GONG FU BASIC TRAINING SERIES
SHUAI JIAO: KUNG FU WRESTLING
SIMPLE QIGONG EXERCISES FOR HEALTH
SIMPLE QIGONG EXERCISES FOR ARTHRITIS RELIEF
SIMPLE QIGONG EXERCISES FOR BACK PAIN RELIEF
SIMPLIFIED TAI CHI CHUAN: 24 & 48 POSTURES
SIMPLIFIED TAI CHI FOR BEGINNERS 48
SPOTTING DANGER BEFORE IT SPOTS YOU
SPOTTING DANGER FOR KIDS
SPOTTING DANGER FOR TEENS
SUN TAI CHI
SWORD: FUNDAMENTAL TRAINING
TAEKWONDO KORYO POOMSAE
TAI CHI BALL QIGONG SERIES
TAI CHI BALL WORKOUT FOR BEGINNERS
TAI CHI CHUAN CLASSICAL YANG STYLE
TAI CHI FIGHTING SET
TAI CHI FIT: 24 FORM
TAI CHI FIT: ALZHEIMER'S PREVENTION
TAI CHI FIT: CANCER PREVENTION
TAI CHI FIT FOR VETERANS
TAI CHI FIT: FOR WOMEN
TAI CHI FIT: FLOW
TAI CHI FIT: FUSION BAMBOO
TAI CHI FIT: FUSION FIRE
TAI CHI FIT: FUSION IRON
TAI CHI FIT: HEALTHY BACK SEATED WORKOUT
TAI CHI FIT: HEALTHY HEART WORKOUT
TAI CHI FIT IN PARADISE
TAI CHI FIT: OVER 50
TAI CHI FIT OVER 50: BALANCE EXERCISES
TAI CHI FIT OVER 50: SEATED WORKOUT
TAI CHI FIT OVER 60: GENTLE EXERCISES
TAI CHI FIT OVER 60: HEALTHY JOINTS
TAI CHI FIT OVER 60: LIVE LONGER
TAI CHI FIT: STRENGTH
TAI CHI FIT: TO GO
TAI CHI FOR WOMEN
TAI CHI FUSION: FIRE
TAI CHI QIGONG
TAI CHI PRINCIPLES FOR HEALTHY AGING
TAI CHI PUSHING HANDS SERIES
TAI CHI SWORD: CLASSICAL YANG STYLE
TAI CHI SWORD FOR BEGINNERS
TAI CHI SYMBOL: YIN YANG STICKING HANDS
TAIJI & SHAOLIN STAFF: FUNDAMENTAL TRAINING
TAIJI CHIN NA IN-DEPTH
TAIJI 37 POSTURES MARTIAL APPLICATIONS
TAIJI SABER CLASSICAL YANG STYLE
TAIJI WRESTLING
TRAINING FOR SUDDEN VIOLENCE
UNDERSTANDING QIGONG SERIES
WHITE CRANE HARD & SOFT QIGONG
YANG TAI CHI FOR BEGINNERS
YOQI: MICROCOSMIC ORBIT QIGONG
YOQI QIGONG FOR A HAPPY HEART
YOQI:QIGONG FLOW FOR HAPPY MIND
YOQI:QIGONG FLOW FOR INTERNAL ALCHEMY
YOQI QIGONG FOR HAPPY SPLEEN & STOMACH
YOQI QIGONG FOR HAPPY KIDNEYS
YOQI QIGONG FLOW FOR HAPPY LUNGS
YOQI QIGONG FLOW FOR STRESS RELIEF
YOQI: QIGONG FLOW TO BOOST IMMUNE SYSTEM
YOQI SIX HEALING SOUNDS
YOQI: YIN YOGA 1
WU TAI CHI FOR BEGINNERS
WUDANG KUNG FU: FUNDAMENTAL TRAINING
WUDANG SWORD
WUDANG TAIJIQUAN
XINGYIQUAN
YANG TAI CHI FOR BEGINNERS

AND MANY MORE . . .

more products available from . . .

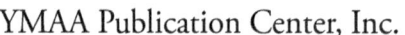 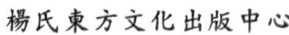 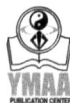

www.ingramcontent.com/pod-product-compliance
Lightning Source LLC
Chambersburg PA
CBHW081103080526
44587CB00021B/3434